DEVELOPMENTAL DISORDERS OF THE BRAIN

Developmental Disorders of the Brain addresses disabilities that occur or have their roots in the early, developmental phase of life which are of utmost concern to parents, siblings, carers and teachers.

This text describes the latest clinical and behavioural findings of disorders which largely or entirely involve the frontostriatal (basal ganglia) system including Tourette's; Obsessive-Compulsive and Attention Deficit Hyperactivity Disorders; Schizophrenia; Autism; gambling and addiction; depression; and Conduct, Developmental Motor Co-ordination and language disorders. Examples of disorders involving the fronto-cerebellar system are also described such as Asperger's disorder, Williams, Fragile X, Cerebellar Cognitive Affective syndromes and Friedreich Ataxia. This book also discusses the relevant anatomy, physiology and pathology, and some of the major functions mediated by affected or relevant structures, together with accounts of the latest recording, brain imaging and stimulating techniques related to these kinds of disorders.

Covering both frontostriatal and fronto-cerebellar systems which control and direct normal behaviour, and which can fail with often distressing consequences during development, as well as addressing behavioural, clinical, pathophysiological and technical aspects, this text is vital to understanding, diagnosis and management of developmental disorders of the brain. This text will be of great interest to clinicians, researchers, teachers and parents.

Nicole J. Rinehart is currently professor of Psychology (Clinical) at Deakin University in Melbourne, Australia.

John L. Bradshaw is Emeritus professor of Psychology and researcher at Monash University, Australia.

Peter G. Enticott is currently associate professor of Psychology (Cognitive Neuroscience) at Deakin University in Melbourne, Australia.

Brain, Behaviour and Cognition

Series editors: Glyn W. Humphreys and Chris Code

Published Titles:

Milestones in the History of Aphasia: Theories and Protagonists
Juergen Tesak and Chris Code

Anomia: Theoretical and Clinical Aspects
Matti Laine and Nadine Martin

Classic Cases in Neuropsychology, Volume II
Chris Code, Yves Joanette, Andre Roch Lecours and Claus-W. Wallesch

Category Specificity in Brain and Mind
Emer Forde and Glyn Humphreys

Neurobehavioural Disability and Social Handicap Following Traumatic Brain Injury
Rodger Ll. Wood and Tom McMillan

Developmental Neuropsychology: A Clinical Approach
Vicki Anderson, Julie Hendy, Elisabeth Northam and Jacquie Wrennall

Developmental Disorders of the Frontostriatal System: Neuropsychological, Neuropsychiatric and Evolutionary Perspectives
John L. Bradshaw

Clinical and Neuropsychological Aspects of Closed Head Injury
J Richardson

Transcortical Aphasias
Marcelo L. Berthier

Spatial Neglect: A Clinical Handbook for Diagnosis and Treatment
Ian H. Robertson and Peter W. Halligan

The Neuropsychology of Smell and Taste
G. Neil Martin

Social and Communication Disorders Following Traumatic Brain Injury 2nd edition
Skye McDonald, Chris Code and Leanne Togher

Clinical Perspectives on Primary Progressive Aphasia
Karen Croot and Lyndsey Nickels

Neuropsychology of Art: Neurological, Cognitive and Evolutionary Perspectives 2nd edition
Dahlia W. Zaidel

DEVELOPMENTAL DISORDERS OF THE BRAIN

2ND EDITION

Edited by Nicole J. Rinehart, John L. Bradshaw, and Peter G. Enticott

Routledge
Taylor & Francis Group
LONDON AND NEW YORK

Second edition published 2017
by Routledge
4 Park Square, Milton Park, Abingdon, Oxon OX14 4RN

and by Routledge
605 Third Avenue, New York, NY 10017

Routledge is an imprint of the Taylor & Francis Group, an informa business

First edition published 2001 by Taylor and Francis

British Library Cataloguing-in-Publication Data
A catalogue record for this book is available from the British Library

Library of Congress Cataloging-in-Publication Data
CIP data has been applied for.

ISBN: 978-1-138-91188-8 (hbk)
ISBN: 978-1-138-91190-1 (pbk)
ISBN: 978-1-315-69228-9 (ebk)

Typeset in Bembo
by codeMantra

CONTENTS

List of affiliations *vii*
Acknowledgement *ix*
Preface *x*
Foreword *xi*

1 The basal ganglia 1
Katherine Johnson

2 The frontal cortex 15
Katherine Johnson

3 Cerebellar cognitive affective syndrome 29
Claudine Kraan

4 New technologies in clinical neuroscience 45
Natalia Albein-Urios and Peter G. Enticott

5 Developmental coordination disorder 63
Christian Hyde, Daniela Rigoli and Jan Piek

6 Language disorder 81
Jarrad A. G. Lum, Michael T. Ullman and Gina Conti-Ramsden

7 Autism spectrum disorder 99
Nicole Rinehart, Jane McGillivray, Melissa Kirkovski and Katrina Williams

8 Attention deficit hyperactivity disorder 119
Janette Tong, Ziarih Hawi and Mark A. Bellgrove

9 Conduct disorder and oppositional defiant disorder 139
Jessica Green, Emma Sciberras and Peter G. Enticott

10 Depression 156
Daphne Voineskos and Zafiris J. Daskalakis

11 Obsessive compulsive disorder 173
Richard Moulding, Matthew. E. Hughes, Linda Byrne, Michael Do and Maja Nedeljkovic

12 Gilles de la Tourette syndrome 191
Dianne M. Sheppard, Nicole Papadopoulos and Valsamma Eapen

13 Addiction 208
Jodie Naim-Feil, Shalini Arunogiri, Primavera A. Spagnolo and Dan I. Lubman

14 Gambling disorder 231
Felicity K. Lorains, Julie C. Stout, Peter G. Enticott and John L. Bradshaw

15 Schizophrenia 251
Tamara May and Paul B. Fitzgerald

16 Williams syndrome 271
Darren R. Hocking

17 Friedreich ataxia 291
Louise A. Corben, Eppie M. Yiu, Marguerite V. Evans-Galea and Martin B. Delatycki

18 Fragile X syndrome and other *FMR1*-related conditions 311
Esther S. Ginsberg and David J. Amor

19 Cerebellar-frontal-parietal axis in developmental disorders 333
Darren R. Hocking

20 Last thoughts 353
John L. Bradshaw, Peter G. Enticott and Nicole J. Rinehart

A postscript *359*
John L. Bradshaw

Subject index *361*

LIST OF AFFILIATIONS

Katherine Johnson, School of Psychological Sciences, University of Melbourne, Australia.
Claudine Kraan, School of Psychological Sciences, Monash University, Australia.
Natalia Albein-Urios, School of Psychology, Deakin University, Australia.
Peter G. Enticott, School of Psychology, Deakin University, Australia.
Christian Hyde, School of Psychology, Deakin University, Australia.
Daniela Rigoli, School of Psychology and Speech Pathology, Curtin University, Western Australia.
Jan Piek, School of Psychology and Speech Pathology, Curtin University, Western Australia.
Jarrad Lum, School of Psychology, Deakin University, Australia.
Michael Ullman, Department of Neuroscience, Georgetown University, United States of America.
Gina Conti-Ramsden, School of Health Sciences, The University of Manchester, United Kingdom.
Nicole J. Rinehart, School of Psychology, Deakin University, Australia.
Jane McGillivray, School of Psychology, Deakin University, Australia.
Melissa Kirkovski, School of Psychology, Deakin University, Australia.
Katrina Williams, Department of Paediatrics, University of Melbourne, Australia.
Janette H.S Tong, School of Psychological Sciences, Monash University, Australia.
Ziarih Hawi, School of Psychological Sciences, Monash University, Australia.
Mark A. Bellgrove, School of Psychological Sciences, Monash University, Australia.
Jessica Green, School of Psychology, Deakin University, Australia
Emma Sciberras, School of Psychology, Deakin University, Australia
Daphne Voineskos, Department of Psychiatry, University of Toronto, Canada.
Zafiris J. Daskalakis, Department of Psychiatry, University of Toronto, Canada
Richard Moulding, School of Psychology, Deakin University, Australia

Matthew E. Hughes, School of Health Sciences, Swinburne University of Technology, Australia
Linda K. Byrne, School of Psychology, Deakin University, Australia
Michael Do, School of Psychology, Deakin University, Australia.
Maja Nedeljkovic, School of Health Sciences, Swinburne University of Technology, Australia.
Dianne M. Sheppard, Monash University Accident Research Centre, Monash University, Australia
Nicole Papadopoulos, School of Psychology, Deakin University, Australia.
Valsamma Eapen, School of Psychiatry, University of New South Wales, Australia.
Jodie Naim-Feil, Department of Physics of Complex Systems, The Weizmann Institute of Science, Israel.
Shalini Arunogiri, School of Psychological Sciences, Monash University, Australia.
Primavera A Spagnolo, National Institute on Alcohol Abuse and Alcoholism, United States of America
Dan I. Lubman, School of Psychological Sciences, Monash University, Australia.
Felicity K. Lorains, School of Psychological Sciences, Monash University, Australia.
Julie C. Stout, School of Psychological Sciences, Monash University, Australia.
John L. Bradshaw, School of Psychological Sciences, Monash University, Australia
Tamara May, Department of Paediatrics, University of Melbourne, Australia.
Paul Fitzgerald, Department of Psychiatry, Monash University, Australia.
Darren R. Hocking, School of Psychology and Public Health, La Trobe University, Australia.
Louise A. Corben, Department of Paediatrics, University of Melbourne, Australia.
Eppie M. Yiu, Department of Paediatrics, University of Melbourne, Australia.
Marguerite V. Evans-Galea, Department of Paediatrics, University of Melbourne, Australia.
Martin B. Delatycki, Department of Paediatrics, University of Melbourne, Australia.
Esther S. Ginsberg, School of Psychological Sciences, Monash University, Australia.
David J. Amor, Department of Developmental Medicine, Murdoch Children's Research Institute, Australia.

ACKNOWLEDGEMENT

John dedicates his contribution to this book to Judy, his beloved spouse of 50 years, now sadly in a nursing home after a catastrophic stroke; she helped him establish and run the Experimental Neuropsychology Research Unit for nearly 20 years, and materially helped so many of our graduate students. Many of the latter are now themselves full professors, and have contributed materially to the preparation and content of this book.

Nicole dedicates her contribution to this book to her husband, Jason, and children, Catherine and Thomas, and to her parents, James and Kathleen. With sincere thanks to her mentors of two decades, John Bradshaw and Bruce Tonge, and to the wonderful families she has had the great privilege of learning from at the Melbourne Children's Clinic. On behalf of the Deakin Child Study Centre team, our sincerest thanks to Moose Toys who have provided considerable support to continue our mission to improve outcomes for all children with developmental challenges. Our gratitude to Jonathan and Simone Wenig for their ongoing support and their vision for a brighter future for all children.

Peter dedicates his contribution to this book to his greatest supports: his wife, Simone, their two boys, Liam and Dylan, and his parents, Liz and Greg. He also expresses his eternal gratitude to John and Nicole, both of whom set an impeccable example in their enthusiasm, empathy and generosity to students, colleagues, patients and participants.

PREFACE

From being an area primarily on the periphery of mainstream behavioural and cognitive science, neuropsychology has developed in recent years into an area of central concern for a range of disciplines. We are witnessing not only a revolution in the way in which brain-behaviour-cognition relationships are viewed, but also a widening of interest concerning developments in neuropsychology on the part of a range of workers in a variety of fields. Major advances in brain-imaging techniques and the cognitive modelling of the impairments following brain injury promise a wider understanding of the nature of the representation of cognition and behaviour in the damaged and undamaged brain.

Neuropsychology is now centrally important for those working with brain-damaged people, but the very rate of expansion in the area makes it difficult to keep with findings from the current research. The aim of the *Brain, Behaviour and Cognition* series is to publish a wide range of books that present comprehensive and up-to-date overviews of current developments in specific areas of interest.

These books will be of particular interest to those working with the brain-damaged. It is the editors' intention that undergraduates, postgraduates, clinicians and researchers in psychology, speech pathology and medicine will find this series a useful source of information on important current developments. The authors and editors of the books in the series are experts in their respective fields, working at the forefront of contemporary research. They have produced texts that are accessible and scholarly. We thank them for their contribution and their hard work in fulfilling the aims of the series.

Chris Code and Glyn Humphreys
University of Exeter, UK and
University of Birmingham, UK
Series Editors

FOREWORD

Until relatively recently, we heard more about, and feared, the neurodegenerative disorders, such as dementia, stroke, Parkinson's and similar if fortunately rarer disorders such as Huntington's and motor neuron diseases, more than disorders which manifest or initially develop early in the developmental phase of life. However, the latter or developmental disorders, possibly with increasing affluence and awareness, have at least over the last half century come ever more to the forefront of concern. In some ways the last decades of the 20th century could be characterised as the period of the basal ganglia/frontostriatal system, as so many disorders of childhood and youth, like autism, attention deficit hyperactivity disorder, Tourette's disorder and schizophrenia either first manifest or have their roots in these early years. However, if there can be seen a turning point, it may be, with the new century, a developing understanding that another great neural system, the fronto-cerebellar, may play an additional, equally important, and largely complementary role. At a purely motor level, and of course we cannot also ignore cognitive and emotional aspects of what it means to be human, we can crudely characterise the frontostriatal system as perhaps more largely responsible for initiating response sequences, and the fronto-cerebellar as fine-tuning end-point accuracy. This book is about the latest findings, neural and behavioural, diagnostic and management, of developmental disorders that have their roots therein in these two great brain systems.

1
THE BASAL GANGLIA

Katherine Johnson

Introduction

The basal ganglia (BG) are a complex set of subcortical nuclei, consisting of the striatum (the caudate nucleus and the putamen), the globus pallidus, the substantia nigra, and the subthalamic nucleus (Redgrave et al., 2010). They are connected with the cerebral cortex in a series of parallel, largely segregated loops that convey limbic (motivation, emotion), associative (cognitive), and sensorimotor information in a topographically organized manner (Draganski et al., 2008; Karachi et al., 2005; Kemp & Powell, 1970; Lambert et al., 2012; Parent & Hazrati, 1995; Postuma & Dagher, 2006; Redgrave et al., 2010). Functional neuroimaging and connectivity studies have provided validation of these circuits in humans, which correspond with evidence from non-human primate lesion and tracing studies (Stoessl, Lehéricy, & Strafella, 2014). Because they receive connections from all areas of the cortex (Kemp & Powell, 1970), and they project back to the motor output regions of the brain, the BG have been proposed to act as a selector of the most appropriate behaviour for a given situation, based on sensory, limbic, and cognitive information (Redgrave et al., 2010). The exact roles of the BG, however, are still under debate.

The BG are "archaic" in evolutionary terms (Redgrave, Prescott, & Gurney, 1999). All jawed vertebrates have an input station (the striatum) and an output station (the pallidum) (Medina, Abellán, Vicario, & Desfilis, 2014). In tetrapods (four-limbed vertebrates), the dorsal BG are associated with somatosensory behaviour, whilst the ventral BG are associated with motivation (Medina et al., 2014). Given the phylogenetic continuity of the BG, much anatomical and physiology research has been conducted on primates and mammals, with magnetic resonance imaging opening the research field for understanding the anatomy and physiology of the BG in humans. Our understanding of how the BG nuclei connect with the rest of the brain has changed considerably over the past 50 years, with advances in research technologies.

This chapter will review the anatomy, connectivity, and the biochemistry of the BG. It will present some of the models of the way the BG connect with the rest of the brain and how the BG nuclei function together. Some of the proposed roles of the BG will be reviewed.

The anatomy of the basal ganglia

The basal ganglia are a set of interconnected nuclei located in the base of the forebrain (Albin, Young, & Penney, 1989). They consist of the ventral striatum (nucleus accumbens and the olfactory tubercle), the dorsal striatum (the caudate nucleus and putamen), the globus pallidus – both the internal (GPi) and external (GPe) sections, the substantia nigra pars compacta (SNc) and the substantia nigra pars reticulata (SNr), and the subthalamic nucleus (STN).

Inputs into the BG

The striatum receives most of the projections from outside of the BG – but not all. The STN receives direct excitatory afferents from the motor and premotor cortices (Albin et al., 1989), and internally from the GPe, whilst the GPi receives excitatory inputs from the thalamus and the pedunculopontine tegmental nucleus (Nelson & Kreitzer, 2014).

The dorsal striatum (caudate nucleus and putamen) receives glutamatergic topographic projections from the entire neocortex (Kemp & Powell, 1970) and from the thalamus (Smith, Raju, Pare, & Sidibe, 2004). It also receives dopaminergic projections from the ventral tegmental area (VTA) and the SNc, and serotonergic and noradrenergic inputs from the raphe and locus coeruleus (Fujiyama, Takahashi, & Karube, 2015). The ventral striatum receives projections from the hippocampal formation, entorhinal cortex, the olfactory cortex, the anterior cingulate, prelimbic and infralimbic cortices, lateral propisocortical areas, the amygdala, the thalamus (Nakano, 2000) and dopaminergic projections from the VTA and SNc (Björklund & Dunnett, 2007).

Outputs from the BG and thalamus

To date, there are three output regions of the BG – the GPi and the SNr complex, the SNc and VTA, and a recently described third output – a direct γ-Aminobutyric acid (GABA)-ergic projection from the GPe to the frontal cortex (Saunders et al., 2015). The GPi and SNr can be considered as parts of a single neuronal system separated by a white matter tract (Albin et al., 1989). This complex sends inhibitory projections to the thalamus and the midbrain tegmentum (Albin et al., 1989). The GPi also projects to the lateral habenula (cells around the pineal gland), whilst the SNr also projects to the superior colliculus (Albin et al., 1989), which is important for eye movements and orienting behaviour (Nelson & Kreitzer, 2014). The GPi and SNr also outputs to the pedunculopontine tegmental nucleus in the brain stem, which is thought to modulate both motor and attention control (Benarroch, 2013).

The SNc and VTA send dopaminergic projections to many brain regions, with prominent projections to the frontal cortex, limbic areas, and within the BG itself (Björklund & Dunnett, 2007). These dopamine projections form three anatomically and functionally discrete paths – the mesostriatal, mesolimbic, and mesocortical paths, but their origins within the SNc and VTA are intermixed (Björklund & Dunnett, 2007).

The newly described direct projection from the GPe to the frontal cortex releases the inhibitory neurotransmitter GABA and to a lesser degree acetylcholine. This projection in turn is inhibited by the striatal projection neurons of the direct and indirect pathways within the dorsal striatum (see below for more details about the direct and indirect pathways), suggesting it is under the control of the striatum (Saunders et al., 2015). The indirect striatal projection that inhibits the GPe projection to the frontal cortex is sensitive to dopamine 2 receptor signaling (Saunders et al., 2015).

The thalamus projects to the prefrontal cortex, with dense projections to the supplementary motor area (Schell & Strick, 1984) and it also projects back to the dorsal striatum (Smith et al., 2014). The center median/parafascicular complex is the main source of connections between the thalamus and the striatum (Smith et al., 2014). About 50% of its neurons are sent to the dorsal striatum, about one third are sents to the primary motor cortex, and the remaining neurons project to both targets. These projections are topographically organized (Smith et al., 2014). The center median/parafascicular complex is activated during the processing of attention-related stimuli. These thalamic inputs may act to gate corticostriatal transmission by regulating striatal cholinergic interneurons – researchers speculate that this may modulate behavioural switching and set-shifting (Kimura, Minamimoto, Matsumoto, & Hori, 2004; Smith et al., 2014). The intralaminar nuclei of the thalamus receive massive ascending projections from reticular formation of the brain stem, and are part of the reticular activating system that regulates arousal and attention (Smith et al., 2014). The outputs of the BG and thalamus remain topographically organized as part of the limbic, associative, and sensorimotor loops (Berendse & Groenewegen, 1990; Redgrave et al., 2010).

Connections within the BG

Within the BG, there are medium spiny GABAergic neuronal connections between the dorsal striatum and the GPi and SNr ("**direct pathway**"). There is a connection between the dorsal striatum and the GPe, which then projects to the STN

(Albin et al., 1989), and the STN sends projections to the GPi and SNr ("**indirect pathway**"). The STN also projects back to the GPe (Albin et al., 1989) and the dorsal striatum (Kita & Kitai, 1987). The striatum and the SNc project to each other (Albin et al., 1989). There is also a "**hyperdirect pathway**" between the cortex, the STN and the GPi, and SNr (Nambu, Tokuno, & Takada, 2002). The GPe neurons send projections to almost every BG nucleus (Nelson & Kreitzer, 2014).

The SNc sends dopaminergic projections to the dorsal and ventral striatum, both the GPi and GPe to the STN, and within the SNc itself (Björklund & Dunnett, 2007). These midbrain dopaminergic neurons can regulate the activity of the dopaminergic neurons themselves and also the release of GABA within the SNr, regulating the activity of its efferent projections (Björklund & Dunnett, 2007).

Dopamine functioning within the BG

The dopaminergic afferents from the SNc modulate the excitatory inputs from the cerebral cortex on the dorsal striatum (Smith et al., 2014). This occurs through a wide variety of pre- and/or post-synaptic mechanisms, depending on the type and the location of the dopamine receptors (Smith et al., 2014). There are two forms of dopamine receptors – the D1 and D2 receptor subtypes. Tonic levels of extracellular dopamine can activate the D2-type receptors (D2, D3, and D4), whilst phasic release of dopamine activates the D1-type receptors (D1, D5) (Da Cunha et al., 2015). All five DA receptors are expressed in the striatum, where D1 and D2 are particularly abundant (Da Cunha et al., 2015). The medium spiny neurons of the striatum predominantly express D1 receptors in the direct, and D2 receptors in the indirect pathways (Da Cunha et al., 2015). D2-like receptors (D2, D3, and D4) are also expressed in the presynaptic terminals of the SNc and VTA dopaminergic neurons and in the terminals of corticostriatal neurons (Da Cunha et al., 2015).

The medium spiny neurons of the dorsal striatum fire only when they are in an "up-state", where their membrane potentials are closer to the depolarization threshold. They phasically release dopamine in amounts that stimulate the D1-like receptors (D1, D5), which is likely to stimulate firing of neurons in the direct pathway (Da Cunha et al., 2015).

Models of how the BG connect with the rest of the brain

The BG receives projections from all over the cortex and relays projections back again. The functional roles of these projections are open to interpretation and modeling. Over time, scientists have forwarded models of BG functioning, and these have changed with improved understanding of the complexity of this system based on animal research, and with the addition of human data from functional and anatomical magnetic resonance imaging. A historical review of the models of how the BG connects with the rest of the brain is presented here below.

Anatomical and physiological research supports the contention that the BG are part of a series of separate but parallel circuits that funnel projections from broad sections of the cortex into discrete sections of the BG and then back to even more discrete sections of the cortex (DeLong & Georgopoulos, 1981). Two distinct loops were first thought to pass through the BG – a motor loop that received projections from the sensorimotor cortex and passed through the putamen, which then sent projections to the premotor areas of the cortex; and an association loop that received projections from the association areas of the cortex and passed through the caudate nucleus, which then sent projections back to the prefrontal cortex (DeLong & Georgopoulos, 1981).

Heimer and colleagues identified that the nucleus accumbens, a region of the basal forebrain associated with limbic function, and its surrounding areas was part of the striatum, and these were relabeled the ventral striatum (Heimer, 1978). Heimer also identified a ventral section of the pallidum, and relabeled this the ventral pallidum. The ventral pallidum sends projections to the medial dorsal thalamus, which then projects back to the frontal cortex. This was the first report of a limbic loop within the BG.

In 1986, Alexander, DeLong, and Strick published a very influential model of BG function detailing five basal ganglia-thalamo-cortical loops (Alexander, DeLong, & Strick, 1986). The authors suggested that similar neuronal operations might occur at each level of the five loops due to the parallel and uniform organization of synapses at each point in the loop. In the motor loop, afferents from the somatosensory, motor, and premotor cortices project to the putamen, which sends projections to both the GPi and GPe, and the SNr, and projections are then sent to the ventrolateral nucleus of the thalamus, which projects to the supplementary motor area (Alexander et al., 1986). In the oculomotor circuit, the frontal eye fields, the dorsolateral prefrontal cortex, and the posterior parietal cortex send projections to the caudate nucleus, which sends projections to the GPi and SNr that in turn project to both the superior colliculus and to the thalamus. The thalamus then projects back to the frontal eye fields (Alexander et al., 1986). In the dorsolateral prefrontal cortex circuit, the DLFPC, the posterior parietal, and the arcuate premotor area send projections to the dorsolateral head of the caudate nucleus around to the tail of the caudate, which projects to the GPi and SNr. Projections are then sent to the thalamus which projects to the prefrontal areas. In the lateral orbitofrontal circuit, projections are sent from the lateral orbitofrontal cortex and the auditory and visual association areas of the temporal cortex to the caudate nucleus, from the head to the tail. The caudate nucleus projects to the SNr, which then projects to the thalamus, and then back to the lateral orbitofrontal cortex. In the anterior cingulate circuit, projections from the anterior cingulate area, the hippocampal cortex, the entorhinal cortex, and the superior and inferior temporal gyri are sent to the ventral striatum, which sends projections to the GPi and SNr, to the mediodorsal nucleus (Alexander et al., 1986).

These hypothesized circuits were rearticulated in 1990 based on updated knowledge of the anatomy of the BG, with four basal ganglia-thalamocortical circuits suggested – motor, oculomotor, prefrontal, and limbic (Alexander, Crutcher, & DeLong, 1990). Researchers noted that although these circuits were segregated, inputs also converged within the BG (Draganski et al., 2008; Takada, Tokuno, Nambu, & Inase, 1998).

The current model of how the BG connects with the rest of the brain holds that there are only three discrete circuits (Lehéricy et al., 2004). These circuits have been determined through anatomical data, tracing studies in non-human primates [e.g. (Künzle, 1975; Middleton & Strick, 2000)], axonal tractography studies using diffusion tensor imaging (Lehéricy et al., 2004; Stoessl et al., 2014), diffusion-weighted imaging (voxel-based connectivity) analyses (Draganski et al., 2008), and with functional neuroimaging studies using behavioural tasks (Postuma & Dagher, 2006). These circuits maintain topographic integrity through each section of the BG (Wiesendanger, Clarke, Kraftsik, & Tardif, 2004). The circuits are the sensorimotor, associative, and limbic (Lehéricy et al., 2004).

The sensorimotor section of the posterior putamen receives afferents from the primary sensory and motor areas and the posterior part of the supplementary motor area (SMA) (Lehéricy et al., 2004). This sensorimotor circuit is similar to that in non-human primates (Lehéricy et al., 2004). Imaging studies have shown involvement of this sensorimotor circuit in the control of habitual movements, such as well learned finger sequences (Lehéricy et al., 2005).

The associative compartment of the anterior section of the striatum, especially the anterior putamen and the head of the caudate nucleus, receives afferents from the prefrontal cortex, the frontal pole, and the pre-SMA (Lehéricy et al., 2004). In this 2004 paper, connections into the anterior striatum from the parietal and temporal cortices were rarely observed in the human participants (Lehéricy et al., 2004), and these connections in the model by Alexander et al. (1986) were minor. It is thought that this section of the circuit is involved in goal-directed behaviour (Redgrave et al., 2010), such as learning new motor sequences, instrumental conditioning, and in complex motor tasks (Lehéricy et al., 2004).

The limbic compartment of the ventral striatum receives afferents from structures associated with the limbic system – the orbitomedial frontal cortex, the amygdala, the hippocampus, and the temporal lobe (Lehéricy et al., 2004). This circuit is involved in understanding when and why rewards occur and how the brain uses reward prediction to improve future decisions (Maia & Frank, 2011; Pessiglione, Seymour, Flandin, Dolan, & Frith, 2006).

Models of how the nuclei of the BG function together

BG functioning is very complex, and as such a number of models exist to explain how this system works. The first functional model of the BG was proposed in the late 1980s (Redgrave et al., 2010). This "direct/indirect" model of the BG (Albin et al., 1989) has been highly influential, especially in terms of understanding the pathophysiology of Parkinson's and Huntington's diseases, and in supporting lesion and deep brain stimulation studies in patients with movement disorders (Calabresi, Picconi, Tozzi, Ghiglieri, & Di Filippo, 2014). Since this model was first proposed, the complexity of the BG structures has become more apparent (Parent & Cicchetti, 1998) and the direct/indirect model has been challenged (Nelson & Kreitzer, 2014). More recent accounts of the structure and function of the BG have been proposed and will be reviewed below. The classic direct/indirect model will be reviewed first.

In the direct/indirect model of the BG, the neurons in the striatum form two separate populations that make direct and indirect projections to the SNr and the GPi. The **direct** pathway describes monosynaptic GABAergic and substance P projections from the putamen to the motor sections of the GPi/SNr output complex (DeLong, 1990). The **indirect** projection arises from putamen neurons containing GABA and encephalin, and its influences are relayed to the GPi/SNr via the GPe and the subthalamic nucleus (STN) (DeLong, 1990). The GPi/SNr GABA neurons project to the thalamus and brain stem.

According to the direct/indirect model, the BG output projections act to keep the thalamus and brain stem under tonic inhibitory control (Redgrave et al., 2010). The SNc modulates activity of the direct and indirect pathways through the phasic release of dopamine (Redgrave et al., 2010). The direct pathway consists of neurons with D1 and D5 receptors, and dopamine activates these neurons, allowing for a release of the tonic inhibitory action of the BG on the thalamus, resulting in action. In contrast, the indirect pathway consists of neurons with D2, D3, and D4 receptors, and the release of dopamine and these D2-like receptors' subsequent activation results in an increase in inhibition and a suppression of behaviour (Chevalier & Deniau, 1990). Shifts in balance between the direct and indirect pathways lead to alterations in the GPi/SNr output to the thalamus, and may result in hypo- and hyperkinetic features of BG disorders, such as Parkinson's and Huntington's diseases, respectively (Albin et al., 1989; DeLong, 1990). In the case of Parkinson's disease, a reduced level of dopamine from the SNc to the putamen has a dual effect – facilitation of neurons in the indirect pathway and reduced activation of neurons in the direct pathway. According to this model, this will result in increased inhibition from the indirect putamen neurons to the GPe, resulting in disinhibition of the STN, which then increases inhibitory output of the GPi and SNr (DeLong, 1990). Decreased activation of the direct pathway reduces the phasic inhibitory influences of the GPi and SNr, contributing to excessive inhibitory output from the BG (Redgrave et al., 2010). In contrast, in Huntington's disease there is a selective loss of enkephalinergic striatal neurons projecting to the GPe (Reiner et al., 1988), which results in decreased activity of the STN, and then a loss of excitatory drive to the GPi and SNr, and reduced inhibition of BG output to the thalamus, resulting in disinhibition of the thalamocortical projections and subsequent hyperkinesia (Albin et al., 1989).

Recent research findings have raised concerns about the anatomical and functional descriptions of the BG in the direct/indirect model. While the direct and indirect pathways remain valid (Redgrave et al., 2010), BG are "a complex and widely distributed neuronal network" (p. 49) (Wu, Richard, & Parent, 2000). The two pathways may not be as anatomically segregated as initially thought – for instance the direct pathway contains branching fibers that project from the putamen to the GPe (Wu et al., 2000). Collateral fibers that bridge the direct and indirect pathways may act as a mechanism of modulation between the two paths (Calabresi et al., 2014). The STN is now considered as a major source of input into the BG with projections from the cortex and subcortical structures. The excitatory **hyperdirect** path links the cortex directly to the STN, which then sends signals through to the GPi/SNr (Nambu et al., 2002). This hyperdirect path may be involved in stopping motor and cognitive commands (Sano, Chiken, Hikida, Kobayashi, & Nambu, 2013). It is now known that the GPe projects directly to the STN, to the GPi and SNr, to the reticular nucleus (Smith, Bevan, Shink, & Bolam, 1998), and to the frontal cortex (Saunders et al., 2015). There are reciprocal connections between the STN and GPe, as noted by Albin et al., 1989, and between the GPe and the striatum (Miwa, Fuwa, Nishi, & Kondo, 2001; Redgrave et al., 2010). Recently, optogenetic activation studies have suggested that both the direct and indirect pathways can have excitatory and inhibitory actions on the GPi and SNr, and that co-ordinated activation of both pathways may be necessary for action selection (Calabresi et al., 2014). Finally, neurons projecting to the GPi show immunolabeling for D1 and D2 receptors, rather than just the D1 receptors as described in the original direct/indirect model (Calabresi et al., 2014).

Calabresi and colleagues suggest that the direct and indirect pathways are functionally and anatomically intertwined. The two pathways may communicate via a complex interneuronal network through GPe collaterals that may allow the direct pathway to directly modulate the indirect pathway (Calabresi et al., 2014).

Recent work using optogenetic manipulations of the direct and indirect pathways in mice has supported the classic direct-indirect model of BG function at the population level of cortical neurons, yet at the individual neuron level it appears that neurons can have heterogeneous, asymmetric, and context-dependent responses when striatal activity is manipulated (Oldenburg & Sabatini, 2015). The researchers suggest that the direct and indirect pathways can have non-antagonistic and selective effects on distinct cortical neurons (Oldenburg & Sabatini, 2015).

One alternative model of BG functioning suggests that two anatomically separate systems work to produce goal-directed and stimulus-response habitual control of behaviour (Redgrave et al., 2010). This model does not differentiate between the direct, indirect, and hyperdirect circuits within the BG, but suggests that the dorsomedial striatum is involved in the acquisition and retention of goal-directed learning, whereas the dorsolateral striatum (posterior putamen) is associated with the development of habit (Redgrave et al., 2010). The loss of dopamine in the sensorimotor areas of the BG in Parkinson's disease is hypothesized to result in a major difficulty with habitual control, whilst pathological output from the sensorimotor circuit will result in distortions of goal-directed responses (Redgrave et al., 2010).

The newly described direct projection from the GPe to the frontal cortex bypasses the thalamus. Saunders and colleagues suggest that this bypassing allows the direct and indirect striatal pathways to directly modulate the frontal cortex (Saunders et al., 2015). In addition, the hyperdirect cortical projection through the STN excites this GPe-frontal cortex circuit directly. This newly described projection, in concert with the hyperdirect pathway, may form a two-synapse loop for ongoing cortical modulation (Saunders et al., 2015). The role of this GPe-frontal cortex projection is being investigated further.

The proposed roles of the BG

The role of the basal ganglia within the brain system has long been a question asked by neuroscientists. From the late 19th century, scientists have focused on the role of the BG in movement control (Redgrave et al., 2010). Many scientists have argued that the BG's main role is that they "are responsible for the automatic execution of learned motor plans" (p. 514) (Marsden, 1982). Indeed, even after reviewing the literature of the time, detailing the sensory and cognitive inputs into the BG, and the negative effects on attention control of lesions to parts of the BG, Marsden still maintained that the BG are concerned with motor control (Marsden, 1982). "… the basal ganglia should still be regarded as organs of motor control" (p. 514) (Marsden, 1982). Scientists argued that because the BG received afferents from the cortex and relayed them through to the motor cortex, the primary role of the BG was to influence the initiation and control of movement.

With further research exploring the large number of projections into the different parts of the BG, the amount of interconnectivity within the BG, and the number of areas of the brain receiving outputs from the BG, the role of the BG has expanded. The current prevalent view of the functions of the BG is that they hold three separate functions – motor control, cognition, and reward processing (Haber, 2014). "… It is clear that the basal ganglia must have a major influence on sensorimotor, limbic, and cognitive information processing …" (p. 7143) (Draganski et al., 2008). Research using functional magnetic resonance imaging (Postuma & Dagher, 2006), and patient group work (Redgrave et al., 2010), has produced results that validate the separation of these three functions. Nevertheless, this separation of functions is one model of how the BG operates, and other models also exist.

Redgrave and colleagues argue that the BG are involved in the **selection** of behaviours, based on both previous experience and expectations of future reward (Redgrave et al., 1999). Behaviours may be either goal-directed or habitual, and the BG are postulated to be involved in switching between these two types of behaviours (Hikosaka & Isoda, 2010). Goal-directed behaviour is under the control of the dorsomedial striatum, whilst habitual behaviour is associated with the dorsolateral striatum (Redgrave et al., 2010). During the explicit learning of a finger movement sequence over a month period, activation in the rostrodorsal region decreased, whilst there was a significant increase in BOLD response in the caudoventral regions of the putamen. This suggests that motor representations shift from the associative to the sensorimotor areas of the BG during explicit motor sequence learning (Lehéricy et al., 2005).

Da Cunha and colleagues argue that unconditioned and conditioned responses, goal-directed actions, and stimulus-response habits are selected in the basal ganglia (Da Cunha, Gómez-A, & Blaha, 2012). These selections occur through the activation of striatal neurons that receive cortical and subcortical neuronal information encoding unconditioned, conditioned, goal, and neutral stimuli (Da Cunha et al., 2012). Variation in extracellular dopamine within the basal ganglia alters the strength of the synapses between the incoming neuronal connections and the striatal neurons, signaling behavioural outcomes that are better or worse than expected (Da Cunha et al., 2012). Salient unconditioned and conditioned stimuli result in the release of dopamine, increasing the signal-to-noise ratio of information from the cortex to the striatum (Da Cunha et al., 2012). Selection occurs when the striatal neurons initiate and cease movement initiation via connections to the supplementary motor area, the premotor, and motor cortices. The BG play a role in the expression of learned responses to stimuli, suggesting a link with the procedural and declarative memory systems (Da Cunha et al., 2012).

Summary

The BG are a complex system of subcortical nuclei involved in the control of movement, cognition, and motivation. The BG receive projections from all areas of the cortex, especially the frontal cortex, and they project to the thalamus, the frontal cortex, the limbic system, the brain stem and back to the BG itself. Within the BG there are the direct, indirect, and the hyperdirect pathways. A number of models exist to explain how the BG system works; however, the exact roles of the BG are still under debate.

Abbreviations

BG: Basal ganglia
Dopamine 1-type receptors: dopamine 1 (D1), dopamine 5 (D5)
Dopamine 2-type receptors: dopamine 2 (D2), dopamine 3 (D3), dopamine 4 (D4)
GABA: γ-Aminobutyric acid
GPe: Globus pallidus - external segment
GPi: Globus pallidus - internal segment
SMA: Supplementary motor area

SNc: Substantia nigra pars compacta
SNr: Substantia nigra pars reticulata
STN: Subthalamic nucleus
VTA: Ventral tegmental area

Further readings

Calabresi, P., Picconi, B., Tozzi, A., Ghiglieri, V., & Di Filippo, M. (2014). Direct and indirect pathways of basal ganglia: A critical reappraisal. *Nature Neuroscience, 17*(8), 1022–1030. doi: 10.1038/nn.3743.

Da Cunha, C., Boschen, S. L., Gómez-A, A., Ross, E. K., Gibson, W. S. J., Min, H.-K., … Blaha, C. D. (2015). Toward sophisticated basal ganglia neuromodulation: Review on basal ganglia deep brain stimulation. *Neuroscience and Biobehavioral Reviews, 58*(November), 186–210. doi: 10.1016/j.neubiorev.2015.02.003.

Nelson, A. B., & Kreitzer, A. C. (2014). Reassessing models of basal ganglia function and dysfunction. *Annual Review of Neuroscience, 37*, 117–135. doi: 10.1146/annurev-neuro-071013-013916.

Obeso, J. A., Rodriguez-Oroz, M. C., Stamelou, M., Bhatia, K. P., & Burn, D. J. (2014). The expanding universe of disorders of the basal ganglia. *The Lancet, 384*(August 9), 523–531. doi: 0.1016/S0140-6736(13)62418-6.

Redgrave, P., Rodriguez, M., Smith, Y., Rodriguez-Oroz, M. C., Lehericy, S., Bergman, H., … Obeso, J. A. (2010). Goal-directed and habitual control in the basal ganglia: Implications for Parkinson's disease. *Nature Reviews Neuroscience, 11*(11), 760–772. doi: 10.1038/nrn2915.

Steiner, H., & Tseng, K.Y. (2010). *Handbook of Basal Ganglia Structure and Function*. London, UK: Academic Press.

References

Albin, R. L., Young, A. B., & Penney, J. B. (1989). The functional anatomy of basal ganglia disorders. *Trends in Neurosciences, 12*(10), 366–375.

Alexander, G. E., Crutcher, M. D., & DeLong, M. R. (1990). Basal ganglia-thalamocortical circuits: parallel substrates for motor, oculomotor, "prefrontal" and "limbic" functions. *Progress in Brain Research, 85*, 119–146. doi:10.1016/S0079-6123(08)62678-3.

Alexander, G. E., DeLong, M. R., & Strick, P. L. (1986). Parallel organization of functionally segregated circuits linking basal ganglia and cortex. *Annual Review of Neuroscience, 9*, 357–381. doi:10.1146/annurev.ne.09.030186.002041.

Benarroch, E. E. (2013). Pedunculopontine nucleus. *Neurology, 80*(12), 1148–1155. doi:10.1212/WNL.0b013e3182886a76.

Berendse, H. W., & Groenewegen, H. J. (1990). Organization of the thalamostriatal projections in the rat, with special emphasis on the ventral striatum. *Journal of Comparative Neurology, 299*(2), 187–228. doi:10.1002/cne.902990206.

Björklund, A., & Dunnett, S. B. (2007). Dopamine neuron systems in the brain: an update. *Trends in Neurosciences, 30*(5), 194–202. doi:10.1016/j.tins.2007.03.006.

Calabresi, P., Picconi, B., Tozzi, A., Ghiglieri, V., & Di Filippo, M. (2014). Direct and indirect pathways of basal ganglia: a critical reappraisal. *Nature Neuroscience, 17*(8), 1022–1030. doi:10.1038/nn.3743.

Chevalier, G., & Deniau, J. M. (1990). Disinhibition as a basic process in the expression of striatal functions. *Trends in Neurosciences, 13*(7), 277–281.

Da Cunha, C., Boschen, S. L., Gómez-A, A., Ross, E. K., Gibson, W. S. J., Min, H.-K., … Blaha, C. D. (2015). Toward sophisticated basal ganglia neuromodulation: Review on basal ganglia deep brain stimulation. *Neuroscience and Biobehavioral Reviews, 58*(November), 186–210. doi:10.1016/j.neubiorev.2015.02.003.

Da Cunha, C., Gómez-A, A., & Blaha, C. D. (2012). The role of the basal ganglia in motivated behavior. *Reviews in the Neurosciences, 23*(5–6), 747–767. doi:10.1515/revneuro-2012-0063.

DeLong, M. R. (1990). Primate models of movement disorders of basal ganglia origin. *Trends in Neurosciences, 13*(7), 281–285.

DeLong, M. R., & Georgopoulos, A. P. (1981). Motor functions of the basal ganglia. In J. M. Brookhart, V. B. Mountcastle, & V. B. Brooks (Eds.), *Handbook of Physiology. The Nervous System. Motor Control.* (Vol. 2, pp. 1017–1061). Bethesda: American Physiological Society.

Draganski, B., Kherif, F., Klöppel, S., Cook, P. A., Alexander, D. C., Parker, G. J. M., … Frackowiak, R. S. J. (2008). Evidence for segregated and integrative connectivity patterns in the human basal ganglia. *Journal of Neuroscience, 28*(28), 7143–7152. doi:10.1523/JNEUROSCI.1486-08.2008.

Fujiyama, F., Takahashi, S., & Karube, F. (2015). Morphological elucidation of basal ganglia circuits contributing reward prediction. *Frontiers in Neuroscience, 9*(6), 1–8. doi:10.3389/fnins.2015.00006.

Haber, S. N. (2014). The place of dopamine in the cortico-basal ganglia circuit. *Neuroscience, 282*, 248–257. doi:10.1016/j.neuroscience.2014.10.008.

Heimer, L. (1978). The olfactory cortex and the ventral striatum. In K. E. Livingston & O. Hornykiewicz (Eds.), *Limbic mechanisms* (pp. 95–187). New York: Plenum Press.

Hikosaka, O., & Isoda, M. (2010). Switching from automatic to controlled behavior: cortico-basal ganglia mechanisms. *Trends in Cognitive Science, 14*(4), 154–161. doi:10.1016/j.tics.2010.01.006.

Karachi, C., Yelnik, J., Tandé, D., Tremblay, L., Hirsch, E. C., & Francois, C. (2005). The pallido-subthalamic projection: an anatomical substrate for nonmotor functions of the subthalamic nucleus in primates. *Movement Disorders, 20*(2), 172–180. doi:10.1002/mds.20302.

Kemp, J. M., & Powell, T. P. S. (1970). The cortico-striate projection in the monkey. *Brain, 93*(3), 525–546. doi:10.1093/brain/93.3.525.

Kimura, M., Minamimoto, T., Matsumoto, N., & Hori, Y. (2004). Monitoring and switching of cortico-basal ganglia loop functions by the thalamo-striatal system. *Neuroscience Research, 48*(4), 355–360. doi:10.1016/j.neures.2003.12.002.

Kita, H., & Kitai, S. T. (1987). Efferent projections of the subthalamic nucleus in the rat: light and electron microscope analysis with the PHA-L method. *Journal of Comparative Neurology, 260*(3), 435–452. doi:10.1002/cne.902600309.

Künzle, H. (1975). Bilateral projections from precentral motor cortex to the putamen and other parts of the basal ganglia. An autoradiographic study in *Macaca fascicularis*. *Brain Research, 88*(2), 195–209. doi:10.1016/0006-8993(75)90384-4.

Lambert, C., Zrinzo, L., Nagy, Z., Lutti, A., Hariz, M., Foltynie, T., … Frackowiak, R. (2012). Confirmation of functional zones within the human subthalamic nucleus: Patterns of connectivity and sub-parcellation using diffusion weighted imaging. *NeuroImage, 60*(1), 83–94. doi:10.1016/j.neuroimage.2011.11.082.

Lehéricy, S., Benali, H., Van de Moortele, P.-F., Pélégrini-Issac, M., Waechter, T., Ugurbil, K., & Doyon, J. (2005). Distinct basal ganglia territories are engaged in early and advanced motor sequence learning. *Proceedings of the National Academy of Sciences, 102*(35), 12566–12571. doi:10.1073/pnas.0502762102.

Lehéricy, S., Ducros, M., Van de Moortele, P.-F., Francois, C., Thivard, L., Poupon, C., … Kim, D.-S. (2004). Diffusion tensor fiber tracking shows distinct corticostriatal circuits in humans. *Annals of Neurology, 55*(4), 522–529. doi:10.1002/ana.20030.

Maia, T. V., & Frank, M. J. (2011). From reinforcement learning models to psychiatric and neurological disorders. *Nature Neuroscience, 14*(2), 154–162. doi:10.1038/nn.2723.

Marsden, C. D. (1982). The mysterious motor function of the basal ganglia: the Robert Wartenberg Lecture. *Neurology, 32*(5), 514–539.

Medina, L., Abellán, A., Vicario, A., & Desfilis, E. (2014). Evolutionary and developmental contributions for understanding the organization of the basal ganglia. *Brain, Behaviour and Evolution, 83*(2), 112–125. doi:10.1159/000357832.

Middleton, F. A., & Strick, P. L. (2000). Basal ganglia and cerebellar loops: motor and cognitive circuits. *Brain Research Reviews, 31*(2–3), 236–250. doi:10.1016/S0165-0173(99)00040-5.

Miwa, H., Fuwa, T., Nishi, K., & Kondo, T. (2001). Subthalamo-pallido-striatal axis: a feedback system in the basal ganglia. *NeuroReport, 12*(17), 3795–3798.

Nakano, K. (2000). Neural circuits and topographic organization of the basal ganglia and related regions. *Brain & Development, 22*(supplement), S5-S16. doi:10.1016/S0387-7604(00)00139-X.

Nambu, A., Tokuno, H., & Takada, M. (2002). Functional significance of the cortico-subthalamo-pallidal 'hyperdirect' pathway. *Neuroscience Research, 43*(2), 111–117. doi:10.1016/S0168-0102(02)00027-5.

Nelson, A. B., & Kreitzer, A. C. (2014). Reassessing models of basal ganglia function and dysfunction. *Annual Review of Neuroscience, 37*, 117–135. doi:10.1146/annurev-neuro-071013-013916.

Oldenburg, I. A., & Sabatini, B. L. (2015). Antagonistic but not symmetric regulation of primary motor cortex by basal ganglia direct and indirect pathways. *Neuron, 86*(5), 1174–1181. doi:10.1016/j.neuron.2015.05.008.

Parent, A., & Cicchetti, F. (1998). The current model of basal ganglia organization under scrutiny. *Movement Disorders, 13*(2), 199–202. doi:10.1002/mds.870130202.

Parent, A., & Hazrati, L.-N. (1995). Functional anatomy of the basal ganglia. I. The cortico-basal ganglia-thalamo-cortical loop. *Brain Research Reviews, 20*(1), 91–127.

Pessiglione, M., Seymour, B., Flandin, G., Dolan, R. J., & Frith, C. D. (2006). Dopamine-dependent prediction errors underpin reward-seeking behaviour in humans. *Nature, 442*(31 August 2006), 1042–1045. doi:10.1038/nature05051.

Postuma, R. B., & Dagher, A. (2006). Basal ganglia functional connectivity based on a meta-analysis of 126 positron emission tomography and functional magnetic resonance imaging publications. *Cerebral Cortex, 16*(10), 1508–1521. doi:10.1093/cercor/bhj088.

Redgrave, P., Prescott, T. J., & Gurney, K. (1999). The basal ganglia: a vertebrate solution to the selection problem? *Neuroscience, 89*(4), 1009–1023. doi:10.1016/S0306-4522(98)00319-4.

Redgrave, P., Rodriguez, M., Smith, Y., Rodriguez-Oroz, M. C., Lehericy, S., Bergman, H., … Obeso, J. A. (2010). Goal-directed and habitual control in the basal ganglia: implications for Parkinson's disease. *Nature Reviews Neuroscience, 11*(11), 760–772. doi:10.1038/nrn2915.

Reiner, A., Albin, R. L., Anderson, K. D., D'Amato, C. J., Penney, J. B., & Young, A. B. (1988). Differential loss of striatal projection neurons in Huntington's disease. *Proceedings of the National Academy of Sciences, 85*(15), 5733–5737. doi:10.1073/pnas.85.15.5733.

Sano, H., Chiken, S., Hikida, T., Kobayashi, K., & Nambu, A. (2013). Signals through the striatopallidal indirect pathway stop movements by phasic excitation in the substantia nigra. *Journal of Neuroscience, 33*(17), 7583–7594. doi:10.1523/JNEUROSCI.4932-12.2013.

Saunders, A., Oldenburg, I. A., Berezovskii, V. K., Johnson, C. A., Kingery, N. D., Elliott, H. L., … Sabatini, B. L. (2015). A direct GABAergic output from the basal ganglia to frontal cortex. *Nature, 521*(7550), 85–89. doi:10.1038/nature14179.

Schell, G. R., & Strick, P. L. (1984). The origin of thalamic inputs to the arcuate premotor and supplmentary motor areas. *Journal of Neuroscience, 4*(2), 539–560.

Smith, Y., Bevan, M. D., Shink, E., & Bolam, J. P. (1998). Microcircuitry of the direct and indirect pathways of the basal ganglia. *Neuroscience, 86*(2), 353–387. doi:10.1016/S0306-4522(98)00047-5.

Smith, Y., Galvan, A., Ellender, T. J., Doig, N., Villalba, R. M., Huerta-Ocampo, I., … Bolam, J. P. (2014). The thalamostriatal system in normal and diseased states. *Frontiers in Systems Neuroscience, 8*(5), 1–18. doi:10.3389/fnsys.2014.00005.

Smith, Y., Raju, D. V., Pare, J.-F., & Sidibe, M. (2004). The thalamostriatal system: a highly specific network of the basal ganglia circuitry. *Trends in Neurosciences, 27*(9), 520–527. doi:10.1016/j.tins.2004.07.004.

Stoessl, A. J., Lehéricy, S., & Strafella, A. P. (2014). Imaging insights into basal ganglia function, Parkinson's disease, and dystonia. *The Lancet, 384*, 532–544. doi:10.1016/S0140-6736(14)60041-6.

Takada, M., Tokuno, H., Nambu, A., & Inase, M. (1998). Corticostriatal projections from the somatic motor areas of the frontal cortex in the macaque monkey: segregation versus overlap of input zones from the primary motor cortex, the supplementary motor area, and the premotor cortex. *Experimental Brain Research, 120*(1), 114–128.

Wiesendanger, E., Clarke, S., Kraftsik, R., & Tardif, E. (2004). Topography of cortico-striatal connections in man: anatomical evidence for parallel organization. *European Journal of Neuroscience, 20*(7), 1915–2004. doi:10.1111/j.1460-9568.2004.03626.x.

Wu, Y., Richard, S., & Parent, A. (2000). The organization of the striatal output system: a single-cell juxtacellular labeling study in the rat. *Neuroscience Research, 38*(1), 49–62. doi:10.1016/S0168-0102(00)00140-1.

2
THE FRONTAL CORTEX

Katherine Johnson

Introduction

Succinctly put, the frontal cortex organizes behaviour, reasoning, and language (Fuster, 2008). Two sections make up the frontal cortex - the prefrontal and the premotor cortices. This section of the brain orchestrates the behaviours associated with the more evolved organisms - attention control, working memory, the integration of perceptions and sensations, learning, monitoring of conflict, planning, making decisions, switching between choices, inhibition of behaviours, and perspective taking and mental relativism (theory of mind) (Fuster, 2008). The prefrontal cortex, in particular, allows one to anticipate future events, and subsequently plan, model, make decisions, and organize appropriate responses to that future event (Fuster, 2013). The frontal cortex is able to play an organizing role because of its connections with a large number of processing nodes spread throughout the other cortices and the subcortical structures (Crossley et al., 2013).

As organisms evolve, they are more likely to behave with greater deliberation and thought. Their reasoning for action may become more covert, and actions may be based on previous experience and delayed gratification rather than being automatic and reflexive (Fuster, 2008). These behaviours are associated with the functioning of the prefrontal cortex. From an evolutionary perspective, the human brain is notable for its size and complexity, especially in the prefrontal cortex (Rakic, 2009), which is one of the latest areas of the brain to evolve (Fuster, 2013). Relative to other orders, the frontal cortex is largest in the primate order, with especially large growth of the lateral prefrontal cortex in the human (Vendetti & Bunge, 2014). This area is essential for intelligent, thoughtful behaviour (Fuster, 2008). In contrast, the phylogenetic growth of the medial and inferior areas of the prefrontal cortex, which are associated with emotional behaviour, is less (Fuster, 2008).

This chapter will review the anatomy, connectivity, and biochemistry of the frontal cortex, the development of this area, what happens when the frontal cortex is damaged, the proposed roles of the frontal cortex, and provide an illustration of the importance of connectivity with the rest of the brain for the frontal cortex, using attention control as an example.

Anatomical description of the frontal cortex

The frontal cortex includes the prefrontal cortex (PFC) and the premotor areas (Fuster, 2008). The **PFC** consists of the lateral PFC (Brodmann areas 8, 9, 10, 44, 45, and 46), the medial PFC (areas 8m, 9m, 10m, 11m, and 12), and the orbitofrontal PFC (areas 10, 11, and 47) (Hélie, Ell, & Ashby, 2015). The neurons within the PFC are either glutaminergic excitatory pyramidal neurons, or GABAergic inhibitory stellate interneurons (Hélie et al., 2015). The PFC may be considered as a single, unified brain region, as many areas within the PFC are heavily connected.

The **premotor areas** (Brodmann area 6) lie between the PFC and the primary motor cortex. There are three separate areas within the premotor area – the ventral (PMv), lateral dorsal (PMd), and medial dorsal premotor areas. The medial dorsal premotor can be further subdivided into rostral [pre-Supplementary Motor Area (pre-SMA)] and caudal (SMA) regions.

Anatomical connections of the frontal cortex

The frontal cortex receives afferents from and projects efferents to most other cortical areas, and therefore is in a position to influence, and be influenced by, other cortical areas of the brain (Hélie et al., 2015).

The **PFC** has connections with all other cortical areas of the brain except the primary sensory and primary motor areas (Miller & Cohen, 2001). The lateral PFC is bidirectionally connected with the sensory association areas of the cortex, especially the visual, auditory, and somatic areas (Hélie et al., 2015). The information received by the lateral PFC is highly processed by these association areas (Hélie et al., 2015). It is also bidirectionally connected with the lateral premotor areas, with the dorsolateral PFC being strongly connected with the lateral premotor areas (Lu, Preston, & Strick, 1994).

The medial PFC receives substantial projections from the auditory association areas, with limited projections from visual and somatosensory areas. The orbitofrontal PFC receives projections from gustatory and olfactory areas, and visual, auditory, and somatosensory areas.

The PFC also sends projections subcortically to the basal ganglia (BG) and the thalamus (Hélie et al., 2015). Specifically, the PFC sends and receives substantial projections to/from the medial dorsal nucleus of the thalamus, and also sends and receives projections to/from the ventrolateral, and ventral anterior nuclei (Hélie et al., 2015). These projections are topographically organized.

The **premotor areas** receive projections from the lateral prefrontal cortex, from the basal ganglia and thalamus. Projections from the premotor area are sent to the primary motor cortex and then onto the spinal cord and the muscle systems involved in producing the movement (Hélie et al., 2015). Projections are also sent back to the premotor area, in a feedback loop. The pre-SMA also projects to the PFC (Hélie et al., 2015). Subcortically, premotor areas project to the ventral lateral and ventral anterior nuclei of the thalamus (Hélie et al., 2015).

Connectivity

The brain has been conceptualized as consisting of networks of neural elements known as the "connectome" (Sporns, Tononi, & Kötter, 2005). This quantitative analysis of complex networks, using graph theory applied to anatomical and functional magnetic imaging brain data, has generated new information about how regions of the brain communicate with each other (Bullmore & Sporns, 2009). "Rich club" hub nodes of neural networks are highly connected, have longer-distance connections than other brain regions, and are involved in integrative processing and adaptive behaviour (Crossley et al., 2014). The prefrontal and parietal cortices house the largest number of rich-club hubs (Crossley et al., 2013). Rich-club hubs, with their higher metabolic demands and longer-distance connections, are more likely to be anatomically abnormal in brain disorders – such as schizophrenia and Alzheimer's disease – than other non-rich-club hubs (Crossley et al., 2014). For example, temporal lobe hubs were associated with a higher lesion probability in Alzheimer's disease, whereas schizophrenia lesions were located in both frontal and temporal cortical hubs (Crossley et al., 2014). Connectivity analyses may provide a clearer understanding of the fundamental mechanisms of brain function, and therefore allow for a better understanding of dysfunction (Deco & Kringelbach, 2014).

The frontal cortex plays a central role in many brain networks. The fronto-striatal network has long been considered a particularly important network, involved in sensorimotor, emotion and motivation, and cognitive control (Redgrave et al., 2010). The fronto-parietal circuit is fundamental for attention control, sustained attention, arousal, response to novelty, and awareness (Robertson, 2014). The fronto-cerebellar circuit plays roles in movement, balance, and cognition (Arnsten & Rubia, 2012). The affective network, incorporating the orbital prefrontal cortex, the limbic cortex, amygdala, and hippocampus is important for emotional regulation and habitual behaviours (Arnsten & Rubia, 2012). The default mode network involves the medial frontal lobe, anterior and posterior cingulate, inferior temporal and parietal areas (Greicius, Krasnow, Reiss, & Menon, 2003); these regions show intercorrelated activation during periods of inactivity, and when a participant is asked to complete a task, this activation is attenuated (Raichle, 2015). There are many different connections between the frontal cortex and other cortical and subcortical areas of the brain. The functions of these different circuits are open to debate and further research. With advancing technologies, our understanding of which circuits play what types of roles in behaviour will become clearer.

Biochemistry of the frontal cortex

The neurotransmitters glutamate, γ-Aminobutyric acid (GABA), acetylcholine, and the monoamines are considered to be the most important of the chemical messenger systems for the functioning of the frontal cortex. Glutamate is the primary excitatory neurotransmitter of the cortex; its N-methyl-D-aspartate (NMDA) receptor is widely distributed through the cortex and hippocampus, and is involved in learning and memory (Fuster, 2008). GABA is the primary inhibitory neurotransmitter of the cortex; it supports local inhibitory control, including lateral inhibition, which enhances the saliency of excitatory responses (Fuster, 2008). The prefrontal cortex also receives diffuse afferents from the subcortical cholinergic system (Fuster, 2008), and these are largely excitatory.

The three monoamine neurotransmitters – dopamine, noradrenaline, and serotonin – are generated in the brainstem structures (the ventral tegmentum, the nucleus coeruleus, and the raphé nuclei, respectively), and have direct pathways into the prefrontal cortex, bypassing the thalamus (Fuster, 2008). The noradrenaline system innervates the neocortex diffusively. The serotonin system innervates mostly sensory areas. The dopamine system innervates the orbitomedial prefrontal cortex, in a discrete manner (Fuster, 2008). This is part of the mesocorticolimbic system, which is involved in reward and motivation (Fuster, 2008).

The prefrontal cortex also contains neuropeptides [e.g., somatostatin, substance P, Cholecystokinin (CCK), angiotensin, neurotensin] that act as neurotransmitters and neuromodulators (Fuster, 2008).

Development of the frontal cortex

In the first trimester, as neurons are produced they migrate to their positions within the brain structure, and connections between neurons start to be made (Marsh, Gerber, & Peterson, 2008). In the second trimester the macro-scale connectome begins to develop with the onset of synaptogenesis. Connections are made between the two hemispheres, between the brain and the spinal cord, between the thalamus and the cortex, and between areas within the cortex (Collin & van den Heuvel, 2013). By birth, the fundamental elements of the connectome are in place – the infant brain has properties of a small-world network, with community structures (brain areas), hubs of highly connected areas, and rich-clubs – hubs that are especially well connected (Di Martino et al., 2014).

At birth, the prefrontal cortex has its basic architecture in place (Stiles & Jernigan, 2010). Around the time of birth, there is an overproduction of neurons, the number of which reduces through apoptosis over time (Marsh et al., 2008). Concurrently, synaptogenesis generates an overproduction of synapses, which also reduce over time. Myelination starts later in the prefrontal cortex than many other regions of the brain, and the finishing of the myelination processes only occurs in the early twenties, coinciding with cognitive maturation (Fuster, 2008; Giedd et al., 2010; Tau & Peterson, 2010). An inverted U shape curve describes changes in grey matter brain development from childhood through adolescence into adulthood (Giedd et al., 2010), with different areas of the brain following different developmental trajectories (Giedd et al., 2010). Grey matter areas in both the cerebral cortex and subcortical structures are larger in older children than young adults and young children (Jernigan & Gamst, 2005). White matter within the lobes shows an increase in volume as the brain matures (Lenroot et al., 2007). Maturation of the commissures and projection fibres occur earliest in development, association fibres continue to mature at later ages, whilst the fronto-temporal connections have the most prolonged development (Lebel & Beaulieu, 2011).

As the brain develops through childhood, there is a shift in the connectome from short- to long-range connectivity, especially within the first two years of life (Fransson et al., 2007). Brain areas are highly connected, and as the child grows, these connections extend to become part of more distributed networks (Fair et al., 2009). Local efficiency of brain networks increases as the child grows; in contrast, it is thought that global efficiency of the brain stays constant throughout life (Di Martino et al., 2014). The structural hubs also appear to remain relatively constant through the lifespan; in contrast, the functional hubs change as the child grows (Di Martino et al., 2014). In the infant brain, the primary motor cortex and primary sensory areas house the hubs and this then shifts in adulthood to heteromodal association cortex (Fransson, Aden, Blennow, & Lagercrantz, 2011). Subcortically, the subcortico-cortico connections tend to be stronger in infancy and childhood, compared with adulthood, whilst cortico-cortical connections tend to increase with age (Di Martino et al., 2014; Superkar, Musen, & Menon, 2009).

Deviations in the development of neural interactions of the connectome can occur through two basic processes – abnormalities associated with **timing** and abnormalities in **shape** (Di Martino et al., 2014). In terms of timing, decelerations in connectome development index immaturity or delay, whilst accelerations index precocious development. Both variations may lead to abnormal connections being made (Di Martino et al., 2014). Attention Deficit Hyperactivity Disorder (ADHD) is associated with delayed cortical development, for example, Shaw et al., (2007). In another example, in adolescents reporting psychotic experiences, abnormal timing of myelination was found in the putamen between the inferior fronto-occipital and the uncinate fasciculi, and in the left parietal regions that include the fibre bundle of the superior longitudinal fasciculus (O'Hanlon et al., 2015). Abnormalities in the shape of the brain may have more severe ramifications for the person. Ectopic, abnormally located connectivity, a failure to make connections, or a halting of development are all examples of problems (and possible compensations) associated with shape abnormalities (Di Martino et al., 2014). For instance, children with autism spectrum disorders (ASD) were found to have ectopic striatal functional connectivity, with increased functional connectivity within the striatum and between the striatum and association and limbic cortices, and hypoconnectivity between the pons and the striatum (Di Martino et al., 2011).

Damage to the frontal cortex

Lesion, disease, transcranial magnetic stimulation (TMS), and magnetic resonance imaging (MRI) studies have incrementally improved our understanding of the physiology and psychology of the frontal cortex. The neuropsychological effects of **prefrontal cortex** damage depend, to a large degree, on the site and the extent of the damage (Fuster, 2008). Large lesions to the prefrontal cortex, especially involving the lateral or medial areas, often result in apathy and general disinterest (Fuster, 2008). Depression may result from damage to the left lateral and polar cortex, and possibly orbital damage. Orbital lesions may result in hyper-reactivity to irrelevant stimuli, but low reactivity to emotional stimuli (Fuster, 2008), and in euphoria, disinhibition, risky decision-making, and blunted moral judgements (Fuster, 2008).

Many executive functions will be affected by damage to the prefrontal cortex. Patients with prefrontal lesions may have difficulties in encoding new memories, and in retrieving old ones, and may show difficulties with working memory (Fuster, 2008). Patients with prefrontal damage, especially laterally, may have difficulties with constructing and executing plans of action. Decision-making may also be affected after prefrontal damage – this can result from working memory and planning deficits, or because of emotional bias and reckless risk-taking (Fuster, 2008). Damage to the frontal cortex may also result in difficulties with the temporal synthesis of language. Patients may suffer from aphasia – a lack of spontaneous speech, diminished verbal expression, and/or loss of verbal fluency (Fuster, 2008). Attention difficulties often arise with prefrontal cortex damage – patients may have difficulties with focusing attention and sustaining it over time, and in inhibiting irrelevant interference (Fuster, 2008).

Damage to specific regions of the prefrontal cortex may result in different syndromes, or clusters of symptoms. Damage to the lateral prefrontal cortex results in problems with sustaining attention, making decisions, initiative, making and executing plans, poor working memory, low verbal fluency, apathy and depression (Fuster, 2008). Damage to the orbital region may result in impulsive, distracted, irritable, and perseverative behaviour that is lacking in moral constraint (Fuster, 2008). Lesions to the medial/anterior prefrontal cortex may result in a lack of initiative and spontaneous behaviour, hypokinesia or akinesia, and apathy (Fuster, 2008).

Lesions to the SMA of the **premotor cortex** can result in alien-limb syndrome, whereby patients make involuntary movements or fail to use a hand, even when they are able to use their hand (Nachev, Kennard, & Husain, 2008). Parkinson's disease has been associated with reduced activity of the SMA and pre-SMA, which may be as a result of reduced dopaminergic input from the basal ganglia to the SMA (Nachev et al., 2008).

Roles of the frontal cortex

Researchers differ in their emphases given to the roles of the frontal cortex. For instance, Stuss and Alexander argue that the frontal cortex plays a role in the cognitive functions of self-awareness, humor, verbal fluency, memory, and attention control (Stuss & Alexander, 2000). Mesulam has argued that the prefrontal cortex has five key roles (Mesulam, 2002). This area of the brain, he says, controls working memory and attention control. It is involved in the inhibition of distractibility, perseveration, and immediate gratification. The prefrontal cortex is in active pursuit of choice and novelty. It performs conditional mapping of emotional significance, and it encodes context, perspective, and mental relativism (Mesulam, 2002). Fuster argues that the frontal cortex is the "action cortex" – it is devoted to action of different kinds – bodily movement, eye movement, the expression of emotion and speech, and reasoning (p. 2) (Fuster, 2008).

Looking at Fuster's suggestions in detail, he argues that the single most important overseeing function of the lateral prefrontal cortex is the ability to organize actions in *time* (Fuster, 2008, 2013). The temporal organizing function of this area of the brain is essential for mammals. It is used for the execution of new, acquired, and elaborate behaviours (Fuster, 2008). A sense of time underpins the coordination of actions, and is essential for speech fluency, higher reasoning, and creative activities (Fuster, 2008).

The three major functions of the prefrontal cortex, according to Fuster, are planning, decision-making, and executive attention (Fuster, 2008). By executive attention, Fuster suggests there are three components – working memory, preparatory set, and inhibitory interference control (Fuster, 2008). The prefrontal cortex orchestrates activities throughout the brain that are involved in executive attention. Working memory is the "temporary activation of updated long-term memory networks for organizing actions in the near term" (p. 4) (Fuster, 2008). Preparatory set is the setting-up of sensory and motor areas for the performance of an upcoming act, which is contingent on previous experience – thus drawing on working memory (Fuster, 2008). Inhibitory control enhances one sensory input and silences other cognitive, emotional, or other operations that may interfere with the purpose at hand (Fuster, 2008). There is a large degree of interdependency and co-operation between the areas of the prefrontal cortex and their roles. There is a sharing of common networks activated during an organism's ongoing cycle of perceiving and acting (Fuster, 2008).

A number of different roles have been suggested for the **premotor cortex**. The PMv contains mirror neurons – neurons that discharge both when a monkey executes a specific motor act and also when it views someone else performing the same motor act (Rizzolatti & Sinigaglia, 2010). Mirror neurons are also present in the parietal cortex, in the inferior parietal lobule, and the anterior intraparietal area in the monkey (Rizzolatti & Sinigaglia, 2010). These parietal areas are heavily connected with the PMv. The PMv is connected with the pre-SMA and the prefrontal cortex (Rizzolatti & Sinigaglia, 2010). A recent meta-analysis of 125 fMRI studies concluded that similar areas are activated in the human brain – the inferior parietal lobule, inferior frontal gyrus, and ventral premotor cortex. In addition, a core network of human brain regions also show mirroring properties – the primary visual cortex, cerebellum, and limbic areas (Molenberghs, Cunnington, & Mattingley, 2012). The human brain has a network of brain areas activated by action observation and execution, and additional areas of the brain are also recruited, such as the somatosensory and affective networks (Molenberghs et al., 2012). The premotor cortex is involved in the mirror neuron system.

Inputs from the premotor cortex control the selection of self-generated and exogenously generated movements (Rizzolatti & Sinigaglia, 2010). The SMA is thought to be involved in the initiation of movements that are internally derived (Cunnington, Iansek, Johnson, & Bradshaw, 1997; Cunnington, Windischberger, Deecke, & Moser, 2002), that may have a temporal component to sequential movement (Cunnington, Iansek, Bradshaw, & Phillips, 1995), and that involve the coordination of the two sides of the body, such as bimanual coordination (Johnson et al., 1998). The SMA and pre-SMA may play roles in learning new associations between stimuli and responses, and learning new sequences of movements. The SMA and pre-SMA may also be involved in switching between movement types, based on monitoring conflicting information (Nachev et al., 2008).

Attention control

The term "attention" refers to a family of cognitive functions that prepare a person to respond quickly and appropriately to information either from the environment or from an internally generated decision (Chica et al., 2012), so that one's mental processes are focused (Luck & Mangun, 2009) and sustained (Robertson, Manly, Andrade, Baddeley, & Yiend, 1997). Attention therefore provides the ability to self-regulate sensory input, motor output, and emotion in the service of internally derived goals (Rothbart & Posner, 2015).

Posner and Peterson's theory of attention networks is a well-subscribed model of attention control (Petersen & Posner, 2012; Posner & Peterson, 1990). This theory has developed over time and has incorporated elements of other theories (e.g., Corbetta & Shulman, 2002) to take into account alternative ideas and research findings, in the scientific process described by Lakatos (1978). This theory of attention describes three separate attention networks – the arousal, orienting, and executive control networks. These networks are separate from the sensory processing systems of the brain and consist of a series of brain regions that each carry out specific processes but that altogether contribute to the functioning of each network (Petersen & Posner, 2012). The alerting network allows a person to acquire and maintain an alert state, ready to accept incoming information from the outside world. This network incorporates parts of the right frontal cortex, parietal cortex, and the locus coeruleus, and operates through noradrenalin release (Posner & Rothbart, 2007). The orienting network allows the selection of information from the senses and for internal direction of attention, and uses acetylcholine as a neurotransmitter (Petersen & Posner, 2012). This network may be split into two parts – the dorsal and ventral attention systems (Corbetta & Shulman, 2002). The dorsal attention system consists of the human analog of the frontal eye fields and the intraparietal sulcus/superior parietal lobe and it modulates voluntary, goal-driven endogenous control of attentional focus (Kincade, Abrams, Asatfiev, Shulman, & Corbetta, 2005). The ventral attention network consists of the temporo-parietal junction and the ventral frontal cortex, including the middle and inferior frontal gyri, frontal operculum, and the anterior insula. The ventral attention network modulates exogenous attention – the involuntary direction of attention to an unexpected stimulus occurring in space, in an automatic and reflexive manner (Kincade et al., 2005). The ventral attention network is thought to act as a 'circuit breaker' for the dorsal system, as it disengages attention from one location and directs it to another (Shulman et al., 2009). Finally, the executive attention network acts to resolve any discrepancies that arise between competing stimuli, and uses dopamine as its neurotransmitter (Petersen & Posner, 2012). This network may also be broken into two parts – the frontoparietal control system and the cingulo-opercular system (Petersen & Posner, 2012). The frontoparietal control system networks the dorsal lateral prefrontal cortex, the precuneus, and the inferior parietal sulcus and lobe, and is involved in moment-to-moment task control (Petersen & Posner, 2012). The cingulo-opercular system networks the thalamus, dorsal anterior cingulate cortex, and the anterior insula/operculum, and is thought to maintain tonic levels of alertness for current processing needs (Sadaghiani & D'Esposito, 2014). The frontal cortex plays a critical role in each of these three attention networks; nevertheless attention control relies on the interactions between the frontal cortex, the parietal cortex, and subcortical regions. Functional connectivity studies, using functional and anatomical magnetic resonance imaging techniques, have provided valuable insights into how these networks function in typically and atypically developing children, adolescents, and adults (e.g., Fitzgerald et al., 2015; Baldassaurre et al., 2014).

Summary

The frontal cortex oversees cognition, language, movement, memory, thinking, planning, and attention control. There are many connections within the frontal cortex itself, and between it and the other cortices and subcortical structures.

A number of neurotransmitters and neuromodulators act within the frontal cortex. The development of the frontal cortex continues into early adulthood. The result of damage to the frontal cortex depends on the site and extent of the damage. The frontal cortex works in conjunction with many other areas of the brain in order to accomplish the behaviours that are associated with *Homo sapiens.*

Abbreviations

BG: Basal Ganglia
CCK: Cholecystokinin
GABA: γ-Aminobutyric acid
NMDA: N-methyl-D-aspartate
PFC: Prefrontal cortex
PMd: Lateral dorsal premotor area
PMv: Ventral premotor area
SMA: Supplementary Motor Area
TMS: Transcranial magnetic stimulation

Further readings

Fuster, J. M. (2008). *The Prefrontal Cortex* (Fourth ed.). London: Academic Press.

Hélie, S., Ell, S. W., & Ashby, F. G. (2015). Learning robust cortico-cortical associations with the basal ganglia: An integrative review. *Cortex, 64*(Mar), 123–135. doi: 10.1016/j.cortex.2014.10.011.

Johnson, M. H., Jones, E. J., & Gliga, T. (2015). Brain adaptation and alternative developmental trajectories. *Development and Psychopathology, 27*(2), 425–442. doi: 10.1017/S0954579415000073.

Raichle, M. E. (2015). The restless brain: How intrinisic activity organizes brain function. *Philosophical Transactions of the Royal Society. Series B, Biological Sciences, 370*(1668), 20140172. doi: 10.1098/rstb.2014.0172.

Stiles, J., & Jernigan, T. L. (2010). The basics of brain development. *Neuropsychology Review, 20*(4), 327–348. doi: 10.1007/s11065-010-9148-4.

Stuss, D. T., & Knight, R. T. (2013). *Principles of Frontal Lobe Function* (Second ed.). New York, NY: Oxford University Press.

Vértes, P. E., & Bullmore, E. T. (2015). Annual research review: Growth connectomics - the organization and reorganization of brain networks during normal and abnormal development. *Journal of Child Psychology and Psychiatry, 56*(3), 299–320. doi: 10.1111/jcpp.12365.

References

Arnsten, A. F. T., & Rubia, K. (2012). Neurobiological circuits regulating attention, cognitive control, motivation, and emotion: Disruptions in neurodevelopmental psychiatric disorders. *Journal of the American Academy of Child and Adolescent Psychiatry, 51*(4), 356–367. doi: 10.1016/j.jaac.2012.01.008.

Baldassaurre, A., Ramsey, L., Hacker, C. L., Callejas, A., Asatfiev, S. V., Metcalf, N. V., … Corbetta, M. (2014). Large-scale changes in network interactions as a physiological signature of spatial neglect. *Brain, 137*(12), 3267–3283. doi: 10.1093/brain/awu297.

Bullmore, E. T., & Sporns, O. (2009). Complex brain networks: Graph theoretical analysis of structural and functional systems. *Nature Reviews. Neuroscience, 10*(3), 186–198. doi: 10.1038/nrn2575.

Chica, A. B., Thiebaut de Schotten, M., Toba, M., Malhotra, P., Lupiáñez, J., & Bartolomeo, P. (2012). Attention networks and their interactions after right-hemisphere damage. *Cortex, 48*(6), 654–663. doi: 10.1016/j.cortex.2011.01.009.

Collin, G., & van den Heuvel, M. P. (2013). The ontogeny of the human connectome: Development and dynamic changes of brain connectivity across the life span. *Neuroscientist, 19*(6), 616–628. doi: 10.1177/1073858413503712.

Corbetta, M., & Shulman, G. L. (2002). Control of goal-directed and stimulus-driven attention in the brain. *Nature Reviews Neuroscience, 3*(3), 201–215. doi: 10.1038/nrn755.

Crossley, N. A., Mechelli, A., Scott, J., Carletti, F., Fox, P. T., McGuire, P., & Bullmore, E. T. (2014). The hubs of the human connectome are generally implicated in the anatomy of brain disorders. *Brain, 137*, 2382–2395. doi: 10.1093/brain/awu132.

Crossley, N. A., Mechelli, A., Vértes, P. E., Winton-Brown, T. T., Patel, A. X., Ginestet, C. E., … Bullmore, E. T. (2013). Cognitive relevance of the community structure of the human brain functional coactivation network. *Proceedings of the National Academy of Sciences, 110*(28), 11583–11588. doi: 10.1073/pnas.1220826110.

Cunnington, R., Iansek, R., Bradshaw, J. L., & Phillips, J. G. (1995). Movement-related potentials in Parkinson's disease: Presence and predictability of temporal and spatial cues. *Brain, 118*, 935–950.

Cunnington, R., Iansek, R., Johnson, K. A., & Bradshaw, J. L. (1997). Movement-related potentials in Parkinson's disease. *Brain, 120*, 1339–1353.

Cunnington, R., Windischberger, C., Deecke, L., & Moser, E. (2002). The preparation and execution of self-intitiated and externally-triggered movement: A study of event-related fMRI. *NeuroImage, 15*(2), 373–385. doi: 10.1006/nimg.2001.0976.

Deco, G., & Kringelbach, M. L. (2014). Great expectations: Using whole-brain computational connectomics for understanding neuropsychiatric disorders. *Neuron, 84*(December 3), 892–905. doi: 10.1016/j.neuron.2014.08.034.

Di Martino, A., Fair, D. A., Kelly, C., Satterthwaite, T. D., Castellanos, F. X., Thomason, M. E., … Milham, M. P. (2014). Unraveling the miswired connectome: A developmental perspective. *Neuron, 83*(6), 1335–1353. doi: 10.1016/j.neuron.2014.08.050.

Di Martino, A., Kelly, C., Grzadzinski, R., Zuo, X. N., Mennes, M., Mairena, M. A., …. Milham, M. P. (2011). Aberrant striatal functional connectivity in children with autism. *Biological Psychiatry, 69*(9), 847–856. doi: 10.1016/j.biopsych.2010.10.029.

Fair, D. A., Cohen, A. L., Power, J. D., Dosenbach, N. U., Church, J. A., Miezin, F. M., … Petersen, S. E. (2009). Functional brain networks develop from a "local to distributed" organization. *PLoS Computational Biology, 5*(5), e1000381. doi: 10.1371/journal.pcbi.1000381.

Fitzgerald, J., Johnson, K. A., Kehoe, E., Bodke, A., Garavan, H., Gallagher, L., & McGrath, J. (2015). Disrupted functional connectivity in dorsal and ventral attention networks during attention orienting in autism spectrum disorders. *Autism Research, 8*(2), 136–152. doi: 10.1002/aur.1430.

Fransson, P., Aden, U., Blennow, M., & Lagercrantz, H. (2011). The functional architecture of the infant brain as revealed by resting-state fMRI. *Cerebral Cortex, 21*(1), 145–154. doi: 10.1093/cercor/bhq071.

Fransson, P., Skiöld, B., Horsch, S., Nordell, A., Blennow, M., Lagercrantz, H., & Aden, U. (2007). Resting-state networks in the infant brain. *Proceedings of the National Academy of Sciences, 104*(39), 15531–15536. doi: 10.1073/pnas.0704380104.

Fuster, J. M. (2008). *The Prefrontal Cortex* (Fourth ed.). London: Academic Press.

Fuster, J. M. (2013). Cognitive functions of the prefrontal cortex. In D. T. Stuss & R. T. Knight (Eds.), *Principles of Frontal Lobe Function* (Second ed., pp. 11–22). New York, NY: Oxford University Press.

Giedd, J. N., Stockman, M., Weddle, C., Liverpool, M., Alexander-Bloch, A. F., Wallace, G. L., … Lenroot, R. K. (2010). Anatomic magnetic resonance imaging of the developing child and adolescent brain and effects of genetic variation. *Neuropsychology Review, 20*(4), 349–361. doi: 10.1007/s11065-010-9151-9.

Greicius, M. D., Krasnow, B., Reiss, A. L., & Menon, V. (2003). Functional connectivity in the resting brain: A network analysis of the default mode hypothesis. *Proceedings of the National Academy of Sciences, 100*(1), 253–258. doi: 10.1073/pnas.0135058100.

Hélie, S., Ell, S. W., & Ashby, F. G. (2015). Learning robust cortico-cortical associations with the basal ganglia: An integrative review. *Cortex, 64*(Mar), 123–135. doi: 10.1016/j.cortex.2014.10.011.

Jernigan, T. L., & Gamst, A. C. (2005). Changes in volume with age—consistency and interpretation of observed effects. *Neurobiology of Aging, 26*(9), 1271–1274. doi: 10.1016/j.neurobiolaging.2005.05.016.

Johnson, K. A., Cunnington, R., Bradshaw, J. L., Phillips, J. G., Iansek, R., & Rogers, M. A. (1998). Bimanual co-ordination in Parkinson's disease. *Brain, 121*, 743–753. doi: 10.1093/brain/121.4.743.

Kincade, J. M., Abrams, R. A., Asatfiev, S. V., Shulman, G. L., & Corbetta, M. (2005). An event-related functional magnetic resonance study of voluntary and stimulus-driven orienting of attention. *Journal of Neuroscience, 25*(18), 4593–4604. doi: 10.1523/JNEUROSCI.0236-05.2005.

Lakatos, I. (1978). *The Methodology of Scientific Research Programmes* (First ed.). London: Cambridge University Press.

Lebel, C., & Beaulieu, C. (2011). Longitudinal development of human brain wiring continues from childhood into adulthood. *The Journal of Neuroscience, 31*(30), 10937–10947. doi: 0.1523/JNEUROSCI.5302-10.2011.

Lenroot, R. K., Gogtay, N., Greenstein, D. K., Wells, E. M., Wallace, G. L., Clasen, L. S., … Giedd, J. N. (2007). Sexual dimorphism of brain developmental trajectories during childhood and adolescence. *NeuroImage, 36*(4), 1065–1073.

Lu, M.-T., Preston, J. B., & Strick, P. L. (1994). Interconections between the prefrontal cortex and the premotor areas in the frontal lobe. *The Journal of Comparative Neurology, 341*(3), 375–392. doi: 10.1002/cne.903410308.

Luck, S. J., & Mangun, S. R. (2009). Introduction. In M. S. Gazzaniga (Ed.), *The Cognitive Neurosciences* (4 ed.). Cambridge: The MIT Press.

Marsh, R., Gerber, A. J., & Peterson, B. S. (2008). Neuroimaging studies of normal brain development and their relevance for understanding childhood neuropsychiatric disorders. *Journal of the American Academy of Child and Adolescent Psychiatry, 47*(11), 1233–1251. doi: 10.1097/CHI.0b013e318185e703.

Mesulam, M. (2002). The human frontal lobes: Transcending the default mode through contingent encoding. In D. T. Stuss & R. T. Knight (Eds.), *Principles of Frontal Lobe Function* (First ed.). New York, NY: Oxford University Press.

Miller, E. K., & Cohen, J. D. (2001). An integrative theory of prefrontal cortex function. *Annual Review of Neuroscience, 24*, 167–202. doi: 10.1146/annurev.neuro.24.1.167.

Molenberghs, P., Cunnington, R., & Mattingley, J. B. (2012). Brain regions with mirror properties: A meta-analysis of 125 human fMRI studies. *Neuroscience and Biobehavioral Reviews, 36*(1), 341–349. doi: 10.1016/j.neubiorev.2011.07.004.

Nachev, P., Kennard, C., & Husain, M. (2008). Functional role of the supplementary and pre-supplementary motor areas. *Nature Reviews. Neuroscience, 9*(11), 856–870. doi: 10.1038/nrn2478.

O'Hanlon, E., Leemans, A., Kelleher, I., Clarke, M. C., Roddy, S., Coughlan, H., … Cannon, M. (2015). White matter differences among adolescents reporting psychotic experiences: A population-based diffusion magnetic resonance imaging study. *JAMA Psychiatry, 72*(7), 668–677. doi: 10.1001/jamapsychiatry.2015.0137.

Petersen, S. E., & Posner, M. I. (2012). The attention system of the human brain: 20 years after. *Annual Review of Neuroscience, 35*, 73–89. doi: 10.1146/annurev-neuro-062111-150525.

Posner, M. I., & Peterson, S. E. (1990). The attention system of the human brain. *Annual Review of Neuroscience, 13*, 35–42. doi: 10.1146/annurev.ne.13.030190.000325.

Posner, M. I., & Rothbart, M. K. (2007). Research on attention networks as a model for the integration of psychological science. *Annual Review of Psychology, 58*(1), 1–23. doi: 10.1146/annurev.psych.58.110405.085516.

Raichle, M. E. (2015). The restless brain: How intrinisic activity organizes brain function. *Philosophical Transactions of the Royal Society. Series B, Biological Sciences, 370*(1668), 20140172. doi: 10.1098/rstb.2014.0172.

Rakic, P. (2009). Evolution of the neocortex: A perspective from developmental biology. *Nature Reviews. Neuroscience, 10*(October 2009), 724–735. doi: 10.1038/nrn2719.

Redgrave, P., Rodriguez, M., Smith, Y., Rodriguez-Oroz, M. C., Lehericy, S., Bergman, H., … Obeso, J. A. (2010). Goal-directed and habitual control in the basal ganglia: Implications for Parkinson's disease. *Nature Reviews. Neuroscience, 11*(11), 760–772. doi: 10.1038/nrn2915.

Rizzolatti, G., & Sinigaglia, C. (2010). The functional role of the parieto-frontal mirror circuit: Interpretations and misinterpretations. *Nature Reviews. Neuroscience, 11*(4), 264–274. doi: 10.1038/nrn2805.

Robertson, I. H. (2014). Right hemisphere role in cognitive reserve. *Neurobiology of Aging, 35*(6), 1375–1385. doi: 10.1016/j.neurobiolaging.2013.11.028.

Robertson, I. H., Manly, T., Andrade, J., Baddeley, B. T., & Yiend, J. (1997). 'Oops!': Performance correlates of everyday attentional failures in traumatic brain injured and normal subjects. *Neuropsychologia, 35*(6), 747–758. doi: 10.1016/S0028-3932(97)00015-8.

Rothbart, M. K., & Posner, M. I. (2015). The developing brain in a multitasking world. *Developmental Review,* in press. doi: 10.1016/j.dr.2014.12.006.

Sadaghiani, S., & D'Esposito, M. (2014). Functional characterization of the cingulo-opercular network in the maintenance of tonic alertness. *Cerebral Cortex,* in press. doi: 10.1093/cercor/bhu072.

Shaw, P., Eckstrand, K., Sharp, W., Blumenthal, J., Lerch, J. P., Greenstein, D., … Rapoport, J. L. (2007). Attention-deficit/hyperactivity disorder is characterized by a delay in cortical maturation. *Proceedings of the National Academy of Science, 104*(49), 19649–19654.

Shulman, G. L., Asatfiev, S. V., Franke, D., Pope, D. L. W., Synder, A. Z., McAvoy, M. P., & Corbetta, M. (2009). Interaction of stimulus-driven reorienting and expectation in ventral and dorsal frontoparietal and basal ganglia-cortical networks. *Journal of Neuroscience, 29*(14), 4392–4407. doi: 10.1523/JNEUROSCI.5609-08.2009.

Sporns, O., Tononi, G., & Kötter, R. (2005). The human connectome: A structural description of the human brain. *PLoS Computational Biology, 1*(4), e42. doi: 10.1371/journal.pcbi.0010042.

Stiles, J., & Jernigan, T. L. (2010). The basics of brain development. *Neuropsychology Review, 20*(4), 327–348. doi: 10.1007/s11065-010-9148-4.

Stuss, D. T., & Alexander, M. P. (2000). Executive functions and the frontal lobes: A conceptual view. *Psychological Research, 63*(2–4), 289–298. doi: 10.1007/s004269900007.

Superkar, K., Musen, M., & Menon, V. (2009). Development of large-scale functional brain networks in children. *PLoS Biology,* 7, e1000157. doi: 10.1371/journal.pbio.1000157.

Tau, G. Z., & Peterson, B. S. (2010). Normal development of brain circuits. *Neuropsychopharmacology, 35*, 147–168. doi: 10.1038/npp.2009.115.

Vendetti, M. S., & Bunge, S. A. (2014). Evolutionary and developmental changes in the lateral frontoparietal network: A little goes a long way for higher-level cognition. *Neuron, 84*(3), 906–917. doi: 10.1016/j.neuron.2014.09.035.

3
CEREBELLAR COGNITIVE AFFECTIVE SYNDROME

Claudine Kraan

Introduction

Schmahmann and colleagues published the first controlled investigation of cognitive and affective deficit following isolated cerebellar injury. This study provided evidence for non-motor clinical features, such as executive dysfunction, impaired spatial cognition, personality change and linguistic difficulties in adult patients with damage to the vermis and/or posterior lobe of the cerebellum. Schmahmann and colleagues named this spectrum of deficits the cerebellar cognitive affective syndrome (hereafter CCAS) and attributed the outcome to "*disruption of the cerebellar modulation of neural circuits that link prefrontal, posterior parietal, superior temporal and limbic cortices with the cerebellum*" (Schmahmann & Sherman, 1998). This work provided a critical contribution to neuroscience as it has significantly enhanced our understanding of how and why cerebellar injury can lead to a variety of cognitive and affective deficits.

The present chapter provides an overview of the CCAS. It begins with discussion of the onset and prevalence of CCAS, highlighting that the location and size of the lesion to the cerebellum is what determines the clinical outcome for the patient. It then discusses neurophysiological and neuroscientific explanations behind CCAS, clinical symptoms and the possible effects of laterality. The second half of the chapter notes that there are actually no guidelines about what diagnostics are to be used when assessing CCAS and few published recommendations for treatments, which almost certainly reflects the infancy of the field of CCAS research.

Onset and prevalence

The onset of CCAS is inherently dependent upon the functional zone of the cerebellum that is injured. Functional zones of the cerebellum have been delineated based on what supratentorial region they are most densely connected to. The posterior region of the cerebellum (mostly lobule VI and VII) receives dense input from the prefrontal and parietal cortices on the contralateral hemispheric side. Coincidentally, injury or damage to the posterior region can lead to deficits of executive function, linguistic function and visuospatial processing. Thus the posterior region is considered to be a 'cognitive zone'. By contrast, the anterior region of the cerebellum (lobule IV-V, extension of lobule VI and parts of VIII) is primarily connected with the motor cortex. Injury to the anterior region will typically result in problems of motor control, postural instability and poor movement coordination (Stoodley, Valera, & Schmahmann, 2012), therefore the anterior region is thought to be a 'motor zone'. Finally, the vermis is a critical node in the cortico-limbic network (Schmahmann, Weilburg, & Sherman, 2007) and injury or damage here leads to communication disorders, autistic-like profiles and affective and behavioural disruptions. Thus, the vermis is largely thought to be an 'affective zone'. Generally speaking, neurological conditions that cause damage to the cerebellar vermis and/or posterior cerebellum have been shown to lead to CCAS.

It is estimated that approximately 30% of children with medulloblastoma removed from a space in the skull near the brainstem and cerebellum called the posterior fossa will develop CCAS, less for astrocytoma (Catsman-Berrevoets & Aarsen, 2010). Cerebellar tumour can occur in adults, though it is far more prevalent in children. Stroke is another common cause of CCAS, usually from infarction of the posterior inferior cerebellar artery which provides the main arterial supply to the posterior cerebellum, although both brainstem stroke and postnatal hemorrhage as a complication of preterm birth have been highlighted in recent publications (Baillieux et al., 2010; Brossard-Racine, du Plessis, & Limperopoulos, 2015). Neurodegenerative conditions characterized by significant neuropathology isolated to the cerebellum are further important etiologies of CCAS. There is also good evidence that children born with congenital malformations of cerebellar development will develop CCAS (Tavano et al., 2007). Furthermore, studies have suggested that congenital malformations of the posterior fossa *bone*, such as Chiari 1 malformations, can also lead to a CCAS-like profile, although this avenue has not been explored in great detail (Kumar et al., 2011). The number of CCAS diagnoses will probably increase over time as medical techniques impacting the likelihood of surviving injury to the cerebellum become more sophisticated. Other etiologies of CCAS are presented in Table 3.1.

Neurophysiology

Many different theories have been proposed to explain CCAS. These include compensatory changes in the cortex through neuroplasticity, vasospasms, disruption of dopaminergic, neuroepinephrine and/or serotonin neurotransmitter

TABLE 3.1 Limited list of disorders/conditions known to lead to CCAS

Type of aetiology	*Name of disorder/condition*	*Description*
Acquired	Surgical resection of cerebellar tumor	Tumour tissue removed from the bone supporting the cerebellum (usually benign astrocytoma or malignant medulloblastoma)
	Cerebellar stroke	Usually infarction of posterior inferior cerebellar artery injuring posterior zone of cerebellum and/or brainstem stroke
	Cerebellar hemorrhage related to premature birth	Hemorrhaged with vermal and/or cerebellar hemisphere damage as a complication of preterm birth (<36 weeks gestational age)
Congenital	Rhombencephalosynapsis	Missing vermis and fusion of hemispheres
	Near-total cerebellar agenesis	Near-total absence of a cerebellum
	Diffuse cerebellar hypoplasia	Cerebellum smaller or incompletely developed
	Agenesis and dysplasia of cerebellar hemisphere(s)	Absence or malformation of cerebellar hemisphere(s)
	Jourbert syndrome	Complete or partial absence of cerebellar vermis
	Chiari 1 malformation	Protrusion of the cerebellum into the foramen magnum (may not become symptomatic until adolescence or adulthood; can emerge following trauma)
	Dandy Walker malformation	Abnormal fourth ventricle, abnormal vermal lobulation and enlarged posterior fossa
Neurodegenerative	Spinocerebellar ataxia	Inherited neurodegenerative disorder leading to atrophy of the cerebellum
	Essential tremor	Inherited movement disorder involving the cerebellum and cortico-cerebellar pathway
	Fragile X-associated tremor ataxia syndrome	Inherited neurodegenerative disorder affecting the cerebellum and white matter throughout the brain
Other	Post-infectious cerebellitis	Inflammatory disorder

systems, hydrocephalus and effects of oedema and tissue swelling on blood flow (Aarsen, Arts, Van Veelen-Vincent, Lequin, & Catsman-Berrevoets, 2014). Adjunct surgical techniques such as radiation, chemotherapy and/or shunts were once thought to be important causes of CCAS, however, while they certainly influence the severity of clinical outcome, CCAS has been observed in patients who did not receive such surgical treatment (Levisohn, Cronin-Golomb, & Schmahmann, 2000).

Today, the foremost model proposed to explain the presence of CCAS following cerebellar or brainstem injury is called diaschesis. Diaschesis is a neurophysiological mechanism whereby inadequate electrical output from the cerebellum caused by injury gradually leads to region specific changes in distally connected supratentorial regions. Over time, this attenuated input leads to a loss of function in the connected region that is reflected as hypoperfusion (reduced blood flow to the region) and hypometabolism (reduced neuronal metabolism), both thought to arise from reduced neuronal and synaptic activity. In support of the diaschisis model, improvement in CCAS symptoms has been found to correlate with improved cerebral blood flow on single-photon emission computerized tomography (SPECT) (De Smet et al., 2009; Maeshima & Osawa, 2007). Similarly, the region of the brain that is hypoperfused will usually correspond with the type of neuropsychological problem (i.e., dysexecutive syndrome with hypoperfusion of the prefrontal cortex) (Baillieux et al., 2010).

More recently, high-end neuroimaging techniques showed that changes within supratentorial regions in CCAS patients may extend well beyond alterations to blood flow normally picked up on SPECT. These studies have found bilateral changes within the white matter bundles of the dentatothalamocortical pathway in children with cerebellar injury and cognitive problems (Morris et al., 2009). Similarly, microstructural abnormalities in white matter tracts within the cortex (especially the corpus callosum, fornix and putamen) have been reported in patients with Chiari 1 malformations (Kumar et al., 2011). Investigations of patients with cerebellar damage have also found grey and white matter microstructural abnormalities throughout the cerebral cortex that are indicative of a combination of both perturbed neurodevelopmental and neurodegenerative processes (Moberget et al., 2015).

Indicating that cerebellar injury could also lead to irreversible changes to the developmental trajectories of other supratentorial regions, studies have shown that the specific characteristics of cortical changes in CCAS patients may differ depending on whether the insult was related to a preterm birth or acquired later. This suggests that developmental stage could determine the characteristics of the supratentorial changes found to follow cerebellar injury. Thus, SPECT results may not provide the whole story behind cognitive and affective deficits arising in CCAS patients.

Posterior fossa syndrome and the acute clinical stage

Children that survive posterior fossa tumour resection may enter an acute clinical stage 0–6 days post-surgery called '**posterior fossa syndrome**'. The posterior fossa syndrome is marked by abrupt '**cerebellar mutism**' (patients will not talk) and highly disruptive changes in emotional regulation. This can also occur in adults, though tumours in this region are less common. Patients with posterior fossa syndrome are described as having a "*decreased initiation of voluntary responses*" with behaviour that can alternate between "*Disinhibited giggling*" and "*inconsolable crying*". These behavioural changes may also include "*Irritability, agitation, whining, a nasal tone during any speech and depressed affect*" (Catsman-Berrevoets & Aarsen, 2010). Between 7 and 35 days post-surgery, these confronting changes will normally resolve, yet consistent with CCAS a proportion will go on to have problems attaining mature speech and will experience chronic cognitive deficits and mood disorder.

The significant cognitive and affective sequelae experienced by patients with posterior fossa syndrome are exemplified within the following clinical vignette. This vignette describes the stages of recovery experienced by a six year old right-handed boy who underwent resection of a large posterior fossa tumour (medulloblastoma) (De Smet et al., 2009).

- <u>Immediately post-surgery:</u> Patient was oriented and able to speak. Mutism developed later that day. Severe apathy, lack of eye contact and paucity of initiation of voluntary movement are noted.
- <u>Five weeks post-surgery:</u> Patient responds verbally but speech is ataxic. Severe apathy is present.
- <u>Eight weeks post-surgery:</u> Patient has verbal intelligence of 105 yet performance intelligence is just 68. Oral output severely lacks vigour (called adynamia) and is still ataxic. A deficit on the semantic verbal fluency task is noted.
- <u>Two years post-surgery:</u> Patient has normal intelligence and language skills. Adynamia, verbal fluency deficit and impairment of executive function remain.

This case clearly highlights the stages that can precede an ongoing case of CCAS. Here the CCAS would be considered the less severe long-term chronic outcome described two years post-surgery.

The relationship between posterior fossa syndrome, cerebellar mutism and CCAS is important to understand. Most evidence suggests that posterior fossa syndrome is an acute post-surgical condition that can precede CCAS. For example, a longer duration of mutism post-injury and hypoperfusion on SPECT during the mute phase has been linked to CCAS severity later in life (Catsman-Berrevoets & Aarsen, 2010). See Table 3.2 for further clarification.

TABLE 3.2 Terminology behind cognitive and affective change after cerebellar injury: a historical perspective

Paper	*Year*	*Terminology*
[1]	1958	Akinetic mutism described after resection of malignant posterior fossa tumour
[2]	1964	'Pseudo-frontal' syndrome proposed to describe the cognitive deficits in a patient with cerebellar tumour (Luria's lab of neuropsychology)
[3]	1972	Mutism and subsequent dysarthia (MSD) named to describe acute symptoms following resection of cerebellar tumour
[4]	1985	Cerebellar mutism introduced to describe acute symptoms following resection of cerebellar tumour
[5]	1994	Cerebellar MSD replaces cerebellar mutism to describe acute symptoms following resection of cerebellar tumour
[6]	1996	Posterior fossa syndrome introduced as an extension of MSD (to cover both cerebellar mutism and acute neuropsychological sequelae)
[7]	1998	Cerebellar cognitive affective syndrome (CCAS) introduced to describe long-term neuropsychological impairments in individuals with cerebellar injury (CCAS is not a replacement of posterior fossa syndrome)

Note: The various terms that have been used to describe cognitive and affective deficits in individuals with cerebellar injury can be confusing in the literature, especially between posterior fossa syndrome and CCAS. To clarify, posterior fossa syndrome is considered an acute manifestation of CCAS and is one of the leading risk factors for CCAS. By contrast, CCAS is understood as the persistent and chronic outcome of cerebellar injury. [1] Daly & Love, 1958; [2] Described in Budisavjevic & Ramnani, 2012; [3] Stein, Fraser, & Tenner, 1972; [4] Rekate, Grubb, Aram, Hahn, & Racheson; [5] van Dongen, Catsman-Berrevoets, & van Mourik, 1994; [6] Schmahmann & Sherman, 1998.

The clinical features of cerebellar cognitive affective syndrome

The various degrees of severity and the different types of deficit observed across patients with CCAS are consistent with the finding that specific zones of the cerebellum are functionally specialised. Clinical outcome is also affected by developmental stage, with CCAS caused by prenatal or congenital injury leading to a more variable and more severe clinical profile than CCAS acquired in adulthood. However, studies of children with acquired injury to the cerebellum have also shown that if no radiation or chemotherapy is employed as an adjunct surgical treatment, then younger age is associated with better outcome. As a result, few CCAS patients have the exact same set of clinical symptoms. The four main domains that cover the spectrum of CCAS are executive dysfunction, visuospatial dysfunction, linguistic deficits and personality and affective change.

Executive dysfunction: This is the most pervasive deficit of CCAS. Though executive function has been explained in the previous chapter, we will briefly review the core executive dysfunctions:

- Sequencing impairment: Difficulty recognizing and reconstructing sequentially organized material.
- Working memory impairment: Poor ability to hold, process and manipulate new and stored information.
- Impaired set-shifting: Difficulty moving back and forth between different cognitive tasks. This makes it effortful to be flexible in an environment where goals and demands are quickly changing.
- Verbal fluency deficit: Poor performance on a demanding 60-second test that asks patients to generate as many words as possible in line with a specific constraint (e.g., words must all start with the same letter; words must all be from the same semantic category – like animals or fruits).
- Inattention: Poor ability to hold focus and attention. Patient is easily distracted.
- Perseveration of actions: Uncontrollable persistence of a thought or action even after the context is appropriate.

This 'pre-frontal-like' profile is thought to reflect disruption of transmission between the posterior cerebellum and contralateral prefrontal and parietal cortices. Unfortunately, these symptoms can significantly and negatively impact daily life functioning by disturbing judgement, multitasking skills, decision making ability, and planning and organizational skills. General cognitive slowing that can occur in CCAS would almost certainly exacerbate any underlying executive deficit.

Visuospatial dysfunction: Patients have difficulty conceptualizing drawn images, and poor performance on tasks of visual spatial planning, mental rotation and block design is observed. However, they perform normally on simpler two-dimensional tests, such as the Benton Line Orientation Test (Lagarde, Hantkie, Hajjioui, & Yelnik, 2009; Molinari, Petrosini, Misciagna, & Leggio, 2004).

Linguistic deficits: The linguistic processes affected by CCAS are considered to be "*high-level non-motor linguistic processes at both the expressive and receptive language level*" (Marien et al., 2014). They are not thought to be simply a consequence of disrupted motor control of speech, nor are they thought to arise from basic semantic and syntactic deficits. Specifically, cerebellar patients have difficulty with meta-linguistic abilities such as those important for using language within the correct context, using the correct social approach, understanding metaphor and interpreting meaning. This together often manifests in patients as a problem "*expressing and grasping complexity*" (Guell, Hoche, & Schmahmann, 2015). Patients may also display mild anomia, dysprosody and agrammatism (Schmahmann & Sherman, 1998). Linguistic deficits in CCAS are consistent with the notion that the cerebellum plays a key role in sequencing operations, timing and skill automatisation. Note that linguistic deficits in CCAS patients could be exacerbated by underlying problems in executive function. This may explain why performance on tasks that have both executive and linguistic components, like verbal fluency, are commonly impaired in CCAS patients.

Personality change: Changes that can be seen in CCAS patients include emotional fragility and oversensitivity, rigidity, uncharacteristic overfamiliarity, verbal disinhibition, irresponsible behaviour, distractibility and hyperactivity (Schmahmann et al., 2007). In extreme cases, children treated for cerebellar tumours may additionally demonstrate psuedo-bulbar like crying and pathological laughter. Individuals have even been found to wake up laughing (Parvizi, Anderson, Martin, Damasio, H. & Damasio, A.R., 2001). Cases of inappropriate laughter or crying may result when the cerebellum has received incomplete information about the situational context, and as a consequence has incorrectly altered its adjustment of the output to the situational context (i.e., execution of laughter/crying). In this respect, cerebellar injury does not cause a disorder of emotions, but instead it causes a disorder of the contextual regulation of emotions by cognition.

> *"She was silly, with disinhibited giggling, but was likable and friendly" (ten year-old girl)*
>
> *"mood was labile and irritable, shifting frequently between anger and crying. Marked difficulty modulating behaviour and sustaining task performance on verbal subtests" (five year-old boy)*

The above clinical vignettes, which are from case studies of children who survived resection of a midline medulloblastoma, are presented to demonstrate the clinical manifestation of this loss of contextual regulation of emotion (Levisohn et al., 2000).

Cross-over between CCAS and symptoms of neuropsychiatric disorders

Many patients with cerebellar injury also have neuropsychiatric symptoms. The most intriguing and well supported example is the cross-over between vermis injury and features of autism spectrum disorder (ASD). For example, Schmahmann et al. (2007) reported an "*inability to appreciate social boundaries and assign ulterior motives*" as well as "*tactile defensiveness and sensory overload*" in adults with CCAS. Ritualistic and stereotypical behaviours and deficits in social emotion recognition are other ASD-like features observed in patients with CCAS. Moreover, investigations of preterm babies and children with congenital malformations of the cerebellum clearly demonstrate a link between vermis injury and positive autism screening (Bolduc et al., 2011; Limperopoulos et al., 2007). Systematic follow-up of patients with cerebellar injury has also revealed significantly increased incidence of bipolar disorder, depression and anxiety traits, and again this was more common when there had been vermal involvement (Lauterbach, Harris, & Bina, 2010; Schmahmann et al., 2007). However, just as individuals with cerebellar injury to the vermis almost always have symptoms of neuropsychiatric disorders, individuals with neuropsychiatric disorders generally have some degree of vermal abnormality. This has been shown for ASD, depression, bipolar disorder and fragile X syndrome, but there are likely to be others (Mostofsky et al., 1998; Phillips, Hewedi, Eissa, & Moustafa, 2015). Thus there could be some cross-over between vermis integrity and neuropsychiatric disorder. Finding out what the common ground is across different disorders and whether the vermis could be investigated as a biomarker for shared symptoms may help to refine diagnostics in neuropsychiatric practice.

Laterality

Studies in support of a lateralization of cerebellar function demonstrated that features which are characteristically "right-hemisphere dominant", such as visuospatial dysfunction and attention deficits, were more common to cases of left-sided cerebellar injury. Alternatively, "left-hemisphere dominant" features, like linguistic and verbal deficits, were more common in instances of right-sided cerebellar injury (Baillieux et al., 2010; Marien, Engelborghs, Fabbro, & De Deyn, 2001). Cerebellar laterality has some support from SPECT investigations which have detected hypoperfusion in specific regions within the cerebral hemisphere contralateral to the cerebellar injury (Sonmezoglu, Sperling, Henriksen, Tfelt-Hansen, & Lassen, 1993). Moreover, neuropsychological testing in children with hypoplasia of the left cerebellar lobe and vermis has revealed in some a 'developmental right-hemisphere syndrome' characterized by impaired visuospatial performances, yet intact language skills (Gross-Tsur, Ben-Bashat, Shalev, Levav, & Sira, 2006). These findings reflect those from anatomical studies demonstrating that the majority of fibres connecting the posterior cerebellar zone with the prefrontal and parietal cortices will cross hemispheric side. However, because cases of contralateral hypoperfusion and/or lateralized neuropsychological deficit are not consistently observed, the notion of cerebellar lateralization does not have full support.

Neuroscientific explanations of CCAS

To understand CCAS, which is a cognitive and affective disorder arising from cerebellar injury, researchers have reappropriated the motor control theory of internal models to that of cognitive and affective control (Ito, 2008). Therefore, this section begins with a brief introduction into the motor control literature. Specifically, computational neuroscientists have suggested that the cerebellum performs important "predictive" neural operations that can smooth over or adjust the program parameters of motor performance (Ito, 2005). This is achieved by adjusting the timing and magnitude of muscle contractions during an action. At a more conceptual level, motor control is understood through the actions of the two main outputs from the cerebellum: (a) an output that holds the code for the actual movement to be read out and actioned by the motor cortex; and (b) an output called an internal model that predicts the sensory outcome of the intended movement based on previous experiences.

The pairing of the motor command with a predictive internal model during movement is likely to have evolved because it offers important functional benefits. For example, it can overcome the need to rely on delayed sensory feedback and thus enables efficient fine targeting of movements (individuals with cerebellar damage are notoriously slow and can experience tremor during voluntary movement). It also enables cancellation of the delayed sensory feedback (disruption leads to sensory integration issues similar to what is observed in children with ASD). Furthermore, it can be used to compute and compare against error codes during motor sequence learning (individuals with cerebellar damage have trouble learning and understanding sequenced events). Over time, this pairing of the motor output with an internal model encourages the cerebellum and other structures to compute codes for the specific expectations of more complex sensory and motor experiences derived from the environment (e.g., hitting a ball, using a tool) (Imamizu et al., 2000).

In the case of cognition and affect, the internal model codes expectations related to mental functions. Examples of mental functions that have been suggested to be facilitated by internal models include language processing, understanding how another is thinking and feeling (i.e., theory of mind) and appreciation of the 'gist' of what's going on. Here, internal models are thought to have the goal of storing properties associated with cortically derived mental states so that they can facilitate prospective mental functions. The core mechanisms are captured within the following quote:

> *"in motor and nonmotor domains, functional state patterns are recorded by cerebellar processing and compared with stored templates. If a match is obtained, then it is assumed that the next incoming event can be predicted from the stored template. Accordingly, the cerebral cortex can be activated in advance, alerting the correct modules".*
>
> *(Leggio & Molinari, 2014)*

These internal model functions of the cerebellum affect how well one can detect changes and patterns within sequential material and how well one can adapt to changing environments or task demands (Ito, 2008; Leggio & Molinari, 2014). Some authors have suggested that the cerebellum may do more than store properties as internal models. For example, researchers have suggested that the cerebellum may utilise the internal models for processing routine aspects of a cognitive task to "free up" the prefrontal cortex for flexible processing of more complex operations (Ramnani et al., 2006; Schweizer et al., 2007). The cerebellum has also been ascribed a role in interpreting and detecting passage of time (Ivry & Keele, 1989), which could explain why patients with cerebellar damage can have difficulties with time perception, music perception and music ability. The internal models of the cerebellum, as well as other important cerebellar functions, appear to be disrupted in CCAS patients.

Diagnostic instruments and clinical rating scales

There are no guidelines about what diagnostic and clinical rating scales are appropriate for assessing and monitoring symptoms of CCAS. Many different neuropsychological tests of intelligence, executive, visuospatial and linguistic function have been cited in CCAS research: Wescheler Adult Intelligence Scale-Revised; Wisconsin Card Sorting Test; Verbal Fluency; Trail Making Test; Stroop Colour Word Test; Rey-Osterrieth Complex Figure Test; Test of Visual-Perceptual Skills; and Boston Naming Test. In congenital cases the Apgar scale can be informative, while in pediatric CCAS the Bayley Scales of Infant Development, Vineland Adaptive Behavioral Scale, Griffiths Mental Developmental Scales and the Achenbach's Child Behaviour checklist can be used to assess developmental stage, adaptive function and problem behaviour. Tools instrumental in making diagnoses for associated neuropsychiatric conditions such as ASD include the Diagnostic and Statistical Manual of Mental Disorders, 4th Edition (DSM-IV), the Frontal Behavioural Inventory and the Structured Clinical Interview for DSM-IV. Magnetic resonance imaging (MRI) and computed tomography are used to determine lesion location; while SPECT provides detailed information about cerebral blood flow and metabolic activity.

Treatment

Unfortunately, there is not a lot of research in this area. An investigation of a patient with CCAS caused by cerebellar hemorrhage revealed improvement from cognitive rehabilitation through real orientation therapy and attention process training, although for unknown reasons his impairment in visuospatial orientation and executive dysfunction persisted (Maeshima & Osawa, 2007). Regarding pharmaceuticals, dopamine agonists (i.e., roprinirole hydrochloride) and anti-convulsant drugs (i.e., carbamazepine) have been shown to be effective at stabilizing mood in cases of posterior fossa syndrome (Marien et al., 2013) and thus may also work in CCAS. There are few investigations in relation to actual pharmaceutical treatment of CCAS. One case study of a patient with ADHD. related to a Chiari 1 malformation published a positive response to ADHD. medication (Adderall) (Eme & Sheffer, 2012) and a series of case study reports of cerebellar patients documented improvement of affect, mood and irritability in patients with cerebellar degeneration treated with serotonin reuptake inhibitors (Schmahmann et al., 2007). An important tool for CCAS treatment is likely to be repetitive Transcranial Magnetic

Stimulation (rTMS), which involves using a "coil" to generate a magnetic field over the skull that can change the likelihood of neural firing within targeted cortical regions. Despite a paucity of investigations in confirmed CCAS cases, rTMS is a well-established approach to correction of imbalance in neural activity within the cortex and cerebellum.

Future directions

It is important that research scientists aim towards improving our understanding of the characteristics and the diagnostic criteria of CCAS. In these investigations, a combination of sophisticated brain imaging techniques (e.g., diffusion tensor imaging, functional MRI) with both neuropsychological tests and tests specifically targeted to operations of internal models of the cerebellum will be needed. In particular, we will need to find a way to distinguish between (a) symptoms related to loss of function by supratentorial structures (i.e., prefrontal cortex dysfunction caused by diaschisis), (b) symptoms related to compensatory changes in neuroplasticity and (c) symptoms arising specifically from improper output from the cerebellum. From this platform, researchers will be able to create a much needed, easy to use and theoretically informed battery of neuropsychological and neurophysiological tests tailored to CCAS that is valid across multiple age groups and etiological cases. With these steps towards better disorder classification and diagnostics, larger cohort investigations can finally take place tracking CCAS-positive cohorts against matched control groups to monitor effectiveness of pharmaceutical, cognitive and neurophysiological interventions.

There is also now the difficult task of understanding the cognitive and affective sequelae of CCAS in terms of known models of lifespan development. This is becoming increasingly important as growing evidence from neurobiological studies indicates that the cerebellum may indeed play a dynamic role in guiding the maturation of remote supratentorial structures, and thus may itself have significant influence over cognitive development (Wang, Kloth, & Badura, 2014).

Summary

CCAS is a newly recognized spectrum condition arising from various forms of cerebellar injury, neurodegeneration or developmental malformation. Patients with CCAS may show bizarre and confronting cognitive and behavioural change, or more subtle executive, visuospatial, linguistic and affective deficit, depending on the type and location of the injury. The type of deficit can usually be traced back to either loss of function in connected supratentorial regions or to impairment of core cerebellar operations and dysmetria of thought. One of the most interesting discoveries is that there are many aspects of CCAS that resemble neuropsychiatric disorders, just as there are many aspects of neuropsychiatric disorders that could be explained by a CCAS model. However, the paucity of treatment is a concern, long term outcome is rather unclear and there are currently no diagnostic scales. Thus, this field which is still in its infancy would greatly benefit from more research.

Glossary

Adynamia: Loss of strength or vigour, usually because of disease.
Agrammatism: A form of aphasia characterized by the inability to produce a grammatical or intelligible sentence.
Anomia: The inability to name objects or to recognize the written or spoken names of objects.
Apathy: Absence of interest in or enthusiasm for things generally considered interesting or moving. Absence of emotion.
Astrocytoma: A malignant tumour of nervous tissue composed of well differentiated astrocytes.
Ataxia: Loss of coordination of the muscles, especially of the extremities.
Diaschisis: Inhibition of function produced by an acute focal disturbance in a portion of the brain at a distance from the original site of injury, but anatomically connected with it through fibre tracts.
Dysmetria: Lack of coordination of movement because of faulty judgement of distance.
Dysplasia: An abnormality of development.
Dysprosody: Lack of the normal rhythm, melody and articulation of speech.
Hypoplasia: Incomplete development of an organ or part.
Medulloblastoma: A rapidly growing brain tumor that develops in children and is responsive to radiotherapy.
Supratentorial: Denoting cranial contents located above the tentorium cerebelli; often used to describe functional symptoms.

References

Aarsen, F. K., Arts, W. F., Van Veelen-Vincent, M. L., Lequin, M. H., & Catsman-Berrevoets, C. E. (2014). Long-term outcome in children with low grade tectal tumours and obstructive hydrocephalus. *European Journal of Paediatric Neurology, 18*(4), 469–474. doi: 10.1016/j.ejpn.2014.03.002.

Baillieux, H., De Smet, H. J., Dobbeleir, A., Paquier, P. F., De Deyn, P. P., & Marien, P. (2010). Cognitive and affective disturbances following focal cerebellar damage in adults: A neuropsychological and SPECT study. *Cortex, 46*(7), 869–879. doi: 10.1016/j.cortex.2009.09.002.

Bolduc, M. E., Du Plessis, A. J., Sullivan, N., Khwaja, O. S., Zhang, X., Barnes, K., … Limperopoulos, C. (2011). Spectrum of neurodevelopmental disabilities in children with cerebellar malformations. *Developmental Medicine and Child Neurology, 53*(5), 409–416. doi: 10.1111/j.1469-8749.2011.03929.x.

Brossard-Racine, M., du Plessis, A. J., & Limperopoulos, C. (2015). Developmental cerebellar cognitive affective syndrome in ex-preterm survivors following cerebellar injury. *Cerebellum, 14*(2), 151–164. doi: 10.1007/s12311-014-0597-9.

Budisavljevic, S., & Ramnani, N. (2012). Cognitive deficits from a cerebellar tumour: A historical case report from Luria's Laboratory. *Cortex, 48*(1), 26–35. doi: 10.1016/j.cortex.2011.07.001.

Catsman-Berrevoets, C. E., & Aarsen, F. K. (2010). The spectrum of neurobehavioural deficits in the Posterior Fossa Syndrome in children after cerebellar tumour surgery. *Cortex, 46*(7), 933–946. doi: 10.1016/j.cortex.2009.10.007.

Daly, D. D., & Love, J. G. (1958). Akinetic mutism. *Neurology, 8*(3), 238–242.

De Smet, H. J., Baillieux, H., Wackenier, P., De Praeter, M., Engelborghs, S., Paquier, P. F., ... Marien, P. (2009). Long-term cognitive deficits following posterior fossa tumor resection: a neuropsychological and functional neuroimaging follow-up study. *Neuropsychology, 23*(6), 694–704. doi: 10.1037/a0016106.

Eme, R., & Sheffer, E. (2012). The cerebellum and attention deficit hyperactivity disorder. A case study of a cerebellar Chiari 1 malformation. *Journal of Counselling and Professional Psychology, 1*.

Gross-Tsur, V., Ben-Bashat, D., Shalev, R. S., Levav, M., & Sira, L. B. (2006). Evidence of a developmental cerebello-cerebral disorder. *Neuropsychologia, 44*(12), 2569–2572. doi: 10.1016/j.neuropsychologia.2006.04.028.

Guell, X., Hoche, F., & Schmahmann, J. D. (2015). Metalinguistic deficits in patients with cerebellar dysfunction: Empirical support for the dysmetria of thought theory. *Cerebellum, 14*(1), 50–58. doi: 10.1007/s12311-014-0630-z.

Imamizu, H., Miyauchi, S., Tamada, T., Sasaki, Y., Takino, R., Putz, B., ... Kawato, M. (2000). Human cerebellar activity reflecting an acquired internal model of a new tool. *Nature, 403*(6766), 192–195.

Ito, M. (2005). Bases and implications of learning in the cerebellum--adaptive control and internal model mechanism. *Progress in Brain Research, 148*, 95–109.

Ito, M. (2008). Control of mental activities by internal models in the cerebellum. *Nature Reviews Neuroscience, 9*(4), 304–313.

Ivry, R. B., & Keele, S. W. (1989). Timing functions of the cerebellum. *Journal of Cognitive Neuroscience, 1*(2), 136–152.

Kumar, M., Rathore, R. K., Srivastava, A., Yadav, S. K., Behari, S., & Gupta, R. K. (2011). Correlation of diffusion tensor imaging metrics with neurocognitive function in Chiari I malformation. *World Neurosurgery, 76*(1–2), 189–194. doi: 10.1016/j.wneu.2011.02.022.

Lagarde, J., Hantkie, O., Hajjioui, A., & Yelnik, A. (2009). Neuropsychological disorders induced by cerebellar damage. *Annals of Physical and Rehabilitation Medicine, 52*(4), 360–370. doi: 10.1016/j.rehab.2009.02.002.

Lauterbach, E. C., Harris, J. B., & Bina, W. F., 3rd. (2010). Mood and neurobehavioral correlates of cerebellar lesions. *Cognitive and Behavioral Neurology, 23*(2), 63–73. doi: 10.1097/WNN.0b013e3181cfb541.

Leggio, M., & Molinari, M. (2014). Cerebellar sequencing: A trick for predicting the future. *Cerebellum*. doi: 10.1007/s12311-014-0616-x.

Levisohn, L., Cronin-Golomb, A., & Schmahmann, J. D. (2000). Neuropsychological consequences of cerebellar tumour resection in children: Cerebellar cognitive affective syndrome in a paediatric population. *Brain, 123*(Pt 5), 1041–1050.

Limperopoulos, C., Bassan, H., Gauvreau, K., Robertson, R. L., Jr., Sullivan, N. R., Benson, C. B., ... duPlessis, A. J. (2007). Does cerebellar injury in premature infants contribute to the high prevalence of long-term cognitive, learning, and behavioral disability in survivors? *Pediatrics, 120*(3), 584–593. doi: 10.1542/peds.2007-1041.

Maeshima, S., & Osawa, A. (2007). Stroke rehabilitation in a patient with cerebellar cognitive affective syndrome. *Brain Injury, 21*(8), 877–883. doi: 10.1080/02699050701504273.

Marien, P., Ackermann, H., Adamaszek, M., Barwood, C. H., Beaton, A., Desmond, J., … Ziegler, W. (2014). Consensus paper: Language and the cerebellum: An ongoing enigma. *Cerebellum, 13*(3), 386–410. doi: 10.1007/s12311-013-0540-5.

Marien, P., De Smet, H. J., Wijgerde, E., Verhoeven, J., Crols, R., & De Deyn, P. P. (2013). Posterior fossa syndrome in adults: A new case and comprehensive survey of the literature. *Cortex, 49*(1), 284–300. doi: 10.1016/j.cortex.2011.06.018.

Marien, P., Engelborghs, S., Fabbro, F., & De Deyn, P. P. (2001). The lateralized linguistic cerebellum: A review and a new hypothesis. *Brain & Language, 79*(3), 580–600. doi: 10.1006/brln.2001.2569.

Moberget, T., Andersson, S., Lundar, T., Due-Tonnessen, B. J., Heldal, A., Endestad, T., & Westlye, L. T. (2015). Long-term supratentorial brain structure and cognitive function following cerebellar tumour resections in childhood. *Neuropsychologia, 69*, 218–231. doi: 10.1016/j.neuropsychologia.2015.02.007.

Molinari, M., Petrosini, L., Misciagna, S., & Leggio, M. G. (2004). Visuospatial abilities in cerebellar disorders. *Journal of Neurology, Neurosurgery, and Psychiatry, 75*(2), 235–240.

Morris, E. B., Phillips, N. S., Laningham, F. H., Patay, Z., Gajjar, A., Wallace, D., … Ogg, R. J. (2009). Proximal dentatothalamocortical tract involvement in posterior fossa syndrome. *Brain, 132*(Pt 11), 3087–3095. doi: 10.1093/brain/awp241.

Mostofsky, S. H., Mazzocco, M. M., Aakalu, G., Warsofsky, I. S., Denckla, M. B., & Reiss, A. L. (1998). Decreased cerebellar posterior vermis size in fragile X syndrome: Correlation with neurocognitive performance. *Neurology, 50*(1), 121–130.

Parvizi, J., Anderson, S. W., Martin, C. O., Damasio, H., & Damasio, A. R. (2001). Pathological laughter and crying: A link to the cerebellum. *Brain, 124*(Pt 9), 1708–1719.

Phillips, J. R., Hewedi, D. H., Eissa, A. M., & Moustafa, A. A. (2015). The cerebellum and psychiatric disorders. *Frontiers in Public Health, 3*, 66. doi: 10.3389/fpubh.2015.00066.

Ramnani, N., Behrens, T. E. J., Johansen-Berg, H., Richter, M. C., Pinsk, M. A., Andersson, J. L. R., … Matthews, P. M. (2006). The evolution of prefrontal inputs to the cortico-pontine system: Diffusion imaging evidence from Macaque monkeys and humans. *Cerebral Cortex, 16*(6), 811–818.

Rekate, H. L., Grubb, R. L., Aram, D. M., Hahn, J. F., & Ratcheson, R. A. (1985). Muteness of cerebellar origin. *Arch Neurol, 42*(7), 697–698.

Schmahmann, J. D., & Sherman, J. C. (1998). The cerebellar cognitive affective syndrome. *Brain, 121*(4), 561–579. doi: 10.1093/brain/121.4.561.

Schmahmann, J. D., Weilburg, J. B., & Sherman, J. C. (2007). The neuropsychiatry of the cerebellum—Insights from the clinic. *Cerebellum, 6*(3), 254–267. doi: 10.1080/14734220701490995.

Schweizer, T. A., Oriet, C., Meiran, N., Alexander, M. P., Cusimano, M., & Stuss, D. T. (2007). The cerebellum mediates conflict resolution. *Journal of Cognitive Neuroscience, 19*(12), 1974–1982.

Sonmezoglu, K., Sperling, B., Henriksen, T., Tfelt-Hansen, P., & Lassen, N. A. (1993). Reduced contralateral hemispheric flow measured by SPECT in cerebellar lesions: Crossed cerebral diaschisis. *Acta Neurologica Scandinavica, 87*(4), 275–280.

Stein, B. M., Fraser, R. A., & Tenner, M. S. (1972). Normal pressure hydrocephalus: Complication of posterior fossa surgery in children. *Pediatrics, 49*(1), 50–58.

Stoodley, C. J., Valera, E. M., & Schmahmann, J. D. (2012). Functional topography of the cerebellum for motor and cognitive tasks: An fMRI study. *Neuroimage, 59*(2), 1560–1570.

Tavano, A., Grasso, R., Gagliardi, C., Triulzi, F., Bresolin, N., Fabbro, F., & Borgatti, R. (2007). Disorders of cognitive and affective development in cerebellar malformations. *Brain, 130*(Pt 10), 2646–2660. doi: 10.1093/brain/awm201.

van Dongen, H. R., Catsman-Berrevoets, C. E., & van Mourik, M. (1994). The syndrome of 'cerebellar' mutism and subsequent dysarthria. *Neurology, 44*(11), 2040–2046.

Wang, S. S., Kloth, A. D., & Badura, A. (2014). The cerebellum, sensitive periods, and autism. *Neuron, 83*(3), 518–532. doi: 10.1016/j.neuron.2014.07.016.

4
NEW TECHNOLOGIES IN CLINICAL NEUROSCIENCE

Natalia Albein-Urios and Peter G. Enticott

Introduction

The development of the nervous system requires a series of complex steps that begin from the earliest stages of embryonic development. Our genetic profile, for instance, is responsible for creating and migrating cells for a range of functions, and that will ultimately form a central nervous system (CNS), including the human brain. To add to this complexity, the interaction between these stages of gene expression and environmental factors will ultimately have a great influence on the function of our CNS, affecting cognitive abilities such as learning, memory, and executive control.

Similarly, any alteration in the stages of brain development can have a major impact and result in significant neurodevelopmental impairments (Meredith, 2015). Such alterations can lead to synaptic dysregulation, abnormal neurochemical function, and changes in CNS plasticity, resulting in deficits to cognitive, behavioural, motor, and emotional processes.

Our understanding of the disorders covered in this volume has typically arisen from largely neuropsychological approaches (e.g., lesion studies, neurobehavioural assessment), but the use of neuroscience techniques has made an enormous contribution to our understanding of the underlying neurobiology of neurodevelopmental disorders. Beyond providing an understanding of group differences in brain structure and function, neuroimaging techniques such as magnetic resonance imaging (MRI), and neurophysiological techniques such as electroencephalography (EEG), have been used as promising tools for the detection of potential biomarkers in neurodevelopmental disorders (Hall, Jiang, Reiss, & Greicius, 2013; Jeste, Frohlich, & Loo, 2015). Although the heterogeneity of certain disorders with complex phenotypic expression (e.g., autism spectrum disorder [ASD]) appears to hinder the identification of specific biomarkers, numerous advances involving neuroscience and genetic techniques are working towards developing clinically useful biomarkers (Reeb-Sutherland & Fox, 2015; Walsh, Elsabbagh, Bolton, & Singh, 2011).

While some neuroscience tools might contribute to the detection and diagnosis of neurodevelopmental disorders, other recently developed neuroscience techniques, including non-invasive brain stimulation, may be useful in the treatment of these disorders (Lefaucheur et al., 2014). For instance, repetitive transcranial magnetic stimulation (rTMS) is now considered a safe and efficacious treatment for treatment-resistant major depressive disorder, and a growing number of clinical trials investigate whether similar techniques could be useful in the treatment of disorders including schizophrenia, obsessive compulsive disorder (OCD), ASD, and Attention Deficit Hyperactivity Disorder (ADHD) (Enticott et al., 2014; Helfrich et al., 2012; Koops, van den Brink, & Sommer, 2015; Senco et al., 2015).

In this chapter we provide an overview of advances in many of the technologies that are currently used to probe the neurobiology of frontostriatal developmental disorders. While this overview will not be exhaustive, we will focus primarily on those techniques that have emerged or developed since the first volume was published in 2001. Despite the important advances that have been made in neuroimaging, genetics, and neuromodulation (and the combination of such methods), there remain a number of significant challenges, particularly around the ability of these techniques to detect, prognosticate, and treat frontostriatal neurodevelopmental disorders.

Neuroimaging and neurophysiology

Neuroimaging approaches have continued to develop at a rapid pace. The resolution at which structural brain images can be acquired has increased substantially, with up to 7 tesla (7T) scanners now used in humans. Diffusion imaging approaches allow not only the mapping of white matter pathways throughout the human brain, but also the integrity of those pathways (Walker et al., 2012). When applied to frontostriatal disorders, we can now access far more detailed information about any disruptions in structures that support neural connectivity.

Functional neuroimaging approaches (e.g., functional magnetic resonance imaging [fMRI]) also offer a number of advances, including new ways of assessing functional connectivity (e.g., connectome analysis; Fornito, Zalesky, & Breakspear, 2015). Some researchers have looked at whether functional neuroimaging patterns might have a predictive or diagnostic utility for neurodevelopmental disorders (Just, Cherkassky, Buchweitz, Keller, & Mitchell, 2014), although at this stage the findings are preliminary and have not influenced methods for clinical diagnosis. It should also be noted that the temporal resolution of neuroimaging techniques continues to be relatively poor, leading to the development of combined, complimentary approaches (e.g., combined fMRI and EEG [Yuan, Zotev, Phillips, Drevets, & Bodurka, 2012], or combined fMRI and TMS [Yau, Jalinous, Cantarero, & Desmond, 2014]).

Other relatively recent techniques for *in vivo*, non-invasive examination of brain function, include functional near infrared spectroscopy (fNIRS), which uses optodes positioned on the scalp to (a) emit near infrared light into the brain and to (b) capture this light reflecting off hemoglobin. When applied at different frequencies, this can give an indication of oxygenation/deoxygenation of hemoglobin with a high degree of temporal (if not spatial) accuracy, thus providing an index of neural activity within specific cortical regions (e.g., Monden et al., 2015).

Despite neuroimaging advances, electrophysiological techniques remain in widespread use. Advancements in EEG include higher-density arrays, new methods for detecting functional connectivity across the cortex, and source reconstruction techniques that allow the determination of the spatial origin of detected electrophysiological activity.

A powerful, related technique is magnetoencephalography (MEG), which uses super-conducting detectors and amplifiers (SQUIDs) to detect magnetic fields within the brain that reflect summed neural activity. MEG has a greater signal-to-noise ratio than EEG and has excellent spatial and temporal resolution; however it requires specialized and expensive equipment and laboratory infrastructure (Khan et al., 2015).

Non-invasive brain stimulation

Among the major technological developments in human neuroscience over the past 15 years has been the widespread uptake of non-invasive brain stimulation techniques. This includes magnetic stimulation techniques, such as transcranial magnetic stimulation (TMS), which can induce electrical current in the brain via a magnetic pulse that is delivered to the scalp. There are also electrical stimulation techniques, such as transcranial direct current stimulation (tDCS), which involves sending weak electrical currents into the brain via two or more electrodes that are placed against the scalp. These techniques are extremely versatile, and there have been many paradigms developed that can be used to not only investigate brain function and brain-behaviour relationships, but also modulate neural activity for therapeutic purposes. Importantly, many of these techniques, both investigative and therapeutic, have recently been applied to individuals with neurodevelopmental disorders including ASD, ADHD, and Tourette's disorder (TD).

Transcranial magnetic stimulation (TMS)

TMS involves stimulation of neural tissue via the administration of one or more magnetic pulses to the scalp. These pulses are delivered via a plastic-coated mental coil. Each pulse is very strong (1.5T+), but also brief and focal. The magnetic pulse is able to travel largely unimpeded to underlying cortical tissue, where it induces electrical current that can cause neural depolarization. TMS is able to act upon both excitatory and inhibitory neurons and interneurons, and several paradigms have been developed to measure, *in vivo*, both cortical excitation (thought to primarily reflect glutamatergic processes, including activity at NMDA receptor sites) and cortical inhibition (thought to reflect primarily GABAergic processes). In neurodevelopmental disorders, TMS has been used to: chart deficits of cortical inhibition in ASD, ADHD, and TS (Bruckmann et al., 2012; Enticott et al., 2013; Enticott, Rinehart, Tonge, Bradshaw, & Fitzgerald, 2010; Gilbert, Isaacs, Augusta, MacNeil, & Mostofsky, 2011; Gilbert et al., 2006; Gilbert, Sallee, Zhang, Lipps, & Wassermann, 2005; Orth, Amann, Robertson, & Rothwell, 2005); demonstrate abnormalities in frontoparietal action observation networks in ASD and schizophrenia (Enticott et al., 2008; Enticott et al., 2012; Theoret et al., 2005); induce atypical neuroplastic processes in ASD (Jung et al., 2013; L. Oberman et al., 2012), and differential effects of TMS on neurocognitive performance in ASD (Fecteau, Agosta, Oberman, & Pascual-Leone, 2011). TMS not only allows *in vivo* probing of neurochemical systems, but its excellent spatial and temporal resolution complements established neuroimaging and electrophysiological techniques. Indeed, combined approaches, such as TMS-EEG, are emerging as new ways to gain a functional understanding of neuroplasticity, and associated neurochemical systems and processes (Rogasch, Daskalakis, & Fitzgerald, 2015; Rogasch et al., 2014).

Repetitive transcranial magnetic stimulation (rTMS)

When applied repeatedly, TMS is able to induce lasting changes in cortical excitability. This is generally termed repetitive transcranial magnetic stimulation (rTMS). This has been useful in targeting neurological and psychiatric disorders where abnormalities of brain function have been identified in specific cortical regions that are accessible via TMS (e.g., dorsolateral prefrontal cortex [DLPFC] in depression; George et al., 2010). A number of recent studies, however, have investigated whether rTMS could be used therapeutically in neurodevelopmental disorders. There is preliminary evidence to suggest that rTMS can improve neurophysiological and clinical aspects of ASD (Oberman, Rotenberg, & Pascual-Leone, 2013), while several preliminary studies suggest that inhibitory rTMS to supplementary motor area can reduce motor tics in TS (Kwon et al., 2011; Le, Liu, Sun, Hu, & Xiao, 2013; Mantovani et al., 2006). Efforts are currently underway to expand this work (Oberman et al., 2015), and it is conceivable that rTMS could be established as a safe and efficacious clinical treatment for one or more neurodevelopmental disorders over the next decade. Recent developments in rTMS technology include "deep rTMS" approaches, which involve specialized coils that generate a magnetic pulse that travels deeper into the brain (raising the prospect of direct non-invasive subcortical stimulation) (Deng, Lisanby, & Peterchev, 2014; Roth & Zangen, 2014), although focality is inevitably reduced, and all tissue between the surface of the coil and the target site will also be stimulated.

Transcranial electrical stimulation (TES)

Unlike TMS, the current induced via TES techniques is not sufficiently strong to cause cell depolarization. It can, however, shift the cellular resting membrane potential, making an action potential either more or less likely (Nitsche et al., 2008). While TES techniques have seen a resurgence in recent decades, TES actually has a rich history in the medical sciences. The application of rudimentary TES in humans dates back to the end of the 18th century, where Giovanni Aldini, Galvani's nephew, one of the pioneers of bioelectricity, used this procedure to treat health mental conditions. More recently, in the 1930s, electroconvulsive therapy (ECT), a form of electrical stimulation, was developed to induce seizures with a view to treat psychiatric illnesses. ECT continues to be used, primarily in the treatment of intractable depression or schizophrenia, and while response rates are high, there are numerous serious side effects (Kellner et al., 2012; Pompili et al., 2013; Sienaert, Dhossche, Vancampfort, De Hert, & Gazdag, 2014).

TES, primarily through tDCS, re-emerged in the 1990s, when work by Priori and colleagues (Priori, Berardelli, Rona, Accornero, & Manfredi, 1998) and Nitsche and Paulus (Nitsche & Paulus, 2000) demonstrated modulation in cortical excitability when applying weak electrical currents through the scalp. These researchers discovered that anodal stimulation of a brain region was facilitatory (i.e., tended to increase excitability), while cathodal stimulation was inhibitory (i.e., reduced cortical excitability).

From a mechanistic perspective, tDCS (unlike TMS) does not cause rapid depolarization (action potential), but rather may modulate spontaneous neuronal system activity. This is achieved by inducing a weak and constant electrical current via scalp electrodes that modifies the resting membrane polarity, either increasing or decreasing neural excitability, and thus making neurons more or less likely to fire. Typically, anodal tDCS provokes a shift toward depolarisation and an increase in neural excitability, while cathodal tDCS induces hyperpolarisation and a decrease in neural excitability (Brunoni et al., 2012; Nitsche et al., 2005). Similar to TMS, these effects are thought to reflect an influence on glutamatergic and GABAergic systems, and reflect long-term potential/long-term depression like mechanisms. It should be noted, however, that effects of TMS and TES on excitability are not seen universally, and are affected by individual factors including neurodevelopmental stage, anatomy, pathology, and neurochemical dynamics. There are also differential effects depending on the stimulation parameters, and it is important to consider factors such as electrode montage, electrode size, stimulation intensity (typically 1–2mA), and duration of stimulation. In the literature, the number of tDCS sessions delivered vary considerably, although it is thought that 10 minutes or more of stimulation is enough to prolong tDCS after-effects (Ardolino, Bossi, Barbieri, & Priori, 2005). Some studies have also shown that the after-effects of tDCS are enhanced when the stimulation interval is prolonged (Boggio et al., 2007; Monte-Silva, Kuo, Liebetanz, Paulus, & Nitsche, 2010). Thus, for clinical purposes, long-term effects using repeated tDCS sessions are critical to increase the duration of behavioural outcomes (Charvet et al., 2015).

The use of tDCS as a clinical tool in mental health disorders has shown promising results (Tortella et al., 2015), although the development of its therapeutic application is well behind that of rTMS. In mood disorders, such as depression and bipolar disorder, anodal tDCS to dorsolateral prefrontal cortex (DLPFC) has demonstrated symptom reduction (Brunoni et al., 2011; Brunoni et al., 2013). Moreover, there is evidence that a combination of tDCS and pharmacological treatment and/or behavioural therapy yields further improved behavioural outcomes (Brunoni et al., 2013). Clinically, tDCS has been also used to treat OCD, where cathodal tDCS stimulation over the pre-supplementary motor area (pre-SMA) significantly reduced OCD-related symptoms (D'Urso et al., 2015; Senco et al., 2015). In schizophrenia, tDCS applied over fronto-temporal regions appears to reduce positive symptoms, while tDCS applied bifrontally reduces negative symptoms (Mondino et al., 2014; Palm, Hasan, Keeser, Falkai, & Padberg, 2013).

There are more recent developments in TES technology. For instance, high definition transcranial current stimulation (HD-tDCS) involves the use of multiple stimulating electrodes to enhance the focality of stimulation. Perhaps the most common configuration is the 4 x 1 ring configuration, where the "active" electrode is usually placed in the centre and is surrounded by four "reference" or return electrodes (Datta, Elwassif, & Bikson, 2009; Edwards et al., 2013; Villamar et al., 2013). Some of the first clinical trials using this technique have shown significant results by reducing symptoms in different disease states, such as in fibromyalgia (Villamar et al., 2013). Another technique is transcranial alternating current stimulation (tACS), which modulates cortical activity by using oscillatory electrical stimulation in different frequency bands (Battleday, Muller, Clayton, & Cohen Kadosh, 2014; Kuo & Nitsche, 2012). This has the potential to entrain specific EEG frequencies/bandwidths, and several studies have found improvements on working memory when applying tACS (Herrmann, Rach, Neuling, & Struber, 2013; Jausovec, N., & Jausovec, K., 2014; Vosskuhl, Huster, & Herrmann, 2015). Finally, transcranial random noise stimulation (tRNS) modulates and desynchronizes specific oscillatory brain activity (Paulus, 2011). To date, the use of this technique for the treatment of psychiatric disorders has not been explored, however, single-case studies in schizophrenia and depression have suggested therapeutic benefits (Chan et al., 2012; Palm, et al., 2013).

Genetics

Significant technological advances to understanding frontostriatal disorders have also been made in areas complimentary to neuroimaging and neurophysiology, particularly in genetics. The heterogeneity of neurodevelopmental disorders may be determined by both heritable and *de novo* genetic variations. In these disorders, a high proportion of genetic variations occur on genes encoding key neurological molecules that modulate synaptic function (Clarke, Lee, & Eapen, 2012; Cristino et al., 2014; Meredith, 2015; O'Roak et al., 2011). Monogenic neurodevelopmental disorders such as Rett, Angelman, or Fragile X syndromes show a more direct relationship between genotype and phenotype, meaning that symptom expression is mainly linked to genetic predisposition rather than environmental factors (Lyst & Bird, 2015). On the other hand, polygenic neurodevelopmental disorders, such as ASD or ADHD, display a more complex interaction between genes and environment, which leads to broader and more complicated phenotypic manifestations (Li, Chang, Zhang, Gao, & Wang, 2014; Loke, Hannan, & Craig, 2015). Some of the environmental factors that may influence the development of these disorders during the early development of the foetus include the intrauterine environment, toxicity exposure (e.g, smoking, valproic acid), viral infection, insufficient maternal nutrition, high levels of stress, obstetric complications, advanced parental age, prematurity, and childhood trauma (Merikangas, Corvin, & Gallagher, 2009).

Our genetic material is inherited from our parents, yet variations in this genetic material are common and can also be affected by environmental factors. Copy number variation (CNV) refers to genomic variations, including insertions, translocations, duplications, and deletions of the chromosomal structure (Merikangas et al., 2009). These variations in repetitive regions of DNA have contributed to evolutionary adaptation and diversity, as well as the development of disease, across species (Asadollahi et al., 2014; Iyer & Girirajan, 2015). Whereas CNVs are largely linked to our inheritance, *de novo* CNVs are genetic variations that can occur spontaneously (e.g., not inherited from parents) and have been recently related with numerous neurodevelopmental disorders, such as schizophrenia, bipolar disorder, ASD, and ADHD (Fromer et al., 2014; Georgieva et al., 2014; Hoischen, Krumm, & Eichler, 2014; Luo et al., 2012; Sanders et al., 2011). Another type of genetic variation is the single nucleotide polymorphism (SNP). These are nucleotide substitutions of one base-pair for another; for instance, SNP may replace the nucleotide cytosine with the nucleotide guanine. These changes in certain parts of our DNA occur with high frequency, and it is estimated that there are around 10 million SNPs in the human genome (Altshuler et al., 2010). Although many of these replacements do not have health-related effects, some are nevertheless related to certain susceptibilities towards environmental factors, or the development of diseases and psychiatric disorders (Cristino et al., 2014).

The fast development of new genetic techniques, together with the implementation of epidemiological genetic studies, have allowed the identification of some of these genetic variations implicated in neurodevelopmental disorders. Some of the most common epidemiological genetic studies associated with these disorders are familial aggregation, linkage, candidate gene association, and genome-wide association studies.

Familial aggregation studies involve procedures that determine the existence of a specific disease or a given trait within a family, comparing the frequency of the disease with the general population (Doherty & Owen, 2014; Mathews et al., 2008). For instance, a recent study has shown that the risk of autism is increased 10 fold if a sibling has the diagnosis, and about 2 fold if a cousin has the diagnosis (Sandin et al., 2014). One of the criticisms that has been made of this technique is that even though a relationship between gene and disease can be found, it is difficult to control for environmental factors (Kim & Leventhal, 2015).

Linkage studies aim to identify genomic regions that contain disease-associated genes. These studies have been successful in identifying novel genes associated with ADHD across the lifespan, as well as in schizophrenia and other neurodevelopmental disorders (Franke et al., 2012; Muraki & Tanigaki, 2015; Ott, Wang, & Leal, 2015; Paschou, 2013).

Candidate gene association studies are focused on the selection of genes that have already been related to a specific disease, and for which we typically have some knowledge about the biological pathway and gene function. For instance, candidate gene association studies have demonstrated that the risk of developing ADHD is associated with genes involved in the noradrenergic pathway (Franke et al., 2012; Hawi et al., 2013). Another example is a recent meta-analysis showing that OCD is mostly associated with polymorphisms involved in serotonin and catecholamine regulation (Taylor, 2013), while dopamine transporter genes have also been implicated (Hawi et al., 2015; Tong et al., 2015).

Genome-wide association studies (GWAS) analyse DNA sequence variations across the human genome to identify genetic risk factors for different diseases (Bush & Moore, 2012; Mullin et al., 2013). An important contribution following this method has been the identification of a protein-protein interaction network for ADHD, which contributes to the understanding of the underlying biological basis and future treatment of this neurodevelopmental disorder (Poelmans, Pauls, Buitelaar, & Franke, 2011).

Another important contribution to the field of behavioural genetics has been twin studies. In these studies, the comparison between monozygotic and dizygotic twins provides a valuable scenario to explore the relationship between gene and environment interaction, as well as to investigate the susceptibility to disease, by evaluating the genetic variations within twins (Boomsma, Busjahn, & Peltonen, 2002). A recent twin study has demonstrated that autism discordant monozygotic twin pairs differ in their DNA methylation patterns, which may provide evidence for the association between epigenetic changes and disease (Wong et al., 2014).

Phenomenal advances are also being seen in genetic studies within animal models. For instance, with *optogenetics* researchers are now able to manipulate, *in vivo*, the activity of specific neurons that have undergone genetic manipulation to be susceptible to light (Fenno, Yizhar, & Deisseroth, 2011). Depending on the wavelength of the light source, the activity of these neurons can be directly modulated, and their activity recorded. Optogentics shows great promise for the continued development of animal models of neurodevelopmental disorders, and could be used to clarify specific neural circuitry associated with these conditions, and perhaps provide new avenues for the development of novel treatments (Halassa et al., 2014).

Computational modelling

Finally, we consider the burgeoning field of computational modelling in neuroscience. These approaches attempt to conceptualise and understand aspects of the nervous system via a series of mathematical equations. These equations not only seek to quantify different parts of the neurobiological system, but also to chart their dynamic interaction, thus providing a functional model by which a given system is thought to operate. This notion of a *system* in computational modelling is quite broad; for instance, it could reflect channel activity within a single neuron, interactions between excitatory neurons and inhibitory interneurons in superficial cortical layers, the activity of a broadly distributed "network" throughout the human brain, or neurocognitive/behavioural aspects linked to a specific symptom or syndrome.

There have been numerous attempts to provide computational modelling accounts of behaviour and neurobiology in relation to frontostriatal neurodevelopmental disorders. For instance, computational modelling has been used to demonstrate impairments in reinforcement learning in ADHD (via a probabilistic reversal learning task) (Hauser et al., 2014). Combined with functional neuroimaging and electrophysiology, these authors also demonstrated that these impairments were linked to impaired activity within medial prefrontal cortex 200–400ms after feedback onset. Similar approaches have yielded advances in a range of psychiatric and neurodevelopmental disorders (for a review, see Wang & Krystal, 2014).

Summary

The development of the technologies and techniques reviewed in this chapter are perhaps the main reason that this is such an exciting time to be working in the neurosciences. We have unprecedented access to the workings of the brain, and some of the many determinants of these processes, both in healthy and pathological states. This is coupled with the emergence of several techniques that are used to modulate brain function, and therefore raise the possibility of new treatments. None of these techniques, however, will be maximally effective when used in isolation; rather, it is likely that the continued efforts to combine these techniques represent our best opportunity for not only understanding neurodevelopmental disorders, but also for finding new ways to determine diagnosis, prognosis, and treatment.

Glossary

Anodal stimulation: Electrode polarity that typically increases cortical excitability.
Cathodal stimulation: Electrode polarity that typically decreases cortical excitability.
Central Nervous System (CNS): Comprising the brain and spinal cord.

Copy number variation (CNV): Genomic variations of the chromosomal structure.

Deep Repetitive Transcranial Magnetic Stimulation (rTMS): rTMS technique that is capable of inducing current in brain regions further away from the scalp.

Electroconvulsive therapy (ECT): Treatment method that uses strong electrical currents via electrodes placed in the scalp to induce a seizure; mainly used in severe forms of depression, schizophrenia, and bipolar disorder.

Electroencephalography (EEG): Electrophysiological technique that measures electrical brain activity via electrodes attached to the scalp.

Functional Magnetic Resonance Imaging (fMRI): Uses MRI technology to provide an index of blood flow, allows inferences of brain activity.

Functional Near-Infrared Spectroscopy (fNIRS): Measures changes in blood (haemoglobin) oxygenation/deoxygenation by using light in the near-infrared range.

Gamma-Aminobutyric acid (GABA): Brain's primary inhibitory neurotransmitter, reduces neural excitability.

Genome-wide association studies (GWAS): Studies that analyse DNA sequence variations across the human genome to identify genetic risk factors for different diseases.

Glutamate: Excitatory neurotransmitter and precursor of GABA.

High definition transcranial current stimulation (HD-tDCS): tDCS technique that involves the use of multiple electrodes to enhance the focality of the stimulation.

Long-term depression (LTD): A mechanism that decreases the efficacy of neural synapses, reducing neural transmission.

Long-term potentiation (LTP): A mechanism that increases the efficacy of neural synapses, increasing neural transmission.

Magnetic Resonance Imaging (MRI): Medical imaging tool that uses a magnetic field and radio frequency pulses to provide structural images inside the body.

Magnetoencephalograhy (MEG): Neuroimaging technique to measure magnetic fields arising from electrical brain activity with high temporal resolution.

N-methyl-D-aspartate (NMDA) receptor: An ionotropic glutamate receptor which allows excitatory neurotransmission.

Optodes: Optical sensors commonly used in fNIRS.

Repetitive Transcranial Magnetic Stimulation (rTMS): TMS applied repeatedly that can induce lasting changes in cortical excitability.

Single nucleotide polymorphism (SNP): Variations of the DNA sequence at particular locations.

Super-conducting detectors and amplifiers (SQUIDs): Highly sensitive detectors to measure magnetic fields.

Transcranial alternating current stimulation (tACS): Brain stimulation technique that modulates cortical activity by using oscillatory electrical stimulation in different frequency bands.

Transcranial direct current stimulation (tDCS): Non-invasive brain stimulation technique that involves delivering weak direct current into the brain via electrodes placed on the scalp.

Transcranial Electrical Stimulation (TES): Non-invasive techniques that uses scalp electrodes to deliver weak electrical currents to the brain to modulate brain activity.

Transcranial magnetic stimulation (TMS): Non-invasive technique that involves the induction of electrical current within the brain via magnetic pulses applied to the scalp, used to study and modulate brain activity.

Transcranial random noise stimulation (tRNS): Brain stimulation technique that modulates and desynchronizes specific oscillatory brain activity.

References

Altshuler, D., Durbin, R. M., Abecasis, G. R., Bentley, D. R., Chakravarti, A., Clark, A. G., ... Consortium, G. P. (2010). A map of human genome variation from population-scale sequencing. *Nature, 467*(7319), 1061–1073. doi: 10.1038/nature09534.

Ardolino, G., Bossi, B., Barbieri, S., & Priori, A. (2005). Non-synaptic mechanisms underlie the after-effects of cathodal transcutaneous direct current stimulation of the human brain. *Physiology Journal, 568*(Pt 2), 653–663. doi: 10.1113/jphysiol.2005.088310.

Asadollahi, R., Oneda, B., Joset, P., Azzarello-Burri, S., Bartholdi, D., Steindl, K., ... Rauch, A. (2014). The clinical significance of small copy number variants in neurodevelopmental disorders. *Journal of Medical Genetics, 51*(10), 677–688. doi: 10.1136/jmedgenet-2014-102588.

Battleday, R. M., Muller, T., Clayton, M. S., & Cohen Kadosh, R. (2014). Mapping the mechanisms of transcranial alternating current stimulation: A pathway from network effects to cognition. *Front Psychiatry, 5*, 162. doi: 10.3389/fpsyt.2014.00162.

Boggio, P. S., Nunes, A., Rigonatti, S. P., Nitsche, M. A., Pascual-Leone, A., & Fregni, F. (2007). Repeated sessions of noninvasive brain DC stimulation is associated with motor function improvement in stroke patients. *Restorative Neurology and Neuroscience, 25*(2), 123–129.

Boomsma, D., Busjahn, A., & Peltonen, L. (2002). Classical twin studies and beyond. *Nature Reviews. Genetics, 3*(11), 872–882. doi: 10.1038/nrg932.

Bruckmann, S., Hauk, D., Roessner, V., Resch, F., Freitag, C. M., Kammer, T., ... Bender, S. (2012). Cortical inhibition in attention deficit hyperactivity disorder: New insights from the electroencephalographic response to transcranial magnetic stimulation. *Brain, 135*(7), 2215–2230. doi: 10.1093/brain/aws071.

Brunoni, A. R., Ferrucci, R., Bortolomasi, M., Vergari, M., Tadini, L., Boggio, P. S., ... Priori, A. (2011). Transcranial direct current stimulation (tDCS) in unipolar vs. bipolar depressive disorder. *Progress in Neuro-Psychopharmacology and Biological Psychiatry, 35*(1), 96–101. doi: 10.1016/j.pnpbp.2010.09.010.

Brunoni, A. R., Kemp, A. H., Shiozawa, P., Cordeiro, Q., Valiengo, L. C., Goulart, A. C., ... Bensenor, I. M. (2013). Impact of 5-HTTLPR and BDNF polymorphisms on response to sertraline versus transcranial direct current stimulation: Implications for the serotonergic system. *European Neuropsychopharmacology, 23*(11), 1530–1540. doi: 10.1016/j.euroneuro.2013.03.009.

Brunoni, A. R., Nitsche, M. A., Bolognini, N., Bikson, M., Wagner, T., Merabet, L., ... Fregni, F. (2012). Clinical research with transcranial direct current stimulation (tDCS): Challenges and future directions. *Brain Stimulation, 5*(3), 175–195. doi: 10.1016/j.brs.2011.03.002.

Bush, W. S., & Moore, J. H. (2012). Chapter 11: Genome-wide association studies. *PLoS Computational Biology, 8*(12), e1002822. doi: 10.1371/journal.pcbi.1002822.

Chan, H. N., Alonzo, A., Martin, D. M., Player, M., Mitchell, P. B., Sachdev, P., & Loo, C. K. (2012). Treatment of major depressive disorder by transcranial random noise stimulation: Case report of a novel treatment. *Biological Psychiatry, 72*(4), e9–e10. doi: 10.1016/j.biopsych.2012.02.009.

Charvet, L. E., Kasschau, M., Datta, A., Knotkova, H., Stevens, M. C., Alonzo, A., ... Bikson, M. (2015). Remotely-supervised transcranial direct current stimulation (tDCS) for clinical trials: Guidelines for technology and protocols. *Fronters in Systems Neuroscience, 9*, 26. doi: 10.3389/fnsys.2015.00026.

Clarke, R. A., Lee, S., & Eapen, V. (2012). Pathogenetic model for Tourette syndrome delineates overlap with related neurodevelopmental disorders including Autism. *Translational Psychiatry, 2*, e158. doi: 10.1038/tp.2012.75.

Cristino, A. S., Williams, S. M., Hawi, Z., An, J. Y., Bellgrove, M. A., Schwartz, C. E., … Claudianos, C. (2014). Neurodevelopmental and neuropsychiatric disorders represent an interconnected molecular system. *Molecular Psychiatry, 19*(3), 294–301. doi: 10.1038/mp.2013.16.

Datta, A., Elwassif, M., & Bikson, M. (2009). Bio-heat transfer model of transcranial DC stimulation: Comparison of conventional pad versus ring electrode. *Conf Proc IEEE Eng Med Biol Soc, 2009*, 670–673. doi: 10.1109/iembs.2009.5333673.

Deng, Z. D., Lisanby, S. H., & Peterchev, A.V. (2014). Coil design considerations for deep transcranial magnetic stimulation. *Clinical Neurophysiology, 125*(6), 1202–1212. doi: 10.1016/j.clinph.2013.11.038.

Doherty, J. L., & Owen, M. J. (2014). Genomic insights into the overlap between psychiatric disorders: Implications for research and clinical practice. *Genome Medicine, 6*(4). doi: 10.1186/gm546.

D'Urso, G., Brunoni, A. R., Anastasia, A., Micillo, M., de Bartolomeis, A., & Mantovani, A. (2015). Polarity-dependent effects of transcranial direct current stimulation in obsessive-compulsive disorder. *Neurocase*, 1–5. doi: 10.1080/13554794.2015.1045522.

Edwards, D., Cortes, M., Datta, A., Minhas, P., Wassermann, E. M., & Bikson, M. (2013). Physiological and modeling evidence for focal transcranial electrical brain stimulation in humans: A basis for high-definition tDCS. *Neuroimage, 74*, 266–275. doi: 10.1016/j.neuroimage.2013.01.042.

Enticott, P. G., Fitzgibbon, B. M., Kennedy, H. A., Arnold, S. L., Elliot, D., Peachey, A., … Fitzgerald, P. B. (2014). A double-blind, randomized trial of deep repetitive transcranial magnetic stimulation (rTMS) for autism spectrum disorder. *Brain Stimulation,* 7(2), 206–211. doi: 10.1016/j.brs.2013.10.004.

Enticott, P. G., Hoy, K. E., Herring, S. E., Johnston, P. J., Daskalakis, J. Z., & Fitzgerald, P. B. (2008). Reduced motor facilitation during action observation in schizophrenia: A mirror neuron deficit? *Schizophrenia Research, 102*(1–3), 116–121.

Enticott, P. G., Kennedy, H. A., Rinehart, N. J., Tonge, B. J., Bradshaw, J. L., & Fitzgerald, P. B. (2013). GABAergic activity in autism spectrum disorders: An investigation of cortical inhibition via transcranial magnetic stimulation. *Neuropharmacology, 68*, 202–209.

Enticott, P. G., Kennedy, H. A., Rinehart, N. J., Tonge, B. J., Bradshaw, J. L., Taffe, J. R., … Fitzgerald, P. B. (2012). Mirror neuron activity associated with social impairments but not age in autism spectrum disorder. *Biological Psychiatry, 71*(5), 427–433.

Enticott, P. G., Rinehart, N. J., Tonge, B. J., Bradshaw, J. L., & Fitzgerald, P. B. (2010). A preliminary transcranial magnetic stimulation study of cortical inhibition and excitability in high-functioning autism and Asperger's disorder. *Developmental Medicine and Child Neurology, 52*(8), e179-e183.

Fecteau, S., Agosta, S., Oberman, L., & Pascual-Leone, A. (2011). Brain stimulation over Broca's area differentially modulates naming skills in neurotypical adults and individuals with Asperger's syndrome. *European Journal of Neuroscience, 34*(1), 158–164. doi: 10.1111/j.1460-9568.2011.07726.x.

Fenno, L., Yizhar, O., & Deisseroth, K. (2011). The development and application of optogenetics. *Vol. 34. Annual Review of Neuroscience,* 389–412.

Fornito, A., Zalesky, A., & Breakspear, M. (2015). The connectomics of brain disorders. *Nature Reviews Neuroscience, 16*(3), 159–172. doi: 10.1038/nrn3901.

Franke, B., Faraone, S.V., Asherson, P., Buitelaar, J., Bau, C. H., Ramos-Quiroga, J. A., … Reif, A. (2012). The genetics of attention deficit/hyperactivity disorder in adults, a review. *Molecular Psychiatry,* 17(10), 960–987. doi: 10.1038/mp.2011.138.

Fromer, M., Pocklington, A. J., Kavanagh, D. H., Williams, H. J., Dwyer, S., Gormley, P., … O'Donovan, M. C. (2014). De novo mutations in schizophrenia implicate synaptic networks. *Nature, 506*(7487), 179–184. doi: 10.1038/nature12929.

George, M. S., Lisanby, S. H., Avery, D., McDonald, W. M., Durkalski, V., Pavlicova, M., … Sackeim, H. A. (2010). Daily left prefrontal transcranial magnetic stimulation therapy for major depressive disorder: A sham-controlled randomized trial. *Archives of General Psychiatry, 67*(5), 507–516. doi: 10.1001/archgenpsychiatry.2010.46.

Georgieva, L., Rees, E., Moran, J. L., Chambert, K. D., Milanova, V., Craddock, N., … Kirov, G. (2014). De novo CNVs in bipolar affective disorder and schizophrenia. *Human Molecular Genetics, 23*(24), 6677–6683. doi: 10.1093/hmg/ddu379.

Gilbert, D. L., Isaacs, K. M., Augusta, M., MacNeil, L. K., & Mostofsky, S. H. (2011). Motor cortex inhibition: A marker of ADHD behavior and motor development in children. *Neurology, 76*(7), 615–621. doi: 10.1212/WNL.0b013e31820c2ebd.

Gilbert, D. L., Ridel, K. R., Sallee, F. R., Zhang, J., Lipps, T. D., & Wassermann, E. M. (2006). Comparison of the inhibitory and excitatory effects of ADHD medications methylphenidate and atomoxetine on motor cortex. *Neuropsychopharmacology, 31*(2), 442–449. doi: 10.1038/sj.npp.1300806.

Gilbert, D. L., Sallee, F. R., Zhang, J., Lipps, T. D., & Wassermann, E. M. (2005). Transcranial magnetic stimulation-evoked cortical inhibition: A consistent marker of attention-deficit/hyperactivity disorder scores in Tourette Syndrome. *Biological Psychiatry, 57*(12), 1597–1600. doi: 10.1016/j.biopsych.2005.02.022.

Halassa, M. M., Chen, Z., Wimmer, R. D., Brunetti, P. M., Zhao, S., Zikopoulos, B., … Wilson, M. A. (2014). State-dependent architecture of thalamic reticular subnetworks. *Cell, 158*(4), 808–821. doi: 10.1016/j.cell.2014.06.025.

Hall, S. S., Jiang, H., Reiss, A. L., & Greicius, M. D. (2013). Identifying large-scale brain networks in fragile X syndrome. *JAMA Psychiatry, 70*(11), 1215–1223. doi: 10.1001/jamapsychiatry.2013.247.

Hauser, T. U., Iannaccone, R., Ball, J., Mathys, C., Brandeis, D., Walitza, S., & Brem, S. (2014). Role of the medial prefrontal cortex in impaired decision making in juvenile attention-deficit/hyperactivity disorder. *JAMA Psychiatry, 71*(10), 1165–1173. doi: 10.1001/jamapsychiatry.2014.1093.

Hawi, Z., Cummins, T. D. R., Tong, J., Johnson, B., Lau, R., Samarrai, W., & Bellgrove, M. A. (2015). The molecular genetic architecture of attention deficit hyperactivity disorder. *Molecular Psychiatry, 20*(3), 289–297. doi: 10.1038/mp.2014.183.

Hawi, Z., Matthews, N., Barry, E., Kirley, A., Wagner, J., Wallace, R. H., … Bellgrove, M. A. (2013). A high density linkage disequilibrium mapping in 14 noradrenergic genes: Evidence of association between SLC6A2, ADRA1B and ADHD. *Psychopharmacology, 225*(4), 895–902. doi: 10.1007/s00213-012-2875-x.

Helfrich, C., Pierau, S. S., Freitag, C. M., Roeper, J., Ziemann, U., & Bender, S. (2012). Monitoring cortical excitability during repetitive transcranial magnetic stimulation in children with ADHD: A single-blind, sham-controlled TMS-EEG study. *PLoS One,* 7(11), e50073. doi: 10.1371/journal.pone.0050073.

Herrmann, C. S., Rach, S., Neuling, T., & Struber, D. (2013). Transcranial alternating current stimulation: A review of the underlying mechanisms and modulation of cognitive processes. *Frontiers in Human Neuroscience,* 7, 279. doi: 10.3389/fnhum.2013.00279.

Hoischen, A., Krumm, N., & Eichler, E. E. (2014). Prioritization of neurodevelopmental disease genes by discovery of new mutations. *Nature Neuroscience, 17*(6), 764–772. doi: 10.1038/nn.3703.

Iyer, J., & Girirajan, S. (2015). Gene discovery and functional assessment of rare copy-number variants in neurodevelopmental disorders. *Briefings in Functional Genomics*. doi: 10.1093/bfgp/elv018.

Jausovec, N., & Jausovec, K. (2014). Increasing working memory capacity with theta transcranial alternating current stimulation (tACS). *Biological Psychology, 96*, 42–47. doi: 10.1016/j.biopsycho.2013.11.006.

Jeste, S. S., Frohlich, J., & Loo, S. K. (2015). Electrophysiological biomarkers of diagnosis and outcome in neurodevelopmental disorders. *Current Opinion in Neurology, 28*(2), 110–116. doi: 10.1097/wco.0000000000000181.

Jung, N. H., Janzarik, W. G., Delvendahl, I., Münchau, A., Biscaldi, M., Mainberger, F., ... Mall, V. (2013). Impaired induction of long-term potentiation-like plasticity in patients with high-functioning autism and Asperger syndrome. *Developmental Medicine and Child Neurology, 55*(1), 83–89. doi: 10.1111/dmcn.12012.

Just, M. A., Cherkassky, V. L., Buchweitz, A., Keller, T. A., & Mitchell, T. M. (2014). Identifying autism from neural representations of social interactions: Neurocognitive markers of autism. *PLoS One, 9*(12). doi: 10.1371/journal.pone.0113879.

Kellner, C. H., Greenberg, R. M., Murrough, J. W., Bryson, E. O., Briggs, M. C., & Pasculli, R. M. (2012). ECT in treatment-resistant depression. *American Journal of Psychiatry, 169*(12), 1238–1244. doi: 10.1176/appi.ajp.2012.12050648.

Khan, S., Michmizos, K., Tommerdahl, M., Ganesan, S., Kitzbichler, M. G., Zetino, M., ... Kenet, T. (2015). Somatosensory cortex functional connectivity abnormalities in autism show opposite trends, depending on direction and spatial scale. *Brain, 138*(5), 1394–1409. doi: 10.1093/brain/awv043.

Kim, Y. S., & Leventhal, B. L. (2015). Genetic epidemiology and insights into interactive genetic and environmental effects in autism spectrum disorders. *Biological Psychiatry,* 77(1), 66–74. doi: 10.1016/j.biopsych.2014.11.001.

Koops, S., van den Brink, H., & Sommer, I. E. (2015). Transcranial direct current stimulation as a treatment for auditory hallucinations. *Frontiers in Psychology, 6*, 244. doi: 10.3389/fpsyg.2015.00244.

Kuo, M. F., & Nitsche, M. A. (2012). Effects of transcranial electrical stimulation on cognition. *Clinical EEG Neuroscience, 43*(3), 192–199. doi: 10.1177/1550059412444975.

Kwon, H. J., Lim, W. S., Lim, M. H., Lee, S. J., Hyun, J. K., Chae, J. H., & Paik, K. C. (2011). 1-Hz low frequency repetitive transcranial magnetic stimulation in children with Tourette's syndrome. *Neuroscience Letters, 492*(1), 1–4. doi: 10.1016/j.neulet.2011.01.007.

Le, K., Liu, L., Sun, M., Hu, L., & Xiao, N. (2013). Transcranial magnetic stimulation at 1 Hertz improves clinical symptoms in children with Tourette syndrome for at least 6 months. *Journal of Clinical Neuroscience, 20*(2), 257–262. doi: 10.1016/j.jocn.2012.01.049.

Lefaucheur, J. P., Andre-Obadia, N., Antal, A., Ayache, S. S., Baeken, C., Benninger, D. H., ... Garcia-Larrea, L. (2014). Evidence-based guidelines on the therapeutic use of repetitive transcranial magnetic stimulation (rTMS). *Clinical Neurophysiology, 125*(11), 2150–2206. doi: 10.1016/j.clinph.2014.05.021.

Li, Z., Chang, S. H., Zhang, L. Y., Gao, L., & Wang, J. (2014). Molecular genetic studies of ADHD and its candidate genes: A review. *Psychiatry Research, 219*(1), 10–24. doi: 10.1016/j.psychres.2014.05.005.

Loke, Y. J., Hannan, A. J., & Craig, J. M. (2015). The role of epigenetic change in autism spectrum disorders. *Frontiers in Neurology, 6*, 107. doi: 10.3389/fneur.2015.00107.

Luo, R., Sanders, S. J., Tian, Y., Voineagu, I., Huang, N., Chu, S. H., ... Geschwind, D. H. (2012). Genome-wide transcriptome profiling reveals the functional impact of rare de novo and recurrent CNVs in autism spectrum disorders. *American Journal of Human Genetics, 91*(1), 38–55. doi: 10.1016/j.ajhg.2012.05.011.

Lyst, M. J., & Bird, A. (2015). Rett syndrome: A complex disorder with simple roots. *Native Reviews. Genetics, 16*(5), 261–275. doi: 10.1038/nrg3897.

Mantovani, A., Lisanby, S. H., Pieraccini, F., Ulivelli, M., Castrogiovanni, P., & Rossi, S. (2006). Repetitive transcranial magnetic stimulation (rTMS) in the treatment of obsessive-compulsive disorder (OCD) and Tourette's syndrome (TS). *International Journal of Neuropsychopharmacology, 9*(1), 95–100. doi: 10.1017/S1461145705005729.

Mathews, C. A., Greenwood, T., Wessel, J., Azzam, A., Garrido, H., Chavira, D. A., … Schork, N. J. (2008). Evidence for a heritable unidimensional symptom factor underlying obsessionality. *American Journal of Medical Genetics, Part B: Neuropsychiatric Genetics, 147*(6), 676–685. doi: 10.1002/ajmg.b.30660.

Meredith, R. M. (2015). Sensitive and critical periods during neurotypical and aberrant neurodevelopment: A framework for neurodevelopmental disorders. *Neuroscience and Biobehavioral Reviews, 50*, 180–188. doi: 10.1016/j.neubiorev.2014.12.001.

Merikangas, A. K., Corvin, A. P., & Gallagher, L. (2009). Copy-number variants in neurodevelopmental disorders: Promises and challenges. *Trends in Genetics, 25*(12), 536–544. doi: 10.1016/j.tig.2009.10.006.

Monden, Y., Dan, I., Nagashima, M., Dan, H., Uga, M., Ikeda, T., … Yamagata, T. (2015). Individual classification of ADHD children by right prefrontal hemodynamic responses during a go/no-go task as assessed by fNIRS. *NeuroImage: Clinical, 9*, 1–12. doi: 10.1016/j.nicl.2015.06.011.

Mondino, M., Bennabi, D., Poulet, E., Galvao, F., Brunelin, J., & Haffen, E. (2014). Can transcranial direct current stimulation (tDCS) alleviate symptoms and improve cognition in psychiatric disorders? *World Journal of Biological Psychiatry, 15*(4), 261–275. doi: 10.3109/15622975.2013.876514.

Monte-Silva, K., Kuo, M. F., Liebetanz, D., Paulus, W., & Nitsche, M. A. (2010). Shaping the optimal repetition interval for cathodal transcranial direct current stimulation (tDCS). *Journal of Neurophysiology, 103*(4), 1735–1740. doi: 10.1152/jn.00924.2009.

Mullin, A. P., Gokhale, A., Moreno-De-Luca, A., Sanyal, S., Waddington, J. L., & Faundez, V. (2013). Neurodevelopmental disorders: Mechanisms and boundary definitions from genomes, interactomes and proteomes. *Translational Psychiatry, 3*, e329. doi: 10.1038/tp.2013.108.

Muraki, K., & Tanigaki, K. (2015). Neuronal migration abnormalities and its possible implications for schizophrenia. *Frontier in Neuroscience, 9*, 74. doi: 10.3389/fnins.2015.00074.

Nitsche, M. A., & Paulus, W. (2000). Excitability changes induced in the human motor cortex by weak transcranial direct current stimulation. *Journal of Physiology, 527 Pt 3*, 633–639.

Nitsche, M. A., Cohen, L. G., Wassermann, E. M., Priori, A., Lang, N., Antal, A., … Pascual-Leone, A. (2008). Transcranial direct current stimulation: State of the art 2008. *Brain Stimulation, 1*(3), 206–223. doi: S1935-861X(08)00040-5 [pii] 10.1016/j.brs.2008.06.004.

Nitsche, M. A., Seeber, A., Frommann, K., Klein, C. C., Rochford, C., Nitsche, M. S., … Tergau, F. (2005). Modulating parameters of excitability during and after transcranial direct current stimulation of the human motor cortex. *Journal of Physiology, 568*(Pt 1), 291–303. doi: 10.1113/jphysiol.2005.092429.

Oberman, L. M., Enticott, P. G., Casanova, M. F., Rotenberg, A., Pascual-Leone, A., & McCracken, J. T. (2015). Transcranial magnetic stimulation (TMS) therapy for autism: An international consensus conference held in conjunction with the international meeting for autism research on May 13th and 14th, 2014. *Frontiers in Human Neuroscience, 8*(JAN). doi: 10.3389/fnhum.2014.01034.

Oberman, L. M., Rotenberg, A., & Pascual-Leone, A. (2013). Use of transcranial magnetic stimulation in autism spectrum disorders. *Journal of Autism and Developmental Disorders*. doi: 10.1007/s10803-013-1960-2.

Oberman, L., Eldaief, M., Fecteau, S., Ifert-Miller, F., Tormos, J. M., & Pascual-Leone, A. (2012). Abnormal modulation of corticospinal excitability in adults with Asperger's syndrome. *European Journal of Neuroscience, 36*(6), 2782–2788. doi: 10.1111/j.1460-9568.2012.08172.x.

O'Roak, B. J., Deriziotis, P., Lee, C., Vives, L., Schwartz, J. J., Girirajan, S., … Eichler, E. E. (2011). Exome sequencing in sporadic autism spectrum disorders identifies severe de novo mutations. *Nature Genetics, 43*(6), 585–589. doi: 10.1038/ng.835.

Orth, M., Amann, B., Robertson, M. M., & Rothwell, J. C. (2005). Excitability of motor cortex inhibitory circuits in Tourette syndrome before and after single dose nicotine. *Brain, 128*(6), 1292–1300. doi: 10.1093/brain/awh473.

Ott, J., Wang, J., & Leal, S. M. (2015). Genetic linkage analysis in the age of whole-genome sequencing. *Nature Reviews. Genetics, 16*(5), 275–284. doi: 10.1038/nrg3908.

Palm, U., Hasan, A., Keeser, D., Falkai, P., & Padberg, F. (2013). Transcranial random noise stimulation for the treatment of negative symptoms in schizophrenia. *Schizophrenia Research, 146*(1–3), 372–373. doi: 10.1016/j.schres.2013.03.003.

Palm, U., Keeser, D., Blautzik, J., Pogarell, O., Ertl-Wagner, B., Kupka, M. J., … Padberg, F. (2013). Prefrontal transcranial direct current stimulation (tDCS) changes negative symptoms and functional connectivity MRI (fcMRI) in a single case of treatment-resistant schizophrenia. *Schizophrenia Research, 150*(2–3), 583–585. doi: 10.1016/j.schres.2013.08.043.

Paschou, P. (2013). The genetic basis of Gilles de la Tourette Syndrome. *Neuroscience and Biobehavioral Reviews, 37*(6), 1026–1039. doi: 10.1016/j.neubiorev.2013.01.016.

Paulus, W. (2011). Transcranial electrical stimulation (tES - tDCS; tRNS, tACS) methods. *Neuropsychological Rehabilitation, 21*(5), 602–617. doi: 10.1080/09602011.2011.557292.

Poelmans, G., Pauls, D. L., Buitelaar, J. K., & Franke, B. (2011). Integrated genome-wide association study findings: Identification of a neurodevelopmental network for attention deficit hyperactivity disorder. *American Journal of Psychiatry, 168*(4), 365–377. doi: 10.1176/appi.ajp.2010.10070948.

Pompili, M., Lester, D., Dominici, G., Longo, L., Marconi, G., Forte, A., … Girardi, P. (2013). Indications for electroconvulsive treatment in schizophrenia: A systematic review. *Schizophrenia Research, 146*(1–3), 1–9. doi: 10.1016/j.schres.2013.02.005.

Priori, A., Berardelli, A., Rona, S., Accornero, N., & Manfredi, M. (1998). Polarization of the human motor cortex through the scalp. *Neuroreport, 9*(10), 2257–2260.

Reeb-Sutherland, B. C., & Fox, N. A. (2015). Eyeblink conditioning: A non-invasive biomarker for neurodevelopmental disorders. *Journal of Autism and Developmental Disorders, 45*(2), 376–394. doi: 10.1007/s10803-013-1905-9.

Rogasch, N. C., Daskalakis, Z. J., & Fitzgerald, P. B. (2015). Cortical inhibition of distinct mechanisms in the dorsolateral prefrontal cortex is related to working memory performance: A TMS-EEG study. *Cortex, 64*, 68–77. doi: 10.1016/j.cortex.2014.10.003.

Rogasch, N. C., Thomson, R. H., Farzan, F., Fitzgibbon, B. M., Bailey, N. W., Hernandez-Pavon, J. C., … Fitzgerald, P. B. (2014). Removing artefacts from TMS-EEG recordings using independent component analysis: Importance for assessing prefrontal and motor cortex network properties. *Neuroimage, 101*, 425–439. doi: 10.1016/j.neuroimage.2014.07.037.

Roth, Y., & Zangen, A. (2014) Reaching deep brain structures: The H-coils. *Vol. 89. Neuromethods* (pp. 57–65).

Sanders, S. J., Ercan-Sencicek, A. G., Hus, V., Luo, R., Murtha, M. T., Moreno-De-Luca, D., … State, M. W. (2011). Multiple recurrent de novo CNVs, including duplications of the 7q11.23 Williams syndrome region, are strongly associated with autism. *Neuron, 70*(5), 863–885. doi: 10.1016/j.neuron.2011.05.002.

Sandin, S., Lichtenstein, P., Kuja-Halkola, R., Larsson, H., Hultman, C. M., & Reichenberg, A. (2014). The familial risk of autism. *Journal of the American Medical Association, 311*(17), 1770–1777. doi: 10.1001/jama.2014.4144.

Senco, N. M., Huang, Y., D'Urso, G., Parra, L. C., Bikson, M., Mantovani, A., … Brunoni, A. R. (2015). Transcranial direct current stimulation in obsessive-compulsive disorder: Emerging clinical evidence and considerations for optimal montage of electrodes. *Expert Review of Medical Devices, 12*(4), 381–391. doi: 10.1586/17434440.2015.1037832.

Sienaert, P., Dhossche, D. M., Vancampfort, D., De Hert, M., & Gazdag, G. (2014). A clinical review of the treatment of catatonia. *Front Psychiatry, 5*, 181. doi: 10.3389/fpsyt.2014.00181.

Taylor, S. (2013). Molecular genetics of obsessive-compulsive disorder: A comprehensive meta-analysis of genetic association studies. *Molecular Psychiatry, 18*(7), 799–805. doi: 10.1038/mp.2012.76.

Theoret, H., Halligan, E., Kobayashi, M., Fregni, F., Tager-Flusberg, H., & Pascual-Leone, A. (2005). Impaired motor facilitation during action observation in individuals with autism spectrum disorder. *Current Biology, 15*(3), R84–R85.

Tong, J. H. S., Cummins, T. D. R., Johnson, B. P., McKinley, L. A., Pickering, H. E., Fanning, P., … Bellgrove, M. A. (2015). An association between a dopamine transporter gene (SLC6A3) haplotype and ADHD symptom measures in nonclinical adults. *American Journal of Medical Genetics, Part B: Neuropsychiatric Genetics, 168*(2), 89–96. doi: 10.1002/ajmg.b.32283.

Tortella, G., Casati, R., Aparicio, L. V., Mantovani, A., Senco, N., D'Urso, G., … Brunoni, A. R. (2015). Transcranial direct current stimulation in psychiatric disorders. *World Journal of Psychiatry, 5*(1), 88–102. doi: 10.5498/wjp.v5.i1.88.

Villamar, M. F., Wivatvongvana, P., Patumanond, J., Bikson, M., Truong, D. Q., Datta, A., & Fregni, F. (2013). Focal modulation of the primary motor cortex in fibromyalgia using 4x1-ring high-definition transcranial direct current stimulation (HD-tDCS): Immediate and delayed analgesic effects of cathodal and anodal stimulation. *The Journal of Pain, 14*(4), 371–383. doi: 10.1016/j.jpain.2012.12.007.

Vosskuhl, J., Huster, R. J., & Herrmann, C. S. (2015). Increase in short-term memory capacity induced by down-regulating individual theta frequency via transcranial alternating current stimulation. *Frontiers in Human Neuroscience, 9*, 257. doi: 10.3389/fnhum.2015.00257.

Walker, L., Gozzi, M., Lenroot, R., Thurm, A., Behseta, B., Swedo, S., & Pierpaoli, C. (2012). Diffusion tensor imaging in young children with autism: Biological effects and potential confounds. *Biological Psychiatry, 72*(12), 1043–1051. doi: 10.1016/j.biopsych.2012.08.001.

Walsh, P., Elsabbagh, M., Bolton, P., & Singh, I. (2011). In search of biomarkers for autism: Scientific, social and ethical challenges. *Nature Reviews. Neuroscience, 12*(10), 603–612. doi: 10.1038/nrn3113.

Wang, X. J., & Krystal, J. H. (2014). Computational psychiatry. *Neuron, 84*(3), 638–654. doi: 10.1016/j.neuron.2014.10.018.

Wong, C. C., Meaburn, E. L., Ronald, A., Price, T. S., Jeffries, A. R., Schalkwyk, L. C., … Mill, J. (2014). Methylomic analysis of monozygotic twins discordant for autism spectrum disorder and related behavioural traits. *Molecular Psychiatry, 19*(4), 495–503. doi: 10.1038/mp.2013.41.

Yau, J. M., Jalinous, R., Cantarero, G. L., & Desmond, J. E. (2014). Static field influences on transcranial magnetic stimulation: Considerations for TMS in the scanner environment. *Brain Stimulation,* 7(3), 388–393. doi: 10.1016/j.brs.2014.02.007.

Yuan, H., Zotev, V., Phillips, R., Drevets, W. C., & Bodurka, J. (2012). Spatiotemporal dynamics of the brain at rest - Exploring EEG microstates as electrophysiological signatures of BOLD resting state networks. *Neuroimage, 60*(4), 2062–2072. doi: 10.1016/j.neuroimage.2012.02.031.

5

DEVELOPMENTAL COORDINATION DISORDER

Christian Hyde, Daniela Rigoli and Jan Piek

Introduction

Historically, Developmental Coordination Disorder (DCD) has perhaps been the most poorly recognized of the neurodevelopmental disorders. As we will canvass in this chapter, the reasons are complex and varied, ranging from considerable variation in the application of diagnostic labelling and criterion, to issues surrounding the appropriateness of assessment methods and the frequent comorbid presentation of DCD with other neurodevelopmental disorders. However, there is a growing awareness of the serious impact that delayed motor development has on the day-to-day lives of these individuals and their broader psycho-social and physical development. While the genetic basis of the disorder has received little attention, the available evidence nonetheless suggests a shared role for familial and environmental factors. Neuropsychological models of the disorder have received greater attention and here we review two particularly promising accounts of motor delay, including impaired internal modelling and executive dysfunction. While each is supported by empirical evidence to some degree, their efficacy will ultimately be judged by their capacity to inform effective treatment. Presently, evidence to this effect is largely lacking. Interestingly, although investigation into the neuropathology of DCD has only recently emerged, there is a strong case that atypical neural activation, white matter microstructure and neural connectivity in critical motor circuitry differentiate children with DCD from typical peers. The suggestion of neural markers for the disorder is interesting, given that neurological impairment is presently an exclusionary criterion for DCD. Taken together, however, despite the continued focus on better understanding the aetiology of DCD, no universal account has emerged. It is perhaps unsurprising then, that evidence as to the efficacy of available intervention methods is mixed, at best.

Preliminary considerations

Developmental Coordination Disorder is a relatively new term, first described in the DSM-III in 1987 (APA, 1987), although cases of children with the same identifying symptoms have appeared in the literature for over a century (e.g., Dupre, 1911; cited in Henderson & Barnett, 1998). Prior to its description in the DSM, DCD was described by a multitude of terms, such as *clumsy* or *developmental clumsiness*, *developmental apraxia*, or simply *physically awkward* or *poorly coordinated* (Henderson & Barnett, 1998), leading to a fragmented approach to research in the area. The World Health Organisation's International Classification of Diseases 10 (ICD 10 Version: 2015) includes *Clumsy Child Syndrome*, *Developmental Coordination Disorder* and *Developmental Dyspraxia* in its definition of *Specific Developmental Disorder of Motor Function*. In 1994, leading researchers in the area of DCD came to a consensus that DCD was the preferred term for the disorder (Polatajko, Fox, & Missiuna, 1995), resulting in a more cohesive approach to research since then.

Onset and prevalence

According to the DSM-IV (APA, 2000), infant motor milestones such as sitting and crawling may be a sign of DCD, suggesting that the disorder affects a child from birth. This view was strengthened in the recent DSM-5 description (APA, 2013), as new diagnostic criteria (criterion C) state that symptoms must appear in the early developmental period. However, DCD is generally diagnosed around school age when the children's poor coordination is seen to impact on a child's activities of daily living, academic achievements or their play and leisure activities (Criterion B: DSM-5). Although earlier reports suggested that children grow out of this disorder (Hall, 1988; Knuckey & Gubbay, 1983), there is now strong evidence that DCD continues into adolescence and adulthood in many cases (Cousins & Smyth, 2003; Tal-Saban, Zarka, Grotto, Ornoy, & Parush, 2012). However, suitable assessments at these ages are still being determined (Hands, Licari, & Piek, 2015).

Prevalence is considered to be between 5 and 6% of children aged between 4 and 11 years (APA, 2013) although this has varied in the literature depending on the interpretation of the criteria given in the DSM. In particular, identification and operationalization of Criterion B, which specifies that motor problems must interfere with activities of daily living and school/academic productivity, differ across studies and have led to much debate in the literature. As a result, prevalence estimates vary considerably, and have been reported to be as low as 1.7% in some cases (Lingam, Hunt, Golding, Jongmans, & Emond, 2009), although this study also acknowledged that a further 4.9% had probable DCD based on less stringent thresholds. Prevalence may also vary between cultures (Tsiotra et al., 2006), with some attributing this to lifestyle differences (Lingam et al., 2009; Pearsall-Jones, Piek, Rigoli, Martin, & Levy, 2009).

As is the case with many neurodevelopmental disorders, most studies have identified a greater prevalence in males. However, the ratio varies substantially across studies, as is highlighted by the large range given in the DSM-5 (males:female between 2:1 and 7:1). This variability may be due to a lack of evidence from studies where stringent inclusion/exclusion criteria have been adopted, including acknowledging factors such as comorbidity or diagnosis. For example, although considerable evidence suggests sex differences in motor ability in all stages of development (e.g., Capute, Shapiro, Palmer, Ross, & Wachtel, 1985; Pedersen, Sigmundsson, Whiting, & Ingvaldsen, 2003; Touwen, 1976), few motor tests have taken this into account (Piek, Hands, and Licari, 2012) despite neurological evidence to support such differences (e.g., Liu et al., 2011). Hence, caution is advised when considering differences in DCD prevalence rates between males and females.

Clinical symptoms

The first symptoms evident for children with DCD are commonly related to gross motor ability. Children may have difficulty achieving early motor milestones such as walking or climbing, or later have a very awkward running style or difficulty catching or kicking a ball. Some of these problems have been linked with postural control, although not all children with DCD have difficulties in this domain (Wann, Mon-Williams, & Rushton, 1998). Other children with DCD may have preserved gross motor functioning, yet experience difficulty with fine motor skills such as drawing, using scissors or eating utensils, and writing. More severe cases of DCD may include all of the above symptoms. Indeed, severe cases of DCD can often be difficult to differentiate from milder forms of neurological motor disorders, such as cerebral palsy (Pearsall-Jones, Piek, & Levy, 2010). Furthermore, given the importance of motor control in speech, this may also be affected in some cases (Bradford & Dodd, 1996).

Importantly, clinical symptomatology associated with DCD extends beyond the motor domain, with these individuals presenting with increased rates of a series of physical and psycho-social problems. Recently, evidence has highlighted a link between DCD and inactivity (Rivilis et al., 2011) and overweight/obesity (Joshi et al., 2015), increasing the risk of cardiovascular disease (Faught, Hay, Cairney, & Flouris, 2005). In turn, these issues have been associated with greater mental health issues in children with DCD (Cairney, Rigoli, & Piek, 2013). For example, studies have found higher levels of depressive and anxiety symptoms compared to those without movement difficulties (Lingam et al., 2012; Pearsall-Jones, Piek, Rigoli, Martin, & Levy, 2011).

Comorbidity

Accumulating research in the past two decades has shown high rates of comorbidity between DCD and other neurodevelopmental disorders, most commonly Attention Deficit Hyperactivity Disorder (ADHD) (e.g., Dewey, Kaplan, Crawford, & Wilson,

2002; Lingam et al., 2010), with up to 50% of children with DCD presenting with comorbid ADHD (Piek, Pitcher, & Hay, 1999; Pitcher, Piek, & Hay, 2003). Other commonly reported comorbidities include Oppositional Defiant Disorder (e.g., Kooistra, Crawford, Dewey, Cantell, & Kaplan, 2005; Martin, Piek, Baynam, Levy, & Hay, 2010), learning difficulties such as reading and spelling deficits (e.g., Dewey et al., 2002; Lingam et al., 2010; Martin et al., 2010), and language and speech impairment (Hill, 2001; Visscher, Houwen, Scherder, Moolenaar, & Hartman, 2007). DCD has also been linked with autism spectrum disorder (e.g., Dyck, Piek, Hay, & Hallmayer, 2007; Reiersen, Constantino, & Todd, 2008).

Although many studies suggest that 'comorbidity is the rule rather than the exception' (Kaplan et al., 1998), the environmental and biological mechanisms subserving this relationship remain unclear. For example, Blank and colleagues (2012) noted that in some cases, it is difficult to establish the extent to which behavioural problems are co-existing disorders or the consequences of the negative environmental experiences associated with DCD. The Environmental Stress Hypothesis (ESH) (Cairney, Rigoli, & Piek 2013; Cairney, Veldhuizen, & Szatmari, 2010) proposes that exposure to personal and interpersonal stressors (e.g., greater peer exclusion, poor self-perceived competence) mediates the relationship between increased emotional symptoms and movement problems. Though largely lacking experimental validation, the ESH provides a promising theoretical framework for understanding the overlap between DCD and emotional outcomes.

Nevertheless, it appears crucial that comorbidity is considered in the assessment and treatment process for individuals presenting with movement problems and vice versa. This is particularly important given evidence of poorer psychosocial, educational and vocational outcomes in individuals who display difficulties in more than one domain (Kadesjö & Gillberg, 1999; Kadesjö & Gillberg, 2001; Piek et al., 2007; Rasmussen & Gillberg, 2000).

Diagnostic instruments and clinical rating scales

The heterogenous and comorbid nature of DCD complicates the selection of appropriate assessment tools for identifying whether an individual's motor performance is "substantially below" that expected for a child's age (DSM-5 criterion A). However, the most common approach is to employ one of the broad-based, norm-referenced tests of motor performance to determine motor ability relative to other individuals of the same age (Barnett, 2008). These tests provide a measure of the severity and extent of the movement difficulties, and also provide indices of someone's 'general' motor ability, while enabling assessment across performance areas (e.g., fine and gross motor skills) (Barnett, 2008). Although no 'gold standard' assessment for DCD has emerged to date, the Movement Assessment Battery for Children-2 (MABC; Henderson, Sugden, & Barnett, 2007), the Bruininks–Oseretsky Test of Motor Proficiency (BOT-2; Bruininks R.H. & Bruininks B.D., 2005), and the McCarron Assessment of Neuromuscular Development (MAND; McCarron, 1997) are used interchangeably to varying degrees. Recent clinical practice guidelines have recommended the use of the MABC-2 (age range three to 16 years) and BOT-2 (four to 21 years of age) given their well-established psychometric properties (Blank et al., 2012).

Still, there remains significant variation in the choice of norm-referenced assessment adopted for DCD, as well as the cut-off scores used in its operationalization. While the ICD-10 suggests a cut-off of two standard deviations below the age-norm on a standardized test of motor skill (World Health Organisation, 1993), the DSM-5 does not specify a cut-off point. However, recommendations from the 2006 consensus statement suggest cut-off scores of performance ≤ the 5th percentile, while scores ≤ 15th percentile may suggest "borderline" or "at-risk" individuals (Sugden, 2006). More recent clinical practice guidelines recommended have adopted the more liberal 15th percentile (Blank et al., 2012).

Equally important when identifying cases of DCD is that symptoms impact an individual's ability to undertake activities of daily living (Criteria B, DSM-5). How Criterion B should be operationalized and assessed remains an issue. To this end, the use of screening questionnaires is becoming more commonplace, particularly in research settings. These not only provide an indication of an individual's motor ability relative to other people their age (A), but also elicit information regarding the quality of everyday life skills requiring movement such as self-care and classroom skills (B) (Barnett, 2008; Barnett, 2014; Blank et al., 2012).

A number of screening questionnaires have been developed to help identify children with DCD, particularly for population screening. Validated Parent or Teacher-rated questionnaires include the revised Developmental Coordination Disorder Questionnaire (DCDQ-2007) (Wilson, Kaplan, Crawford, & Roberts, 2007) and the MABC-2 checklist. Whilst these show adequate psychometric properties, their low sensitivity indicates that they may not be useful for population based screening (Blank et al., 2012). Acknowledging the enduring nature of DCD, a number of self-report measures have also been developed for identifying DCD in adolescents and young-adults, including the Adolescent and Adults Coordination Questionnaire (AAC-Q: Tal-Saban, Ornoy, Grotto, & Parush, 2012), the Functional Difficulties Questionnaire (FDQ: Clark, Thomas, Khattab, & Carr, 2013) and the Adult Dyspraxia and Developmental Coordination Disorder Questionnaire (ADC: Kirby, Edwards, Sugden, & Rosenblum, 2010). Despite showing some promise, limitations relating to poor sensitivity of the questionnaires have also been noted (see Barnett, 2014).

Importantly, the use of "multiple sources" of information in the assessment of DCD (Missiuna & Pollock, 1995) also appears to be a generally accepted recommendation, including information relating to developmental and medical history, physical examination, and school-based or work reports (APA, 2013).

Clinical vignette

Jack is 10 years old and is in his fifth year of school. The school psychologist has recently identified him as being within the clinical range for anxiety. He is having some difficulties academically, although his verbal IQ score puts him in the above average range. His performance IQ, however, is below average. His teachers complain that he is not trying. He often doesn't finish his work in class, and needs to complete it at home. His work is always untidy and he has very poor handwriting. He often loses things needed for particular tasks (e.g., pens, assignments, etc). He is messy and disorganized at home, and has few friends. He prefers to play computer games in his leisure time and refuses to join any sports or athletic organisations. This appears to have contributed to his problem with being overweight. An assessment of his motor skills puts him below the 5th percentile, suggesting he has a motor coordination problem. Furthermore, an assessment for ADHD identified a low score on hyperactivity/impulsivity but a high score on inattention, although not enough to give a diagnosis of ADHD. As a result, Jack was identified with DCD, and a program to improve his motor and social competence was recommended involving a multidisciplinary team including physiotherapist, occupational therapist and clinical psychologist.

Genetics and epigenetics

Although familial factors have been implicated in DCD symptomatology (Fliers et al., 2009), it is generally agreed that DCD is a multifactorial disorder in which both genetic and environmental factors play a role. However, research regarding specific genetic factors and their possible interactions is very limited. It has been argued that multiple genes likely act together, each contributing to the presentation of the disorder (Sugden, Kirby, & Dunford, 2008). Recently, a genome-wide association study suggested that motor coordination problems are associated with genes expressed in both nerve tissue and skeletal muscle. However, these did not reach genome-wide significance (Fliers et al., 2012). Further, children with DCD were primarily selected as having ADHD.

The high rates of comorbidity further complicate investigation of the genetic basis of DCD. Many studies have investigated the genetic basis of motor difficulties in association with other disorders such as ADHD (Martin, Piek, and Hay, 2006), autism (Lichtenstein, Carlström, Råstam, Gillberg, & Anckarsäter, 2010), reading (Francks et al., 2014) and language problems (Bishop, 2002), with diverse findings. For example, twin research has suggested a common aetiology between motor development and language impairment in children (Bishop, 2002), as well as a strong shared additive genetic component between ADHD and DCD (Martin et al., 2006). Further, a recent population-based study (N=10,895) examined the heritability of DCD and other neuropsychiatric disorders and found a heritability estimate of 70% for DCD and higher concordance rates in monozygotic twins than dizygotic twins for the disorder. High comorbidity was found across the different neuropsychiatric disorders (namely DCD, autism spectrum disorder, ADHD, tic disorder, and learning disorders), with genetic effects having a significant role in explaining these relationships (Lichtenstein et al., 2010). Conversely, although Francks et al. (2014) found strong familial effects on motor coordination and reading ability, these were largely distinct.

Overview of neuropsychology of DCD

The issue of aetiology has been the subject of considerable experimental investigation since the initial acceptance of DCD as a distinct diagnostic entity some three decades ago. During this period, the neuropsychological basis of poor motor skill has been hotly debated, with the resultant evidence the subject of two seminal meta-analyses undertaken 15 years apart (Wilson & McKenzie, 1998; Wilson, Ruddock, Smits-Engelsman, Polatajko, & Blank, 2013). Both reviews suggest that individuals with DCD demonstrate broad perceptuo- and visuo-motor deficits. However, Wilson and colleagues' (2013) most recent review highlights an array of general neuropsychological domains for which there is strong evidence of deficit. These include:

Internal modeling of action: there is mounting evidence that individuals with DCD experience difficulties generating and/or using predictive estimates of action (i.e., internal 'neural' representations of action) to plan and control their actions (for a review, see Adams, Lust, Wilson, & Steenbergen, 2014). The action representation forms part of an internal feedback loop thought to be critical to motor planning and control, and learning (Desmurget & Grafton, 2000; Hyde, Willmut, Fuelscher, & Williams, 2013). Hence, a deficit in internal modeling has the potential to impact not just an individuals' immediate motor competence, but also their ability to adapt and improve the quality and repertoire of action across longer timescales (Wilson et al., 2013). Interestingly, a number of studies noted similarities in performance between children with DCD and parietal and cerebellar patients (Hyde & Wilson, 2011; Kagerer, Contreras-Vidal, Bo, & Clark, 2006; Zwicker, Missiuna, & Boyd, 2009), suggesting possible fronto-parieto-cerebellar involvement in DCD. While the bulk of the available evidence involves primary-school aged children, there is recent evidence to suggest that where motor difficulties persist into adulthood, so too do difficulties using the internal action representation (Hyde et al., 2014).

Executive functioning. Evidence from a variety of experimental and standardized neuropsychological assessments suggests executive dysfunction is common in individuals with DCD, specifically in the domains of working memory (WM), inhibitory and cognitive flexibility (see Leonard and Hill, 2015, for a review). While executive dysfunction is a relatively stable property of developmental disorders, some evidence suggests that children with DCD show a unique profile of deficits, at least with respect to WM, typified by poor visuo-spatial working memory and processing (Alloway, Rajendran, & Archibald, 2009; Piek, Dyck, Francis, & Conwell, 2007). Hence, the profile of WM deficits observed in DCD appears to be consistent with the core deficit of the disorder, highlighting the relationship between poor motor skill and broader cognitive development (Alloway et. al., 2009; Rigoli, Piek, & Kane, 2012). However, as argued by Leonard and Hill (2015), the complex nature of many neuropsychological and experimental tests of executive function makes it difficult to determine whether group differences between DCD and controls are related to executive function as purported, or alternative cognitive mechanisms (e.g., intelligence). Further, many of the tasks adopted place demands, to varying degrees, on motor systems themselves. In these instances, it is difficult to determine the degree to which poor motor control contributed to atypical executive performance.

The capacity of neuropsychological accounts to inform effective intervention remains largely unknown and this will ultimately dictate their efficacy. Further, possibly as a consequence of the heterogeneity of the disorder, no theory is universally supported by the available evidence, nor provides a comprehensive account of atypical motor development. With this in mind, rather than a 'typical' neuropsychological profile of deficit existing for DCD, it seems more likely that each symptom type, or cluster, may be subserved by a separable neuropsychological substrate. Accordingly, future aetiological investigations may be better focused on identifying the neuropsychological basis of specific symptoms, or clusters. This approach has recently been adopted in the study of the neuropathology of DCD (Licari et al., 2015).

Overview of neuropathology/neurochemistry of DCD

Until recently, the neurological basis of DCD had received very little interest in the experimental literature, with the first published study reporting neuroimaging data in DCD only emerging in 2008 (Querne et al., 2008). Since then, there has been a limited yet steady flow of studies reporting on function, connectivity and structure of the DCD brain (see Brown-Lum & Zwicker, 2015 for a review).

Neuroimaging. A small group of studies investigating cortical activation in DCD during cognitive (Debrabant, Gheysen, Caeyenberghs, van Waelvelde, & Vingerhoets, 2013; Querne et al., 2008) and visuomotor tasks (Kashiwagi, Iwaki, Narumi, Tamai, & Suzuki, 2009; Licari et al., 2015; Querne et al., 2008; Zwicker, Missiuna, Harris, & Boyd, 2010; Zwicker, Missiuna, Harris, & Boyd, 2011) suggest differential neural activation compared to typical controls broadly consistent with the core motor and cognitive symptoms of DCD. Querne et al. (2008) found that children with DCD demonstrated differential hemispheric specialization during a classic task of inhibition, the go-no-go task, suggesting atypical neural activation during executive functioning. Similarly, Debrabant et al. (2013) observed hypoactivation of the dorsolateral prefrontal cortex (DLPFC) during a predictive timing task, a region known to support executive functions such as inhibition and working memory (see also Querne et al., 2008; Zwicker et al., 2011). Further evidence of differential activation of executive networks has been reported by Licari and colleagues (2015) and

Zwicker et al. (2010), who observed decreased activation of the left superior frontal gyrus (SFG) and the left inferior frontal gyrus (IFG) during finger-sequencing and trail-tracing tasks respectively.

Interestingly, while the IFG supports executive processes, it is also a critical node within the mirror neuron system (MNS), a finely-tuned network of neurons thought to subserve action execution, interpretation, imitation and learning (Rizzolatti & Craighero, 2004; Werner, Cermak, & Aziz-Zadeh, 2012). Connectivity studies suggest weaker connections between the IFG and the primary motor cortex in children with DCD (McLeod, Langevin, Goodyear, & Dewey, 2014). Other work has reported differential activation of downstream nodes within the MNS, including the inferior parietal cortex (IPC) (Kashiwagi et al., 2009; Zwicker et al., 2010; Zwicker et al., 2011). Further, connectivity between the IPC and action and attentional structures (e.g., the striatum) is reportedly weaker in DCD (Querne et al., 2008). This work supports earlier research, directly or indirectly implicating dysfunction of the MNS in DCD symptomatology (see Werner et al., 2012) and key neuropsychological markers including internal modeling of action. While the evidence for the latter is only indirect at present, there is a case for involvement of fronto-parietal and fronto-cerebellar circuitry at some level (see also Kashiwagi et al., 2009; Zwicker et al., 2010; Zwicker et al., 2011).

Two studies of functional connectivity during cognitively demanding tasks (Querne et al., 2008) and at rest (McLeod et al., 2014) provide additional evidence of atypical function in networks critical for motor control, cognition, and executive control. For example, Querne et al. (2008) demonstrated atypical connectivity within attentional and inhibitory networks in children with DCD, including the middle-frontal cortex, striatum, anterior cingulate and IPC. McLeod and colleagues (2014) reported that functional connectivity was either reduced or atypical between the primary motor cortex and cortices that support sensorimotor processing (posterior insular cortex), motor planning and executive functioning (prefrontal cortex; IFG), and fine motor skill (IFG). They also reported atypical connectivity between the primary motor cortex and subcortical structures critical for motor execution (e.g., caudate, putamen and globus pallidus).

At a *structural* level, neuroimaging studies on the morphological underpinnings of poor motor skill point towards a number of neurobiological markers for atypical motor development. Cortical thickness appears to be reduced in fronto-parietal and temporal regions involved in action and attention in children with combined DCD and ADHD (Langevin, Macmaster, and Dewey, 2015). This study also showed that decreases in cortical thickness correlated with reduced motor and executive functioning. Furthermore, atypical fissuration of the cerebellar anterior vermis has also been documented in a case study of a 19 year-old with DCD (Mariën, Wacknier, De Surgeloose, De Deyn, & Verhoeven, 2010). This structural abnormality is consistent with the common view of cerebellar involvement in DCD (Lundy-Ekman, Ivry, Keele, & Woollacott, 1991; Piek & Dyck, 2004).

Finally, it appears that atypical white matter architecture may be associated with poor motor skill in children with DCD. For example, Langevin, Macmaster, Crawford, Level, & Dewey (2014) showed decreased fractional anisotropy (FA) in parietal regions of the corpus callosum in children with DCD and the left superior longitudinal fasciculus. Decreased FA values correlated with poor motor function and executive functioning. Furthermore, De Kieviet and colleagues (2014) found that diffuse decreased FA differentiated school-aged children born very preterm who met the research criteria for DCD from pre-term children with normal motor abilities and age-matched term-birth children. Here, correlations between decreased FA and poorer motor function were also observed across multiple tracts. In contrast, early pilot work failed to observe differences in FA in the cortico-spinal tract, posterior thalamic radiation and superior and middle cerebellar peduncles between DCD and control groups (Zwicker, Missiuna, Harris, & Boyd, 2012). However, lower mean diffusity was observed in the cortico-spinal tract.

In summary, while the limited evidence available provides strong support for the view that children with DCD activate sensorimotor cortices differentially to typical children and may possess differential white matter micro-architecture, those networks implicated are widespread and often differ across studies. This is likely a consequence of the small sample sizes adopted in most studies, the complexity and heterogeneity of symptom expression across samples, and in the case of functional imaging, differences in the motor and cognitive demands of the tasks adopted.

Treatment

Cognitive and Behavioural treatments. There are three main approaches to intervention (see Smits-Engelsman et al., 2013): process-oriented (or deficit-oriented), task-oriented, and conventional physical and occupational therapy. *Process-oriented* approaches target a child's competence in sensory or neural areas understood to be responsible for motor delays (Sugden, 2007). It is assumed that improvements will then transfer to skills subserved by these processes. Although this has been a popular approach, it appears to have little empirical support, with an outdated neuromaturational and hierarchical theoretical basis (Wilson, 2005). Conversely, *task-oriented* approaches tend to focus on learning specific motor and functional skills based on goal-setting (e.g., essential activities of daily living). Based on popular theories of motor control and motor learning such as dynamical systems (Thelen, 1995) and the neuronal group selection theory (Pearson, Finkel, & Edelman, 1987), task-oriented approaches aim to enhance a child's participation at home, school, leisure, and sports (Blank et al., 2012; Smits-Engelsman et al., 2013). Finally, traditional physical therapy or occupational therapy has been described as combining process-oriented approaches with direct skills training in order to teach important fundamental gross and fine motor skills (hopping, jumping, throwing, catching, cutting, drawing, writing), as well as training basic motor abilities that are understood to be prerequisite for skills (e.g., trunk stability) (Smits-Engelsman et al., 2013).

As it stands, there is no universally favoured or effective approach to treatment. In a recent comprehensive systematic review, Blank et al. (2012) found sufficient evidence to suggest that physiotherapy and/or occupational therapy intervention is better than no intervention for children with DCD. Furthermore, task-oriented approaches were found to be effective in treating children with DCD, and appear to be more successful than process-oriented approaches (Blank et al., 2012). While reducing primary impairment may no longer be an appropriate goal, intervention is perhaps best aimed at preventing secondary difficulties (e.g., strength, fitness and endurance) by improving performance of, and participation in, motor activities (Missiuna, Rivard, & Bartlett, 2006). This approach may in turn address the cycle of withdrawal and diminished opportunities for physical development typical of DCD, and promote psychosocial areas such as self-efficacy (Missiuna et al., 2006).

Pharmacological treatment. Although there is some evidence to suggest that methylphenidate may be useful in children with comorbid ADHD and DCD (particularly for fine-motor issues like handwriting), very little is known regarding pharmacological intervention for DCD (Flapper, Houwen, & Schoemaker, 2006). However, pharmacological intervention alone should not be considered for children with combined DCD and ADHD, and additional treatment and support is recommended (Blank et al., 2012). It is also important to note that given the comorbidity associated with DCD, different approaches to intervention may be required.

Summary

Though variability persists, consensus statements in 1994 and 2006 have seen a more uniform approach to identifying and monitoring DCD. Given the heterogeneous and comorbid nature of DCD, it is perhaps unsurprising that efforts to develop effective treatment have been mixed at best. Our scope for developing more effective intervention may depend largely on how well we are able to elucidate the genetic, neuropsychological and neuropathological bases of what is a complex and multifactorial disorder. While we should be buoyed by recent advances, particularly in our understanding of the neuropathology of the disorder, we are still far from developing a unified account of DCD. As we have argued, given that a 'prototypical' case of DCD does not exist, it is similarly unlikely that a 'prototypical' cause exists. Instead, we have argued that it is likely that symptom types, or clusters, may be subserved by distinct (even if overlapping) aetiologies. With this in mind, the neuropsychology and neuropathology responsible for an individual case of delayed motor skill may differ according to the array of symptoms. Given this, future research may be better served mapping the genetic, cognitive and neurological correlates of specific symptom types rather than the omnibus DCD diagnosis.

Abbreviations

AAC-Q: Adolescent and Adults Coordination Questionnaire
ADC: Adult Dyspraxia and Developmental Coordination Disorder Questionnaire
ADHD: Attention Deficit/Hyperactivity Disorder
BOT: Bruininks–Oseretsky Test of Motor Proficiency
DCD: Developmental Coordination Disorder
DCD-Q 2007: Developmental Coordination Disorder Questionnaire
DFC: Dorsolateral prefrontal cortex
ESH: Environmental Stress Hypothesis
FA: Fractional anisotropy
FDQ: Functional Difficulties Questionnaire
ICD 10: International Classification of Diseases 10
IFG: Inferior frontal gyrus
MABC-2: Movement Assessment Battery for Children-2
MNS: Mirror neuron system
SFG: Superior frontal gyrus

Further readings

Cairney, J. (2015) *Developmental Coordination Disorder in Children: Consequences and Concurrent Problems*. University of Toronto Press.

Geuze, R. H. (2007). *Developmental Coordination Disorder: A Review of Current Approaches.* Groupe de Boeck.

References

Adams, I., Lust, J., Wilson, P., & Steenbergen, B. (2014). Compromised motor control in children with DCD: A deficit in the internal model? A systematic review. *Neuroscience & Biobehavioral Reviews, 47*, 225–244.

Alloway, T., Rajendran, G., & Archibald, L. (2009). Working memory in children with developmental disorders. *Journal of Learning Disabilities, 42*(4), 372–382.

American Psychiatric Association. (1987). *Diagnostic and Statistical Manual of Mental Disorders. 3rd edition-revised.* Washington, DC: American Psychiatric Association.

American Psychiatric Association. (2013). *Diagnostic and Statistical Manual of Mental Disorders. 5th edition.* Arlington, VA: American Psychiatric Association.

American Psychiatric Association. (2000). *Diagnostic and Statistical Manual of Mental Disorders: Text revision (4th ed.).* Washington, DC: Author.

Barnett, A. L. (2008). Motor assessment in developmental coordination disorder: From identification to intervention. *International Journal of Disability, Development and Education, 55*(2), 113–129.

Barnett, A. L. (2014). Is there a 'Movement Thermometer' for developmental coordination disorder? *Current Developmental Disorder Reports, 1*, 132–139.

Bishop, D. V. (2002). Motor immaturity and specific speech and language impairment: Evidence for a common genetic basis. *American Journal of Medical Genetics, 114*(1), 56–63.

Blank, R., Smits-Engelsman, B., Polatajko, H., & Wilson, P. (2012). European Academy for Childhood Disability (EACD): Recommendations on the definition, diagnosis and intervention of developmental coordination disorder (long version). *Developmental Medicine & Child Neurology, 54*(1), 54–93.

Bradford, A., & Dodd, B. (1996). Do all speech-disordered children have motor deficits? *Clinical Linguistics & Phonetics, 10*(2), 77–101.

Brown-Lum, M., & Zwicker, J. (2015). Brain imaging increases our understanding of developmental coordination disorder: A review of literature and future directions. *Current Developmental Disorder Reports, 2,* 131–140.

Bruininks, R. H., & Bruininks, B. D. (2005). *Bruininks-Oseretsky Test of Motor Proficiency 2nd Edition.* Windsor: NFER-Nelson.

Cairney, J., Rigoli, D., & Piek, J. (2013). Developmental coordination disorder and internalizing problems in children: The environmental stress hypothesis elaborated. *Developmental Review, 33,* 224–238.

Cairney, J., Veldhuizen, S., & Szatmari, P. (2010). Motor coordination and emotional-behavioral problems in children. *Current Opinion in Psychiatry, 23*(4), 324–329.

Capute, A. J., Shapiro, B. K., Palmer, F. B., Ross, A., & Wachtel, R. C. (1985). Normal gross motor development: The influences of race, sex and socio-economic status. *Developmental Medicine & Child Neurology, 27*(5), 635–643.

Clarke, C., Thomas, S., Khattab, A., & Carr, E. (2013). Development and psychometric properties of a screening tool for assessing developmental coordination disorder in adults. *International Journal of Physical Medicine & Rehabilitation, 1*(5). doi: 10.4172/2329-9096.1000145.

Cousins, M., & Smyth, M. M. (2003). Developmental coordination impairments in adulthood. *Human Movement Science, 22*(4), 433–459.

De Kieviet, J., Pouwels, P., Lafeber, H., Vermeulen, R., van Elburg, R., & Oosterlaan, J. (2014). A crucial role of altered fractional anisotropy in motor problems of very preterm children. *European Journal of Paediatric Neurology, 18,* 126–133.

Debrabant, J., Gheysen, F., Caeyensberghs, K., van Waelvelde, H., & Vingerhoets, G. (2013). Neural underpinnings of impaired predictive motor timing in children with developmental coordination disorder. *Research in Developmental Disabilities, 34,* 1478–1487.

Desmurget, M., & Grafton, S. (2000). Forward modeling allows feedback control for fast reaching movements. *Trends in Cognitive Sciences, 4*(11), 423–431.

Dewey, D., Kaplan, B. J., Crawford, S. G., & Wilson, B. N. (2002). Developmental coordination disorder: Associated problems in attention, learning, and psychosocial adjustment. *Human Movement Science, 21*(5), 905–918.

Dyck, M., Piek, J., Hay, D., & Hallmayer. (2007). The relationship between symptoms and abilities in autism. *Journal of Developmental and Physical Disabilities, 19,* 251–261.

Faught, B. E., Hay, J. A., Cairney, J., & Flouris, A. (2005). Increased risk for coronary vascular disease in children with developmental coordination disorder. *Journal of Adolescent Health, 37*(5), 376–380.

Flapper, B. C., Houwen, S., & Schoemaker, M. M. (2006). Fine motor skills and effects of methylphenidate in children with attention-deficit–hyperactivity disorder and developmental coordination disorder. *Developmental Medicine & Child Neurology, 48*(3), 165–169.

Fliers, E. A., Vasquez, A. A., Poelmans, G., Rommelse, N., Altink, M., Buschgens, C., … Franke, B. (2012). Genome-wide association study of motor coordination problems in ADHD identifies genes for brain and muscle function. *The World Journal of Biological Psychiatry, 13*(3), 211–222.

Fliers, E., Vermeulen, S., Rijsdijk, F., Altink, M., Buschgens, C., Rommelse, N., … Franke, B. (2009). ADHD and poor motor performance from a family genetic perspective. *Journal of the American Academy of Child & Adolescent Psychiatry, 48*(1), 25–34.

Francks, C., Fisher, S. E., Marlow, A. J., MacPhie, I. L., Taylor, K. E., Richardson, A. J., … Monaco, A. P. (2014). Familial and genetic effects on motor coordination, laterality, and reading-related cognition. *American Journal of Psychiatry, 160* (11), 1970–1977.

Hall, D. M. B. (1988). Clumsy children. *British Medical Journal, 296*, 375–376.

Hands, B., Licari, M., & Piek, J. P. (2015). A review of five tests to identify motor coordination difficulties in young adults. *Research in Developmental Disabilities, 41–42*, 40–51.

Henderson, S. E., & Barnett, A. L. (1998). The classification of specific motor coordination disorders in children: Some problems to be solved. *Human Movement Science, 17*, 449–469.

Henderson, S. E., Sugden, D. A., & Barnett, A. L. (2007). *Movement Assessment Battery for Children – 2 second edition*. London: Harcourt Assessment.

Hill, E. L. (2001). Non-specific nature of specific language impairment: A review of the literature with regard to concomitant motor impairments. *International Journal of Language & Communication Disorders, 36*(2), 149–171.

Hyde, C., & Wilson, P. E. (2011). Dissecting online control in children with developmental coordination disorder: A kinematic analysis of double-step reaching. *Brain and Cognition, 75*(3), 232–241.

Hyde, C., Fueslcher, I., Buckthought, K., Enticott, P., Gitay, M., & Williams, J. (2014). Motor imagery is less efficient in adults with probable developmental coordination disorder: Evidence from the hand rotation task. *Research in Developmental Disabilities, 35*(11), 3062–3070.

Hyde, C., Wilmut, K., Fuelscher, I., & Williams, J. (2013). Does implicit motor imagery ability predict reaching correction efficiency? A test of recent models of human motor control. *Journal of Motor Behavior, 43*(3), 259–269.

Joshi, D., Missiuna, C., Hanna, S., Hay, J., Faught, B., & Cairney, J. (2015). Relationship between BMI, waist circumference, physical activity and probable developmental coordination disorder over time. *Human Movement Science, 40*, 237–247.

Kadesjö, B., & Gillberg, C. (1999). Developmental coordination disorder in Swedish 7-year-old children. *Journal of the American Academy of Child & Adolescent Psychiatry, 38*(7), 820–828.

Kadesjö, B., & Gillberg, C. (2001). The comorbidity of ADHD in the general population of Swedish school-age children. *Journal of Child Psychology and Psychiatry, 42*(4), 487–492.

Kagerer, F., Contreras-Vidal, Bo, J., & Clark, J. (2006). Abrupt, but not gradual visuomotor distortion facilitates adaptation in children with developmental coordination disorder. *Human Movement Science, 25*, 622–633.

Kaplan, B. J., Wilson, B. N., Dewey, D., & Crawford, S. G. (1998). DCD may not be a discrete disorder. *Human Movement Science, 17*(4), 471–490.

Kashiwagi, M., Iwaki, S., Narumi, Y., Tamai, H., & Suzuki, S. (2009). Parietal dysfunction in developmental coordination disorder: A functional MRI study. *Brain Imaging, 20*, 1319–1324.

Kirby, A., Edwards, L., Sugden, D., & Rosenblum, S. (2010). The development and standardization of the adult developmental coordination disorders/dyspraxia checklist (ADC). *Research in Developmental Disabilities, 31*(1), 131–139.

Knuckey, N. W., & Gubbay, S. S. (1983). Clumsy children: A prognostic study. *Journal of Paediatrics and Child Health, 19*(1), 9–13.

Kooistra, L., Crawford, S., Dewey, D., Cantell, M., & Kaplan, B. J. (2005). Motor correlates of ADHD contribution of reading disability and oppositional defiant disorder. *Journal of Learning Disabilities, 38*(3), 195–206.

Langevin, L., Macmaster, F., & Dewey, D. (2015). Distinct patterns of cortical thinning in concurrent motor and attention disorder. *Developmental Medicine and Child Neurology, 57,* 257–264.

Langevin, L., Macmaster, F., Crawford, S., Lebel, C., & Dewey, D. (2014). Common white matter microstructure alterations in pediatric motor and attention disorder. *The Journal of Pediatrics, 164,* 1157–64.

Leonard, H., & Hill, E. (2015). Executive difficulties in developmental coordination disorder: Methodological issues and future directions. *Current Developmental Disorder Reports, 2,* 141–149.

Licari, M., Billington, J., Reid, S., Wann, J., Elliott, C., Winsor, A., … Bynevolt, M. (2015). Cortical functioning in children with developmental coordination disorder: A motor overflow study. *Experimental Brain Research, 233*(6), 1703–1710.

Lichtenstein, P., Carlström, E., Råstam, M., Gillberg, C., & Anckarsäter, H. (2010). The genetics of autism spectrum disorders and related neuropsychiatric disorders in childhood. *American Journal of Psychiatry, 167*(11), 1357–1363.

Lingam, R., Golding, J., Jongmans, M. J., Hunt, L. P., Ellis, M., & Emond, A. (2010). The association between developmental coordination disorder and other developmental traits. *Pediatrics, 126*(5), e1109-e1118.

Lingam, R., Hunt, L., Golding, J., Jongmans, M., & Emond, A. (2009). Prevalence of developmental coordination disorder using the DSM-IV at 7 years of age: A UK population-based study. *Pediatrics, 123,* e693–700.

Lingam, R., Jongmans, M. J., Ellis, M., Hunt, L. P., Golding, J., & Emond, A. (2012). Mental health difficulties in children with developmental coordination disorder. *Pediatrics, 129*(4), e882-e891.

Liu, Y., Metems, T., Absil, J., De Maertelaer, V., Balériaux, D., David, P., … Aeby, A. (2011). Gender differences in language and motor-related fibers in a population of healthy preterm neonates at term-equivalent age: A diffusion tensor and probablistic tractography study. *American Journal of Neuroradiology, 32,* 2011–2016.

Lundy-Ekman, L., Ivry, R., Keele, S. W., & Woollacott, M. (1991). Timing and force control deficits in clumsy children. *Journal of Cognitive Neuroscience, 3,* 367–376.

Mariën, P., Wacknier, P., De Surgeloose, D., De Deyn, P., & Verhoeven, J. (2010). Developmental coordination disorder: Disruption of the cerebello-cerebral network evidence by SPECT. *Cerebellum, 9,* 405–510.

Martin, N. C., Piek, J. P., Baynam, G., Levy, F., & Hay, D. (2010). An examination of the relationship between movement problems and four common developmental disorders. *Human Movement Science,* 29, 799–808.

Martin, N., Piek, J. P., & Hay, D. (2006). DCD and ADHD: A genetic study of their shared aetiology. *Human Movement Science, 25,* 110–124.

McCarron, L. T. (1997). *MAND: McCarron Assessment of Neuromuscular Development, Fine and Gross Motor Abilities.* McCarron-Dial Systems, Incorporated.

McLeod, K., Langevin, L., Goodyear, B., & Dewey, D. (2014). Functional connectivity of neural motor networks is disrupted in children with developmental coordination disorder and attention-deficit/hyperactivity disorder. *Neuroimage: Clinical, 4,* 566–575.

Missiuna, C., & Pollock, N. (1995). Beyond the norms: Need for multiple sources of data in the assessment of children. *Physical & Occupational Therapy in Pediatrics, 15*(4), 57–74.

Missiuna, C., Rivard, L., & Bartlett, D. (2006). Exploring assessment tools and the target of intervention for children with developmental coordination disorder. *Physical & Occupational Therapy in Pediatrics, 26*(1–2), 71–89.

Pearsall-Jones, J. G., Piek, J. P., Rigoli, D., Martin, N., & Levy, F. (2009). An investigation into etiological pathways of DCD and ADHD using a monozygotic twin design. *Twin Research & Human Genetics*, *12*, 381–391.

Pearsall-Jones, J. G., Piek, J. P., & Levy, F. (2010). Developmental coordination disorder and cerebral palsy: Categories or a continuum? *Human Movement Science*, *29*, 787–798.

Pearsall-Jones, J. G., Piek, J. P., Rigoli, D., Martin, N., & Levy, F. (2011). Motor disorder and anxiety and depressive symptomatology: A monozygotic co-twin control approach. *Research in Developmental Disabilities*, *32*, 1245–1252.

Pearson, J. C., Finkel, L. H., & Edelman, G. M. (1987). Plasticity in the organization of adult cerebral cortical maps: A computer simulation based on neuronal group selection. *The Journal of Neuroscience*, 7(12), 4209–4223.

Pedersen, A. V., Sigmundsson, H., Whiting, H. T. A., & Ingvaldsen, R. P. (2003). Sex differences in lateralisation of fine manual skills in children. *Experimental Brain Research*, *149*(2), 249–251.

Piek, J. P. & Dyck, M. J. (2004). Sensory-motor deficits in children with developmental coordination disorder, attention deficit hyperactivity disorder and autistic disorder. *Human Movement Science*, *23*, 475–488.

Piek, J. P., Dyck, M. J., Francis, M., & Conwell, A. (2007). Working memory, processing speed and set-shifting in children with developmental coordination disorder and attention deficit hyperactivity disorder. *Developmental Medicine & Child Neurology*, *49*, 678–683.

Piek, J. P., Hands, B., & Licari, M. K. (2012). Assessment of motor functioning in the preschool period. *Neuropsychology Review*, *22*, 402–413. doi: 10.1007/s11065-012-9211-4.

Piek, J. P., Pitcher, T., & Hay, D. A. (1999). Motor coordination and kinaesthesis in boys with attention deficit hyperactivity disorder. *Developmental Medicine & Child Neurology*, *41*, 159–165.

Piek, J. P., Rigoli, D., Pearsall-Jones, J. G., Martin, N. C., Hay, D. A., Bennett, K. S., & Levy, F. (2007). Depressive symptomatology in child and adolescent twins with attention deficit hyperactivity disorder and/or developmental coordination disorder. *Twin Research and Human Genetics*, *10*, 587–596.

Pitcher, T. M., Piek, J. P., & Hay, D. A. (2003). Fine and gross motor ability in boys with attention deficit hyperactivity disorder. *Developmental Medicine & Child Neurology*, *45*, 525–535.

Polatajko, H. J., Fox, M., & Missiuna, C. (1995). An international consensus on children with developmental coordination disorder. *Canadian Journal of Occupational Therapy*, *62*, 3–6.

Querne, L., Berquin, P., Vernier-Hauvette, M., Fall, S., Deltour, L., Meyer, M., & Marco, G. (2008). Dysfunction of the attentional brain network in children with developmental coordination disorder: A *f*MRI study. *Brain Research*, *1244*, 89–102.

Rasmussen, P., & Gillberg, C. (2000). Natural outcome of ADHD with developmental coordination disorder at age 22 years: A controlled, longitudinal, community-based study. *Journal of the American Academy of Child & Adolescent Psychiatry*, *39*(11), 1424–1431.

Reiersen, A. M., Constantino, J. N., & Todd, R. D. (2008). Co-occurrence of motor problems and autistic symptoms in attention-deficit/hyperactivity disorder. *Journal of the American Academy of Child & Adolescent Psychiatry*, *47*(6), 662–672.

Rigoli, D., Piek, J. P., & Kane, R. (2012). Motor coordination and psychosocial correlates in a normal adolescent sample. *Pediatrics*, *129*, e892-e900. doi: 10.1542/peds.2011-1237.

Rivilis, I., Hay, J., Cairney, J., Klentrou, P., Liu, J., & Faught, B. E. (2011). Physical activity and fitness in children with developmental coordination disorder: A systematic review. *Research in Developmental Disabilities*, *32*(3), 894–910.

Rizzolatti, G., & Craighero, L. (2004). The mirror-neuron system. *Annual Reviews Neuroscience*, *27*, 169–192.

Smits-Engelsman., Blank, R., van der Kaay, A. C., Mosterd-van der Meijs, R., Vlugt-van den Brand, E., Polatajko, H. J., & Wilson, P. H. (2013). Efficacy of interventions to improve motor performance in children with developmental coordination disorder: A combined systematic review and meta-analysis. *Developmental Medicine & Child Neurology*, *55*(3), 229–237.

Sugden, D. (2007). Current approaches to intervention in children with developmental coordination disorder. *Developmental Medicine & Child Neurology*, *49*(6), 467–471.

Sugden, D. A. (2006). Development Coordination Disorder as a specific learning difficulty. *Leeds Consensus Statement ESRC*, 2004–2005.

Sugden, D., Kirby, A., & Dunford, C. (2008). Issues surrounding children with developmental coordination disorder. *International Journal of Disability, Development and Education*, *55*(2), 173–187.

Tal-Saban, M., Ornoy, A., Grotto, I., & Parush, S. (2012). Adolescents and adults coordination questionnaire: Development and psychometric properties. *The American Journal of Occupational Therapy*, *66*(4), 406–413.

Tal-Saban, M., Zarka, S., Grotto, I., Ornoy, A., & Parush, S. (2012). The functional profile of young adults with suspected Developmental Coordination Disorder (DCD). *Research in Developmental Disabilities*, *33*(6), 2193–2202.

Thelen, E. (1995). Motor development: A new synthesis. *American Psychologist*, *50*(2), 79.

Touwen, B. C. L. (1976). *Neurological Development in Infancy* (Vol. 58). Heinemann Educational Books.

Tsiotra, G. D., Flouris, A. D., Koutedakis, Y., Faught, B. E., Nevill, A. M., Lane, A. M., & Skenteris, N. (2006). A comparison of developmental coordination disorder prevalence rates in Canadian and Greek children. *Journal of Adolescent Health*, *39*(1), 125–127.

Visscher, C., Houwen, S., Scherder, E. J., Moolenaar, B., & Hartman, E. (2007). Motor profile of children with developmental speech and language disorders. *Pediatrics*, *120*(1), e158–e163.

Wann, J. P., Mon-Williams, M., & Rushton, K. (1998). Postural control and co-ordination disorders: The swinging room revisited. *Human Movement Science*, *17*, 491–513.

Werner, J., Cermak, S., & Aziz-Zadeh, L. (2012). Neural correlates of developmental coordination disorder: The mirror neuron system hypothesis. *Journal of Behavioral and Brain Science*, *2*, 258–268.

Wilson, B. N., Kaplan, B. J., Crawford, S. G., & Roberts, G. (2007). Developmental coordination questionnaire 2007 (DCDQ'07). *Alberta Children Hospital.*

Wilson, P. H. (2005). Practitioner review: Approaches to assessment and treatment of children with DCD: An evaluative review. *Journal of Child Psychology and Psychiatry*, *46*(8), 806–823.

Wilson, P.H., & McKenzie, B. (1998). Information processing deficits association with developmental coordination disorder: A meta analysis of research findings. *The Journal of Child Psychology and Psychiatry*, *39*(6), 829–840.

Wilson, P.H., Ruddock, S., Smits-Engelsman, B., Polatajko, H., & Blank, R. (2013). Understanding performance deficits in developmental coordination disorder: A meta-analysis of recent research. *Developmental Medicine & Child Neurology*, *55*(3), 217–228.

Wisdom, S., Dyck, M.J., Piek, J.P., Hay, D., & Hallmayer, J. (2007). Can autism, language and coordination disorders be differentiated based on ability profiles? *European Child and Adolescent Psychiatry*, *16*, 178–186.

World Health Organisation. (1993). *The ICD-10 Classification of Mental and Behavioural Disorders: Clinical Descriptions and Diagnostic Guidelines*. Geneva: World Health Organisation.

Zwicker, J., Missiuana, C., & Boyd, L. (2009). Neural correlates of developmental coordination disorder: A review of hypotheses. *Journal of Child Neurology, 24*(20), 1273–1281.

Zwicker, J., Missiuana, C., Harris, S., & Boyd, L. (2010). Brain activation of children with developmental coordination disorder is different than peers. *Pediatrics, 126*, 678–686.

Zwicker, J., Missiuana, C., Harris, S., & Boyd, L. (2011). Brain activation associated with motor skill practice in children with developmental coordination disorder: An fMRI study. *International Journal of Developmental Neuroscience, 29*, 145–152.

Zwicker, J., Missiuana, C., Harris, S., & Boyd, L. (2012). Developmental coordination disorder: A pilot diffusion tensor imaging study. *Pediatric Neurology, 46*, 162–167.

6
LANGUAGE DISORDER

Jarrad A. G. Lum, Michael T. Ullman and Gina Conti-Ramsden

Introduction

For most children, the ability to learn and use language to communicate appears to be a feat that is easily accomplished. Without any formal instruction children are able to learn the various aspects of language, for example grammar and phonology, so they can communicate with others. Typically, by the time children are around 5 years of age, their mastery of language begins to approach adult like levels (Gleason & Ratner, 2012). However, this is not the case for children who meet the criteria for Language Disorder (LD; American Psychiatric Association, 2013), also commonly referred to as developmental language disorder, language impairment or specific language impairment (SLI; Bishop, 2014). These children have clinically significant problems with the production and/or comprehension of language.

A curious feature of the language problems in this population is the absence of a clear identifiable cause. By definition, children with LD do not have hearing, sensory or intellectual impairments. Similarly, there is no separate medical condition or diagnosable neurological problem that accounts for these children's difficulty with language. Thus, with the exception of language, these children are otherwise typical. However, since proficient language skills are required in nearly all aspects of life, affected children will likely experience social (Durkin & Conti-Ramsden, 2007) and educational problems (Snowling, Adams, Bishop, & Stothard, 2001). Childhood language problems can also lead to negative impacts in adults, who can experience psychosocial, vocational and mental health problems (Beitchman et al., 2001; Rutter & Mawhood, 1991; Voci, Beitchman, Brownlie, & Wilson, 2006).

The idea that LD might be conceptualised as a frontostriatal disorder has only appeared in relatively recent times (Ullman, 2004; Ullman & Pierpont, 2005). Nevertheless, substantial research has already been presented that is consistent with this proposal (e.g., Hsu & Bishop, 2014b; Lee, Nopoulos, & Tomblin, 2013; Lum, Conti-Ramsden, Morgan, & Ullman, 2014).

Preliminary considerations

LD has been described as a "hidden disability" (Bishop, Clark, Conti-Ramsden, Norbury, & Snowling, 2012) with respect to the identification of affected children and the attention it receives in research and clinical settings. This may be partly due to the fact that LD is not characterised by the absence of language. Children with the disorder are able to talk and interact with others with varying degrees of success, which may lead to language problems being overlooked, and its importance minimised (Conti-Ramsden, 2013). An interesting analysis by Bishop (2010) indicated that LD receives less research funding and appears in fewer peer reviewed journals in comparison to other disorders of comparable prevalence and severity. Thus, more work needs to be done to understand the underlying nature of the problems and the best methods for identification and intervention.

Perhaps contributing to the aforementioned problems is the lack of a universally agreed label for children with LD. In the introduction of this chapter, the label 'Language Disorder' or LD was used to describe the syndrome. This term was assigned in the DSM-5 (American Psychiatric Association, 2013). However, as indicated above, other terms are also used, in particular specific language impairment (SLI). In addition, in the current edition of the International Classification of Diseases (World Health Organization, 2010), the terms "Expressive Language Disorder" and "Receptive Language Disorder" are used to refer to describe the same set of individuals. This taxonomy distinguishes between individuals with mainly expressive language problem and those who have both expressive and receptive language problems. The term(s) that should be used for this group have been debated in the literature (Bishop, 2014; Ebbels, 2014; Reilly et al., 2014). For the purposes of this chapter we adopt the DSM-5 label of "Language Disorder" (LD).

Diagnostic considerations

The diagnosis of LD is based on exclusionary criteria. Specifically, once any clinically significant language problems have been identified, additional assessment is required to discount identifiable causes of the language difficulties such as hearing deficits, deprivation of language input, social or emotional problems, low IQ, or another medical condition that might be causing the communication difficulties (American Psychiatric Association, 2013).

At a practical level, the diagnosis of LD may require assessments from a range of experts. For instance, a speech-language pathologist may undertake a formal assessment of language skills using a standardised language test. A psychologist may assess whether an intellectual disability is present. An audiologist and optometrist might be called upon to screen for hearing or visual impairments. Potentially, a paediatrician might be involved to determine the presence of any other medical problems.

Another challenge associated with diagnosing LD is the absence of universally accepted psychometric criteria with respect to determining the presence of a language impairment. A core feature of LD is that the ability to produce and/or understand language is below levels expected for a child's age. However, there is no gold standard concerning how to operationalise this level of functioning on the basis of scores derived from standardised language tests (Reilly et al., 2014; Spaulding, Plante, & Farinella, 2006). As a consequence, the number of standard deviations below the normative mean required before language skills are considered below age appropriate levels often varies among clinicians and researchers. Thus, in the research described in this chapter, it needs to be appreciated that the methods and criteria used to identify LD are not always the same.

Clinical vignette

The following case is fictitious, but describes some of the common problems found in children with LD. Parents were concerned about their child, who at 2-years of age had only recently started speaking. After a check-up from a paediatrician, no medical problems were identified. A subsequent audiological examination did not reveal any hearing problems. At age 4-years, the child is friendly and sociable and has a group friends at day care. However, there are some differences in the way the child speaks compared to others of the same age. Perhaps most noticeable are the omission of function words (e.g., articles, auxillary verbs) and inflections (i.e., past tense *–ed*) from speech. For example, the child might say "It go this way" and "Him lost it"[1]. These difficulties with grammar are one of the key deficits associated with LD. When the child begins primary school, both teachers and parents notice the child has a poor short-term memory and has difficulty following instructions. Academically, the child is not only learning slower than others in the class, but also struggles with some rudimentary skills such as holding and using a pencil. Following parent and teacher concerns, the child is referred to a psychologist for an IQ assessment. However, the child's intelligence is within normal limits. A language problem is eventually identified following an assessment by the school speech pathologist.

Prevalence and onset

The absence of gold standard diagnostic criteria for LD impacts estimates concerning the prevalence of the condition. Not surprisingly, Law, Boyle, Harris, Harkness, and Nye's (2000) systematic review found studies that utilised more stringent criteria to define LD typically observed lower prevalence rates. Estimates of prevalence also tend to be influenced by psychometric instrumentation. Keeping these points in mind, one of the most widely cited estimates of LD is based on Tomblin et al.'s (1997) epidemiological study of over 7000 children. In that study, a combination of standardised tests and clinical judgement was used to determine whether children met the criteria for LD. Using this methodology, the prevalence rate was found to be 7.4% amongst kindergarten-aged children. The prevalence rate for males (8%) was slightly higher than that of females (6%). Other prevalence estimates for LD have ranged between 2 (Silva, McGee, & Williams, 1983) and 19% (Rescorla, Hadicke-Wiley, & Escarce, 1993).

It has been difficult to determine the age of onset for LD. At least one factor may be that during early years of development, especially before age 4, there is considerable variability in children's language skills (e.g., Lahey, Liebergott, Chesnick, Menyuk, & Adams, 1992). Thus, language functioning during infancy and early childhood is not a strong predictor of long-term language outcomes (Reilly et al., 2010). For example, a child who is a late talker is not necessarily going to have long-term language problems. Alternatively, a toddler with precocious language skills may go on to experience language problems later in development (Ukoumunne et al., 2012). However, the evidence does appear to indicate that LD diagnosed after 4-years of age is likely to persist into adolescence and adulthood (e.g., Bishop & Edmundson, 1987).

Comorbidity

In the beginning of this chapter, we presented LD as a condition whereby language functioning is dissociated from other problems. Nevertheless, further assessment of affected children often reveals a number of co-occurring deficits (e.g., Cohen et al., 2000; Flapper & Schoemaker, 2013). For example, behavioural and social problems are common (McCabe, 2005), and both verbal and non-verbal cognitive impairments (Leonard, 2014; Ullman & Pierpont, 2005) as well as motor problems (Hill, 2001) may be observed. Increasing evidence suggests that children with LD generally, if not always, have deficits beyond the domain of language (Ullman and Pierpont, 2005).

Indeed, LD is in fact commonly diagnosed alongside other conditions. Four commonly reported conditions found in these children are Attention-Deficit Hyperactivity Disorder (ADHD), Developmental Coordination Disorder (DCD), Dyslexia and autism spectrum disorder. For instance, Cohen, Barwick, Horodezky, Vallance, and Im (1998) found that 46% of children with LD referred to a paediatric mental health service also met the diagnostic criteria for ADHD. Similarly, Love and Thompson (1988) found that 85% of children with a diagnosis of ADHD were also diagnosed with a language or speech disorder. LD and DCD also co-occurs at high rates (e.g., Flapper & Schoemaker, 2013). Therefore it is not surprising to find that children with LD also perform poorly on standardised tests of motor functioning. Webster, Majnemer, Platt, and Shevell (2005) found that 52% (22/70) of children with LD were impaired on at least one aspect of motor functioning. Dyslexia (Specific Reading Disability) is identified when a child fails to obtain age appropriate reading levels despite appropriate input and educational instruction. Reading difficulties often co-occur with language problems. To illustrate, McArthur, Hogben, Edwards, Heath, and Mengler (2000) found that 51% of children with LD also met the criteria for dyslexia. There has been debate about whether language and reading problems are the same or a different disorder (Bishop & Snowling, 2004; Catts, Adlof, Hogan, & Weismer, 2005). Finally, symptoms associated with autism spectrum disorder are also commonly found in children with language problems (Conti-Ramsden, Simkin, & Botting, 2006; Verhoeven et al., 2012). For example, in Leyfer, Tager-Flusberg, Dowd, Tomblin, and Folstein (2008) 41% of children with LD met the criteria for autism spectrum disorder.

The preceding discussion serves to highlight the heterogeneous nature of LD. Affected children not only vary with respect to the nature and severity of the language problems, but also in the extent and severity of problems in other domains. Indeed, it is currently an ongoing subject of research whether or not the relationship between the language and comorbid problems reflect a common deficit (Sanjeevan et al., 2015; Williams, Botting, & Boucher, 2008). One possibility is that LD may even be describing a group with a range of comorbid conditions (e.g., autism, ADHD) that also have language problems, rather than as an independently occurring syndrome. Relevant to this discussion also is Ullman and Pierpont's (2005) proposal that LD is caused by dysfunction of the basal ganglia-frontal circuitry. A prediction of this model is that other functions dependent on this network (e.g., motor, attention) may also be compromised, either because they depend on the same circuits that underlie language, or because the abnormalities may extend to other circuits. Since the extent and degree of these abnormalities may vary across individuals, heterogeneity of other impairments may be expected (Ullman and Pierpont, 2005). Theoretical issues aside, from a clinical viewpoint, the presence of comorbid disorders and co-occurring problems will mean a child diagnosed with a LD will likely have additional problems. Thus, further assessment will be required along with additional therapy and support.

Genetics

It has been known for some time that LD has a genetic component. One source of evidence emerged from studies examining familial aggregation (Neils & Aram, 1986; Tomblin, 1989). This research demonstrated that the rate of the disorder in children was higher in families when one or both parents also had LD or related problems. For instance, Tallal et al. (2001) found the rate of LD to be 71.4% in cases where both biological parents also had the same diagnosis or similar language problems. As a comparison, when neither parent had language problems the rate was 13%. The extent that transmission of the disorder could be attributed to environmental influences alone was discounted in twin studies (Bishop, 2006). In this research, the concordance rate for the disorder was compared between pairs of monozygotic twins, who are genetically identical, to dizygotic twins, who on average share 50% of their genes. Using this design, if environmental influences were responsible for the disorder, one would expect concordance rates to be similar across mono- and dizygotic twins. However, concordance rates are typically higher in monozygotic twins (e.g., Lewis & Thompson, 1992; Spinath, Price, Dale, & Plomin, 2004). To illustrate, Bishop, North, and Donlan (1995) observed the concordance rate to be .70 in monozygotic twins and .46 in dizygotic twins.

Research has also begun to elucidate specific genes associated with LD. Genome-wide linkage studies, first undertaken by the SLI Consortium (SLI Consortium, 2002, 2004), identified regions on Chromosomes 16 and 19 to be associated with common phenotypic deficits. These findings led to the identification of the SLI1 (Chromosomes 16) and SLI2 (Chromosomes 19) genes. An additional set of genes identified in LD arose from the study of the KE Family, who presented with severe speech, motor and language problems (Alcock, Passingham, Watkins, & Vargha-Khadem, 2000; Vargha-Khadem, Watkins, Alcock, Fletcher, & Passingham, 1995). Molecular genetic research later identified a mutation on Chromosome 7 (location 7q31), in the FOXP2 gene (Fisher, Vargha-Khadem, Watkins, Monaco, & Pembrey, 1998). Although some evidence suggests that the FOXP2 gene does not appear to play a key role in the language problems associated with children diagnosed with LD (Newbury et al., 2002), the presence of language problems (amongst other difficulties) found in the KE Family led to the hypothesis that one or more genes regulated by FOXP2 might play a role in LD (Vernes et al., 2008). This approach has led to the identification of a range of genes on Chromosome 7 that are reliably associated with a diagnosis of LD. Chief amongst these includes CNTNAP2, ATP2C2 and CMIP genes (Newbury, Fisher, & Monaco, 2010; Nudel, Ceroni, Simpson, & Newbury, 2015). Discovery of the CNTNAP2 gene might be of particular interest in understanding the origins of the comorbid problems in LD. This gene has also been implicated in autism and dyslexia (Rodenas-Cuadrado, Ho, & Vernes, 2014).

Neuropsychology

A key feature of the diagnostic criteria of LD is that communication impairments occur in the absence of intellectual, sensory or medical problems (American Psychiatric Association, 2013). That is, there is no clear cause of the difficulty learning and using language. However, the diagnostic criteria do not preclude the presence of cognitive and/or motor problems. Indeed, in LD, a wide range of problems in the cognitive and motor domain have been reported (see Leonard, 2014). Children with LD have been found to have slower processing speeds (Miller, Kail, Leonard, & Tomblin, 2001), executive dysfunction (Williams, Stott, Goodyer, & Sahakian, 2000), poorer fine and gross motor skills (Hill, 1998) and attention (Stevens, Sanders, & Neville, 2006).

Two well-researched cognitive deficits repeatedly found in LD are of auditory processing (Tallal, 2004) and nonword repetition (Gathercole & Baddeley, 1990). In relation to auditory processing impairments, research by Tallal and colleagues (Tallal, 1976; Tallal & Piercy, 1974) initially found children with LD had problems detecting differences between rapidly presented sounds. A subsequent finding suggested the auditory processing problems might be better conceptualised as an impairment discriminating between different frequencies (McArthur & Bishop, 2004). One hypothesised consequence of the auditory processing problems were difficulties acquiring the sounds of a language (i.e., phonology) which, in turn, impacted on the ability to understand and produce language (Tallal, 2000). However, a number of studies have since questioned this claim. First, not all children with LD have been found to have poor auditory processing problems (Rosen, 2003). Second, and perhaps the strongest challenge, comes from intervention studies showing that improving auditory processing skills does not lead to improvements in language (Strong, Torgerson, C.J. & Torgerson, D., & Hulme, 2011).

Gathercole and Baddeley (1990) identified nonword repetition deficits in LD. The findings revealed that children with the disorder had more difficulty repeating nonwords (e.g., blonterstaping, skilticult) of increasing syllabic length as compared to controls. This finding is one of the most widely replicated in the literature (Estes, Evans, & Else-Quest, 2007). Poor nonword repetition has been interpreted to suggest impaired phonological short-term memory (Gathercole, Willis, Baddeley, & Emslie, 1994). Performance on non-word repetition tests appears to predict word learning (Gathercole, 2006) and is related to expressive language skills (Adams & Gathercole, 1995). Interestingly, nonword repetition deficits have a genetic component (Bishop et al., 1995). Research by the SLI Consortium, described earlier, found significant linkage between nonword repetition and a site on Chromosome 16 (SLI Consortium, 2002).

The memory problems in LD might not be confined to short-term storage. Children with LD have more general problems with tasks requiring both the short-term storage and also the processing (or manipulation) of information. That is, working memory. This includes tasks such as the Backward Digit Span (e.g., Wechsler, 2003) and Competing Language Processing (Gaulin & Campbell, 1994) Tasks. On the Competing Language Processing Task children are auditorily presented with a sentence (e.g., 'Roses smell nice'). They are asked whether the sentence is true or false (e.g., true) and then recall the sentences' final word (e.g., nice). Children with LD perform poorer on these types of tasks compared to age matched controls, even after statistically controlling for language skills (Lum, Conti-Ramsden, Page, & Ullman, 2012). It is not clear whether working memory problems extend to non-verbal information. Several investigators (Archibald & Gathercole, 2006; Lum et al., 2012) have reported no significant differences between language disordered children and controls on nonverbal working memory tasks. However, results from a meta-analysis reported that overall, children with LD performed poorer on short-term visuo-spatial memory tasks as well (Vugs, Cuperus, Hendriks, & Verhoeven, 2013).

Children with LD also perform poorly on tasks probing procedural memory, that is the frontal/basal-ganglia based implicit learning of skills and habits. Much of this work was undertaken to investigate Ullman and Pierpont's (2005) claim that abnormalities of the basal ganglia and/or frontal areas play a key role in LD. On this view, frontal/basal-ganglia abnormalities lead to grammar and other language problems in LD, especially due to the dependence of some of these functions on procedural memory. Since procedural memory depends on these circuits, this model (the Procedural Deficit Hypothesis) predicted that children with LD should perform poorly on tasks that assess procedural memory.

To date, children with LD have been presented with a wide range of tasks that are known to be supported by the procedural memory system. This includes tasks that assess the statistical learning of verbal information (Evans, Saffran, & Robe-Torres, 2009; Mayor-Dubois, Zesiger, Van der Linden, & Roulet-Perez, 2014), artificial grammar (Lukács & Kemény, 2014), probabilistic classification (Kemény & Lukács, 2010), motor skill learning (Hsu & Bishop, 2014) and implicit learning of a visuo-motor sequence (Lum et al., 2012; Tomblin, Mainela-Arnold, & Zhang, 2007). A meta-analysis revealed that, across studies, children with LD perform poorly on procedural memory tasks (Lum et al., 2014), even including studies not reporting this pattern (e.g., Gabriel, Maillart, Guillaume, Stefaniak, & Meulemans, 2011). Although some correlational evidence has linked procedural memory deficits with language problems (Hedenius et al., 2011), additional work is still required to determine if problems with procedural memory are causally related to the language problems.

However, not all long-term memory systems appear to be impaired or compromised in LD. In particular, the hippocampus-supported declarative memory system appears to be intact (Lum & Conti-Ramsden, 2013; Ullman & Pierpont, 2005). For instance, children with LD perform as well as non-disordered children learning and remembering faces and abstract shapes (Lum et al., 2012). Although children with LD do appear to struggle with learning and remembering verbal information, such as a word list or short story (Riccio, Cash, & Cohen, 2007; Wulfeck, Bates, Krupa-Kwiatkowski, & Saltzman, 2004), and visual information that can be verbally encoded (Lum, Conti-Ramsden, & Ullman, 2013), these difficulties appear to be attributable to co-occurring language or working memory problems (Lum et al., Cortex 2012). Lum, Ullman, & Conti-Ramsden (2015) found that among children with LD, only those with working memory problems showed deficits on a word list learning task. A recent study suggests that consolidation of information (the stabilisation of memories over time) in declarative memory may actually be enhanced in children with LD compared to controls (Agnes et al., under review).

Since declarative memory seems to be largely spared, if not enhanced, in the disorder, it has been suggested that it may compensate for impairments in procedural memory (Ullman & Pierpont, 2005; Ullman & Pullman, 2015).

Neuropathology

Neuroimaging studies investigating the neural basis of LD have reported a wide range of grey and white matter abnormalities in this condition (e.g., Badcock, Bishop, Hardiman, Barry, & Watkins, 2012; Herbert et al., 2003). However, as noted in recent reviews, this literature is characterised by inconsistencies in findings (Liégeois, Mayes, & Morgan, 2014; Mayes, Reilly, & Morgan, 2015). For instance, structural differences between individuals with and without LD have been reported in cortical areas known to support language such as the inferior frontal gyrus and temporal gyrus. But variability in findings has emerged with reports of both increased (Badcock et al., 2012) and decreased grey matter (Gauger, Lombardino, & Leonard, 1997) in language disordered participants. A similar trend has emerged from studies investigating white matter density. Results indicate both increased and decreased (Herbert et al., 2004) white matter volumes in frontal and temporal areas. Liégeois, Mayes, & Morgan (2014) suggest that structural differences in temporal regions may contribute to auditory processing problems in the group.

Subcortical anomalies in LD are common. Following their review of the literature, Ullman and Pierpiont (2005) note that nearly all studies investigating subcortical structures in LD report basal ganglia, in particular the caudate nucleus, anomalies (Badcock et al., 2012; Jernigan, Hesselink, Sowell, & Tallal, 1991; Tallal, Jernigan, & Trauner, 1994). The body of research showing structural differences in the caudate nucleus in language disordered may explain the procedural memory problems in this group (Lum et al., 2014). This is because the learning and consolidation in procedural memory occurs via spiny cells in the caudate and putamen that are sensitive to sequential or pattern like information arriving from the neocortex (Carrillo-Reid et al., 2008; Houk, Davis, & Beiser, 1995; Rauch et al., 1997). It is also possible that caudate anomalies may reflect genetic influence, given that the FOXP2 gene is expressed in this region of the brain (e.g., Lai, Gerrelli, Monaco, Fisher, & Copp, 2003).

The evidence indicates neurological differences between individuals with and without LD. As to be expected, differences in brain structure are found in areas known to support language; although research has also revealed differences in non-language centres as well (see Mayes et al., 2015). An outstanding issue to be resolved is the heterogeneity in structural findings. One possibility is that the differences reflect variability in the diagnostic criteria used to identify LD. Another is that differences in findings may reflect the developmental nature of LD (Karmiloff-Smith, 1998). Thus the variability in findings may arise from neurological compensatory mechanism/s as the brain tries to learn language. From this perspective, individual differences may be a product of the child's genetic endowment and interactions with the environment.

Treatment

There are a number of challenges that exist with the provision of treatment and support for children with LD. Ideally, diagnosis and treatment should take place early in development. However, as mentioned above, at present it is not yet possible to reliably diagnose language problems within the 0 – 3 year age range. Reilly, McKean, Morgan, & Wake (2015) highlight that during this age range it is therefore important that children suspected of language problems are continuously exposed to environments that facilitate language development. Indeed, there are a number of empirically supported strategies for achieving this goal at preschool (Fricke, Bowyer-Crane, Haley, Hulme, & Snowling, 2013) and at home (Mol, Bus, de Jong, & Smeets, 2008; Roberts & Kaiser, 2015).

For school-aged children who are diagnosed with LD, therapy provided by a speech pathologist, and in some instances trained parents, has been shown to improve language. Law, Garrett, & Nye's (2003) Cochrane review of randomised controlled trials indicates that improvements can be made in the area of expressive vocabulary and syntax. However, this review revealed that not all aspects of LD appear to be modifiable via therapy. Receptive language or oral comprehension skills are resistant to intervention. It has also been suggested that, given the possible role of declarative memory as a compensatory system, therapy might target compensatory learning of language in this system (Ullman and Pullman, 2015).

The treatment of LD may also extend beyond targeting communication problems. Intact language skills are essential in order to advance in educational, psychosocial and vocational domains. As noted earlier, individuals with LD may need support or treatment in addition to the communication problems. Children with language problems often struggle academically, socially and may have mental health problems such as anxiety disorder (Conti-Ramsden & Botting, 2008; Voci, Beitchman, Brownlie, & Wilson, 2006). Subsequently, treatments aimed at resolving non-language aspects of the disorder may be required.

Summary

LD is diagnosed on the basis that the ability to produce and/or understand language is below-age expected levels, in the absence of other explanations. Not surprisingly, given this broad exclusionary definition, the presentation of the disorder varies considerably between individuals. This is seen with respect to the severity of the expressive and receptive language problems. However, it is interesting to note that despite the variability in language functioning, neurological data appears to be consistently on striatal abnormalities in LD. Thus, frontostriatal problems might be at least one origin of the subsequent problems found in this group. While the disorder clearly has a genetic component, the variability observed at various endpoints highlights the complex nature of the language learning process. That is, learning and using language occurs through reciprocal interactions with the environment and other cognitive systems. In providing support to affected individuals, the best approach currently involves being able to identify affected individuals as early as possible. Through this approach, the negative impact of language problems can be reduced, affording children a more positive future.

Abbreviations

ADHD: Attention Deficit Hyperactivity Disorder
DCD: Developmental Coordination Disorder
LD: Language Disorder
SLI: Specific Language Impairment

Further readings

Bishop, D.V., & Leonard, L. (2014). *Speech and Language Impairments in Children: Causes, Characteristics, Intervention and Outcome*. New York: Psychology Press.

Brinton, B., Fujiki, M., & Robinson, L. A. (2005). Life on a tricycle: A case study of language impairment from 4 to 19. *Topics in Language Disorders, 25*(4), 338–352.

Leonard, L. B. (2014). *Children with Specific Language Impairment* (2nd ed.). Cambridge: The MIT Press.

Lum, J. A., & Conti-Ramsden, G. (2013). Long-term memory: A review and meta-analysis of studies of declarative and procedural memory in specific language impairment. *Topics in Language Disorders, 33*(4), 282.

Stavrakaki, S. (2015). *Specific Language Impairment: Current Trends in Research*. Amsterdam: John Benjamins Publishing Company.

Ullman, M. T., & Pierpont, E. I. (2005). Specific language impairment is not specific to language: The procedural deficit hypothesis. *Cortex, 41*(3), 399–433.

Verhoeven, L., & van Balkom, H. (2003). *Classification of Developmental Language Disorders: Theoretical Issues and Clinical Implications*. Psychology Press.

Note

1. Examples from Leonard (2014).

References

Adams, A.-M., & Gathercole, S. E. (1995). Phonological working memory and speech production in preschool children. *Journal of Speech, Language, and Hearing Research, 38*(2), 403–414.

Alcock, K. J., Passingham, R. E., Watkins, K. E., & Vargha-Khadem, F. (2000). Oral dyspraxia in inherited speech and language impairment and acquired dysphasia. *Brain and Language, 75*(1), 17–33.

American Psychiatric Association. (2013). *Diagnostic and Statistical Manual of Mental Disorders (DSM-5)* (5th ed.). Washington, DC: American Psychiatric Association.

Archibald, L. M., & Gathercole, S. E. (2006). Visuospatial immediate memory in specific language impairment. *Journal of Speech, Language, and Hearing Research, 49*(2), 265–277.

Badcock, N. A., Bishop, D. V., Hardiman, M. J., Barry, J. G., & Watkins, K. E. (2012). Co-localisation of abnormal brain structure and function in specific language impairment. *Brain and Language, 120*(3), 310–320.

Beitchman, J. H., Wilson, B., Johnson, C. J., Atkinson, L., Young, A., Adlaf, E., ... Douglas, L. (2001). Fourteen-year follow-up of speech/language-impaired and control children: Psychiatric outcome. *Journal of the American Academy of Child & Adolescent Psychiatry, 40*(1), 75–82.

Bishop, D., & Edmundson, A. (1987). Language-impaired 4-year-olds distinguishing transient from persistent impairment. *Journal of Speech and Hearing Disorders, 52*(2), 156–173.

Bishop, D.V. (2006). What causes specific language impairment in children? *Current Directions in Psychological Science, 15*(5), 217–221.

Bishop, D. V. (2010). Which neurodevelopmental disorders get researched and why? *PLoS One, 5*(11), e15112.

Bishop, D.V., Clark, B., Conti-Ramsden, G., Norbury, C. F., & Snowling, M. J. (2012). RALLI: An internet campaign for raising awareness of language learning impairments. *Child Language Teaching and Therapy, 28*(3), 259–262.

Bishop, D.V., North, T., & Donlan, C. (1995). Genetic basis of specific language impairment: Evidence from a twin study. *Developmental Medicine & Child Neurology, 37*(1), 56–71.

Bishop, D.V., & Snowling, M. J. (2004). Developmental dyslexia and specific language impairment: Same or different? *Psychological Bulletin, 130*(6), 858.

Bishop, D.V. M. (2014). Ten questions about terminology for children with unexplained language problems. *International Journal of Language & Communication Disorders, 49*(4), 381–415. doi: 10.1111/1460-6984.12101.

Carrillo-Reid, L., Tecuapetla, F., Tapia, D., Hernández-Cruz, A., Galarraga, E., Drucker-Colin, R., & Bargas, J. (2008). Encoding network states by striatal cell assemblies. *Journal of Neurophysiology, 99*(3), 1435–1450.

Catts, H. W., Adlof, S. M., Hogan, T. P., & Weismer, S. E. (2005). Are specific language impairment and dyslexia distinct disorders? *Journal of Speech, Language, and Hearing Research, 48*(6), 1378–1396.

Cohen, N. J., Barwick, M. A., Horodezky, N. B., Vallance, D. D., & Im, N. (1998). Language, achievement, and cognitive processing in psychiatrically disturbed children with previously identified and unsuspected language impairments. *Journal of Child Psychology and Psychiatry, 39*(06), 865–877.

Cohen, N. J., Vallance, D. D., Barwick, M., Im, N., Menna, R., Horodezky, N. B., & Isaacson, L. (2000). The interface between ADHD and language impairment: An examination of language, achievement, and cognitive processing. *Journal of Child Psychology and Psychiatry, 41*(3), 353–362. doi: 10.1111/1469-7610.00619.

Conti-Ramsden, G. (2013). Commentary: Increased risk of later emotional and behavioural problems in children with SLI–reflections on Yew and O'Kearney (2013). *Journal of Child Psychology and Psychiatry, 54*(5), 525–526.

Conti-Ramsden, G., & Botting, N. (2008). Emotional health in adolescents with and without a history of specific language impairment (SLI). *Journal of Child Psychology and Psychiatry, 49*(5), 516–525.

Conti-Ramsden, G., Simkin, Z., & Botting, N. (2006). The prevalence of autistic spectrum disorders in adolescents with a history of specific language impairment (SLI). *Journal of Child Psychology and Psychiatry, 47*(6), 621–628.

Durkin, K., & Conti-Ramsden, G. (2007). Language, social behavior, and the quality of friendships in adolescents with and without a history of specific language impairment. *Child Development, 78*(5), 1441–1457.

Ebbels, S. (2014). Introducing the SLI debate. *International Journal of Language & Communication Disorders, 49*(4), 377–380. doi: 10.1111/1460-6984.12119.

Estes, K. G., Evans, J. L., & Else-Quest, N. M. (2007). Differences in the nonword repetition performance of children with and without specific language impairment: A meta-analysis. *Journal of Speech, Language, and Hearing Research, 50*(1), 177–195.

Evans, J. L., Saffran, J. R., & Robe-Torres, K. (2009). Statistical learning in children with specific language impairment. *Journal of Speech, Language, and Hearing Research, 52*(2), 321–335.

Fisher, S. E., Vargha-Khadem, F., Watkins, K. E., Monaco, A. P., & Pembrey, M. E. (1998). Localisation of a gene implicated in a severe speech and language disorder. *Nature Genetics, 18*, 168–170.

Flapper, B. C. T., & Schoemaker, M. M. (2013). Developmental coordination disorder in children with specific language impairment: Co-morbidity and impact on quality of life. *Research in Developmental Disabilities, 34*(2), 756–763. doi: 10.1016/j.ridd.2012.10.014.

Fricke, S., Bowyer-Crane, C., Haley, A. J., Hulme, C., & Snowling, M. J. (2013). Efficacy of language intervention in the early years. *Journal of Child Psychology and Psychiatry, 54*(3), 280–290.

Gabriel, A., Maillart, C., Guillaume, M., Stefaniak, N., & Meulemans, T. (2011). Exploration of serial structure procedural learning in children with language impairment. *Journal of the International Neuropsychological Society, 17*(2), 336–343.

Gathercole, S. E. (2006). Nonword repetition and word learning: The nature of the relationship. *Applied Psycholinguistics, 27*(4), 513–543.

Gathercole, S. E., & Baddeley, A. D. (1990). Phonological memory deficits in language disordered children: Is there a causal connection? *Journal of Memory and Language, 29*(3), 336–360.

Gathercole, S. E., Willis, C. S., Baddeley, A. D., & Emslie, H. (1994). The children's test of nonword repetition: A test of phonological working memory. *Memory, 2*(2), 103–127.

Gauger, L. M., Lombardino, L. J., & Leonard, C. M. (1997). Brain morphology in children with specific language impairment. *Journal of Speech, Language, and Hearing Research, 40*(6), 1272–1284.

Gaulin, C. A., & Campbell, T. F. (1994). Procedure for assessing verbal working memory in normal school-age children: Some preliminary data. *Perceptual and Motor Skills, 79*(1), 55–64.

Gleason, J. B., & Ratner, N. B. (2012). *The Development of Language* (8th ed.). Boston: Allyn & Bacon.

Hedenius, M., Persson, J., Tremblay, A., Adi-Japha, E., Veríssimo, J., Dye, C. D., … Ullman, M. T. (2011). Grammar predicts procedural learning and consolidation deficits in children with specific language impairment. *Research in Developmental Disabilities, 32*(6), 2362–2375.

Herbert, M. R., Ziegler, D. A., Makris, N., Bakardjiev, A., Hodgson, J., Adrien, K. T., … Caviness, V. S. (2003). Larger brain and white matter volumes in children with developmental language disorder. *Developmental Science, 6*(4), F11-F22.

Herbert, M. R., Ziegler, D. A., Makris, N., Filipek, P. A., Kemper, T. L., Normandin, J. J., ... Caviness, V. S. (2004). Localization of white matter volume increase in autism and developmental language disorder. *Annals of Neurology, 55*(4), 530–540.

Hill, E. L. (1998). A dyspraxic deficit in specific language impairment and developmental coordination disorder? Evidence from hand and arm movements. *Developmental Medicine & Child Neurology, 40*(6), 388–395.

Hill, E. L. (2001). Non-specific nature of specific language impairment: A review of the literature with regard to concomitant motor impairments. *International Journal of Language & Communication Disorders, 36*(2), 149–171.

Houk, J. C., Davis, J. L., & Beiser, D. G. (1995). *Models of Information Processing in the Basal Ganglia.* Cambridge: MIT Press.

Hsu, H. J., & Bishop, D.V. (2014). Sequence-specific procedural learning deficits in children with specific language impairment. *Developmental Science, 17*(3), 352–365.

Jernigan, T. L., Hesselink, J. R., Sowell, E., & Tallal, P. A. (1991). Cerebral structure on magnetic resonance imaging in language-and learning-impaired children. *Archives of Neurology, 48*(5), 539–545.

Karmiloff-Smith, A. (1998). Development itself is the key to understanding developmental disorders. *Trends in Cognitive Sciences, 2*(10), 389–398.

Kemény, F., & Lukács, Á. (2010). Impaired procedural learning in language impairment: Results from probabilistic categorization. *Journal of Clinical and Experimental Neuropsychology, 32*(3), 249–258.

Lahey, M., Liebergott, J., Chesnick, M., Menyuk, P., & Adams, J. (1992). Variability in children's use of grammatical morphemes. *Applied Psycholinguistics, 13*(03), 373–398.

Lai, C. S., Gerrelli, D., Monaco, A. P., Fisher, S. E., & Copp, A. J. (2003). FOXP2 expression during brain development coincides with adult sites of pathology in a severe speech and language disorder. *Brain, 126*(11), 2455–2462.

Law, J., Boyle, J., Harris, F., Harkness, A., & Nye, C. (2000). Prevalence and natural history of primary speech and language delay: Findings from a systematic review of the literature. *International Journal of Language and Communication Disorders, 35*(2), 165–188.

Law, J., Garrett, Z., & Nye, C. (2003). Speech and language therapy interventions for children with primary speech and language delay or disorder. *Cochrane Database of Systematic Reviews,* (3), CD004110.

Lee, J. C., Nopoulos, P. C., & Tomblin, J. B. (2013). Abnormal subcortical components of the corticostriatal system in young adults with DLI: A combined structural MRI and DTI study. *Neuropsychologia, 51*(11), 2154–2161.

Leonard, L. B. (2014). *Children with Specific Language Impairment.* Cambridge: MIT press.

Lewis, B. A., & Thompson, L. A. (1992). A study of developmental speech and language disorders in twins. *Journal of Speech, Language, and Hearing Research, 35*(5), 1086–1094.

Leyfer, O. T., Tager-Flusberg, H., Dowd, M., Tomblin, J. B., & Folstein, S. E. (2008). Overlap between autism and specific language impairment: Comparison of autism diagnostic interview and autism diagnostic observation schedule scores. *Autism Research, 1*(5), 284–296.

Liégeois, F., Mayes, A., & Morgan, A. (2014). Neural correlates of developmental speech and language disorders: Evidence from neuroimaging. *Current Developmental Disorders Reports, 1*(3), 215–227.

Love, A. J., & Thompson, M. G. (1988). Language disorders and attention deficit disorders in young children referred for psychiatric services: Analysis of prevalence and a conceptual synthesis. *American Journal of Orthopsychiatry, 58*(1), 52.

Lukács, Á., & Kemény, F. (2014). Domain-general sequence learning deficit in specific language impairment. *Neuropsychology, 28*(3), 472.

Lum, J. A., & Conti-Ramsden, G. (2013). Long-term memory: A review and meta-analysis of studies of declarative and procedural memory in specific language impairment. *Topics in Language Disorders, 33*(4), 282–297.

Lum, J. A., Conti-Ramsden, G., Morgan, A. T., & Ullman, M. T. (2014). Procedural learning deficits in specific language impairment (SLI): A meta-analysis of serial reaction time task performance. *Cortex, 51*, 1–10.

Lum, J. A., Conti-Ramsden, G., Page, D., & Ullman, M. T. (2012). Working, declarative and procedural memory in specific language impairment. *Cortex, 48*(9), 1138–1154.

Lum, J. A., Conti-Ramsden, G., & Ullman, M. T. (2013). The role of verbal and nonverbal memory in the Family Pictures Subtest: Data from children with specific language impairment. *Child Neuropsychology, 19*(6), 648–661.

Lum, J. A., Ullman, M. T., & Conti-Ramsden, G. (2015). Verbal declarative memory impairments in specific language impairment are related to working memory deficits. *Brain and Language, 142*, 76–85.

Mayes, A. K., Reilly, S., & Morgan, A. T. (2015). Neural correlates of childhood language disorder: A systematic review. *Developmental Medicine & Child Neurology*.

Mayor-Dubois, C., Zesiger, P., Van der Linden, M., & Roulet-Perez, E. (2014). Nondeclarative learning in children with specific language impairment: Predicting regularities in the visuomotor, phonological, and cognitive domains. *Child Neuropsychology, 20*(1), 14–22.

McArthur, G., & Bishop, D. (2004). Frequency discrimination deficits in people with specific language impairment reliability, validity, and linguistic correlates. *Journal of Speech, Language, and Hearing Research, 47*(3), 527–541.

McArthur, G. M., Hogben, J. H., Edwards, V. T., Heath, S. M., & Mengler, E. D. (2000). On the "specifics" of specific reading disability and specific language impairment. *Journal of Child Psychology and Psychiatry, 41*(07), 869–874.

McCabe, P. C. (2005). Social and behavioral correlates of preschoolers with specific language impairment. *Psychology in the Schools, 42*(4), 373–387. doi: 10.1002/pits.20064.

Miller, C. A., Kail, R., Leonard, L. B., & Tomblin, J. B. (2001). Speed of processing in children with specific language impairment. *Journal of Speech, Language, and Hearing Research, 44*(2), 416–433.

Mol, S. E., Bus, A. G., de Jong, M. T., & Smeets, D. J. (2008). Added value of dialogic parent–child book readings: A meta-analysis. *Early Education and Development, 19*(1), 7–26.

Neils, J., & Aram, D. M. (1986). Family history of children with developmental language disorders. *Perceptual and Motor Skills, 63*(2), 655–658.

Newbury, D. F., Bonora, E., Lamb, J. A., Fisher, S. E., Lai, C. S., Baird, G., … Merricks, M. J. (2002). FOXP2 is not a major susceptibility gene for autism or specific language impairment. *The American Journal of Human Genetics, 70*(5), 1318–1327.

Newbury, D. F., Fisher, S. E., & Monaco, A. P. (2010). Recent advances in the genetics of language impairment. *Genome Medicine, 2*(6), doi:10.1186/gm1127.

Nudel, R., Ceroni, F., Simpson, N. H., & Newbury, D. F. (2015). The genetics of specific language impairment. In S. Stavrakaki (Ed.), *Specific Language Impairment: Current Trends in Research* (pp. 7–34). Amsterdam: John Benjamins Publishing Company.

Rauch, S. L., Whalen, P. J., Savage, C. R., Curran, T., Kendrick, A., Brown, H. D., … Rosen, B. R. (1997). Striatal recruitment during an implicit sequence learning task as measured by functional magnetic resonance imaging. *Human Brain Mapping, 5*(2), 124–132.

Reilly, S., McKean, C., Morgan, A., & Wake, M. (2015). Identifying and managing common childhood language and speech impairments. *British Medical Journal, 350*, h2318.

Reilly, S., Tomblin, B., Law, J., McKean, C., Mensah, F. K., Morgan, A., … Wake, M. (2014). Specific language impairment: A convenient label for whom? *International Journal of Language & Communication Disorders, 49*(4), 416–451. doi: 10.1111/1460-6984.12102.

Reilly, S., Wake, M., Ukoumunne, O. C., Bavin, E., Prior, M., Cini, E., … Bretherton, L. (2010). Predicting language outcomes at 4 years of age: Findings from Early Language in Victoria Study. *Pediatrics, 126*(6), e1530-e1537.

Rescorla, L., Hadicke-Wiley, M., & Escarce, E. (1993). Epidemiological investigation of expressive language delay at age two. *First Language, 13*(37), 5–22. doi: 10.1177/014272379301303702.

Riccio, C. A., Cash, D. L., & Cohen, M. J. (2007). Learning and memory performance of children with specific language impairment (SLI). *Applied Neuropsychology, 14*(4), 255–261.

Roberts, M. Y., & Kaiser, A. P. (2015). Early intervention for toddlers with language delays: A randomized controlled trial. *Pediatrics, 135*(4), 686–693.

Rodenas-Cuadrado, P., Ho, J., & Vernes, S. C. (2014). Shining a light on CNTNAP2: Complex functions to complex disorders. *European Journal of Human Genetics, 22*(2), 171–178.

Rosen, S. (2003). Auditory processing in dyslexia and specific language impairment: Is there a deficit? What is its nature? Does it explain anything? *Journal of Phonetics, 31*(3), 509–527.

Rutter, M., & Mawhood, L. (1991). The long-term psychosocial sequelae of specific developmental disorders of speech and language. *Biological Risk Factors for Psychosocial Disorders* (pp. 233–259). Cambridge: Cambridge University Press.

Sanjeevan, T., Rosenbaum, D. A., Miller, C., van Hell, J. G., Weiss, D. J., & Mainela-Arnold, E. (2015). Motor issues in specific language impairment: A window into the underlying impairment. *Current Developmental Disorders Reports, 2*(3), 228–236.

Silva, P. A., McGee, R., & Williams, S. M. (1983). Developmental language delay from three to seven years and its significance for low intelligence and reading difficulties at age seven. *Developmental Medicine & Child Neurology, 25*(6), 783–793. doi: 10.1111/j.1469-8749.1983.tb13847.x.

SLI Consortium. (2002). A genomewide scan identifies two novel loci involved in specific language impairment. *The American Journal of Human Genetics, 70*(2), 384–398.

SLI Consortium. (2004). Highly significant linkage to the SLI1 locus in an expanded sample of individuals affected by specific language impairment. *The American Journal of Human Genetics, 74*(6), 1225–1238.

Snowling, M. J., Adams, J. W., Bishop, D. V. M., & Stothard, S. E. (2001). Educational attainments of school leavers with a preschool history of speech-language impairments. *International Journal of Language & Communication Disorders, 36*(2), 173–183.

Spaulding, T. J., Plante, E., & Farinella, K. A. (2006). Eligibility criteria for language impairment: Is the low end of normal always appropriate? *Language, Speech, and Hearing Services in Schools, 37*(1), 61–72.

Spinath, F. M., Price, T. S., Dale, P. S., & Plomin, R. (2004). The genetic and environmental origins of language disability and ability. *Child Development*, 445–454.

Stevens, C., Sanders, L., & Neville, H. (2006). Neurophysiological evidence for selective auditory attention deficits in children with specific language impairment. *Brain Research, 1111*(1), 143–152.

Strong, G. K., Torgerson, C. J., Torgerson, D., & Hulme, C. (2011). A systematic meta-analytic review of evidence for the effectiveness of the 'Fast For Word' language intervention program. *Journal of Child Psychology and Psychiatry, 52*(3), 224–235.

Tallal, P. (1976). Rapid auditory processing in normal and disordered language development. *Journal of Speech, Language, and Hearing Research, 19*(3), 561–571.

Tallal, P. (2000). Experimental studies of language learning impairments: From research to remediation. In D.V. M. Bishop & L. B. Leonard (Eds.), *Speech and Language Impairments in Children: Causes, Characteristics, Intervention and Uutcome* (pp. 131–155). Hove: Psychology Press.

Tallal, P. (2004). Improving language and literacy is a matter of time. *Nature Reviews Neuroscience, 5*(9), 721–728.

Tallal, P., Hirsch, L. S., Realpe-Bonilla, T., Miller, S., Brzustowicz, L. M., Bartlett, C., & Flax, J. F. (2001). Familial aggregation in specific language impairment. *Journal of Speech, Language, and Hearing Research, 44*(5), 1172–1182.

Tallal, P., Jernigan, T., & Trauner, D. (1994). Developmental bilateral damage to the head of the caudate nuclei: Implications for speech-language pathology. *Journal of Medical Speech-Language Pathology, 2*(1), 23–28.

Tallal, P., & Piercy, M. (1974). Developmental aphasia: Rate of auditory processing and selective impairment of consonant perception. *Neuropsychologia, 12*(1), 83–93.

Tomblin, J. B. (1989). Familial concentration of developmental language impairment. *Journal of Speech and Hearing Disorders, 54*(2), 287–295.

Tomblin, J. B., Mainela-Arnold, E., & Zhang, X. (2007). Procedural learning in adolescents with and without specific language impairment. *Language Learning and Development, 3*(4), 269–293.

Tomblin, J. B., Records, N. L., Buckwalter, P., Zhang, X., Smith, E., & O'Brien, M. (1997). Prevalence of specific language impairment in kindergarten children. *Journal of Speech, Language, and Hearing Research, 40*(6), 1245–1260.

Ukoumunne, O., Wake, M., Carlin, J., Bavin, E., Lum, J., Skeat, J., … Reilly, S. (2012). Profiles of language development in pre-school children: A longitudinal latent class analysis of data from the Early Language in Victoria Study. *Child: Care, Health and Development, 38*(3), 341–349.

Ullman, M. T. (2004). Contributions of memory circuits to language: The declarative/procedural model. *Cognition, 92*(1), 231–270.

Ullman, M. T., & Pierpont, E. I. (2005). Specific language impairment is not specific to language: The procedural deficit hypothesis. *Cortex, 41*(3), 399–433.

Ullman, M. T., & Pullman, M. Y. (2015). A compensatory role for declarative memory in neurodevelopmental disorders. *Neuroscience & Biobehavioral Reviews, 51*, 205–222.

Vargha-Khadem, F., Watkins, K., Alcock, K., Fletcher, P., & Passingham, R. (1995). Praxic and nonverbal cognitive deficits in a large family with a genetically transmitted speech and language disorder. *Proceedings of the National Academy of Sciences, 92*(3), 930–933.

Verhoeven, J. S., Rommel, N., Prodi, E., Leemans, A., Zink, I., Vandewalle, E., … Boets, B. (2012). Is there a common neuroanatomical substrate of language deficit between autism spectrum disorder and specific language impairment? *Cerebral Cortex, 22*(10), 2263–2271.

Vernes, S. C., Newbury, D. F., Abrahams, B. S., Winchester, L., Nicod, J., Groszer, M., … Geschwind, D. H. (2008). A functional genetic link between distinct developmental language disorders. *New England Journal of Medicine, 359*(22), 2337–2345.

Voci, S. C., Beitchman, J. H., Brownlie, E. B., & Wilson, B. (2006). Social anxiety in late adolescence: The importance of early childhood language impairment. *Journal of Anxiety Disorders, 20*(7), 915–930. doi: 10.1016/j.janxdis.2006.01.007.

Vugs, B., Cuperus, J., Hendriks, M., & Verhoeven, L. (2013). Visuospatial working memory in specific language impairment: A meta-analysis. *Research in Developmental Disabilities, 34*(9), 2586–2597.

Webster, R. I., Majnemer, A., Platt, R. W., & Shevell, M. I. (2005). Motor function at school age in children with a preschool diagnosis of developmental language impairment. *The Journal of Pediatrics, 146*(1), 80–85.

Wechsler, D. (2003). *Wechsler Intelligence Scale for Children–Fourth Edition (WISC-IV)*. San Antonio, TX: The Psychological Corporation.

Williams, D., Botting, N., & Boucher, J. (2008). Language in autism and specific language impairment: Where are the links? *Psychological Bulletin, 134*(6), 944.

Williams, D., Stott, C., Goodyer, I., & Sahakian, B. (2000). Specific language impairment with or without hyperactivity: Neuropsychological evidence for frontostriatal dysfunction. *Developmental Medicine & Child Neurology, 42*(06), 368–375.

World Health Organization. (2010). *International Classification of Diseases (ICD-10)*. Geneva: World Health Organization.

Wulfeck, B., Bates, E., Krupa-Kwiatkowski, M., & Saltzman, D. (2004). Grammaticality sensitivity in children with early focal brain injury and children with specific language impairment. *Brain and Language, 88*(2), 215–228.

7
AUTISM SPECTRUM DISORDER

Nicole Rinehart, Jane McGillivray, Melissa Kirkovski and Katrina Williams

Introduction

Autism Spectrum Disorder (ASD) is a complex neurodevelopmental condition characterised by impairments in social communication and behaviour. While ASD genetics and neuroimaging research are progressing, the search for the identification of objective phenotypic features and biomarkers continues. Individuals with ASD can be significantly disadvantaged in regard to social relationships, physical and mental health, and quality of life (Howlin & Moss, 2012). ASD is associated with significant cost to families and society with an estimated $3 million spent by families of individuals with ASD beyond the ordinary costs of raising a child (Knapp, Romeo, & Beecham, 2009). Intervention can reduce the level of impairment faced by children with ASD (Elberling et al., 2014), with the aim to start intervention as soon as difficulties are identified.

Preliminary considerations

Throughout history there have been many terms to describe what we now know as Autism Spectrum Disorder. DSM-IV-TR (American Psychiatric Association, 2000) and ICD-10 (WHO, 1992) included the terms to 'Autistic Disorder' and 'Asperger's Disorder or Syndrome' as separate disorders under the category of pervasive developmental disorder. In DSM-5 (American Psychiatric Association, 2013), these diagnoses have been incorporated together under the category of Autism Spectrum Disorder (ASD). As foreshadowed by Bradshaw (2001), our diagnostic manuals now recognise ASD as a neurodevelopmental disorder, which commonly overlaps with disorders such as Attention Deficit Hyperactivity Disorder (ADHD). It is well known that ASD is far from homogeneous. For example, while Asperger's disorder is no longer included in Diagnostic and Statistical Manual of Mental Disorders (DSM), the clinical and neurobiological differences that have been identified between 'Autistic disorder' and 'Asperger' disorder' (Rinehart, Bradshaw, Brereton, & Tonge, 2002) may provide important clues about whether there are common or different causal pathways to these different phenotypes. It is also likely that other important phenotypic differences will emerge that will also point to different causal pathways and intervention response. This chapter will use terms consistent with both DSM-IV-TR and DSM-5 throughout.

Prevalence

Most recent prevalence studies estimate over 1 in 100 children will be diagnosed with ASD (CDC, 2014; Elsabbagh et al., 2012). In recent years there has been a greater increase in 'cognitively able' or 'high-functioning' children diagnosed with ASD compared to the increase in those diagnosed with both ASD and intellectual disability (historically referred to as 'low functioning autism'; Van Naarden et al., 2015).

Clinical characteristics

The essential clinical features of ASD involve impairments in social communication and interaction and repetitive, restricted and stereotypical behavioural patterns that interfere with everyday life. More males are diagnosed with ASD compared to females (4.3:1), with the preponderance of males to females greater amongst individuals with intact cognitive ability (May, Cornish, & Rinehart, 2014). It has been suggested that females require a greater burden of genetic abnormality or neuropathology to develop ASD (Jacquemont et al., 2014) or that they could be undiagnosed or misdiagnosed, potentially due to the presence of less severe externalising behavioural deficits (May et al., 2014; see also Kirkovski, Enticott, & Fitzgerald, 2013).

Diagnostic instruments and clinical rating scales

Accurate and timely identification of ASD is critical to enabling appropriate support for the child and family, including early intervention. However, the process involved in conducting an assessment for ASD is complex and dependent on information derived from different settings, and a range of different tools that use different methods. Clinical multidisciplinary assessment may involve the use of assessment tools like the Autism Diagnostic Observations Scale (ADOS-2; Lord et al., 2012), the Childhood Autism Rating Scale (CARS-2; Schopler et al., 2010), or the Autism Diagnostic Interview (ADI-R; Lord, Rutter, & Le Couteur, 1994; see also Kim et al., 2013). Gold standard assessment involves medical (including genetic testing where indicated), cognitive and language assessment. Other assessments, such as sensory, motor and adaptive functioning, can also add to the understanding of each individual, both for diagnosis and future planning. In best practice, the information is synthesised by an experienced clinical team who make the final decision regarding a diagnosis according to current classification systems (American Psychiatric Association, 2013; WHO, 1992).

Clinical vignette

Phillip was described as a child who was 'always on the go'. He was unable to stay seated during mealtime, and constantly moved his hands or legs. He was diagnosed with ADHD at the age of 8 years by his paediatrician, commenced on a trial of dexamphetamine and subsequently referred to a clinical psychologist for further developmental assessment and behavioural management input. The severity of his behavioural symptoms, which included running away, violent temper tantrums and fighting with other children, escalated when academic demands at school increased in Grade 3. Further observation revealed he had an 'odd' gait that made him the subject of teasing by his peers. Handwriting problems were also apparent and contributed to his academic struggles. Teacher's reports indicated Phillip rarely spoke in class and avoided eye contact with peers. Insomnia, hypersensitivity to clothing and a preference for only eating white, soft food were also noted. Transition periods between home and school frequently triggered behavioural outbursts. At school Philip played only with his younger brother, re-enacting scenes from their favourite video games and avoiding interactions with his same-aged peers. Intellectual assessment indicated an uneven cognitive profile characterised by high-average perceptual reasoning skills, and low-average verbal comprehension ability. Phillip's working memory and processing abilities were well below average (below the 5th percentile). Phillip was subsequently diagnosed according to DSM-5 criteria with ASD and comorbid ADHD, and referred to a specialist intervention team, with continued follow up and input from both the paediatrician and psychologist to manage comorbidities. Later that year, Philip's younger brother was referred for assessment due to concerns about problems concentrating in class.

* Clinical Vignette also relates to Chapter 8.

Co-occurring neurological, behavioural, and mental health problems

There are many different types of comorbidities: those that share a common underlying causal pathway with ASD; those that occur because having ASD increases their likelihood; and those that occur in many other individuals but are more common or more difficult to manage in ASD. Gillberg (2010) notes that 'comorbidity is the rule rather than the exception in child psychiatry and developmental medicine' (p. 1543) and coined the acronym ESSENCE to refer to 'Early Symptomatic Syndromes Eliciting Neurodevelopmental Clinical Examinations' (p. 1543) to highlight the co-existence of ASD with other conditions including ADHD, epilepsy, tic disorder, sleep and feeding problems, learning problems and developmental coordination disorder. Gillberg and others have highlighted that it is often not the diagnosis of ASD alone that is associated with poor outcomes, but the type and nature of comorbidity. In particular, children with more severe intellectual disability tend to have the poorest life outcomes (Matson & Goldin, 2014).

Attention Deficit Hyperactivity Disorder and other learning related problems

It has been estimated that over 50% of children with ASD will experience clinically significant ADHD (Simonoff et al., 2008). How ASD and ADHD are related and possible common causal underpinnings are being explored (Gargaro, Rinehart, Bradshaw, Tonge, & Sheppard, 2011). Emerging evidence suggests that children with ASD and ADHD have more disturbed emotional-behavioural profiles and poorer quality of life than children with ASD alone. Information relevant to ADHD and other learning problems is usually better understood when intelligence has been assessed (Gargaro et al., 2011) (see also Chapter 8 for a comprehensive overview of ADHD).

Epilepsy

An increased occurrence of epilepsy in children with ASD has long been reported, but the presence of epilepsy is not increased compared to the general population if estimates are adjusted for intellectual disability (Woolfenden, Sarkozy, Ridley, Coory, & Williams, 2012). Important considerations specific to ASD are that epilepsy could be a cause of ASD behaviours, especially in the setting of marked communication disorder, a loss of previously acquired skills or reports of "funny turns". Also, amongst other ASD behaviours it may be more difficult to distinguish seizures from other behaviours, so a high index of suspicion is needed. Finally, the co-occurrence of ASD and epilepsy warrants genetic investigation beyond usual recommendations for ASD (Lee, Smith, & Paciorkowski, 2015).

Sleeping and eating problems

Many problems that are not uncommon in other children are reported in children with ASD, including sleep disturbance and eating problems, most commonly fussy eating. There are not thought to be any specific differences in neurological processes that underpin these behavioural problems. Instead, these problems are thought to be similar but more exaggerated and more difficult to change due to ASD characteristics, notably resistance to change. To illustrate, sensory sensitivities complicate eating problems, and a lack of interest in usual rewards and natural social reinforcers, complicate management of sleeping problems. Melatonin is commonly prescribed to treat sleep disorder in children with ASD and has been shown to be effective in reducing sleep onset latency, but not behavioural sleep disturbances such as night-time waking (Gringras et al., 2012).

Stereotypes and tics

Stereotypical movements seen in ASD are still not well explained in terms of their underpinning mechanism or their purpose, which is often thought to be self-soothing or enjoyable (see Chapter 12, Tourette syndrome). Movements that can be difficult to distinguish from stereotypies, including vocal and motor tics, are more common in ASD. Motor and vocal tics that are sufficiently varied in type and frequency are diagnosed as Tourette syndrome, which is also more common in ASD. Whether a stereotypy or tic should be managed depends on the impact it is having on the person with ASD and those around them, either directly, for example causing them harm, or indirectly, by limiting their engagement in social and learning opportunities. Because the function of stereotypies is often not clear, their disruption can cause unexpected consequences which may be worse than the primary behaviour. Behavioural interventions and medication can be trialled for tics, but they are not always effective and may have side effects. Optimal management involves increasing the understanding of the movement or vocalization for those around the person with ASD, so it does not disrupt interactions and does not increase stress for the individual.

Mental health problems

Comorbid anxiety is common, with a synthesis of the literature identifying a diagnosis of one or more anxiety disorders in 40% of young people with ASD (van Steensel, Bögels, & Perrin, 2011). Current thinking endorses the likelihood of multiple pathways to the co-occurrence of ASD and anxiety, with some fundamental to ASD and others with ASD as a secondary occurrence. For example, for some individuals anxiety may contribute to difficulties with social communication and other behaviours. For others, anxiety may be secondary to a lack of understanding of social communication, making everyday encounters stressful because they require considerable cognitive effort and can result in public ridicule if they don't go well. Regardless, the families of individuals with ASD rate anxiety as one of the major issues requiring attention (McConachie et al., 2015). Management is based on evidence-informed strategies for individuals with anxiety who do not have ASD (NICE, 2014), management and intervention being tailored to the diagnosed type of anxiety disorder, age and ability, with further adaptations so the intervention is appropriate to each individual's needs, strengths and difficulties.

Depression and other mood disorders can also co-occur with ASD (Bitsika & Sharpley, 2015) and should be considered if there are behaviour changes, because low mood may not be expressed. There is an increased risk of psychosis in ASD, although the overall risk is still low (3%; Jones, Thapar, Lewis, & Zammit, 2012). The co-occurrence of psychosis and ASD is not yet understood for all instances, but a gene that increases risk of both ASD and psychosis, either in isolation or combination, has now been identified (see Chapter Psychosis and Depression).

Neuropsychology

In general, the cognitive profile of ASD tends to be characterised by uneven verbal and non-verbal profiles, with intact, or superior, ability for tasks requiring a high degree of attention to detail, such as visuospatial processing, matrix reasoning and block design tasks. Tasks demanding a high degree of abstract processing, such as language comprehension and the use of pragmatic language, are often considered to be impaired in children with ASD. Attention is one factor that plays an important role in these processes. Individuals with ASD are generally able to demonstrate sustained attention, yet have difficulty with reorienting attention (Casey, Gordon, Mannheim, & Rumsey, 1993). This can be exemplified by individual's ability to be heavily focused on a particular aspect of their environment (e.g., restricted and repetitive behaviours) and also having difficulty in orientating attention (e.g., re-orientating attentional gaze) to another stimulus (see Sanders, Johnson, Garavan, Gill, & Gallagher, 2008 for a review). Motivational factors may also contribute. Reduced social motivation, for example, may explain (at least to some degree) fixation or restricted interest toward non-social stimuli and also difficulty in re-orienting attention to social-stimuli (Chevallier, Kohls, Troiani, Brodkin, & Schultz, 2012). There is, however, considerably less research investigating attentional and motivational factors (Chevallier et al., 2012; Sanders et al., 2008) in comparison to the cognitive theories discussed below. From a neuropsychological perspective, there have traditionally been three prominent, and overlapping, cognitive theories associated with both clinical and non-clinical features of the ASD: Theory of Mind (ToM), Weak Central Coherence (WCC), and Executive Dysfunction (Rajendran & Mitchell, 2007). It is important to note that these theories do not provide mutually exclusive accounts of the neuropsychological profile of ASD, nor are they found in all individuals with a diagnosis of ASD.

ToM (or mentalising), a concept predominantly associated with social impairment, is the ability to understand the thoughts and feelings of others (Baron-Cohen, 2001), which also requires understanding your own thoughts and feelings. While there are many accounts of individuals with ASD being able to pass ToM tests in a laboratory setting (Rajendran & Mitchell, 2007), this does not directly translate to improved behaviours requiring ToM for all of these individuals who are able to pass ToM tasks (Frith, 1994).

The WCC theory reflects a preference towards processing of small details rather than global processing (Happé, 2005), having implications for impairments as well as savant abilities seen in ASD (Frith & Happé, 1994). WCC has been linked to superior performances in tasks requiring detail-focused processing such as mathematics, memory or visuo-spatial ability (Howlin, Goode, Hutton, & Rutter, 2009).

The Executive Dysfunction (EF) theory originally explained the difficulties individuals with ASD experience in higher-order cognitive processes such as planning, mental flexibility, impulse control and behavioural inhibition (Hill, 2004a, 2004b). In considering the role of EF in relation to characteristics of ASD, it has been suggested that poor inhibitory control may underpin the restricted and repetitive behaviours and interests which form part of the core diagnostic criteria for ASD (Lopez, Lincoln, Ozonoff, & Lai, 2005; Sanders et al., 2008). Further, planning and shifting (mental flexibility) have recently been suggested to play an important role in ToM (Kimhi, Shoam-Kugelmas, Ben-Artzi, Ben-Moshe, & Bauminger-Zviely, 2014) and therefore may have implications for social deficits.

Neurocognitive difficulties may also impact on academic performance in this population. Children with ASD generally show academic performance commensurate with their cognitive functioning; however, similar to their uneven cognitive profiles, academic profiles are often idiosyncratic and uneven (Mayes & Calhoun, 2003). Difficulties with switching attention have been associated with poorer mathematics performance in children with ASD (May, Rinehart, Wilding, & Cornish, 2013). Other common areas of academic difficulty include reading comprehension, abstract reasoning related tasks and handwriting (Mayes & Calhoun, 2003; Whitby & Mancil, 2009).

Neuropathology

There has been an intense focus on ASD neurobiological investigations in the last decade. Investigations of head-circumference, as well as neuroimaging studies, have suggested that children with ASD display an atypical brain growth trajectory during early childhood, with early brain overgrowth followed by a hasty cessation of growth (Redcay & Courchesne, 2005). However, a meta-analysis of the head-circumference literature in ASD cautions that the use of population norms may yield biased results (Raznahan et al., 2013).

Many studies have identified atypical neural connectivity in ASD, both structurally and functionally (Wass, 2011). Broadly, atypical connectivity in ASD is characterised by long-distance hypo-connectivity and short distance hyper-connectivity (Vissers, Cohen, & Geurts, 2012). Connections with, and within, the frontal lobe have been reported to be most severely atypical (Carper & Courchesne, 2005; Courchesne & Pierce, 2005). The fronto-striatal and fronto-parietal networks have also been implicated in higher order cognitive functions (Geurts, Corbett, & Solomon, 2009; Minshew & Keller, 2010; Sanders et al., 2008). Atypical structure (Langen et al., 2014) and function (Delmonte, Gallagher, O'Hanlon, McGrath, & Balsters, 2013) of the fronto-striatal network have long been suggested to be related to the core characteristics of ASD (see Bradshaw, 2001). The neuroanatomical findings from neuroimaging in older individuals suggests slight or no differences between individuals with and without ASD (Aylward, Minshew, Field, Sparks, & Singh, 2002; Haar, Berman, Behrmann, & Dinstein, 2014; Tepest et al., 2010).

Post-mortem research supports microstructural abnormality (Amaral, Schumann, & Nordahl, 2008; Hutsler & Casanova, 2015) characterised by an increased number of minicolumns (albeit narrower) in individuals with ASD (Casanova, Buxhoeveden, Switala, & Roy, 2002; Casanova, El-Baz, Vanbogaert, Narahari, & Switala, 2010). Minicolumnar pathology in ASD is most consistently noted in the frontal regions of the brain (Buxhoeveden et al., 2006), and has also been reported in the temporal cortices (Casanova et al., 2002). Functionally, and from a neurochemical perspective, minicolumnar pathology in ASD may be associated with inhibitory dysfunction and the gamma-aminobutyric acid (GABA) system (Casanova, 2006).

Neuropathology in ASD is not limited to the cerebrum, with reports that the cerebellum is enlarged in ASD, although this may be proportional to cerebral volume, and reduced anatomical volume has been identified for some cerebellar structures (Amaral et al., 2008; Fatemi et al., 2012; Stanfield et al., 2008). Post-mortem (Skefos et al., 2014; Whitney, Kemper, Rosene, Bauman, & Blatt, 2009) and in-vivo (Jeong, Tiwari, Behen, Chugani, H.T., & Chugani, D.C., 2014) investigations provide strong evidence for smaller, and a reduced number of, Purkinje cells in the cerebella of individuals with ASD. Moreover, using mouse models, Tsai et al. (2012) demonstrate that loss of the TSC1 gene (mutation of which is related to tuberous sclerosis complex, a disorder for which ASD is a common comorbidity) in cerebellar Purkinje cells may result in both social and behavioural impairments akin to autistic symptomatology.

Atypical cerebellar anatomy may be related to characteristics of ASD including higher-order cognitive/affective deficits in ASD (D'Mello, Crocetti, Mostofsky, & Stoodley, 2015; Jeong et al., 2014, Wang, Kloth, & Badura, 2014). Wang et al. (2014) highlights that there may be critical time points in life during which cerebellar perturbation can impact upon cognitive and social processes associated with ASD. Impaired functional connectivity has been noted in both sensorimotor as well as supramodal cerebro-cerebellar pathways in ASD (Khan et al., 2015) with atypical cerebellar function present during motor (Allen & Courchesne, 2014; Mostofsky et al., 2009) and cognitive tasks (attention; Allen & Courchesne, 2014; Murphy et al., 2014) in individuals with ASD. See Sivaratnam, Newman, Tonge, and Rinehart (2015) for a review of non-biological determinants of social and communication impairments in children and considerations in assessment.

Neuromotor profile

From an early age children with ASD show delays in fine and gross motor development compared to typically developing children (Landa & Garrett-Mayer, 2006; Ozonoff et al., 2008). The recent inclusion of the term "odd gait" (Associated features supporting diagnosis; p. 55) in DSM-5 does not do justice to the extent of motor problems that some children with ASD experience. Observational and instrumented gait studies have suggested that movement disturbance may be an early ASD diagnostic sign (Teitelbaum, P., Teitelbaum, O., Nye, Fryman, & Maurer, 1998) with evidence of cerebellar-related gait anomalies that distinguished children with ASD from non-ASD children (Nayate, Bradshaw, & Rinehart, 2005; Rinehart et al., 2006). The most recent systematic reviews have confirmed motor variability and motor planning difficulties as the main characteristics in children with ASD (Fournier, Hass, Naik, Lodha, & Cauraugh, 2010). The motor literature has yielded consistent biomarkers for differentiating ASD from non-ASD cohorts (Dowd, Rinehart, & McGinley, 2010), while sibling cohort studies using measures associated with diagnostic differentiation, such as language and cognitive functioning, have been much less clear (Durand, 2014; Ozonoff et al., 2014; Sharma, Woolfson, & Hunter, 2012). There is emerging evidence that the gait of children with ASD may differ from those with ADHD (Nayate et al., 2012; Papadopoulos, McGinley, Bradshaw, & Rinehart, 2014). While the emergence and presence of motor problems affecting gait in ASD is now well recognised, the pattern and relative stability of these impairments over early childhood is not yet known, limiting their application to screening or intervention programs.

Genetics and Epigenetics

In recent years there has been an explosion in publications about the genetics of ASD, bringing an increased understanding of the genetic pathways to ASD for an increasing minority of those given the diagnosis. One of the first findings that put genetics at the top of the list of causes for ASD was a high concordance in monozygotic twins (Folstein & Rutter, 1977). Subsequent publications have confirmed that concordance for a diagnosis of ASD in monozygotic twins ranges from 70–90% (Hallmayer et al., 2011).

Four main types of genetic underpinnings of ASD are now well described. The most well-known are specific genetic problems associated with a known phenotype that incurs an increased risk of ASD compared to the general population, for example tuberous sclerosis. Recently new genetic testing techniques have identified single gene mutations. These single gene mutations are often referred to as copy number variants (CNV) or single nucleotide polymorphisms (SNP). Single gene mutations can be inherited or occur during the first stages of development in pregnancy. They are often a deletion or a duplication of a DNA sequence. The Simons Foundation Autism Research Initiative (SFARI) is now collating genetic findings for ASD and community scoring that indicates the confidence with which reported genes are likely to be associated with autism spectrum disorder. Results are available at this website (https://gene.sfari.org/autdb/GS_Home.do). Researchers are now trying to establish common pathways through which different gene mutations could act to produce problems of the type seen in ASD (Pinto et al., 2014).

There is also emerging evidence about common variant mutations. One study (Gaugler et al., 2014), awaiting replication, found that nearly 50% of all individuals diagnosed with ASD had multiple common variant gene mutations. In other words, individuals with ASD had gene mutations that many of us would also have, but more of them. Common variant genes as a cause of ASD could explain some of the heterogeneity of ASD, and also why individuals without ASD can have one or more behaviours that are similar to individuals with ASD.

As our ability to identify small genetic changes has increased, so too has our ability to assess genetic changes in different cell types from different organ systems, like blood and the brain. A genetic change in one, but not all, cells is known as a somatic cell line mutation, with the gene altered after some differentiation of cells to different organ types has occurred. It is possible that there are yet unidentified genetic mutations present only in the brain of people with ASD, but advancement in this area is limited by availability of brain tissue.

Finally, an understanding of how regions that are part of our DNA but are not genes can influence the way genes work is emerging. This field is known as epigenetics, with regions of DNA around genes sometimes thought of as "gene switches". The role of epigenetics in ASD is still being explored. If epigenetic differences are found, they could provide one pathway through which experiences during pregnancy and delivery could influence whether a person develops ASD, and explain the between twin differences already identified. For example, there is some speculation that maternal stress occurring in the pre-, peri-, and postnatal stages of development can influence the onset and clinical severity of ASD through epigenetic changes (see Kinney, Munir, Crowley, & Miller, 2008; O'Connor, Heron, Golding, & Glover, 2003).

Interventions

There have been many suggested interventions for ASD. Most tested and widely used are those that incorporate behavioural, developmental and/or communication strategies aimed at increasing learning, communication, and improving function and participation. There are also widely used interventions available for comorbid conditions, such as anxiety disorders, with adaptation required for individuals with ASD.

Psychopharmacology is widely used for ASD with reports that at least one medication is taken by a substantial number of children and young people with ASD (Rosenberg et al., 2010; van Steensel et al., 2011). No medication has been proven to change the core features of ASD with Level 1 or 2 evidence. Some medications have been proven to change behaviours that challenge or positively influence restricted or repetitive behaviours, mood or anxiety, but not without side effects (risperidone, other antipsychotics, selective serotonin reuptake inhibitors SSRIs). In general, medication is appropriate when behaviours place the individual with ASD or their family at risk, or when behavioural interventions have not been successful and a behaviour needs to change to allow other important interventions to proceed and/or to improve quality of life for the individual or family. Clear goals to be achieved by the introduction of the medication should be established prior to commencement of a medication, and risks and benefits monitored to inform decisions about continuation or cessation (NICE, 2013). Medications that improve cognition in adults, such as N-methyl d-aspartate (NMDA) receptor antagonists and cholinesterase inhibitors, are now being trialled in individuals with ASD, but are not proven to be effective. Biological therapies that are used in mental health disorders, like transcranial magnetic stimulation, are also being explored as interventions for ASD (Enticott et al., 2014). Preliminary findings from therapeutic agents such as oxytocin have been mixed in showing clinical efficacy (Dadds et al., 2014; Yatawara, Einfeld, Hickie, Davenport, & Guastella, 2015). There is increasing evidence that parent-focused interventions that involve education and behaviour management can improve child adaptive behaviour and symptoms of ASD (McConachie & Diggle, 2007), sleep disorder (Papadopoulos et al., 2015) and the mental health and adjustment of parents with children, particularly those with associated intellectual disability (Tonge et al., 2014).

It is important to note that many interventions available for neurodevelopmental disorders today are currently considered as complementary and alternative therapies. Despite widespread availability and uptake, there is no evidence for their effectiveness in improving the core features of ASD. A number have been proven not to work for improving core features of ASD, and/or are considered to have too many potential risks to be used. Secretin and chelation therapy should not be used for any autism characteristics. Exclusion diets (like gluten and casein free diets) and hyperbaric oxygen should not be used for core features of ASD. Neurofeedback and auditory integration therapy do not improve speech and language, and omega-3-fatty acids do not help sleep problems (NICE, 2013).

With gene discovery and the advent of functional MRI has come hope that a clearer understanding of the mechanisms for ASD will facilitate rapid development of drugs that are able to act in a way that is targeted to the particular genetic or neurological deficit and personalised for each individual's needs, medication processing and tolerance profiles. However, we have not yet achieved this for many conditions that have well understood and less complex mechanisms than ASD, so the timeframe for this is still uncertain.

Summary

While ASD was once referred to as 'the dementia of childhood' and 'the most destructive disorder of youth' (Bradshaw, 2001, p. 167), recent research has highlighted that ASD is a heterogeneous disorder, with many comorbidities at play that give rise to a large variation of health and well-being and considerable variation in outcomes. We now understand that motor impairment, sleep disorder and epilepsy are common complications in children with ASD (Jeste, 2011). Awareness of the multi-dimensional, multi-brain system conceptualization of ASD has seen intervention frameworks move away from the notion of 'curing ASD' toward interventions that enable individuals with ASD to adjust to their environment and delivering targeted interventions tailored to each individual's unique clinical presentation and their family's needs and preferences. Social frameworks and intervention approaches have also made us aware that adjustment of the environment and our acceptance of difference can maximise participation for individuals with ASD.

Further readings

Lenroot, Rhoshel K., & Yeung, Pui Ka. (2013). Heterogeneity within autism spectrum disorders: What have we learned from neuroimaging studies? *Frontiers in Human Neuroscience*, 7. doi: 10.3389/fnhum.2013.00733.

Mayes, S. D., & Calhoun, S. L. (2003). Ability profiles in children with autism influence of age and IQ. *Autism*, 7(1), 65–80.

NHS. (2013). Autism spectrum disorder - Treatment. From http://www.nhs.uk/conditions/autistic-spectrum-disorder/pages/treatment.aspx.

NHS. (2013). Treatment options for tics. From http://www.nhs.uk/conditions/tics/pages/treatmentoptions.aspx.

Weitlauf, A., McPheeters, M., Peters, B., Sathe, N., Travis, R., Aiello, R., … Warren, Z. (2014). Therapies for Children with Autism Spectrum Disorder: Behavioral Interventions Update. from http://effectivehealthcare.ahrq.gov/index.cfm/search-for-guides-reviews-and-reports/?productid=1945&pageaction=displayproduct.

Whitby, P. J. S., & Mancil, G. R. (2009). Academic achievement profiles of children with high functioning autism and Asperger syndrome: A review of the literature. *Education & Training in Developmental Disabilities*, 551–560. doi: 10.1177/1362361303007001006.

References

Allen, G., & Courchesne, E. (2014). Differential effects of developmental cerebellar abnormality on cognitive and motor functions in the cerebellum: An fMRI study of autism. *American Journal of Psychiatry, 160*(2), 262–273. doi: 10.1176/appi.ajp.160.2.262.

Amaral, D. G., Schumann, C. M., & Nordahl, C. W. (2008). Neuroanatomy of autism. *Trends in Neurosciences, 31*(3), 137–145. doi: 10.1016/j.tins.2007.12.005.

American Psychiatric Association. (2000). *Diagnostic & Statistical Manual of Mental Disorders - Text Revision* (4 ed.). Washington, DC: Author.

American Psychiatric Association. (2013). *Diagnostic & Statistical Manual of Mental Disorders* (5 ed.). Washington, DC: American Psychiatric Publishing.

Aylward, E. H., Minshew, N. J., Field, K., Sparks, B. F., & Singh, N. (2002). Effects of age on brain volume and head circumference in autism. *Neurology, 59*(2), 175–183. doi: 10.1212/WNL.59.2.175.

Baron-Cohen, S. (2001). Theory of mind in autism: A review. *Special Issue of the International Review of Mental Retardation, 23*. doi: 10.1016/S0074-7750(00)80010-5.

Bitsika, V., & Sharpley, C. F. (2015). Differences in the prevalence, severity and symptom profiles of depression in boys and adolescents with an autism spectrum disorder versus normally developing controls. *International Journal of Disability, Development & Education, 62*(2), 158–167. doi: 10.1080/1034912X.2014.998179.

Bradshaw, J. L. (2001). Developmental disorders of the frontostriatal system. *Neuropsychological Neuropsychiatric & Evolutionary Perspectives, Psychology Press/Taylor & Francis, Hove.*

Bryson, S. E. (1996). Brief report: Epidemiology of autism. *Journal of Autism and Developmental Disorders, 26*(2), 165–167. doi: 10.1007/BF02172005.

Buxhoeveden, D., Semendeferi, K., Buckwalter, J., Schenker, N., Switzer, R., & Courchesne, E. (2006). Reduced minicolumns in the frontal cortex of patients with autism. *Neuropathology & Applied Neurobiology, 32*(5), 483–491. doi: 10.1111/j.1365-2990.2006.00745.x.

Carper, R. A., & Courchesne, E. (2005). Localized enlargement of the frontal cortex in early autism. *Biological Psychiatry, 57*(2), 126–133. doi: 10.1016/j.biopsych.2004.11.005.

Casanova, M. F. (2006). Neuropathological and genetic findings in autism: The significance of a putative minicolumnopathy. *The Neuroscientist, 12*(5), 435–441. doi: 10.1177/1073858406290375.

Casanova, M. F., Buxhoeveden, D. P., Switala, A. E., & Roy, E. (2002). Minicolumnar pathology in autism. *Neurology, 58*(3), 428–432. doi: 10.1212/WNL.58.3.428.

Casanova, M. F., El-Baz, A., Vanbogaert, E., Narahari, P., & Switala, A. (2010). A topographic study of minicolumnar core width by lamina comparison between autistic subjects and controls: Possible minicolumnar disruption due to an anatomical element in-common to multiple laminae. *Brain Pathology, 20*(2), 451–458. doi: 10.1111/j.1750-3639.2009.00319.x.

Casey, B., Gordon, C., Mannheim, G. B., & Rumsey, J. M. (1993). Dysfunctional attention in autistic savants. *Journal of Clinical & Experimental Neuropsychology, 15*(6), 933–946. doi: 10.1080/01688639308402609.

CDC. (2014). Prevalence of autism spectrum disorders among children aged 8 years - Autism and developmental diabilities monitoring network, 11 sites, United States, 2010. *Morbidity & Mortality Weekly Report, 63*(2), 1–22.

Chevallier, C., Kohls, G., Troiani, V., Brodkin, E. S., & Schultz, R. T. (2012). The social motivation theory of autism. *Trends in Cognitive Sciences, 16*(4), 231–239. doi: 10.1016/j.tics.2012.02.007.

Courchesne, E., & Pierce, K. (2005). Why the frontal cortex in autism might be talking only to itself: Local over-connectivity but long-distance disconnection. *Current Opinion in Neurobiology, 15*(2), 225–230. doi: 10.1016/j.conb.2005.03.001.

D'Mello, A. M., Crocetti, D., Mostofsky, S. H., & Stoodley, C. J. (2015). Cerebellar gray matter and lobular volumes correlate with core autism symptoms. *NeuroImage: Clinical, 7*, 631–639. doi: 10.1016/j.nicl.2015.02.007.

Dadds, M. R., MacDonald, E., Cauchi, A., Williams, K., Levy, F., & Brennan, J. (2014). Nasal oxytocin for social deficits in childhood autism: A randomized controlled trial. *Journal of Autism & Developmental Disorders, 44*(3), 521–531. doi: 10.1007/s10803-013-1899-3.

Delmonte, S., Gallagher, L., O'Hanlon, E., McGrath, J., & Balsters, J. H. (2013). Functional and structural connectivity of frontostriatal circuitry in Autism Spectrum Disorder. *Frontiers in Human Neuroscience, 7*. doi: 10.3389/fnhum.2013.00430.

Dowd, A. M., Rinehart, N. J., & McGinley, J. (2010). Motor function in children with autism: Why is this relevant to psychologists? *Clinical Psychologist, 14*(3), 90–96. doi: 10.1080/13284207.2010.525532.

Durand, V. M. (2014). *Screening, Diagnosis, and Assessment, in Autism Spectrum Disorder: A Clinical Guide for General Practitioners.* Washington, DC: American Psychological Association.

Elberling, H., Linneberg, A., Olsen, E. M., Houmann, T., Rask, C. U., Goodman, R., & Skovgaard, A. M. (2014). Infancy predictors of hyperkinetic and pervasive developmental disorders at ages 5–7 years: Results from the Copenhagen Child Cohort CCC2000. *Journal of Child Psychology & Psychiatry, 55*(12), 1328–1335. doi: 10.1111/jcpp.12256.

Elsabbagh, M., Divan, G., Koh, Y. J., Kim, Y. S., Kauchali, S., Marcín, C., … Wang, C. (2012). Global prevalence of autism and other pervasive developmental disorders. *Autism Research, 5*(3), 160–179. doi: 10.1002/aur.239.

Enticott, P. G., Fitzgibbon, B. M., Kennedy, H. A., Arnold, S. L., Elliot, D., Peachey, A., … Fitzgerald, P. B. (2014). A double-blind, randomized trial of deep repetitive transcranial magnetic stimulation (rTMS) for autism spectrum disorder. *Brain Stimulation, 7*(2), 206–211. doi: 10.1016/j.brs.2013.10.004.

Fatemi, S. H., Aldinger, K. A., Ashwood, P., Bauman, M. L., Blaha, C. D., Blatt, G. J., … Dickson, P. E. (2012). Consensus paper: Pathological role of the cerebellum in autism. *The Cerebellum, 11*(3), 777–807. doi: 10.1007/s12311-012-0355-9.

Folstein, S., & Rutter, M. (1977). Infantile autism: A genetic study of 21 twin pairs. *Journal of Child Psychology & Psychiatry, 18*(4), 297–321. doi: 10.1111/j.1469-7610.1977.tb00443.x.

Fournier, K. A., Hass, C. J., Naik, S. K., Lodha, N., & Cauraugh, J. H. (2010). Motor coordination in autism spectrum disorders: A synthesis and meta-analysis. *Journal of Autism & Developmental Disorders, 40*(10), 1227–1240. doi: 10.1007/s10803-010-0981-3.

Frith, U. (1994). Autism and theory of mind in everyday life. *Social Development, 3*(2), 108–124. doi: 10.1111/j.1467-9507.1994.tb00031.x.

Frith, U., & Happé, F. (1994). Autism: Beyond "theory of mind". *Cognition, 50*(1), 115–132. doi: 10.1016/0010-0277(94)90024-8.

Gargaro, B. A., Rinehart, N. J., Bradshaw, J. L., Tonge, B. J., & Sheppard, D. M. (2011). Autism and ADHD: How far have we come in the comorbidity debate? *Neuroscience & Biobehavioral Reviews, 35*(5), 1081–1088. doi: 10.1016/j.neubiorev.2010.11.002.

Gaugler, T., Klei, L., Sanders, S. J., Bodea, C. A., Goldberg, A. P., Lee, A. B., … Reichert, J. (2014). Most genetic risk for autism resides with common variation. *Nature Genetics, 46*(8), 881–885. doi: 10.1038/ng.3039.

Geurts, H. M., Corbett, B., & Solomon, M. (2009). The paradox of cognitive flexibility in autism. *Trends in Cognitive Sciences, 13*(2), 74–82. doi: 10.1016/j.tics.2008.11.006.

Gillberg, C. (2010). The ESSENCE in child psychiatry: Early symptomatic syndromes eliciting neurodevelopmental clinical examinations. *Research in Developmental Disabilities, 31*(6), 1543–1551. doi: 10.1016/j.ridd.2010.06.002.

Gillberg, C., & Wing, L. (1999). Autism: Not an extremely rare disorder. *Acta Psychiatrica Scandinavica, 99*(6), 399–406. doi: 10.1111/j.1600-0447.1999.tb00984.x.

Gringras, P., Gamble, C., Jones, A., Wiggs, L., Williamson, P., Sutcliffe, A., … Allport, T. (2012). Melatonin for sleep problems in children with neurodevelopmental disorders: Randomised double masked placebo controlled trial. *British Medical Journal, 345*, e6664. doi: http://dx.doi.org/10.1136/bmj.e6664.

Haar, S., Berman, S., Behrmann, M., & Dinstein, I. (2014). Anatomical abnormalities in autism? *Cerebral Cortex*. doi: 10.1093/cercor/bhu242.

Hallmayer, J., Cleveland, S., Torres, A., Phillips, J., Cohen, B., Torigoe, T., … Smith, K. (2011). Genetic heritability and shared environmental factors among twin pairs with autism. *Archives of General Psychiatry, 68*(11), 1095–1102. doi: 10.1001/archgenpsychiatry.2011.76.

Happé, F. (2005). The weak central coherence account of autism. *Handbook of Autism & Pervasive Developmental Disorders, Volume 1, Third Edition*, 640–649.

Hill, E. L. (2004a). Evaluating the theory of executive dysfunction in autism. *Developmental Review, 24*(2), 189–233. doi:10.1016/j.dr.2004.01.001.

Hill, E. L. (2004b). Executive dysfunction in autism. *Trends in Cognitive Sciences, 8*(1), 26–32. doi: 10.1016/j.tics.2003.11.003.

Howlin, P., Goode, S., Hutton, J., & Rutter, M. (2009). Savant skills in autism: Psychometric approaches and parental reports. *Philosophical Transactions of the Royal Society B: Biological Sciences, 364*(1522), 1359–1367. doi: 10.1098/rstb.2008.0328.

Howlin, P., & Moss, P. (2012). Adults with autism spectrum disorders. *Canadian Journal of Psychiatry, 57*(5), 275–283.

Hutsler, J. J., & Casanova, M. F. (2015). Review: Cortical construction in autism spectrum disorder: Columns, connectivity and the subplate. *Neuropathology & Applied Neurobiology*. doi: 10.1111/nan.12227.

Jacquemont, S., Coe, B. P., Hersch, M., Duyzend, M. H., Krumm, N., Bergmann, S., … Eichler, E. E. (2014). A higher mutational burden in females supports a "female protective model" in neurodevelopmental disorders. *The American Journal of Human Genetics, 94*(3), 415–425. doi: 10.1016/j.ajhg.2014.02.001.

Jeong, J. W., Tiwari, V. N., Behen, M. E., Chugani, H. T., & Chugani, D. C. (2014). In vivo detection of reduced Purkinje cell fibers with diffusion MRI tractography in children with autistic spectrum disorders. *Frontiers in Human Neuroscience, 8*. doi: 10.3389/fnhum.2014.00110.

Jeste, S. S. (2011). The neurology of autism spectrum disorders. *Current Opinion in Neurology, 24*(2), 132–139. doi: 10.1097/WCO.0b013e3283446450.

Jones, R. B., Thapar, A., Lewis, G., & Zammit, S. (2012). The association between early autistic traits and psychotic experiences in adolescence. *Schizophrenia Research, 135*(1), 164–169. doi: 10.1016/j.schres.2011.11.037.

Khan, A. J., Nair, A., Keown, C. L., Datko, M. C., Lincoln, A. J., & Müller, R. A. (2015). Cerebro-cerebellar resting-state functional connectivity in children and adolescents with autism spectrum disorder. *Biological Psychiatry*. doi: 10.1016/j.biopsych.2015.03.024.

Kim, S. H., Thurm, A., Shumway, S., & Lord, C. (2013). Multisite study of new autism diagnostic interview-revised (ADI-R) algorithms for toddlers and young preschoolers. *Journal of Autism & Developmental Disorders, 43*(7), 1527–1538. doi: 10.1007/s10803-012-1696-4.

Kimhi, Y., Shoam-Kugelmas, D., Ben-Artzi, G. A., Ben-Moshe, I., & Bauminger-Zviely, N. (2014). Theory of mind and executive function in preschoolers with typical development versus intellectually able preschoolers with autism spectrum disorder. *Journal of Autism & Developmental Disorders, 44*(9), 2341–2354.

Kinney, D. K., Munir, K. M., Crowley, D. J., & Miller, A. M. (2008). Prenatal stress and risk for autism. *Neuroscience & Biobehavioral Reviews, 32*(8), 1519–1532. doi: 10.1016/j.neubiorev.2008.06.004.

Kirkovski, M., Enticott, P. G., & Fitzgerald, P. B. (2013). A review of the role of female gender in autism spectrum disorders. *Journal of Autism & Developmental Disorders, 43*, 2584–2603. doi: 10.1007/s10803-013-1811-1.

Knapp, M., Romeo, R., & Beecham, J. (2009). Economic cost of autism in the UK. *Autism, 13*(3), 317–336. doi: 10.1177/1362361309104246.

Landa, R., & Garrett-Mayer, E. (2006). Development in infants with autism spectrum disorders: A prospective study. *Journal of Child Psychology & Psychiatry, 47*(6), 629–638. doi: 10.1111/j.1469-7610.2006.01531.x.

Langen, M., Bos, D., Noordermeer, S. D., Nederveen, H., van Engeland, H., & Durston, S. (2014). Changes in the development of striatum are involved in repetitive behavior in autism. *Biological Psychiatry, 76*(5), 405–411. doi: 10.1016/j.biopsych.2013.08.013.

Lee, B. H., Smith, T., & Paciorkowski, A. R. (2015). Autism spectrum disorder and epilepsy: Disorders with a shared biology. *Epilepsy & Behavior, 47*, 191–201. doi: 10.1016/j.yebeh.2015.03.017.

Lopez, B. R., Lincoln, A. J., Ozonoff, S., & Lai, Z. (2005). Examining the relationship between executive functions and restricted, repetitive symptoms of autistic disorder. *Journal of Autism & Developmental Disorders, 35*(4), 445–460. doi: 10.1007/s10803-005-5035-x.

Lord, C., Rutter, M., DiLavore, P. C., Risi, S., Gotham, K., & Bishop, S. L. (2012). *Autism Diagnostic Observation Schedule: ADOS-2*. Los Angeles, CA: Western Psychological Services.

Lord, C., Rutter, M., & Le Couteur, A. (1994). Autism diagnostic interview-revised: A revised version of a diagnostic interview for caregivers of individuals with possible pervasive developmental disorders. *Journal of Autism & Developmental Disorders, 24*(5), 659–685. doi: 10.1007/BF02172145.

Matson, J. L., & Goldin, R. L. (2014). Diagnosing young children with autism. *International Journal of Developmental Neuroscience, 39*, 44–48. doi: 10.1016/j.ijdevneu.2014.02.003.

May, T., Cornish, K., & Rinehart, N. (2014). Does gender matter? A one year follow-up of autistic, attention and anxiety symptoms in high-functioning children with autism spectrum disorder. *Journal of Autism & Developmental Disorders, 44*(5), 1077–1086. doi: 10.1007/s10803-013-1964-y.

May, T., Rinehart, N., Wilding, J., & Cornish, K. (2013). The role of attention in the academic attainment of children with autism spectrum disorder. *Journal of Autism & Developmental Disorders, 43*(9), 2147–2158. doi: 10.1007/s10803-013-1766-2.

Mayes, S. D., & Calhoun, S. L. (2003). Ability profiles in children with autism influence of age and IQ. *Autism, 7*(1), 65–80. doi: 10.1177/1362361303007001006.

McConachie, H., & Diggle, T. (2007). Parent implemented early intervention for young children with autism spectrum disorder: A systematic review. *Journal of Evaluation in Clinical Practice, 13*(1), 120–129. doi: 10.1111/j.1365-2753.2006.00674.x.

McConachie, H., Parr, J. R., Glod, M., Hanratty, J., Livingstone, N., Oono, I. P., … Williams, K. (2015). Systematic review of tools to measure outcomes for young children with autism spectrum disorder. *Health Technology Assessment, 19*(41), 1–538. doi: 10.3310/hta19410.

Minshew, N. J., & Keller, T. A. (2010). The nature of brain dysfunction in autism: Functional brain imaging studies. *Current Opinion in Neurology, 23*(2), 124–130. doi: 10.1097/WCO.0b013e32833782d4.

Mostofsky, S. H., Powell, S. K., Simmonds, D. J., Goldberg, M. C., Caffo, B., & Pekar, J. J. (2009). Decreased connectivity and cerebellar activity in autism during motor task performance. *Brain*, awp088. doi: http://dx.doi.org/10.1093/brain/awp088.

Murphy, C. M., Christakou, A., Daly, E. M., Ecker, C., Giampietro, V., Brammer, M., … Murphy, D. G. (2014). Abnormal functional activation and maturation of fronto-striato-temporal and cerebellar regions during sustained attention in autism spectrum disorder. *American Journal of Psychiatry, 171*(10), 1107–1116. doi: http://dx.doi.org/10.1176/appi.ajp.2014.12030352.

Nayate, A., Bradshaw, J. L., & Rinehart, N. J. (2005). Autism and Asperger's disorder: Are they movement disorders involving the cerebellum and/or basal ganglia? *Brain Research Bulletin, 67*(4), 327–334. doi: 10.1016/j.brainresbull.2005.07.011.

Nayate, A., Tonge, B. J., Bradshaw, J. L., McGinley, J. L., Iansek, R., & Rinehart, N. J. (2012). Differentiation of high-functioning autism and Asperger's disorder based on neuromotor behaviour. *Journal of Autism & Developmental Disorders, 42*(5), 707–717. doi: 10.1007/s10803-011-1299-5.

NICE. (2013, August). *Autism: The Management and Support of Children and Young People on the Autism Spectrum.* from https://www.nice.org.uk/guidance/cg170/chapter/1-Recommendations.

NICE. (2014, February). *Anxiety Disorders.* from https://www.nice.org.uk/guidance/qs53.

O'Connor, T. G., Heron, J., Golding, J., & Glover, V. (2003). Maternal antenatal anxiety and behavioural/emotional problems in children: A test of a programming hypothesis. *Journal of Child Psychology & Psychiatry, 44*(7), 1025–1036. doi: 10.1111/1469-7610.00187.

Ozonoff, S., Young, G. S., Belding, A., Hill, M., Hill, A., Hutman, T., ... Schwichtenberg, A. (2014). The broader autism phenotype in infancy: When does it emerge? *Journal of the American Academy of Child & Adolescent Psychiatry, 53*(4), 398–407. e392. doi: doi:10.1016/j.jaac.2013.12.020.

Ozonoff, S., Young, G. S., Goldring, S., Greiss-Hess, L., Herrera, A. M., Steele, J., ... Rogers, S. J. (2008). Gross motor development, movement abnormalities, and early identification of autism. *Journal of Autism & Developmental Disorders, 38*(4), 644–656. doi: 10.1007/s10803-007-0430-0.

Papadopoulos, N., McGinley, J. L., Bradshaw, J. L., & Rinehart, N. J. (2014). An investigation of gait in children with Attention Deficit Hyperactivity Disorder: A case controlled study. *Psychiatry Research, 218*(3), 319–323. doi: 10.1016/j.psychres.2014.04.037.

Papadopoulos, N., Sciberras, E., Hiscock, H., Mulraney, M., McGillivray, J., & Rinehart, N. (2015). The efficacy of a brief behavioral sleep intervention in school-aged children with ADHD and comorbid autism spectrum disorder. *Journal of Attention Disorders*. doi: 10.1177/1087054714568565.

Pinto, D., Delaby, E., Merico, D., Barbosa, M., Merikangas, A., Klei, L., ... Wang, Z. (2014). Convergence of genes and cellular pathways dysregulated in autism spectrum disorders. *The American Journal of Human Genetics, 94*(5), 677–694. doi: 10.1016/j.ajhg.2014.03.018.

Rajendran, G., & Mitchell, P. (2007). Cognitive theories of autism. *Developmental Review, 27*(2), 224–260. doi: 10.1016/j.dr.2007.02.001.

Raznahan, A., Wallace, G. L., Antezana, L., Greenstein, D., Lenroot, R., Thurm, A., ... Swedo, S. E. (2013). Compared to what? Early brain overgrowth in autism and the perils of population norms. *Biological Psychiatry, 74*(8), 563–575. doi: 10.1016/j.biopsych.2013.03.022.

Redcay, E., & Courchesne, E. (2005). When is the brain enlarged in autism? A meta-analysis of all brain size reports. *Biological Psychiatry, 58*(1), 1–9. doi: 10.1016/j.biopsych.2005.03.026.

Rinehart, N. J., Bradshaw, J. L., Brereton, A. V., & Tonge, B. J. (2002). A clinical and neurobehavioural review of high-functioning autism and Asperger's disorder. *Australian & New Zealand Journal of Psychiatry, 36*(6), 762–770. doi: 10.1046/j.1440-1614.2002.01097.x.

Rinehart, N. J., Tonge, B. J., Iansek, R., McGinley, J., Brereton, A. V., Enticott, P. G., & Bradshaw, J. L. (2006). Gait function in newly diagnosed children with autism: Cerebellar and basal ganglia related motor disorder. *Developmental Medicine & Child Neurology, 48*(10), 819–824. doi: http://dx.doi.org/10.1017/S0012162206001769.

Rosenberg, R. E., Mandell, D. S., Farmer, J. E., Law, J. K., Marvin, A. R., & Law, P. A. (2010). Psychotropic medication use among children with autism spectrum disorders enrolled in a national registry, 2007–2008. *Journal of Autism & Developmental Disorders, 40*(3), 342–351. doi: 10.1007/s10803-009-0878-1.

Sanders, J., Johnson, K. A., Garavan, H., Gill, M., & Gallagher, L. (2008). A review of neuropsychological and neuroimaging research in autistic spectrum disorders: Attention, inhibition and cognitive flexibility. *Research in Autism Spectrum Disorders, 2*(1), 1–16. doi: 10.1016/j.rasd.2007.03.005.

Schopler, E., Van Bourgondien, M. E., Wellman, G. J., & Love, S. R. (2010). *The Childhood Autism Rating Scale (CARS2)*. Los Angeles, CA: Western Psychological Services.

Sharma, S., Woolfson, L. M., & Hunter, S. C. (2012). Confusion and inconsistency in diagnosis of Asperger syndrome: A review of studies from 1981 to 2010. *Autism, 16*(5), 465–486. doi: 10.1177/1362361311411935.

Simonoff, E., Pickles, A., Charman, T., Chandler, S., Loucas, T., & Baird, G. (2008). Psychiatric disorders in children with autism spectrum disorders: Prevalence, comorbidity, and associated factors in a population-derived sample. *Journal of the American Academy of Child & Adolescent Psychiatry, 47*(8), 921–929. doi: 10.1097/CHI.0b013e318179964f.

Sivaratnam, C. S., Newman, L. K., Tonge, B. J., & Rinehart, N. J. (2015). Attachment and emotion processing in children with autism spectrum disorders: Neurobiological, neuroendocrine, and neurocognitive considerations. *Review Journal of Autism & Developmental Disorders, 2*(2), 222–242. doi: 10.1007/s40489-015-0048-7.

Skefos, J., Cummings, C., Enzer, K., Holiday, J., Weed, K., Levy, E., … Bauman, M. (2014). Regional alterations in Purkinje cell density in patients with autism. *PloS one, 9*(2), e81255. doi: 10.1371/journal.pone.0081255.

Stanfield, A. C., McIntosh, A. M., Spencer, M. D., Philip, R., Gaur, S., & Lawrie, S. M. (2008). Towards a neuroanatomy of autism: A systematic review and meta-analysis of structural magnetic resonance imaging studies. *European Psychiatry, 23*(4), 289–299. doi: 10.1016/j.eurpsy.2007.05.006.

Teitelbaum, P., Teitelbaum, O., Nye, J., Fryman, J., & Maurer, R. G. (1998). Movement analysis in infancy may be useful for early diagnosis of autism. *Proceedings of the National Academy of Sciences, 95*(23), 13982–13987. doi: 10.1073/pnas.95.23.13982.

Tepest, R., Jacobi, E., Gawronski, A., Krug, B., Moller-Hartmann, W., Lehnhardt, F. G., & Vogeley, K. (2010). Corpus callosum size in adults with high-functioning autism and the relevance of gender. *Psychiatry Research, 183*(1), 38–43. doi: 10.1016/j.pscychresns.2010.04.007.

Tonge, B., Brereton, A., Kiomall, M., MacKinnon, A., & Rinehart, N. J. (2014). A randomised group comparison controlled trial of 'preschoolers with autism': A parent education and skills training intervention for young children with autistic disorder. *Autism, 18*(2), 166–177. doi: 10.1177/1362361312458186.

Tsai, P. T., Chu, Y., Greene-Colozzi, E., Sadowski, A. R., Leech, J. M., Steinberg, J., … Sahin, M. (2012). Autistic-like behaviour and cerebellar dysfunction in Purkinje cell TSC1 mutant mice. *Nature, 488*(7413), 647–651.

Van Naarden Braun, K., Christensen, D., Doernberg, N., Schieve, L., Rice, C., Wiggins, L., … Yeargin-Allsopp, M. (2015). Trends in the prevalence of autism spectrum disorder, cerebral palsy, hearing loss, intellectual disability, and vision impairment, Metropolitan Atlanta, 1991–2010. *PloS one, 10*(4). doi: 10.1371/journal.pone.0124120.

van Steensel, F. J., Bögels, S. M., & Perrin, S. (2011). Anxiety disorders in children and adolescents with autistic spectrum disorders: A meta-analysis. *Clinical Child and Family Psychology Review, 14*(3), 302–317. doi: 10.1007/s10567-011-0097-0.

Vissers, M. E., Cohen, M., & Geurts, H. M. (2012). Brain connectivity and high functioning autism: A promising path of research that needs refined models, methodological convergence, and stronger behavioral links. *Neuroscience & Biobehavioral Reviews, 36*(1), 604–625. doi: 10.1016/j.neubiorev.2011.09.003.

Wang, S. S.-H., Kloth, A. D., & Badura, A. (2014). The cerebellum, sensitive periods, and autism. *Neuron, 83*(3), 518–532. doi: 10.1016/j.neuron.2014.07.016.

Wass, S. (2011). Distortions and disconnections: Disrupted brain connectivity in autism. *Brain and Cognition, 75*(1), 18–28. doi: 10.1016/j.bandc.2010.10.005.

Whitby, P. J. S., & Mancil, G. R. (2009). Academic achievement profiles of children with high functioning autism and Asperger syndrome: A review of the literature. *Education and Training in Developmental Disabilities*, 551–560.

Whitney, E. R., Kemper, T. L., Rosene, D. L., Bauman, M. L., & Blatt, G. J. (2009). Density of cerebellar basket and stellate cells in autism: Evidence for a late developmental loss of Purkinje cells. *Journal of Neuroscience Research, 87*(10), 2245–2254. doi: 10.1002/jnr.22056.

WHO. (1992). *ICD-10: International Statistical Classification of Diseases and Related Health Problems: 10th Revision.* World Health Organization.

Woolfenden, S., Sarkozy, V., Ridley, G., Coory, M., & Williams, K. (2012). A systematic review of two outcomes in autism spectrum disorder–epilepsy and mortality. *Developmental Medicine & Child Neurology, 54*(4), 306–312. doi: 10.1111/j.1469-8749.2012.04223.x.

Yatawara, C. J., Einfeld, S. L., Hickie, I. B., Davenport, T. A., & Guastella, A. J. (2015). The effect of oxytocin nasal spray on social interaction deficits observed in young children with autism: A randomized clinical crossover trial. *Molecular Psychiatry*. Advanced online publication. doi: 10.1038/mp.2015.162.

8

ATTENTION DEFICIT HYPERACTIVITY DISORDER

Janette Tong, Ziarih Hawi and Mark A. Bellgrove

Aspects of this chapter are based on work presented in Hawi et al. Mol Psychiatry. 2015 Mar; 20(3): 289–97

Introduction

Attention Deficit Hyperactivity Disorder (ADHD) is a heterogeneous neurodevelopmental disorder. It is characterized by symptoms of inattention and/or hyperactivity-impulsivity that interferes with the functioning and development of affected individuals. The disorder affects 5.3–7.1% of school age children worldwide (Polanczyk, de Lima, Horta, Biederman, & Rohde, 2007; Willcutt, 2012). Although a diagnosis of ADHD is frequently made in childhood, the persistence of symptoms and neuropsychological impairments into adulthood in approximately 50% of cases supports the notion that ADHD is a chronic neurobiological condition (Goodman, 2007; Simon, Czobor, Bálint, Mészáros, & Bitter, 2009). The disorder is more prevalent in boys compared to girls with ratios ranging from 2.4:1 in population based surveys and 4:1 in clinical cohorts (Polanczyk et al., 2007). Children with ADHD frequently underachieve at school and have family, social and emotional dysfunction (Harpin, 2005). Adults with ADHD are at high risk of substance abuse and risk taking behaviours such as reckless driving (Mannuzza, Klein, Bessler, Malloy, & LaPadula, 1993). Children and adults with ADHD are commonly co-diagnosed with one or more other psychiatric conditions. Available evidence suggests that the incidence of comorbidity is higher in adults with ADHD than in children. Recent evidence showed that ADHD is associated with dramatic increases in mortality (Dalsgaard, Østergaard, Leckman, Mortensen, & Pedersen, 2015), underscoring the pressing need for a greater understanding of the neurobiology of ADHD, which may drive improved diagnosis and tailored treatment options.

Comorbidity of ADHD

Population-based twin and epidemiological studies report symptom overlap and high rates of ADHD with many psychiatric conditions (Reiersen, Constantino, Volk, & Todd, 2007). The two most commonly diagnosed comorbidities with ADHD are oppositional defiant disorder (ODD) and conduct disorder (CD). ODD (behavioural patterns including irritability, defiance, arguing, anger/resentfulness or vindictiveness) is present in 50–60% of individuals diagnosed with ADHD. The average age at onset of ODD in ADHD subjects is reported to be younger (5.3 years) compared to controls recruited from paediatric and psychiatric clinics (Biederman et al., 2008). A significant overlap between ADHD and CD (disruptive behaviour disorders involve violating the rights of others) is also well documented with up to 30% of those diagnosed with ADHD having comorbid CD. As with ODD, the age of onset for CD was found to be lower (8.9 years) in ADHD cases compared to controls recruited from paediatric and psychiatric clinics. The co-occurrence of ODD and particularly CD with ADHD is associated with higher rates of school suspensions. Further, individuals with CD are at increased risk for substance use disorders, smoking, criminal convictions and job loss. High comorbidity is also reported between ADHD and autism spectrum disorder (ASD). Twin-based questionnaire data showed that a significant proportion of the co-variation of ADHD and ASD symptomatology can be explained by shared additive genetic factors (Rommelse, Franke, Geurts, Hartman, & Buitelaar, 2010; Ronald, Simonoff, Kuntsi, Asherson, & Plomin, 2008). High rates of anxiety, learning disability and depression have also been reported in childhood and adult ADHD (Larson et al., 2011 and The Multimodal Treatment Study of ADHD Cooperative Group, 1999).

The high rates of comorbidity between psychiatric conditions generally suggest a common spectrum of psychopathology. Genetic mapping in five psychiatric conditions (ADHD, ASD, schizophrenia, bipolar disorder and major depressive disorder) reported significant association of two chromosomal regions (3p21 and 10q24) and single nucleotide polymorphisms (SNPs) mapped to two L-type voltage-gated calcium channel subunits genes (CACNA1C and CACNB) with these conditions (Cross-Disorder Group of the Psychiatric Genomics Consortium, 2013). This suggests that a shared genetic origin exists for a range of psychopathological traits.

The aetiology of ADHD

Complications during pregnancy and birth and exposure to environmental toxins can increase risk for psychiatric conditions through disturbance of common pathway(s) in the nervous system. Although environmental contributions to ADHD have been identified and are reviewed below, genetic factors appear to explain a greater proportion of the liability for developing ADHD.

Familial, twin and adoption studies

Familial, twin and adoption studies have demonstrated increased risk for individuals related to those with a diagnosis of ADHD. Diagnostic concordance for ADHD was estimated at 15–20% for maternal, 25–30% for paternal and 32% for sibling relationships (Biederman et al., 2008). A decline in the concordance for the disorder was reported in the second degree relatives of ADHD probands, indicating the importance of inherited factors in the aetiology of ADHD (Faraone, Biederman, & Milberger, 1994). The classical twin study design separates the familial risk into that accounted for by shared genes versus shared environment. In ADHD, large-scale twin studies have consistently demonstrated higher concordance rates (heritability estimates ~75–90%) for ADHD in monozygotic (MZ) twins (share 100% of their DNA) compared to a modest (~20%) in dizygotic (DZ) twins (share 50% of their DNA) (Levy, Hay, McStephen, Wood, & Waldman, 1997). Despite being limited, adoption studies provide additional support for the genetic predisposition to ADHD. For example, Sprich, Biederman, Crawford, Mundy, & Faraone (2000) reported that 6% of the adoptive parents of ADHD probands met diagnosis for ADHD compared to 18% of biological parents.

The genetic architecture of ADHD

In contrast to monogenic diseases (identified with clear patterns of inheritance caused by one or a few highly penetrant gene variants), common diseases including psychiatric conditions have no clear mode of inheritance. In ADHD, a polygenic model is proposed whereby risk is conferred by a number of genes, each with a relatively small/modest effect. This proposal is consistent with the high prevalence of ADHD and high concordance in monozygotic twins (68–81%) but modest risk to first-degree relatives. Although our knowledge of the molecular genetic architecture of ADHD remains incomplete, replicable genetic signals have been identified using candidate and genome wide association studies (GWAS). A brief review of the most replicated findings from candidate gene and GWAS literatures is presented below. The interested reader is referred to Hawi et al. (2015) for a fuller discussion of the genetics of ADHD including the role of rare DNA variations, such as copy number variants (CNVs).

Candidate genes in ADHD

A substantial body of evidence has implicated dysregulation of catecholamine (and more generally monoamines such as serotonin) neurotransmission in the pathophysiology of ADHD. More specifically, animal models, pharmacological and molecular genetic studies all point to a fundamental disturbance in extracellular dopamine and noradrenaline levels as contributing factors to ADHD. For example, the clinical effectiveness of stimulant medications such as methylphenidate, which increase dopamine and noradrenaline concentrations in the synapse (Barry, Hawi, & Kirley, 2007), provides firm support for dysregulation of these neurotransmitters. Moreover, candidate gene-based association studies have established that common variants (population frequency ≥5%) in catecholamine system genes are predisposing factors for ADHD. These include the dopamine transporter gene (DAT1; *SLC6A3*) and the dopamine D4 and D5 receptor genes (*DRD4*; *DRD5*) (Hawi et al., 2003; Lowe et al., 2004). DNA variations of the genes encoding the serotonin system including *SLC6A4* and *5-HT1B* have also been implicated (Kent et al., 2002; Hawi et al., 2002).

DNA variations mapped to genes that are functionally related to neurotransmitters have also been reported to increase risk for ADHD. These include the genes encoding latrophilin 3 (*LPHN3*), nitric oxide synthase1 (*NOS1*), synaptosomal-associated protein 25 (*SNAP25*) and the G protein-coupled receptor kinase interacting protein ArfGAP 1 (*GIT1*) (see Hawi et al., 2015 for a full discussion).

Genome wide association studies (GWAS)

Although candidate gene studies have shed light on the molecular genetic architecture of ADHD, they are inherently narrow in their approach. In contrast, several ADHD GWAS have now been conducted, assessing hundreds of thousands of variants across the genome for genetic association. To date, six case-control, two family-based and a quantitative trait loci (QTL) GWAS have been performed in children. Another case-control and QTL-GWAS have been performed in adults (see Hawi et al., 2015). Disappointingly, only two QTL-GWAS hits have been observed thus far, involving the Cadherin13 and glucose-fructose oxidoreductase domain 1 genes (Lasky-Su et al., 2008). The low yield of significant associations from GWAS in ADHD likely reflects a lack of statistical power that arises from both the small effect size of likely associations and the stringent corrections required to maintain Type 1 error rate at an appropriate level. In schizophrenia genetics, 47% of single nucleotide polymorphisms (SNPs) that were identified as being of potential interest but failed to attain genome-wide significance in the original studies ($5\times10-8\leq p\leq8.40\times10-5$) were subsequently found to be statistically associated in a replication study that carried greater power (Hamshere et al., 2013). Recent sample size increases for ADHD in the Psychiatric Genetic Consortium (PGC) are likely to drive a flurry of new associations for ADHD that attain GWAS significance levels. These novel gene associations will, in time, shed new light on the neurobiology of ADHD.

Environmental risk factors for ADHD

Although genetic factors are strongly implicated in the aetiology of ADHD, evidence also suggests a role for environmental factors. These include low birth weight (LBW), maternal alcohol consumption and maternal tobacco use, maternal substance abuse, socioeconomic adversity and exposure to toxins. Establishing causal links between environmental factors and risk for ADHD remains complex. This is particularly so since alcohol, tobacco or substance use in the mother, for example, may be influenced by an underlying genetic predisposition itself, thereby making it difficult to discern genetic versus environmental effects in the offspring. It may also be the case that environmental factors may only exert their influence in individuals carrying a particular genetic predisposition- so called gene-environment interactions. Below we provide a brief account of the environmental factors that are thought to increase the risk for ADHD. The interested reader is directed to Thapar et al. (Thapar, Cooper, Jefferies, & Stergiakouli, 2011) and Tarver et al. (Tarver, Daley, & Sayal, 2014) for a considerable discussion of this literature.

Low weight birth

Negative outcomes, such as neurocognitive dysfunction, are well correlated with premature/low birth weight (LBW). Poor attention and increased hyperactivity are well-defined behavioural correlates of LBW in children. In a comprehensive review of the literature, Bhutta, Cleves, Casey, Cradock, & Anand (2002) reported that the cognitive scores of preterm born children and full term born controls were directly proportionate to their birth weight and gestation age. Moreover, preterm infants who experienced less negative parenting had higher IQs at 36 months, with the greatest effects seen in very-preterm infants (VPIs; <30 weeks) compared with late preterm infants (LPIs; 34–36). LPIs manifested similar IQ, but more externalizing, oppositional and aggressive behaviours compared to VPIs. Overall, LBW children were likely to show hyperactive behaviour relative to normal birth weight children if they were brought up in a negative family environment (Shah et al., 2013). The relationship between LBW and symptom severity in children with ADHD may also be influenced by genetic factors. For instance, Jackson & Beaver (2015) reported that irrespective of ADHD subtype, LBW was found to increase the severity of ADHD symptoms. Further, possession of ADHD genetic risk variants mapped to dopaminergic genes (DAT1, DRD2 and DRD4) was found to increase the differences in ADHD symptomatology in LBW siblings relative to those with normal birth weight (Jackson & Beaver, 2015).

Exposure to alcohol

Prenatal exposure to significant amounts of alcohol during a mother's pregnancy has been reported as a predisposing factor in the aetiology of ADHD. It has also been implicated in the development of foetal alcohol syndrome (FAS). Assessment of ADHD core symptoms in FAS individuals demonstrated significant phenotypic similarity to ADHD. These two conditions significantly overlap and ADHD is diagnosed in 73–81% of children with FAS (Burd, Klug, Martsolf, & Kerbeshian, 2003;

Infante et al., 2014). Regardless of diagnosis, individuals exposed to a high level of alcohol were found to be significantly less accurate and made increased number of omission errors, had longer response latencies and increased variability in response time on the "Quotient ADHD System" (Infante et al., 2014). Like those with ADHD, individuals with FAS often perform well in language tests (Kodituwakku, Handmaker N.S., Cutler, Weathersby, & Handmaker S.D., 1995), but not in arithmetic (Clarren, Shurtleff, Unis, Astley, & Clarren, 1994; Kopera-Frye, Dehaene, & Streissguth, 1996) and attentional domains (Kodituwakku et al., 1995). The hyperactivity in FAS was found to be the less severe among other problems associated with phenotype by Nanson & Hiscock (1990).

Maternal smoking and drug exposure during pregnancy

Higher rates of hyperactive/inattentive symptoms are overrepresented in children born to smoking mothers (Keyes, Davey Smith, & Susser, 2014; Langley, Heron, Smith, & Thapar, 2012). It is, however, not clear whether the association with exposure to tobacco is a causal or cofounding factor that enhances the effect of the genetic risk variant on ADHD. As most of the published literature focuses on the influence of smoking during pregnancy and are retrospective in nature, establishing the actual timing of any effect (pre-, during or post-pregnancy) on the development of ADHD is important. The outcome of prenatal cocaine exposure in early childhood on many domains including motor function, attention and neurophysiology has been comprehensively reviewed (Frank, Augustyn, Knight, Pell, & Zuckerman, 2001). Despite the perception that drugs of abuse are a uniformly dangerous teratogen, there is as yet no convincing evidence that prenatal exposure to cocaine, for example, is associated with developmental toxic effects that give rise to behavioural traits such as inattention and/or hyperactivity/impulsivity (Linnet et al., 2003).

Exposure to toxins

Exposures to organophosphate pesticides (OPs), lead and polychlorinated biphenyl (PCBs) have been implicated as risk factors for ADHD, although the findings are not always consistent. OP measurements using urinary dialkyl phosphate (DAP) metabolites in Mexican-American pregnant women and their children showed a significant association with ADHD for children at the age of 5 years (Marks et al., 2010). Prenatal exposure to PCB has also been associated with cognitive impairments, including deficits on tests of working memory, response inhibition, vigilance and alertness (Eubig, Aguiar, & Schantz, 2010). Lead may be associated with poorer attention and response inhibition, whereas PCBs may impair response inhibition to a greater degree than attention (Eubig et al., 2010; Kim et al., 2010).

In summary, although the study of the influence of environmental factors on the development of ADHD is clearly an important area of study, firm conclusions remain premature and could be of small effect sizes. The literature suffers from a range of methodological shortcomings, including poorly powered studies, use of retrospective designs and the difficulty in establishing causal relationships between exposure to the environmental factor and the risk of developing ADHD. Further, the psychopathological history of the mother and families needs to be documented rigorously, so that one can determine whether any reported associations represent a true causal risk factor or a maternal genetic inheritance factor. Finally, the influence of gene by environmental interactions on the development of ADHD remains largely unknown.

Neurochemistry of ADHD

Despite the promising advances in identifying risk genes and pathways for ADHD, neurobiological research has focused on alterations within chemical signalling pathways, particularly the monoamine (dopamine, noradrenaline and serotonin) system that is influential in modulating transmission within the fronto-striatal system of the brain. The monoamines have been extensively examined as they are the targets for the pharmacological agents that regulate attention and hyperactivity (Purper-ouakil, Ramoz, Gorwood, & Simonneau, 2011). One of the most frequently prescribed medications for ADHD is methylphenidate. It is a psychostimulant which acts on dopamine and noradrenaline. The efficacy of methylphenidate in ameliorating the symptoms of ADHD has been attributed to its ability to inhibit the reuptake of dopamine and noradrenaline via their respective transporters (the dopamine transporter-DAT; the noradrenaline transporter-NET), with subsequent receptor level effects occurring via D1 and alpha2a receptors in regions such as the prefrontal cortex. Although paradoxical to the action of methylphenidate, genetically engineered mice lacking the dopamine transporter (DAT1-knockout; DAT-KO) are characterized by spontaneous hyper-locomotion, impaired cognition and deficient spatial learning (Giros et al., 1996).

Atomoxetine, a re-uptake inhibitor of noradrenaline, is known to be effective in treating the impulsivity of ADHD (Wehmeier et al., 2011). Further, administration of nisoxetine [noradrenergic transporter (NET) blocker] into DAT-KO mice significantly improved impulsivity in the cliff-avoidance test (Yamashita et al., 2013), presumably by increasing the extracellular noradrenaline levels in the prefrontal cortex (PFC). Further, administration of fluoxetine (a serotonin reuptake inhibitor) was found to ameliorate the hyperactivity phenotype of the DAT1-KO mouse with no significant alteration in the striatal dopamine concentrations. Treatment of DAT1-KO with 5-hydroxytryptophan or with the dietary 5-HT precursor (L-tryptophan) profoundly reduced the hyperactivity of these mice. These findings demonstrated that the serotonergic neurotransmission can modulate hyperactivity independent of changes in extracellular striatal DA concentrations (Gainetdinov et al., 1999). Although the exact mechanism remains unclear, alteration in the concentrations of one of the above neurotransmitters appears to cause significant changes in the others and is likely necessary for the efficacy of ADHD treatment (Bortolozzi & Artigas, 2003).

Promising biomarkers

Despite intensive research activity at the molecular level, no biomarker has been identified to diagnose or predict treatment efficacy in ADHD. This could be in part due to the clinical and etiological heterogeneity of ADHD, with no single biomarker being able to capture the complexity of the underlying aetiology of ADHD. However, DNA variations of the dopamine transporter gene (SLC6A3) and the dopamine receptor 4 (DRD4) have emerged as potential biomarkers for predicting treatment response in ADHD (Faraone et al., 2014). Earlier attempts predicting dose-response to methylphenidate treatment were based on the association of ADHD with the variable number of tandem repeats (VNTR) variants mapped to the 3' region of DAT1. Broadly speaking, the 10-repeat risk allele is associated with increased MPH response, enhanced activation of inhibition tasks and smaller caudate volume in the left hemisphere, whereas the 9-repeat allele is involved with greater neural activation and increased DAT1 activity in striatum (Falcone et al., 2013; Faraone et al., 2014).

Neuroimaging and ADHD

Accumulating evidence from neuropsychological, genetic and neurochemical studies has implicated deficits in fronto-striatal neural networks as an important contributing factor in the pathophysiology of ADHD. Early hypotheses were built on brain regions supporting higher level cognitive functions such as attention, working memory, motor control and response inhibition. The vast majority of neuroimaging studies have been conducted with structural imaging (for example Magnetic Resonance Imaging [sMRI] and diffusion tensor imaging [DTI]) and functional brain imaging using functional MRI (fMRI) and positron emission tomography (PET). sMRI studies focus on the volume and shape of various brain regions and compare these differences between ADHD cases and typically developing children. A large array of structural MRI studies, including meta-analyses in children with ADHD relative to controls, reported consistent reductions in total and right cerebral volumes, cortical thickness in the basal ganglia, the cerebellum, the frontal lobes (dorsolateral prefrontal cortex; DLPFC) and striatum (right caudate) (Cubillo, Halari, Smith, Taylor, & Rubia, 2012; Valera, Faraone, Biederman, Poldrack, & Seidman, 2005). Although fewer sMRI studies have been published in adults with ADHD, relatively similar regions of structural abnormalities were observed, including the prefrontal cortex (inferior- and orbito- frontal cortex, DLPFC), anterior cingulate cortex (ACC) and cerebellar regions (Almeida Montes et al., 2013; Cortese, Klein, Mannuzza, Ramos-olazagasti, & Castellanos, 2014; Proal et al., 2011; Shaw et al., 2013). DLPFC maintains strong neural circuitry with dACC, the parietal cortex and striatum. This network is believed to play roles in complex cognitive processes, including response selection and inhibition, as well as performance monitoring and motivation (Bush et al., 2002).

Another sMRI method, diffusion tensor imaging, is a non-invasive approach which relies on the translational motion of water molecules that provides an assessment of white matter organization within the brain (Mori & Zhang, 2006). Using a commonly used DTI index "fractional anisotropy or FA", several studies have reported white matter differences in children, adolescents and adults with ADHD (Ashtari et al., 2005; Konrad & Eickhoff, 2010a; Pavuluri et al., 2009; Silk, Vance, Rinehart, Bradshaw, & Cunnington, 2009a, 2009b). Fractional anisotropy dictates axonal density and branching in white matter, while higher FA values suggest an increase in white matter density or decrease in white matter branching. Consistent with the hypothesis that ADHD is associated with developmental delay, white matter organization within the caudate is different in adolescents with ADHD than controls over ages 8–18 years which eventually appeared to catch up to normal levels by the age of 18 years (Silk et al., 2009a). Further, higher FA values with white matter regions underlying the inferior parietal, occipito-parietal, inferior frontal and inferior temporal cortex were observed in a group of 15 ADHD individuals when compared with an equal number of age-matched controls (Silk et al., 2009b). This is consistent with previous findings of fronto-striatial and parietal dysfunction in ADHD.

Contrary to sMRI studies, which provide information about brain structure, functional brain imaging studies have being used to examine brain functioning and connectivity patterns in ADHD individuals. By monitoring changes in oxygenated and deoxygenated blood flow, fMRI allows researchers to trace metabolic activities in brain regions across time (Weyandt, 2006). fMRI enables examination of neural connectivity patterns, not only during performance of cognitive tasks, but also across time and between proximal and distal regions (Konrad & Eickhoff, 2010b). Under the cognitive control Go/No-Go task, children with ADHD (6 to 10 years old) showed marked decreases in blood oxygenation level when compared to controls in basal ganglia, ventral prefrontal cortex and the anterior cingulate gyrus, while significant increases in activity were observed in posterior parietal lobe, posterior cingulate and regions of DLPFC (Durston et al., 2003). The distinctive activation patterns in children with ADHD led to the proposal of compensatory hyper-activation mechanisms in response to impairment within the fronto-striatal network. Similar brain activation patterns were reported using a rewarded continuous performance task in medication naïve children with ADHD (Rubia, Halari, Cubillo, et al., 2009), and an N-back task in adults with ADHD (Valera et al., 2005). Decreased fronto-parietal activation was also found in boys with ADHD during a spatial working memory task (Vance et al., 2007), as well as adults with ADHD during No-Go conditions of Go/No-Go task (Schneider et al., 2010). Further supportive evidence for the hypo-functioning/activation of fronto-striatal-parietal network came from a meta-analysis of 13 fMRI studies conducted by Dickstein and colleagues (Dickstein, Bannon, Xavier Castellanos, & Milham, 2006). Consistent evidence of abnormal activation was found in fronto-parietal and fronto-striato-parieto-cerebellar networks of ADHD individuals when compared to controls (Rubia, Halari, Cubillo, et al., 2009; Rubia, Halari, Smith, et al., 2009; Wolf et al., 2009).

Dysconnectivity of the default mode network (DMN) has also been implicated in children with ADHD (Fassbender et al., 2009). DMN encompasses the posterior cingulate cortex, the medial prefrontal cortex and the lateral and inferior parietal cortex, which is associated with task-irrelevant mental processes and mind wandering. The DMN is therefore believed to be deactivated for successful cognitive functioning, as demonstrated by increased attentional lapses being associated with failure to deactivate the DMN. Methylphenidate administration enabled inhibition of the DMN activity in a group of children and adolescents with ADHD (Peterson et al., 2009). Medication naïve adolescents showed an inverse connectivity between dACC and regions within the DMN including the posterior cingulate cortex (Sun et al., 2012). Such relationship was attenuated in adolescents with ADHD (Castellanos et al., 2008). Thus, connectivity between dACC and some DMN regions in adults with ADHD were reported to be more similar to that of developing children than healthy adults, which suggests a potential maturation delay in neural development (Sato, Hoexter, Castellanos, & Rohde, 2012).

Previous SPECT and PET studies in ADHD have suggested changes of DAT availability in the striatum; however, the direction of this effect is inconclusive with increased, decreased and no differences reported (Rubia et al., 2014; Spencer et al., 2005, 2007; Volkow et al., 2007). Differences in these results across studies could be due to developmental stages of participants, gender or medication status of the patients under study. For instance, it is known that the DAT is highly plastic and can be up- or down-regulated by changes in its neurochemical environment, thereby significantly influencing the results of molecular imaging studies.

Neuroimaging studies in ADHD have therefore shown multiple functional and structural neural abnormalities in the fronto-striatal, fronto-parietal and fronto-cellebellar networks. Studies including those in children, adolescents and adults with ADHD have found that anti-correlations between default mode and cognitive control activations are either reduced or absent in ADHD. The inability to suppress the DMN is thought to impede sustained attention by interfering with the normal functioning of the cognitive control network, which is thought to underlie ADHD (Castellanos et al., 2008).

An alternative approach towards understanding the aetiology of ADHD – endophenotypes

Deciphering the genetic architecture of psychiatric disorders is a challenging task which is complicated by clinical and aetiological heterogeneity (Almasy & Blangero, 2001; Castellanos & Tannock, 2002; Gottesman & Gould, 2003; Robinson et al., 2014). Despite this broad acknowledgement, each of the case-control SNP or CNV-GWAS studies of ADHD performed thus far has adopted a unitary view of the disorder, comparing large heterogeneous samples of individuals with ADHD to control samples. Although this approach is pragmatic as neither individual ADHD nor consortia cohorts have the sample size to parse by DSM subtype or the presence of comorbidity, for example, it undoubtedly introduces noise and places an upper limit on the gene discovery potential of these case-control studies. Although latent classes derived from quantitative symptom counts, for example, have been shown to be heritable and may offer greater gene discovery potential than DSM-defined subtypes, in general there has been little application of these symptom-based approaches within ADHD GWAS (Rasmussen et al., 2004). The study by Lasky-Su et al. (2008) is a notable exception that suggests that gains in power may be afforded by adopting a quantitative trait, as opposed to case-control methodology (Almasy & Blangero, 2001; Wijsman & Amos, 1997). Quantitative symptom-based approaches have also been employed in both child and adult population-based cohorts (Ebejer et al., 2013; Groen-Blokhuis et al., 2014). Groen-Blokhuis et al. (2014) recently tested the hypothesis that a polygenic risk score derived from GWAS meta-analysis of clinically defined childhood ADHD could predict continuous scores of inattention and hyperactivity rated using the Attention Problems (APs) scale of the Child Behaviour Checklist (CBCL) in a population-based child cohort (N = 2437). Polygenic risk scores predicted both maternal (pre-school and school age) and teacher (school age) ratings of AP, highlighting both the fact that APs exist on a continuum in the normal population, and the potential value of dimensional ratings for genetic studies of ADHD behaviour.

Although a shift from categorical diagnoses to quantitative symptom measures is encouraging, we argue that the use of intermediate traits, or endophenotypes, may hold greater promise for gene discovery in ADHD (Castellanos & Tannock, 2002; Doyle et al., 2005; Waldman, 2005). Although the study of susceptibility genes is a valid and reliable method for improving biological understanding, its power is limited by several factors: the small size of likely individual gene effects, the heterogeneity of genetic effects, reduced gene penetrance and the presence of phenocopies within the sample. For these reasons, studies of susceptibility genes for psychiatric disorders have emphasized the utility of quantitative indices of disease risk or liability, termed endophenotypes (Almasy & Blangero, 2001; Gottesman & Gould, 2003).

Endophenotypes are traits—cognitive or physiological—for example, that may be closer to dysfunction in discrete neural systems than in the broad phenotype. Since the endophenotype is thought to be less removed from the relevant gene action than diagnosis, the genetic architecture of the endophenotype may be simpler than that for a complex disorder such as ADHD (Castellanos & Tannock, 2002; Gottesman & Gould, 2003; Waldman, 2005). Arguably the best evidence for an endophenotype for ADHD exists for a number of neurocognitive measures, for example, response time variability (Andreou et al., 2007; Kuntsi & Stevenson, 2001), response inhibition (Crosbie & Schachar, 2001; Crosbie et al., 2013; McAuley et al., 2014) and temporal processing (Himpel et al., 2009; Nikolas & Nigg, 2014). Detailed reviews of the endophenotype approach in ADHD can be found elsewhere (Castellanos & Tannock, 2002; Doyle et al., 2005; Franke et al., 2012;

Waldman, 2005). Broadly speaking, studies have now demonstrated that these cognitive measures are heritable, associated with ADHD and often exhibit a familial risk profile, with the performance of unaffected siblings lying intermediate between that of ADHD probands and unrelated controls. Neurocognitive measures also have the added advantage of being readily scalable to the large sample sizes that are required for gene discovery. A number of physiological measures, derived either from human electroencephalography (for example, low frequency EEG oscillations) (Tye et al., 2012) or functional brain imaging (for example, resting-state functional MRI [rsfMRI]) (Fair et al., 2010; Glahn et al., 2010), may relate to these cognitive measures and show tremendous promise for indexing liability to ADHD. The challenge is now for such measures to be implemented in a cohesive fashion across sufficiently large populations of patients with ADHD to drive new biological knowledge.

Summary

ADHD is a highly heritable mental disorder which is now appreciated to be lifelong in many cases, with dramatic increases in morbidity and mortality particularly when left untreated and poorly managed. The early phases of neurobiological research have focused on the relationship between the monoamines (dopamine, noradrenaline and serotonin) and the cognitive and symptomatic features of ADHD, mediated in large part via the effects of these chemicals on the development of fronto-striatal and associated parietal and cerebellar circuits. Although this hypothesis has served ADHD well, the next phase of neurobiological research will surely encompass a systems biology approach, where genes acting within connected biological networks will be seen to influence both short- and longer-range communications within neural networks that represent attention and cognitive control, for example. The next tranche of GWAS studies will surely identify significant genome wide associations which may be used to anchor these systems biology approaches to bona fide genetic risk signals. As with many neuropsychiatric conditions, heterogeneity in ADHD is the rule rather than the exception, and dimensional rather than categorical approaches, as enshrined for example within NIMH's research domain criteria (RDoc) approach, must now be employed to drive new biological knowledge and novel treatment pathways.

Glossary

Biomarker: an objective measure of physiological processes

Comorbidity: co-occurrence of two or more disorders within an individual

Dizygotic: two zygotes, each egg fertilized by separate sperm, giving rise to two individuals sharing about 50% of their genetic make-up

Monozygotic: one zygote, originated from one egg and one sperm, giving rise to two individuals sharing identical genes

Psychostimulant: compound with the capacity to stimulate the activity of the central nervous system thereby relieving symptoms

Further readings

Chandler, C. (2010). *The Science of ADHD: A Guide for Parents & Professionals*. Wiley-Blackwell: West Sussex, UK.

Cornish, K., & Wilding, J. (eds.). (2010). *Attention, Genes & Developmental Disorders*. Oxford University Press: Oxford, UK.

Friedman, L. A., & Rapoport, J. L. (2015). Brain development in ADHD. *Current Opinion in Neurobiology, 30*, 106–111.

van Ewijk, H., Heslenfeld, D. J., Zwiers, M. P., Buitelaar, J. K., Oosterlaan, J. (2012). Diffusion tensor imaging in attention deficit/hyperactivity disorder: A systematic review and meta-analysis. *Neuroscience and Biobehavioral Reviews, 36*, 1093–1106.

References

Almasy, L., & Blangero, J. (2001). Endophenotypes as quantitative risk factors for psychiatric disease: Rationale and study design. *American Journal of Medical Genetics, 105*(1), 42–4.

Almeida Montes, L., Prado Alcantara, H., Martinez Garcia, R., De La Torre, L., Avila Acosta, D., & Duarte, M. (2013). Brain cortical thickness in ADHD: Age, sex, and clinical correlations. *Journal of Attention Disorders, 17*(8), 641–54. http://doi.org/10.1177/1087054711434351.

Andreou, P., Neale, B. M., Chen, W., Christiansen, H., Gabriels, I., Heise, A., … Kuntsi, J. (2007). Reaction time performance in ADHD: Improvement under fast-incentive condition and familial effects. *Psychological Medicine, 37*(12), 1703–15. http://doi.org/10.1017/S0033291707000815.

Ashtari, M., Kumra, S., Bhaskar, S. L., Clarke, T., Thaden, E., Cervellione, K. L., … Ardekani, B. A. (2005). Attention-deficit/hyperactivity disorder: A preliminary diffusion tensor imaging study. *Biological Psychiatry, 57*(5), 448–55.

Barry, E., Hawi, Z., & Kirley, A. (2007). Avenues for pharmacogenetic research in ADHD. In *Handbook of Attention Deficit Hyperactivity Disorder* (pp. 355–71).

Bhutta, A., Cleves, M., Casey, P., Cradock, M., & Anand, K. (2002). Cognitive and behavioral outcomes of school-aged children who were born preterm: A meta-analysis. *Journal of the American Medical Association, 288*, 728–37. http://doi.org/jma10039 [pii].

Biederman, J., Petty, C. R., Dolan, C., Hughes, S., Mick, E., Monuteaux, M. C., & Faraone, S.V. (2008). The long-term longitudinal course of oppositional defiant disorder and conduct disorder in ADHD boys: Findings from a controlled 10-year prospective longitudinal follow-up study. *Psychological Medicine, 38*(7), 1027–36. http://doi.org/10.1016/S0084-3970(08)79233-8.

Bortolozzi, A., & Artigas, F. (2003). Control of 5-hydroxytryptamine release in the dorsal raphe nucleus by the noradrenergic system in rat brain. Role of alpha-adrenoceptors. *Neuropsychopharmacology: Official Publication of the American College of Neuropsychopharmacology, 28*(3), 421–34. http://doi.org/10.1038/sj.npp.1300061.

Burd, L., Klug, M. G., Martsolf, J. T., & Kerbeshian, J. (2003). Fetal alcohol syndrome: Neuropsychiatric phenomics. *Neurotoxicology and Teratology, 25*(6), 697–705. http://doi.org/10.1016/j.ntt.2003.07.014.

Bush, G., Vogt, B., Holmes, J., Dale, A., Greve, D., Jenike, M., & Rosen, B. (2002). Dorsal anterior cingulate cortex: A role in reward-based decision making. *Proceedings of the National Academy of Sciences of the United States of America, 99*(1), 523–8. http://doi.org/10.1073/pnas.012470999.

Castellanos, F. X., Margulies, D. S., Kelly, C., Uddin, L. Q., Ghaffari, M., Kirsch, A., … Milham, M. P. (2008). Cingulate-precuneus interactions: A new locus of dysfunction in adult attention-deficit/hyperactivity disorder. *Biological Psychiatry*, *63*(3), 332–7.

Castellanos, F. X., & Tannock, R. (2002). Neuroscience of attention-deficit/hyperactivity disorder: The search for endophenotypes. *Nature Reviews. Neuroscience*, *3*(8), 617–28. http://doi.org/10.1038/nrn896.

Clarren, S. G.B., Shurtleff, H., Unis, A., Astley, S., & Clarren, S. K. (1994). Comprehensive educational, psychologic, and psychiatric profiles of children with fetal alcohol syndrome. In *Alcoholism: Clinical and Experimental Research 1994;18(2), 502.*

Cortese, S., Klein, R., Mannuzza, S., Ramos-olazagasti, M., & Castellanos, F. (2014). White matter alterations at 33-year follow-up in adults with childhood ADHD. *Biological Psychiatry*, *74*(8), 591–8. http://doi.org/10.1016/j.biopsych.2013.02.025.White.

Crosbie, J., Arnold, P., Paterson, A., Swanson, J., Dupuis, A., Li, X., … Schachar, R. J. (2013). Response inhibition and ADHD traits: Correlates and heritability in a community sample. *Journal of Abnormal Child Psychology*, *41*(3), 497–507. http://doi.org/10.1007/s10802-012-9693-9.

Crosbie, J., & Schachar, R. (2001). Deficient inhibition as a marker for familial ADHD. *The American Journal of Psychiatry*, *158*(11), 1884–90.

Cubillo, A., Halari, R., Smith, A., Taylor, E., & Rubia, K. (2012). A review of fronto-striatal and fronto-cortical brain abnormalities in children and adults with Attention Deficit Hyperactivity Disorder (ADHD) and new evidence for dysfunction in adults with ADHD during motivation and attention. *Cortex*. http://doi.org/10.1016/j.cortex.2011.04.007.

Dalsgaard, S., Østergaard, S. D., Leckman, J. F., Mortensen, P. B., & Pedersen, M. G. (2015). Mortality in children, adolescents, and adults with attention deficit hyperactivity disorder: A nationwide cohort study. *The Lancet*. http://doi.org/10.1016/S0140-6736(14)61684-6.

Dickstein, S. G., Bannon, K., Xavier Castellanos, F., & Milham, M. P. (2006). The neural correlates of attention deficit hyperactivity disorder: An ALE meta-analysis. *Journal of Child Psychology & Psychiatry and Allied Disciplines*, *47*(10), 1051–62. http://doi.org/10.1111/j.1469-7610.2006.01671.x.

Doyle, A. E., Willcutt, E. G., Seidman, L. J., Biederman, J., Chouinard, V. A., Silva, J., & Faraone, S. V. (2005). Attention-deficit/hyperactivity disorder endophenotypes. *Biological Psychiatry*, *57*(11), 1324–35. http://doi.org/10.1016/j.biopsych.2005.03.015.

Durston, S., Tottenham, N. T., Thomas, K. M., Davidson, M. C., Eigsti, I. M., Yang, Y., … Casey, B. J. (2003). Differential patterns of striatal activation in young children with and without ADHD. *Biological Psychiatry*, *53*(10), 871–8. http://doi.org/10.1016/S0006-3223(02)01904-2.

Ebejer, J. L., Duffy, D. L., van der Werf, J., Wright, M. J., Montgomery, G., Gillespie, N. A, … Medland, S. E. (2013). Genome-wide association study of inattention and hyperactivity-impulsivity measured as quantitative traits. *Twin Research and Human Genetics: The Official Journal of the International Society for Twin Studies*, *16*(2), 560–74. http://doi.org/10.1017/thg.2013.12.

Eubig, P., Aguiar, A., & Schantz, S. (2010). Lead and PCBs as risk factors for attention deficit/hyperactivity disorder. *Environmental Health Perspectives*, *118*(12), 1654–67. http://doi.org/10.1289/ehp.0901852.

Fair, D. A., Posner, J., Nagel, B. J., Bathula, D., Dias, T. G. C., Mills, K. L., … Nigg, J. T. (2010). Atypical default network connectivity in youth with attention-deficit/hyperactivity disorder. *Biological Psychiatry*, *68*(12), 1084–91. http://doi.org/10.1016/j.biopsych.2010.07.003.

Falcone, M., Smith, R. M., Chenoweth, M. J., Kumar Bhattacharjee, A., Kelsoe, J. R., Tyndale, R. F., & Lerman, C. (2013). Neuroimaging in psychiatric pharmacogenetics research: The promise and pitfalls. *Neuropsychopharmacology: Official Publication of the American College of Neuropsychopharmacology*, *38*(12), 2327–37. http://doi.org/10.1038/npp.2013.152.

Faraone, S., Biederman, J., & Milberger, S. (1994). An exploratory study of ADHD among second-degree relatives of ADHD children. *Biological Psychiatry*, *35*(6), 398–402. http://doi.org/10.1016/0006-3223(94)90006-X.

Faraone, S.V., Bonvicini, C., & Scassellati, C. (2014). Biomarkers in the diagnosis of ADHD – Promising directions. *Current Psychiatry Reports*, *16*(11), 497. http://doi.org/10.1007/s11920-014-0497-1.

Fassbender, C., Zhang, H., Buzy, W. M., Cortes, C. R., Mizuiri, D., Beckett, L., & Schweitzer, J. B. (2009). A lack of default network suppression is linked to increased distractibility in ADHD. *Brain Research*, *1273*, 114–28.

Frank, D. A., Augustyn, M., Knight, W. G., Pell, T., & Zuckerman, B. (2001). Growth, development, and behavior in early childhood following prenatal cocaine exposure: A systematic review. *JAMA*, *285*(12), 1613–25.

Franke, B., Faraone, S.V, Asherson, P., Buitelaar, J., Bau, C. H. D., Ramos-Quiroga, J. A, … Reif, A. (2012). The genetics of attention deficit/hyperactivity disorder in adults, a review. *Molecular Psychiatry*, *17*(10), 960–87. http://doi.org/10.1038/mp.2011.138.

Gainetdinov, R. R., Wetsel, W. C., Jones, S. R., Levin, E. D., Jaber, M., & Caron, M. G. (1999). Role of serotonin in the paradoxical calming effect of psychostimulants on hyperactivity. *Science (New York, N.Y.)*, *283*(5400), 397–401. http://doi.org/10.1126/science.283.5400.397.

Giros, B., Jaber, M., Jones, S. R., Wightman, R. M., & Caron, M. G. (1996). Hyperlocomotion and indifference to cocaine and amphetamine in mice lacking the dopamine transporter. *Nature*, *379*(6566), 606–12. http://doi.org/10.1038/379606a0.

Glahn, D. C., Winkler, A. M., Kochunov, P., Almasy, L., Duggirala, R., Carless, M. A., … Blangero, J. (2010). Genetic control over the resting brain. *Proceedings of the National Academy of Sciences of the United States of America*, *107*(3), 1223–8. http://doi.org/10.1073/pnas.0909969107.

Goodman, D. W. (2007). The consequences of attention-deficit/hyperactivity disorder in adults. *Journal of Psychiatric Practice*, *13*(5), 318–27.

Gottesman, I. I., & Gould, T. D. (2003). The endophenotype concept in psychiatry: Etymology and strategic intentions. *The American Journal of Psychiatry*, *160*(4), 636–45.

Groen-Blokhuis, M. M., Middeldorp, C. M., Kan, K. J., Abdellaoui, A., van Beijsterveldt, C. E. M., Ehli, E. A., … Boomsma, D. I. (2014). Attention-deficit/hyperactivity disorder polygenic risk scores predict attention problems in a population-based sample of children. *Journal of the American Academy of Child & Adolescent Psychiatry*, *53*(10), 1123–9. http://doi.org/10.1016/j.jaac.2014.06.014.

Group, C., & Consortium, P. G. (2013). Identification of risk loci with shared effects on five major psychiatric disorders: A genome-wide analysis. *The Lancet*, *381*, 1371–1379. http://doi.org/10.1016/S0140-6736(12)62129-1.

Group, T. M. C. (1999). A 14-month randomized clinical trial of treatment strategies for attention-deficit/hyperactivity disorder. *Archives of General Psychiatry*, *56*(12), 1073–86.

Hamshere, M. L., Walters, J. T. R., Smith, R., Richards, A., Green, E. K., Grozeva, D.V., … O'Donovan, M. C. (2013). Genome-wide significant associations in schizophrenia to ITIH3/4, CACNA1C and SDCCAG8, and extensive replication of associations reported by the Schizophrenia PGC. *Molecular Psychiatry*, *18*(6), 708–12. http://doi.org/10.1038/mp.2012.67.

Harpin, V. A. (2005). The effect of ADHD on the life of an individual, their family, and community from preschool to adult life. *Archives of Disease in Childhood*. http://doi.org/10.1136/adc.2004.059006.

Hawi, Z., Cummins, T. D. R., Tong, J., Johnson, B., Lau, R., Samarrai, W., & Bellgrove, M. A. (2015). The molecular genetic architecture of attention deficit hyperactivity disorder. *Molecular Psychiatry*, *20*(3), 289–97. http://doi.org/10.1038/mp.2014.183.

Hawi, Z., Dring, M., Kirley, A., Foley, D., Kent, L., Craddock, N., … Gill, M. (2002). Serotonergic system and attention deficit hyperactivity disorder (ADHD): A potential susceptibility locus at the 5-HT(1B) receptor gene in 273 nuclear families from a multi-centre sample. *Molecular Psychiatry*, 7(7), 718–25. http://doi.org/10.1038/sj.mp.4001048.

Hawi, Z., Lowe, N., Kirley, A., Gruenhage, F., Nöthen, M., Greenwood, T., … Gill, M. (2003). Linkage disequilibrium mapping at DAT1, DRD5 and DBH narrows the search for ADHD susceptibility alleles at these loci. *Molecular Psychiatry*, *8*(3), 299–308.

Himpel, S., Banaschewski, T., Grüttner, A., Becker, A., Heise, A., Uebel, H., … Rammsayer, T. (2009). Duration discrimination in the range of milliseconds and seconds in children with ADHD and their unaffected siblings. *Psychological Medicine*, *39*(10), 1745–51. http://doi.org/10.1017/S003329170900542X.

Infante, M. A., Moore, E. M., Nguyen, T. T., Fourligas, N., Mattson, S. N., & Riley, E. P. (2014). Objective assessment of ADHD core symptoms in children with heavy prenatal alcohol exposure. *Physiology & Behavior*, *148*, 45–50. http://doi.org/10.1016/j.physbeh.2014.10.014.

Jackson, D. B., & Beaver, K. M. (2015). Sibling differences in low birth weight, dopaminergic polymorphisms, and ADHD symptomatology: Evidence of GxE. *Psychiatry Research*, *226*(2–3), 467–73. http://doi.org/10.1016/j.psychres.2015.01.025.

Kent, L., Doerry, U., Hardy, E., Parmar, R., Gingell, K., Hawi, Z., … Craddock, N. (2002). Evidence that variation at the serotonin transporter gene influences susceptibility to attention deficit hyperactivity disorder (ADHD): Analysis and pooled analysis. *Molecular Psychiatry*, 7(8), 908–12.

Keyes, K. M., Davey Smith, G., & Susser, E. (2014). Associations of prenatal maternal smoking with offspring hyperactivity: Causal or confounded? *Psychological Medicine*, *44*(4), 857–67.

Kim, Y., Cho, S. C., Kim, B. N., Hong, Y. C., Shin, M. S., Yoo, H. J., … Bhang, S. Y. (2010). Association between blood lead levels (<5 μg/dL) and inattention-hyperactivity and neurocognitive profiles in school-aged Korean children. *The Science of the Total Environment*, *408*(23), 5737–43. http://doi.org/10.1016/j.scitotenv.2010.07.070.

Kodituwakku, P. W., Handmaker, N. S., Cutler, S. K., Weathersby, E. K., & Handmaker, S. D. (1995). Specific impairments in self-regulation in children exposed to alcohol prenatally. *Alcoholism: Clinical & Experimental Research*, *19*(6), 1558–64.

Konrad, K., & Eickhoff, S. B. (2010a). Is the ADHD brain wired differently? A review on structural and functional connectivity in attention deficit hyperactivity disorder. *Human Brain Mapping*. http://doi.org/10.1002/hbm.21058.

Konrad, K., & Eickhoff, S. B. (2010b). Is the ADHD brain wired differently? A review on structural and functional connectivity in attention deficit hyperactivity disorder. *Human Brain Mapping*, *31*(6), 904–16. http://doi.org/10.1002/hbm.21058.

Kopera-Frye, K., Dehaene, S., & Streissguth, A. P. (1996). Impairments of number processing induced by prenatal alcohol exposure. *Neuropsychologia*, *34*(12), 1187–96.

Kuntsi, J., & Stevenson, J. (2001). Psychological mechanisms in hyperactivity: II. The role of genetic factors. *Journal of Child Psychology & Psychiatry, & Allied Disciplines*, *42*(2), 211–9.

Langley, K., Heron, J., Smith, G. D., & Thapar, A. (2012). Maternal and paternal smoking during pregnancy and risk of ADHD symptoms in offspring: Testing for intrauterine effects. *American Journal of Epidemiology, 176*(3), 261–8.

Larson, K., Russ, S., Kahn, R., & Halfon, N. (2011). Patterns of comorbidity, functioning, and service use for US children with ADHD, 2007. *Pediatrics, 127*(3), 462–70. http://doi.org/10.1542/peds.2010-0165.

Lasky-Su, J., Neale, B. M., Franke, B., Anney, R. J. L., Zhou, K., Maller, J. B., … Faraone, S.V. (2008). Genome-wide association scan of quantitative traits for attention deficit hyperactivity disorder identifies novel associations and confirms candidate gene associations. *American Journal of Medical Genetics. Part B, Neuropsychiatric Genetics, 147B*(8), 1345–54. http://doi.org/10.1002/ajmg.b.30867.

Levy, F., Hay, D. A., McStephen, M., Wood, C., & Waldman, I. (1997). Attention-deficit hyperactivity disorder: A category or a continuum? Genetic analysis of a large-scale twin study. *Journal of the American Academy of Child & Adolescent Psychiatry*. http://doi.org/10.1097/00004583-199706000-00009.

Linnet, K., Dalsgaard, S., Obel, C., Wisborg, K., Henriksen, T., Rodriguez, A., … Jarvelin, M. (2003). Maternal lifestyle factors in pregnancy risk of attention deficit hyperactivity disorder and associated behaviors: Review of the current evidence. *American Journal of Psychiatry, 160*(6), 1028–40.

Lowe, N., Kirley, A., Hawi, Z., Sham, P., Wickham, H., Kratochvil, C. J., … Gill, M. (2004). Joint analysis of the DRD5 marker concludes association with attention-deficit/hyperactivity disorder confined to the predominantly inattentive and combined subtypes. *American Journal of Human Genetics, 74*(2), 348–356.

Mannuzza, S., Klein, R. G., Bessler, A., Malloy, P., & LaPadula, M. (1993). Adult outcome of hyperactive boys. Educational achievement, occupational rank, and psychiatric status. *Archives of General Psychiatry, 50*(7), 565–76.

Marks, A. R., Harley, K., Bradman, A., Kogut, K., Barr, D. B., Johnson, C., … Eskenazi, B. (2010). Organophosphate pesticide exposure and attention in young Mexican-American children: The CHAMACOS study. *Environmental Health Perspectives, 118*(12), 1768–74. http://doi.org/10.1289/ehp.1002056.

McAuley, T., Crosbie, J., Charach, A., & Schachar, R. (2014). The persistence of cognitive deficits in remitted and unremitted ADHD: A case for the state-independence of response inhibition. *Journal of Child Psychology & Psychiatry, & Allied Disciplines, 55*(3), 292–300. http://doi.org/10.1111/jcpp.12160.

Mori, S., & Zhang, J. (2006). Principles of diffusion tensor imaging and its applications to basic neuroscience approach. *Neuron, 51*(5), 527–539.

Nanson, J. L., & Hiscock, M. (1990). Attention deficits in children exposed to alcohol prenatally. *Alcoholism, Clinical & Experimental Research, 14*(5), 656–61.

Nikolas, M. A., & Nigg, J. T. (2014). Moderators of neuropsychological mechanism in attention-deficit hyperactivity disorder. *Journal of Abnormal Child Psychology, 43*(2), 271–81. http://doi.org/10.1007/s10802-014-9904-7.

Pavuluri, M. N., Yang, S., Kamineni, K., Passarotti, A. M., Srinivasan, G., Harral, E. M., … Zhou, X. J. (2009). Diffusion tensor imaging study of white matter fiber tracts in pediatric bipolar disorder and attention-deficit/hyperactivity disorder. *Biological Psychiatry, 65*(7), 586–93.

Peterson, B. S., Potenza, M. N., Wang, Z., Zhu, H., Martin, A., Marsh, R., … Yu, S. (2009). An FMRI study of the effects of psychostimulants on default-mode processing during Stroop task performance in youths with ADHD. *The American Journal of Psychiatry, 166*(11), 1286–94.

Polanczyk, G., de Lima, M. S., Horta, B. L., Biederman, J., & Rohde, L. A. (2007). The worldwide prevalence of ADHD: A systematic review and metaregression analysis. *The American Journal of Psychiatry*. http://doi.org/10.1176/ajp.2007.164.6.942.

Proal, E., Reiss, P., Klein, R., Mannuzza, S., Gotimer, K., Ramos-Olazagasti, M., ... Castellanos, F. (2011). Brain gray matter deficits at 33-year follow-up in adults with attention-deficit/hyperactivity disorder established in childhood. *Archives of General Psychiatry*, *68*(11), 1122–34. http://doi.org/10.1001/archgenpsychiatry.2011.117.

Purper-ouakil, D., Ramoz, N., Gorwood, P., & Simonneau, M. (2011). Neurobiology of attention deficit/hyperactivity disorder. *Pediatric Research*, *69*(5 Pt 2), 69R–76R.

Rasmussen, E. R., Neuman, R. J., Heath, A. C., Levy, F., Hay, D. A., & Todd, R. D. (2004). Familial clustering of latent class and DSM-IV defined attention-deficit/hyperactivity disorder (ADHD) subtypes. *Journal of Child Psychology & Psychiatry, & Allied Disciplines*, *45*(3), 589–98.

Reiersen, A. M., Constantino, J. N., Volk, H. E., & Todd, R. D. (2007). Autistic traits in a population-based ADHD twin sample. *Journal of Child Psychology & Psychiatry, & Allied Disciplines*. http://doi.org/10.1111/j.1469-7610.2006.01720.x.

Robinson, M. R., Wray, N. R., & Visscher, P. M. (2014). Explaining additional genetic variation in complex traits. *Trends in Genetics: TIG*, *30*(4), 124–32. http://doi.org/10.1016/j.tig.2014.02.003.

Rommelse, N., Franke, B., Geurts, H., Hartman, C., & Buitelaar, J. (2010). Shared heritability of attention-deficit/hyperactivity disorder and autism spectrum disorder. *European Child & Adolescent Psychiatry*, *19*(3), 281–95. http://doi.org/10.1007/s00787-010-0092-x.

Ronald, A., Simonoff, E., Kuntsi, J., Asherson, P., & Plomin, R. (2008). Evidence for overlapping genetic influences on autistic and ADHD behaviours in a community twin sample. *Journal of Child Psychology & Psychiatry, & Allied Disciplines*. http://doi.org/10.1111/j.1469-7610.2007.01857.x.

Rubia, K., Alegria, A. A., Cubillo, A. I., Smith, A. B., Brammer, M. J., & Radua, J. (2014). Effects of stimulants on brain function in attention-deficit/hyperactivity disorder: A systematic review and meta-analysis. *Biological Psychiatry*, *76*(8), 616–28. Retrieved from http://www.pubmedcentral.nih.gov/articlerender.fcgi?artid=4183380&tool=pmcentrez&rendertype=abstract.

Rubia, K., Halari, R., Cubillo, A., Mohammad, A. M., Brammer, M., & Taylor, E. (2009). Methylphenidate normalises activation and functional connectivity deficits in attention and motivation networks in medication-naïve children with ADHD during a rewarded continuous performance task. *Neuropharmacology*, *57*(7–8), 640–52. http://doi.org/10.1016/j.neuropharm.2009.08.013.

Rubia, K., Halari, R., Smith, A. B., Mohammad, M., Scott, S., & Brammer, M. J. (2009). Shared and disorder-specific prefrontal abnormalities in boys with pure attention-deficit/hyperactivity disorder compared to boys with pure CD during interference inhibition and attention allocation. *Journal of Child Psychology & Psychiatry & Allied Disciplines*, *50*(6), 669–78. http://doi.org/10.1111/j.1469-7610.2008.02022.x.

Sato, J. R., Hoexter, M. Q., Castellanos, X. F., & Rohde, L. A. (2012). Abnormal brain connectivity patterns in adults with ADHD: A coherence study. *PloS One*, 7(9), e45671.

Schneider, M. F., Krick, C. M., Retz, W., Hengesch, G., Retz-Junginger, P., Reith, W., & Rösler, M. (2010). Impairment of fronto-striatal and parietal cerebral networks correlates with attention deficit hyperactivity disorder (ADHD) psychopathology in adults - A functional magnetic resonance imaging (fMRI) study. *Psychiatry Research - Neuroimaging*, *183*(1), 75–84. http://doi.org/10.1016/j.pscychresns.2010.04.005.

Shah, P. E., Robbins, N., Coelho, R. B., & Poehlmann, J. (2013). The paradox of prematurity: The behavioral vulnerability of late preterm infants and the cognitive susceptibility of very preterm infants at 36 months post-term. *Infant Behaviour & Development*, *36*(1), 50–62.

Shaw, P., Malek, M., Watson, B., Greenstein, D., De Rossi, P., & Sharp, W. (2013). Trajectories of cerebral cortical development in childhood and adolescence and adult attention-deficit/hyperactivity disorder. *Biological Psychiatry*, *74*(8), 599–606. http://doi.org/10.1016/j.biopsych.2013.04.007.

Silk, T. J., Vance, A., Rinehart, N., Bradshaw, J. L., & Cunnington, R. (2009a). Structural development of the basal ganglia in attention deficit hyperactivity disorder: A diffusion tensor imaging study. *Psychiatry Research*, *172*(3), 220–5.

Silk, T. J., Vance, A., Rinehart, N., Bradshaw, J. L., & Cunnington, R. (2009b). White-matter abnormalities in attention deficit hyperactivity disorder: A diffusion tensor imaging study. *Human Brain Mapping*, *30*(9), 2757–65.

Simon, V., Czobor, P., Bálint, S., Mészáros, A., & Bitter, I. (2009). Prevalence and correlates of adult attention-deficit hyperactivity disorder: Meta-analysis. *The British Journal of Psychiatry: The Journal of Mental Science*, *194*(3), 204–11. Retrieved from http://www.ncbi.nlm.nih.gov/pubmed/19252145.

Spencer, T. J., Biederman, J., Madras, B. K., Dougherty, D. D., Bonab, A. A., Livni, E., … Fischman, A. J. (2007). Further evidence of dopamine transporter dysregulation in ADHD: A controlled PET imaging study using altropane. *Biological Psychiatry*, *62*(9), 1059–61.

Spencer, T. J., Biederman, J., Madras, B. K., Faraone, S. V, Dougherty, D. D., Bonab, A. A., & Fischman, A. J. (2005). In vivo neuroreceptor imaging in attention-deficit/hyperactivity disorder: A focus on the dopamine transporter. *Biological Psychiatry*, *57*(11), 1293–300.

Sprich, S., Biederman, J., Crawford, M. H., Mundy, E., & Faraone, S. V. (2000). Adoptive and biological families of children and adolescents with ADHD. *Journal of the American Academy of Child & Adolescent Psychiatry*, *39*(11), 1432–7. http://doi.org/10.1097/00004583-200011000-00018.

Sun, L., Cao, Q., Long, X., Sui, M., Cao, X., Zhu, C., … Wang, Y. (2012). Abnormal functional connectivity between the anterior cingulate and the default mode network in drug-naïve boys with attention deficit hyperactivity disorder. *Psychiatry Research*, *201*(2), 120–7.

Tarver, J., Daley, D., & Sayal, K. (2014). Attention-deficit hyperactivity disorder (ADHD): An updated review of the essential facts. *Child: Care, Health & Development*, *40*(6), 762–74. http://doi.org/10.1111/cch.12139.

Thapar, A., Cooper, M., Jefferies, R., & Stergiakouli, E. (2011). What causes attention deficit hyperactivity disorder? *Archives of Disease in Childhood*, *97*(3), 260–5. http://doi.org/10.1136/archdischild-2011-300482.

Tye, C., Rijsdijk, F., Greven, C. U., Kuntsi, J., Asherson, P., & McLoughlin, G. (2012). Shared genetic influences on ADHD symptoms and very low-frequency EEG activity: A twin study. *Journal of Child Psychology & Psychiatry, & Allied Disciplines*, *53*(6), 706–15. http://doi.org/10.1111/j.1469-7610.2011.02501.x.

Valera, E. M., Faraone, S.V., Biederman, J., Poldrack, R.A., & Seidman, L. J. (2005). Functional neuroanatomy of working memory in adults with attention-deficit/hyperactivity disorder. *Biological Psychiatry*, *57*(5), 439–47.

Vance, A., Silk, T., Casey, M., Rinehart, N., Bradshaw, J., Bellgrove, M., & Cunnington, R. (2007). Right parietal dysfunction in children with attention deficit hyperactivity disorder, combined type: A functional MRI study. *Molecular Psychiatry*, *12*(9), 826–32. http://doi.org/10.1038/sj.mp.4001999.

Volkow, N. D., Wang, G.-J., Newcorn, J., Fowler, J. S., Telang, F., Solanto, M.V, … Pradhan, K. (2007). Brain dopamine transporter levels in treatment and drug naïve adults with ADHD. *NeuroImage*, *34*(3), 1182–90.

Waldman, I. D. (2005). Statistical approaches to complex phenotypes: Evaluating neuropsychological endophenotypes for attention-deficit/hyperactivity disorder. *Biological Psychiatry*, *57*(11), 1347–56. http://doi.org/10.1016/j.biopsych.2005.03.002.

Wehmeier, P. M., Schacht, A., Wolff, C., Otto, W. R., Dittmann, R. W., & Banaschewski, T. (2011). Neuropsychological outcomes across the day in children with attention-deficit/hyperactivity disorder treated with atomoxetine: Results from a placebo-controlled study using a computer-based continuous performance test combined with an infra-red motion-tra. *Journal of Child & Adolescent Psychopharmacology*, *21*(5), 433–44. http://doi.org/10.1089/cap.2010.0142.

Weyandt, L. (2006). *The Physiological Bases of Cognitive and Behavioral Disorders.* Mahwah, NJ: Lawrence Erlbaum and Associates.

Wijsman, E. M., & Amos, C. I. (1997). Genetic analysis of simulated oligogenic traits in nuclear and extended pedigrees: Summary of GAW10 contributions. *Genetic Epidemiology*, *14*(6), 719–35. http://doi.org/10.1002/(SICI)1098-2272(1997)14:6<719::AID-GEPI28>3.0.CO;2-S.

Willcutt, E. G. (2012). The prevalence of DSM-IV attention-deficit/hyperactivity disorder: A meta-analytic review. *Neurotherapeutics*, *9*(3), 490–9. http://doi.org/10.1007/s13311-012-0135-8.

Wolf, R. C., Plichta, M. M., Sambataro, F., Fallgatter, A. J., Jacob, C., Lesch, K. P., … Vasic, N. (2009). Regional brain activation changes and abnormal functional connectivity of the ventrolateral prefrontal cortex during working memory processing in adults with attention-deficit/hyperactivity disorder. *Human Brain Mapping*, *30*(7), 2252–66. http://doi.org/10.1002/hbm.20665.

Yamashita, M., Sakakibara, Y., Hall, F. S., Numachi, Y., Yoshida, S., Kobayashi, H., … Sora, I. (2013). Impaired cliff avoidance reaction in dopamine transporter knockout mice. *Psychopharmacology*, *227*(4), 741–9. http://doi.org/10.1007/s00213-013-3009-9.

9
CONDUCT DISORDER AND OPPOSITIONAL DEFIANT DISORDER

Jessica Green, Emma Sciberras and Peter G. Enticott

Introduction

Antisocial behaviour, including aggression and frequent interpersonal conflict, has long been observed as a common feature of frontostriatal impairment. Following Phineas Gage's famous accident, which involved extensive damage to ventral and dorsal aspects of the frontal lobe, friends and colleagues noted his tendency toward aggressive, offensive, and generally antisocial behaviour (although this account is potentially somewhat apocryphal; Horn et al., 2012). Unlike many of the disorders presented in this volume, those with Oppositional Defiant Disorder (ODD) or Conduct Disorder (CD), particularly childhood onset CD, can have involvement with the criminal justice system from an early age. While perhaps not as widely studied as other neurodevelopmental disorders, there is evidence for a range of neuropsychological and neurobiological impairments in ODD/CD that are closely related to frontostriatal circuitry.

Clinical vignette

Max, an eight-year-old boy, was referred for a clinical psychology assessment by his pediatrician. Max's parents reported frequent occasions where Max would lose his temper with his parents and sisters, often without a clear trigger, and that he often blamed others for his mistakes. They also noted that Max rarely did what he was asked to the point in which it was having a great impact on Max and the family's functioning. Max's two older sisters described how Max would deliberately annoy them while they were doing their homework almost every day and that he had been observed to ruin family property on multiple occasions.

Max's classroom teacher reported a similar history of oppositional behaviour and property destruction at school over the past year, with these behaviours contributing to academic and social difficulties. She said that Max persistently annoyed his peers, leading him to become increasingly isolated from them. He had also initiated four physical fights with peers over the past year. A cognitive assessment showed that Max's intellectual abilities were in the High Average Range, with superior abilities in perceptual reasoning.

Following assessment, Max was diagnosed with moderate ODD according to DSM-5 criteria. The psychologist noted that Max also exhibited early signs of CD (e.g., deliberate destruction of property and initiating physical fights), but this was not sufficient for a diagnosis. Parent training with a clinical psychologist was recommended for his parents and ongoing pediatrician review.

When Max was in Year 7, he was re-referred to the psychology service. The referring pediatrician noted that Max had deteriorating academic and social functioning. He had initiated a number of physical fights with peers at high school leading to significant injuries, made daily verbal threats to his teachers and parents, and had stayed out past midnight on four occasions, despite a 9 pm curfew set by his parents. Max's daily verbal threats led his classroom teacher to become visually upset, eventually needing to take sick leave from her work at the school. Max was reported to be cold and uncaring in response to his teacher's distress. They were also concerned by the number of suspensions he had received, with the most recent suspension given when Max graffitied the school hall. The pediatrician also noted that Max's school was concerned about his unexplained absences from school, which had occurred consistently throughout the year, with a week long absence in fourth term. Max was reported to consistently show a similar lack of remorse and empathy towards his peers and his mother. Max was diagnosed with moderate DSM-5 CD, Childhood-Onset type, with limited prosocial emotions, specifically a lack of empathy and a lack of remorse.

Clinical description, etiology, and epidemiology

ODD and CD are described in the 'Disruptive, Impulse-Control, and Conduct Disorders' section of the Diagnostic and Statistical Manual of Mental Disorders Version 5 (DSM-5; American Psychiatric Association, 2013). The hallmark features of these disorders are difficulties in emotional and behavioural self-control, which manifest in behaviours that violate the rights of others (Klahr & Burt, 2014). These are disorders that have their origins in childhood or adolescence; it is rare for either of these disorders to appear for the first time in adulthood (Blair, Leibenluft, & Pine, 2014). Most adolescents with CD have previously met criteria for ODD, however, it is important to note that the majority of children with ODD do not go on to meet the full criteria for CD (Rowe, Costello, Angold, Copeland, & Maughan, 2010).

Clinical presentation and diagnosis

Within DSM-5, ODD is diagnosed on the basis of a pattern of 'angry/irritable mood' (e.g., often loses temper), 'argumentative/defiant behaviour' (e.g., often argues with authority figures), or vindictiveness (American Psychiatric Association, 2013). Symptoms need to be present for 6 months and occur during interactions with at least one person that is not a sibling. In order to meet diagnostic criteria, the behaviours must result in distress to the individual or others or need to have a negative impact on daily functioning. ODD behaviours may only manifest in one setting, typically home, however, the pervasiveness of symptoms is usually reflective of the severity of the disorder (American Psychiatric Association, 2013).

CD is a more severe behavioural disorder characterized by repetitive and persistent behaviour that violates the basic rights of others or major age-appropriate societal norms (American Psychiatric Association, 2013). Fifteen CD symptoms are included in the diagnostic criteria, categorised across four domains including aggression to people and animals, destruction of property, deceitfulness or theft, and serious violations of rules. However, only three behaviours need to be present over the past 12 months (with at least one in the past 6 months) in order to make a diagnosis, which makes the clinical presentation of CD quite heterogeneous (Klahr & Burt, 2014). For example, physical or overtly aggressive behaviour appears to be distinct from non-aggressive rule-breaking behaviour (Frick et al., 1993). Physical aggression seems to be a more stable interpersonal trait with early physical aggression being predictive of later physical aggression (Blair et al., 2014). While physical aggression generally tends to decline with age, nonaggressive rule breaking behaviour sharply increases from childhood to adolescence (Maughan, Rowe, Messer, Goodman, & Meltzer, 2004).

In order to diagnose CD, the behaviours must cause clinically significant impairment in functioning and the pattern of behaviour needs to be present across multiple settings (American Psychiatric Association, 2013). The DSM-5 criteria include two important specifiers, which are likely to be important when considering the neuropsychological and neurobiological underpinning of CD, namely age of onset and the presence of callous and unemotional (CU) traits.

Developmental progression and outcomes

Although CD can occur during the early preschool years, the first signs of the condition typically emerge from middle childhood through to middle adolescence. Based on age of onset, CD can be classified according to two main subtypes, childhood onset subtype, with at least one behaviour present prior to age 10 years, and adolescent onset subtype (American Psychiatric Association, 2013). Adolescents with the childhood onset type are more likely to have a history of ODD (American Psychiatric Association, 2013). The less serious symptoms of CD tend to emerge first (e.g., lying, shoplifting), with more severe symptoms emerging later in its developmental progression (e.g., rape, theft while confronting victim). Nevertheless, there is a great deal of heterogeneity in the presentation and course of CD.

For most, the disorder remits in adulthood, particularly for those presenting with the adolescent type, but those with childhood onset CD carry a poorer prognosis including increased physical aggression, poorer social relationships, elevated comorbid disorders, and increased persistence into adulthood, in comparison to the adolescent onset subtype (Klahr & Burt, 2014). As a group, youth with CD are at risk for multiple psychiatric disorders in adulthood including anxiety, mood, impulse-control, and psychotic and substance-related disorders in adulthood (Morcillo et al., 2012).

More broadly, CD is associated with a number of negative functional outcomes including school suspension/expulsion, risky sexual behaviour (e.g., sexually transmitted diseases, unplanned pregnancies), physical injuries from accidents/fights, contact with the criminal justice system, earlier onset of sexual behaviour and substance abuse (Burke, Rowe, & Boylan, 2014).

ODD symptoms often emerge during preschool and it is rare for symptoms to first emerge later in adolescence. Although most children with ODD do not go on to have CD, the disorder is not benign (Rowe et al., 2010). Children with ODD are at later risk for anxiety and mood disorders even in the absence of CD (Rowe et al., 2010). The presence of defiant, argumentative, and vindictive ODD symptoms conveys the most risk for CD, whereas the angry-irritable mood ODD symptoms place children at particular risk of internalizing disorders (Leadbeater & Homel, 2015). As a group, children with ODD are also at risk of poorer adult outcomes, including antisocial behaviour, impulse-control problems, and substance abuse (Morcillo et al., 2012).

ODD and CD are considered to be developmental precursors to diagnoses made in adulthood, such as antisocial personality disorder and psychopathy (Blair et al., 2014). Similar to ODD and CD, these conditions involve a high level of interpersonal conflict and a violation of the rights of others. Unsurprisingly, prevalence rates among incarcerated populations are high (Boduszek, Belsher, Dhingra, & Ioannou, 2013).

Presence of callous and unemotional (CU) traits

CU traits, including a lack of empathy and guilt, are present in 10–50% of youth with CD (Kahn, Frick, Youngstrom, Findling, & Youngstrom, 2012). The presence of CU traits, for both males and females with CD, is more likely predictive of a poorer prognosis, characterized by a more severe, aggressive, and persistent pattern of antisocial behaviour compared to youth with CD without CU traits (Blair et al., 2014; Frick & White, 2008; Kahn et al., 2012). CU traits appear to be more elevated in the childhood onset version of the disorder and may have stronger neurocognitive underpinnings (Blair et al., 2014).

The 'limited prosocial emotions' specifier can be used to note the presence of CU traits in youth with CD (American Psychiatric Association, 2013). This specifier was an important addition to the DSM-5 that recognised the differential presentation and prognosis of CD in the presence or absence of CU. This specifier can be applied if two or more of the following characteristics have been present over the past 12 months across multiple relationships and settings (American Psychiatric Association, 2013, p. 470):

1. Lack of remorse or guilt (e.g., general lack of concern about negative consequences of actions);
2. Callousness or lack of empathy (e.g., disregards and unconcerned about feelings of others);
3. Being unconcerned about poor or problematic performance; and
4. Shallow or deficient affect (e.g., does not express feelings or show emotions to others except in ways that may be shallow or superficial).

Prevalence

DSM-5 reports the prevalence of ODD and CD to be 3% (range: 1–11%) and 4% (range: 2–10%), respectively (American Psychiatric Association, 2013). A recent meta-analysis examining the worldwide prevalence of mental health disorders in 41 studies across 27 countries reported the prevalence of disruptive behaviour disorders (ODD/CD) to be 5.7% (CI 95% 4.0–8.1) and 3.6% (CI 95% 2.8–4.7) for ODD and 2.1% for CD (95% CI 1.6–2.9) (Polanczyk et al., 2015). The prevalence of ODD and CD is higher in males; accordingly, the majority of previous research has centered on males with these disorders, leaving females with CD a particularly under-researched group. There are more notable gender differences for physically aggressive behaviours than for non-aggressive rule breaking behaviour (Blair et al., 2014).

Comorbidity

ODD and CD rarely occur in isolation; the most common comorbidity is Attention Deficit/Hyperactivity Disorder (ADHD) (Efron et al., 2014). Approximately one-third of children with severe ADHD go on to have CD (Beauchaine, Hinshaw, & Pang, 2010). ADHD symptoms often precede the development of ODD symptoms, which in turn increases the risk for CD symptoms (Beauchaine et al., 2010). ADHD appears to be more strongly correlated with childhood onset CD and is more generally associated with greater impairment compared to CD alone (Pardini & Fite, 2010). Mood disorders, anxiety disorders, non-suicidal self-injury, substance use, and learning disorders are also commonly associated with ODD and CD (Preyde et al., 2012).

Aetiology

A number of risk factors have been implicated in the development of ODD including harsh, inconsistent, or neglectful parenting behaviours, a child temperament characterized by high emotional reactivity, and poor frustration tolerance (American Psychiatric Association, 2013). Similarly, CD has been associated with a number of child factors including difficult infant temperament and cognitive and neuropsychological deficits, which are reviewed in the latter part of this chapter (Stringaris, Maughan, & Goodman, 2010). Indeed, dysfunction within several frontostriatal circuits appears to be associated with both ODD and CD, and this is likely a result of the influence of both genetic and environmental factors on developmental of the central nervous system. A number of family and community level factors have also been linked with CD including parental rejection and neglect, hostile parenting practices, abuse history (physical and/or sexual), large family size, parental criminality, and a family history of psychopathology (e.g., CD, substance use disorders, mood disorders, or ADHD) (Burke et al., 2002). Community level factors include a history of peer rejection, association with delinquent peer groups, and neighbourhood violence. The presence of multiple individual and family risk factors is particularly predictive of the childhood onset subtype (Fairchild, van Goozen, Calder, & Goodyer, 2013) as opposed to the adolescent onset subtype.

The aetiology of CD may also differ depending on the presence of CU traits. Whilst aggression and CU traits have moderate-high heritability, CD without CU is more modestly influenced by genetics (Tuvblad & Beaver, 2013). Moreover, although positive and negative parenting practices have been longitudinally associated with CU (Waller, Gardner, & Hyde, 2013), it has been suggested that the association between parenting practices and CD is not as strong when high CU traits are present (Klahr & Burt, 2014). It is likely that the relationship between parenting behaviours and CD and CU is bidirectional, as CU traits in youth are likely to elicit more negative parenting behaviours (Klahr & Burt, 2014).

Evidence-based treatment for Oppositional Defiant Disorder and Conduct Disorder

Treatment for Oppositional Defiant Disorder (ODD)

Evidence based psychosocial interventions, such as Parent Child Interaction Therapy (PCIT), which is a parent training program, are the gold standard treatment for children and adolescents with ODD (Kapalka, 2015). Medication is sometimes used to treat comorbid conditions, or to manage aggression, but is not recommended as the sole intervention for ODD (Steiner & Remsing, 2007). The first line psychosocial treatment for children with ODD is parent training (Eyberg, Nelson, & Boggs, 2008). Established evidence based programs include Parent Child Interaction

Therapy (McNeil & Hembree-Kigin, 2010), The Incredible Years (IY), Triple P Positive Parenting Program (Sanders, 1999), Parent Management Training – Oregon model (PMTO; Patterson & Reid, 1975) and Helping the Non-Compliant Child (HNC; McMahon & Forehand, 2003). Treatment for adolescents typically focuses on individual or group treatment for the child, with an adjunct of parent training (Wu et al., 2015). Current evidence based programs include Problem Solving Skills training (PSST; Kazdin, 2010), a cognitive behavioural individual therapy program, with a focus on cognitive restructuring and problem solving, and Anger Control Training (ACT; Larson & Lochman, 2002), a group school based program targeting defiance towards teachers, with an individual and parent adjunct called Coping Power (Larson & Lochman, 2002). Randomised controlled trials of these programs show superior outcomes to waitlist and control groups, with significant reductions in ODD symptoms following treatment.

Treatment for Conduct Disorder (CD)

Guidelines for treating CD in children and adolescents suggest creating an individual treatment plan based on the type of CD symptoms and the age of symptom onset (Pardini & Frick, 2013). Behavioural parent-management training is recommended across all subtypes of CD, however, the specific emphasis within parent training, and the selection of appropriate adjunct treatments, can be informed by the presenting CD subtype (Henggeler & Sheidow, 2012; Klahr & Burt, 2014). Specific evidence based programs for CD include PSST (Kazdin, 2010), Parent Management Training (PMT; (Kazdin, 2005), PCIT (McNeil & Hembree-Kigin, 2010), Multi-systemic therapy (Henggeler & Borduin, 1990), functional family therapy (Alexander, 1994) and brief strategic family therapy (Szapocznik, Hervis, & Schwartz, 2003).

Behavioural parent-management training is effective for those with CD and callous-unemotional traits (CU), with some additional requirements (Klahr & Burt, 2014). Research suggests that treatment needs to focus on intensive highly structured positive reinforcement plans that are implemented across all settings (e.g., home and school; Klahr & Burt, 2014). It is recommended that psychotropic medication be considered for children with CD + CU traits at the commencement of therapy (Wu et al., 2015), together with multi-systemic therapy, given its comprehensive and intensive approach (Wagner, Borduin, Sawyer, & Dopp, 2014).

Any treatment plan needs to also consider intervention for comorbid conditions and difficulties that children with ODD or CD may present with. This commonly includes ADHD, social difficulties, internalising symptoms, or academic problems (Pardini & Frick, 2013).

A limitation of treatment studies in this area is that outcome evaluations do not specifically measure changes in frontostriatal deficits. Whilst a number of the treatment programs specifically target frontostriatal deficits, such as poor problem solving and impulsivity, treatment outcome studies rarely examine changes in these skills from a neuropsychological or physiological perspective. Future research would benefit from including this within treatment outcome evaluations.

Neuropsychology of Oppositional Defiant Disorder/ Conduct Disorder

As noted above, psychosocial risk factors for ODD/CD have been explored at length (e.g., poor attachment, reduced academic performance, rearing within criminogenic environments, early aggressive behaviour (Bassarath, 2001), but in this section we examine the likely frontostriatal contribution from a neuropsychological perspective. These studies of ODD/CD can be difficult to interpret, largely because of the aforementioned common comorbidities, and require careful study design to ensure that specific contributions from ODD/CD to neuropsychological impairment can be ascertained. This might involve, for instance, a matched ADHD group which is not comorbid for ODD/CD, or careful use of ADHD symptom measures that are then accounted for during statistical analyses. It is also apparent that despite a number of group-level trends, neuropsychological aspects of CD/ODD are highly heterogeneous (Närhi, Lehto-Salo, Ahonen, & Marttunen, 2010). There is also a lack of longitudinal data on the neuropsychology/neurobiology of these conditions (Blair et al., 2014), which is critical considering the developmental trajectory of ODD/CD.

Verbal ability

Historically, perhaps the most commonly reported neuropsychological impairment in CD is reduced verbal ability (Närhi et al., 2010). Verbal ability has been measured in various ways, including the verbal scales of the Wechsler Intelligence Scale for Children (WISC) and more detailed language/verbal assessment. Importantly, these verbal deficits in CD are evident even after controlling for the influence of ADHD symptomatology/comorbidity (Déry, Toupin, Pauzé, Mercier, & Fortin, 1999), and have been associated with increased physical aggression and theft (Barker et al., 2011).

Executive function

As noted, CD/ODD are typically comorbid with a range of other conditions for which developmental frontostriatal dysfunction is evident, most notably ADHD. Nevertheless, where CD/ODD have been examined, there is evidence for specific neuropsychological impairments in these conditions (Pajer et al., 2008).

Many of the studies conducted have examined executive abilities relevant to externalizing behaviours; for instance, response inhibition and emotional regulation. These are often interpreted in the context of characteristic behaviours, including impulsiveness, aggression, and violence. For instance, children with CD demonstrate impaired delay of gratification (Dolan & Lennox, 2013), response disinhibition (Nigg, 2003), faster responding (Dougherty, Bjork, Marsh, & Moeller, 2000), and poor cognitive control for emotive stimuli (Euler, Sterzer, & Stadler, 2014). Increased response perseveration has also been reported in "pure" CD, but this was less impaired than among those with CD/ADHD (Matthys, Van Goozen, De Vries, Cohen-Kettenis, & Van Engeland, 1998), while Toupin, Déry, Pauzé, Mercier, & Fortin (2000) found a range of executive impairments (e.g., perseveration, poor planning, impaired conflict resolution) in CD after controlling for ADHD symptoms. When accounting for comorbid intellectual disability, Van Der Meer and Van Der Meere (2004) still found evidence for go/no go response disinhibition in CD.

Nevertheless, there is evidence to suggest that many executive deficits that might be seen in CD/ODD are attributable to comorbid ADHD (Clark, Prior, & Kinsella, 2000; Déry et al., 1999; Dolan & Lennox, 2013), and thus not attributable to CD/ODD per se, while Narhi et al. (2010) suggest that CD is not associated with either visuospatial or memory impairments. Some authors have also warned against the use of many of these measures in clinical settings (Frick & Loney, 2000).

Social cognition: Facial emotion recognition, theory of mind, and empathy

As children with CD consistently violate the rights of others, they can appear to have reduced empathy and a bias toward misinterpreting others' emotions (e.g., attribution of hostility). Accordingly, most recent studies examining neuropsychological function in these groups have focused primarily on social cognitive abilities. Perhaps unsurprisingly, children with CD have been found to have reduced empathy and automatic facial mimicry, yet this is not identical to the social cognitive impairments seen in autism spectrum disorder (ASD; Bons et al., 2013). Children with CD also show deficits in facial affect recognition (Fairchild, Stobbe, Van Goozen, Calder, & Goodyer, 2010), particularly for negative emotions (Bowen, Morgan, Moore, & Van Goozen, 2014), which may lead to attribution errors in interpersonal settings. Results, however, are not consistent across all studies (Schepman, Taylor, Collishaw, & Fombonne, 2012), and an examination of girls with CD revealed no impairments in facial affect recognition (Pajer, Leininger, & Gardner, 2010), suggesting possible differential gender effects on CD. Children with CD have shown impairment on "theory of mind" tasks assessing false beliefs (i.e., recognition that another individual can hold a belief that you know is factually incorrect), which is typically linked to dorsomedial prefrontal and temporoparietal regions, and considered characteristic of ASD (Frith & Happé, 1994).

Developmental neurobiology: Frontostriatal impairments

Relative to other neurodevelopmental disorders addressed in this volume, there have been relatively few neuroimaging and neurophysiological investigations of CD/ODD. Early studies employing electroencephalography (EEG) revealed a reduced P300 amplitude in children with CD (Bauer & Hesselbrock 2003), which was broadly interpreted as reflecting delayed maturation of prefrontal regions critical for executive abilities. There is also evidence to suggest altered autonomic arousal in CD/ODD (Fairchild et al., 2010), which has been related to deficits in motivation and social cognitive responsiveness.

Structural neuroimaging (magnetic resonance imaging [MRI]) studies have revealed several anatomical differences in CD. Compared to healthy controls, boys with CD (some of which have comorbid ADHD) have shown reduced grey matter volume in the orbitofrontal cortex, amygdala, and hippocampus (Huebner et al., 2008), while boys with CD/ODD also show evidence of a larger cavum septum pellucidum (indicative of abnormal brain development) (White et al., 2013) and reduced grey matter volume in the temporal cortex (Michalska, Decety, Zeffiro, & Lahey, 2014) (although the latter study failed to replicate earlier studies demonstrating more widespread grey matter reductions in CD). Examining "pure" CD and ADHD groups, Stevens and Haney-Caron (2012) found extensive reductions in grey matter volume in children with CD, including frontostriatal regions. Diffusion tensor imaging (DTI), which maps and assesses the integrity of white matter pathways in the brain, has revealed white matter abnormalities, with adolescents with CD showing increased fractional anisotropy (FA) in the uncinate fascicle, which links amygdala with orbitofrontal regions, even after accounting for comorbid ADHD (Passamonti et al., 2012). Such abnormalities in limbic-prefrontal circuitry may relate to difficulties in regulating behaviour in the context of strong emotionality, which is consistent with some of the neuropsychological data (Euler et al., 2014). By contrast, however, McAlonan et al. (2007) found that, among a small sample of children with ADHD, comorbid CD/ODD did not have a significant effect on grey and white matter volume, while Hummer et al. (Hummer, Wang, Kronenberger, Dunn, & Mathews, 2015) found that children with CD/ODD did not show grey matter volume or FA differences after accounting for ADHD.

Functional neuroimaging studies of CD/ODD have also demonstrated specific evidence for neurobiological impairment. Children with CD/ODD display reduced amygdala activation when viewing fearful faces, and reduced functional connectivity between the ventromedial cortex and amygdala (perhaps consistent with structural abnormalities in the uncinate fascicle) (Passamonti et al., 2012). In a series of studies involving "pure" groups of children with CD and ADHD, boys with CD demonstrated less activation in posterior cingulate and inferior parietal/superior temporal cortical regions during failed response inhibition (Rubia et al., 2008), reduced activity in the frontal cortex, insula, hippocampus, and cerebellum during a sustained attention task (Rubia et al., 2009), and reduced activity in the temporal, parietal, and occipital cortices during a cognitive flexibility task (Rubia et al., 2010). More recently, adolescent females with CD have shown reduced activity with the orbitofrontal cortex and insula during facial emotion processing, yet these did not remain when controlling for ADHD symptoms (Fairchild et al., 2014). Although not examining CD/ODD per se, Cohn et al. (2015) found associations between abnormal resting-state connections and psychopathic traits among adolescents who had had contact with the juvenile criminal justice system, including a link between enhanced connectivity in a frontal pole region and increased callous-unemotional traits (Cohn et al., 2015).

Summary

Children with CD/ODD show deficits in a range of abilities that are typically mediated by frontostriatal networks, including verbal ability, inhibitory control, facial emotion recognition, theory of mind, and verbal intelligence. Many of these impairments are evident even after accounting for comorbidities including ADHD and intellectual disability, although there remains much controversy as to the specific contribution of neuropsychological impairments to the cognitive profile of CD/ODD. Data from neurophysiological and neuroimaging studies provides evidence for impairments in a range of networks of the brain, including prefrontal and limbic structures.

Despite these studies, our neuropsychological and neurobiological understanding of CD/ODD remains quite limited. The research to date is characterised by small and confounded samples, a limited number of experimental paradigms, and somewhat inconsistent findings. Even where "pure" samples of CD/ODD are employed, this is generally a less representative sample and it is unclear whether the findings will generalize to those with, for example CD and ADHD, or CD and mood/anxiety disorder. The sheer variety of measures employed, even within a specific domain (e.g., response inhibition), also makes it difficult to summarise these studies. In addition, while there are several neuropsychological and neurobiological studies of CD, there are very few such studies of ODD.

Abbreviations

ADHD: Attention Deficit/Hyperactivity Disorder
ASD: Autism Spectrum Disorder
CD: Conduct Disorder
CI: Confidence interval
CU: Callous and unemotional traits
DSM-5: Diagnostic and Statistical Manual of Mental Disorders, 5th Edition
FA: Fractional anisotropy
ODD: Oppositional Defiant Disorder

PCIT: Parent Child Interaction Therapy
PMT: Parent Management Training
PSST: Problem Solving Skills Training
WISC: Wechsler Intelligence Scale for Children

Further readings

Kapalka, G. M. (Ed.). (2015). *Treating Disruptive Disorders: A Guide to Psychological, Pharmacological, and Combined Therapies*. New York: Routledge.

Klahr, A. M., & Burt, S. A. (2014). Practitioner review: Evaluation of the known behavioral heterogeneity in conduct disorder to improve its assessment and treatment. *Journal of Child Psychology & Psychiatry, 55*(12), 1300–1310. doi: 10.1111/jcpp.12268.

Steiner, H., & Remsing, L. (2007). Practice parameter for the assessment and treatment of children and adolescents with Oppositional Defiant Disorder. *Journal of the American Academy of Child & Adolescent Psychiatry, 46*(1), 126–141. doi: 10.1097/01.chi.0000246060.62706.af.

References

Alexander, J. F. (1994). The process and outcome of marital and family therapy research: Review and evaluation. In A. E. Bergin & S. L. Garfield (Eds.), *Handbook of Behavior Therapy and Behavior Change* (4th edition ed., pp. 595–630). New York: Wiley.

American Psychiatric Association. (2013). *The Diagnostic and Statistical Manual of Mental Disorders (5th Ed.)*. Arlington, VA: American Psychiatric Publishing.

Barker, E. D., Tremblay, R. E., Van Lier, P. A., Vitaro, F., Nagin, D. S., Assaad, J. M., & Séguin, J. R. (2011). The neurocognition of conduct disorder behaviors: Specificity to physical aggression and theft after controlling for ADHD symptoms. *Aggressive Behavior, 37*(1), 63–72. doi: 10.1002/ab.20373.

Bassarath, L. (2001). Conduct disorder: A biopsychosocial review. *Canadian Journal of Psychiatry, 46*(7), 609–616.

Bauer, L. O., & Hesselbrock, V. M. (2003). Brain maturation and subtypes of conduct disorder: Interactive effects on P300 amplitude and topography in male adolescents. *Journal of the American Academy of Child & Adolescent Psychiatry, 42*(1), 106–115. doi: 10.1097/00004583-200301000-00017.

Beauchaine, T. P., Hinshaw, S. P., & Pang, K. L. (2010). Comorbidity of attention-deficit/hyperactivity disorder and early-onset conduct disorder: Biological, environmental, and developmental mechanisms. *Clinical Psychology: Science & Practice, 17*(4), 327–336. doi: 10.1111/j.1468-2850.2010.01224.x.

Blair, R. J. R., Leibenluft, E., & Pine, D. S. (2014). Conduct disorder and callous-unemotional traits in youth. *New England Journal of Medicine, 371*(23), 2207–2216. doi: 10.1056/NEJMra1315612.

Boduszek, D., Belsher, R., Dhingra, K., & Ioannou, M. (2013). Psychosocial correlates of recidivism in a sample of ex-prisoners: The role of oppositional defiant disorder and conduct disorder. *The Journal of Forensic Psychiatry & Psychology, 25*(1), 61–76. doi: 10.1080/14789949.2013.862293.

Bons, D., Van Den Broek, E., Scheepers, F., Herpers, P., Rommelse, N., & Buitelaaar, J. K. (2013). Motor, emotional, and cognitive empathy in children and adolescents with autism spectrum disorder and conduct disorder. *Journal of Abnormal Child Psychology, 41*(3), 425–443. doi: 10.1007/s10802-012-9689-5.

Bowen, K. L., Morgan, J. E., Moore, S. C., & Van Goozen, S. H. M. (2014). Young offenders' emotion recognition dysfunction across emotion intensities: Explaining variation using psychopathic traits, conduct disorder and offense severity. *Journal of Psychopathology & Behavioral Assessment, 36*(1), 60–73. doi: 10.1007/s10862-013-9368-z.

Burke, J. D., Loeber, R., & Birmaher, B. (2002). Oppositional defiant disorder and conduct disorder: A review of the past 10 years, Part II. *Journal of the American Academy of Child & Adolescent Psychiatry, 41*(11), 1275–1293. doi: 10.1097/00004583-200211000-00009.

Burke, J. D., Rowe, R., & Boylan, K. (2014). Functional outcomes of child and adolescent oppositional defiant disorder symptoms in young adult men. *Journal of Child Psychology & Psychiatry, 55*(3), 264–272. doi: 10.1111/jcpp.12150.

Clark, C., Prior, M., & Kinsella, G. J. (2000). Do executive function deficits differentiate between adolescents with ADHD and oppositional defiant/conduct disorder? A neuropsychological study using the Six Elements Test and Hayling Sentence Completion Test. *Journal of Abnormal Child Psychology, 28*(5), 403–414. doi: 10.1023/A:1005176320912.

Cohn, M. D., Pape, L. E., Schmaal, L., van den Brink, W., van Wingen, G., Vermeiren, R. R. J. M., … Popma, A. (2015). Differential relations between juvenile psychopathic traits and resting state network connectivity. *Human Brain Mapping, 36*(6), 2396–2405. doi: 10.1002/hbm.22779.

Déry, M., Toupin, J., Pauzé, R., Mercier, H., & Fortin, L. (1999). Neuropsychological characteristics of adolescents with conduct disorder: Association with attention-deficit-hyperactivity and aggression. *Journal of Abnormal Child Psychology, 27*(3), 225–236. doi: 10.1023/A:1021904523912.

Dolan, M., & Lennox, C. (2013). Cool and hot executive function in conduct-disordered adolescents with and without co-morbid attention deficit hyperactivity disorder: Relationships with externalizing behaviours. *Psychological Medicine, 43*(11), 2427–2436. doi: 10.1017/S0033291712003078.

Dougherty, D. M., Bjork, J. M., Marsh, D. M., & Moeller, G. F. (2000). A comparison between adults with conduct disorder and normal controls on a continuous performance test: Differences in impulsive response characteristics. *Psychological Record, 50*(2), 203–219.

Efron, D., Sciberras, E., Anderson, V., Hazell, P., Ukoumunne, O. C., Jongeling, B., … Nicholson, J. M. (2014). Functional status in children with ADHD at age 6–8: A controlled community study. *Pediatrics*. doi: 10.1542/peds.2014-1027.

Euler, F., Sterzer, P., & Stadler, C. (2014). Cognitive control under distressing emotional stimulation in adolescents with conduct disorder. *Aggressive Behavior, 40*(2), 109–119. doi: 10.1002/ab.21508.

Eyberg, S. M., Nelson, M. M., & Boggs, S. R. (2008). Evidence-based psychosocial treatments for children and adolescents with disruptive behavior. *Journal of Clinical Child & Adolescent Psychology, 37*(1), 215–237. doi: 10.1080/15374410701820117.

Fairchild, G., Hagan, C. C., Passamonti, L., Walsh, N. D., Goodyer, I. M., & Calder, A. J. (2014). Atypical neural responses during face processing in female adolescents with conduct disorder. *Journal of the American Academy of Child & Adolescent Psychiatry, 53*(6), 677–687.E675. doi: 10.1016/j.jaac.2014.02.009.

Fairchild, G., Stobbe, Y., Van Goozen, S. H. M., Calder, A. J., & Goodyer, I. M. (2010). Facial expression recognition, fear conditioning, and startle modulation in female subjects with conduct disorder. *Biological Psychiatry, 68*(3), 272–279. doi: 10.1016/j.biopsych.2010.02.019.

Fairchild, G., van Goozen, S. H., Calder, A. J., & Goodyer, I. M. (2013). Research review: Evaluating and reformulating the developmental taxonomic theory of antisocial behaviour. *Journal of Child Psychology & Psychiatry, 54*(9), 924–940. doi: 10.1111/jcpp.12102.

Frick, P. J., & Loney, B. R. (2000). The use of laboratory and performance-based measures in the assessment of children and adolescents with Conduct Disorders. *Journal of Clinical Child & Adolescent Psychology, 29*(4), 540–554.

Frick, P. J., & White, S. F. (2008). Research review: The importance of callous-unemotional traits for developmental models of aggressive and antisocial behavior. *Journal of Child Psychology & Psychiatry, 49*(4), 359–375. doi: 10.1111/j.1469-7610.2007.01862.x.

Frick, P. J., Lahey, B. B., Loeber, R., Tannenbaum, L., Vanhorn, Y., Christ, M. A. G., … Hanson, K. (1993). Oppostional defiant disorder and conduct disorder - A meta-analytic review of factor-analyses and cross-validation in a clinic sample. *Clinical Psychology Review, 13*(4), 319–340. doi: 10.1016/0272-7358(93)90016-f.

Frith, U., & Happé, F. (1994). Autism: Beyond "theory of mind". *Cognition, 50*(1), 115–132. doi: 10.1016/0010-0277(94)90024-8.

Henggeler, S. W., & Borduin, C. M. (1990). *Family Therapy and Beyond: A Multisystemic Approach to Teaching the Behavior Problems of Children and Adolescents.* Pacific Grove, CA: Brooks/Cole.

Henggeler, S. W., & Sheidow, A. J. (2012). Empirically supported family-based treatments for conduct disorder and delinquency in adolescents. *Journal of Marital & Family Therapy, 38*(1), 30–58. doi: 10.1111/j.1752-0606.2011.00244.x.

Horn, J. D., Irimia, A., Torgerson, C. M., Chambers, M. C., Kikinis, R., & Toga, A. W. (2012). Mapping connectivity damage in the case of Phineas Gage. *PLoS One,* 7(5). doi: 10.1371/journal.pone.0037454.

Huebner, T., Vloet, T. D., Marx, I., Konrad, K., Fink, G. R., Herpertz, S. C., & Herpertz-Dahlmann, B. (2008). Morphometric brain abnormalities in boys with conduct disorder. *Journal of the American Academy of Child & Adolescent Psychiatry, 47*(5), 540–547. doi: 10.1097/CHI.0b013e3181676545.

Hummer, T. A., Wang, Y., Kronenberger, W. G., Dunn, D. W., & Mathews, V. P. (2015). The relationship of brain structure to age and executive functioning in adolescent disruptive behavior disorder. *Psychiatry Research—Neuroimaging, 231*(3), 210–217. doi: 10.1016/j.pscychresns.2014.11.009.

Kahn, R. E., Frick, P. J., Youngstrom, E., Findling, R. L., & Youngstrom, J. K. (2012). The effects of including a callous-unemotional specifier for the diagnosis of conduct disorder. *Journal of Child Psychology & Psychiatry, 53*(3), 271–282. doi: 10.1111/j.1469-7610.2011.02463.x.

Kapalka, G. M. (Ed.). (2015). *Treating Disruptive Disorders: A Guide to Psychological, Pharmacological, & Combined Therapies.* New York: Routledge.

Kazdin, A. E. (2005). *Parent Management Training: Treatment for Oppositional, Aggressive and Antisocial Behavior in Children and Adolescents.* New York: Oxford University Press.

Kazdin, A. E. (2010). Problem-solving skills training and parent management training for oppositional defiant disorder and conduct disorder. In A. E. Kazdin & J. R. Weisz (Eds.), *Evidence-Based Psychotherapies for Children and Adolescents* (2nd edition ed., pp. 211–226). New York: Guilford Press.

Klahr, A. M., & Burt, S. A. (2014). Practitioner review: Evaluation of the known behavioral heterogeneity in conduct disorder to improve its assessment and treatment. *Journal of Child Psychology & Psychiatry, 55*(12), 1300–1310. doi: 10.1111/jcpp.12268.

Larson, J., & Lochman, J. E. (2002). *Helping School Children Cope with Anger: A Cognitive Behavioral Intervention.* New York: Guilford Press.

Leadbeater, B., & Homel, J. (2015). Irritable and defiant sub-dimensions of ODD: Their stability and prediction of internalizing symptoms and conduct problems from adolescence to young adulthood. *Journal of Abnormal Child Psychology, 43*(3), 407–421.

Matthys, W., Van Goozen, S. H. M., De Vries, H., Cohen-Kettenis, P. T., & Van Engeland, H. (1998). The dominance of behavioural activation over behavioural inhibition in conduct disordered boys with or without attention deficit hyperactivity disorder. *Journal of Child Psychology & Psychiatry & Allied Disciplines, 39*(5), 643–651. doi: 10.1017/S0021963098002534.

Maughan, B., Rowe, R., Messer, J., Goodman, R., & Meltzer, H. (2004). Conduct disorder and oppositional defiant disorder in a national sample: Developmental epidemiology. *Journal of Child Psychology & Psychiatry, 45*(3), 609–621. doi: 10.1111/j.1469-7610.2004.00250.x.

McAlonan, G. M., Cheung, V., Cheung, C., Chua, S. E., Murphy, D. G. M., Suckling, J., … Ho, T. P. (2007). Mapping brain structure in attention deficit-hyperactivity disorder: A voxel-based MRI study of regional grey and white matter volume. *Psychiatry Research—Neuroimaging, 154*(2), 171–180. doi: 10.1016/j.pscychresns.2006.09.006.

McMahon, R. J., & Forehand, R. (2003). *Helping the Noncompliant Child: Family-Based Treatment for Oppositional Behavior* (2nd edition ed.). New York: Guilford Press.

McNeil, C. B., & Hembree-Kigin, T. L. (2010). *Parent-Child Interaction Therapy* (2nd edition ed.). New York: Springer.

Michalska, K. J., Decety, J., Zeffiro, T. A., & Lahey, B. B. (2014). Association of regional gray matter volumes in the brain with disruptive behavior disorders in male and female children. *NeuroImage: Clinical, 7*, 252–257. doi: 10.1016/j.nicl.2014.12.012.

Morcillo, C., Duarte, C. S., Sala, R., Wang, S., Lejuez, C. W., Kerridge, B. T., & Blanco, C. (2012). Conduct disorder and adult psychiatric diagnoses: Associations and gender differences in the U.S. adult population. *Journal of Psychiatric Research, 46*(3), 323–330.

Närhi, V., Lehto-Salo, P., Ahonen, R., & Marttunen, M. (2010). Neuropsychological subgroups of adolescents with conduct disorder. *Scandinavian Journal of Psychology, 51*(3), 278–284. doi: 10.1111/j.1467-9450.2009.00767.x.

Nigg, J. T. (2003) Response inhibition and disruptive behaviors: Toward a multiprocess conception of etiological heterogeneity for ADHD combined type and conduct disorder early-onset type. *Annals of the New York Academy of Sciences*, 1008, 170–182.

Pajer, K., Chung, J., Leininger, L., Wang, W., Gardner, W., & Yeates, K. (2008). Neuropsychological function in adolescent girls with conduct disorder. *Journal of the American Academy of Child & Adolescent Psychiatry, 47*(4), 416–425. doi: 10.1097/CHI.0b013e3181640828.

Pajer, K., Leininger, L., & Gardner, W. (2010). Recognition of facial affect in girls with conduct disorder. *Psychiatry Research, 175*(3), 244–251. doi: 10.1016/j.psychres.2009.06.003.

Pardini, D. A., & Fite, P. J. (2010). Symptoms of conduct disorder, oppositional defiant disorder, attention-deficit/hyperactivity disorder, and callous-unemotional traits as unique predictors of psychosocial maladjustment in boys: Advancing an evidence base for DSM-V. *Journal of the American Academy of Child & Adolescent Psychiatry, 49*(11), 1134–1144. doi: 10.1016/j.jaac.2010.07.010.

Pardini, D., & Frick, P. J. (2013). Multiple developmental pathways to conduct disorder: Current conceptualizations and clinical implications. *Journal of the Canadian Academy of Child & Adolescent Psychiatry, 22*(1), 20–25.

Passamonti, L., Fairchild, G., Fornito, A., Goodyer, I. M., Nimmo-Smith, I., Hagan, C. C., & Calder, A. J. (2012). Abnormal anatomical connectivity between the amygdala and orbitofrontal cortex in conduct disorder. *PLoS One, 7*(11). doi: 10.1371/journal.pone.0048789.

Patterson, G., & Reid, J. B. (1975). *A Social Learning Approach to Family Intervention: Families with Aggressive Children* (Vol. 1). Eugene, OR: Castalia Pub. Co.

Polanczyk, G.V., Salum, G. A., Sugaya, L. S., Cave, A. & Rohde, L.A. (2015). Annual research review: A meta-analysis of the worldwide prevalence of mental disorders in children and adolescents. *Journal of Child Psychology & Psychiatry, 56*, 345–365.

Preyde, M., Watkins, H., Csuzdi, N., Carter, J., Lazure, K., White, S., … Frensch, K. (2012). Non-suicidal self-injury and suicidal behaviour in children and adolescents accessing residential or intensive home-based mental health services. *Journal of the Canadian Academy of Child & Adolescent Psychiatry, 21*(4), 270–281.

Rowe, R., Costello, E. J., Angold, A., Copeland, W. E., & Maughan, B. (2010). Developmental pathways in oppositional defiant disorder and conduct disorder. *Journal of Abnormal Psychology, 119*(4), 726–738. doi: 10.1037/a0020798.

Rubia, K., Halari, R., Cubillo, A., Mohammad, A. M., Scott, S., & Brammer, M. (2010). Disorder-specific inferior prefrontal hypofunction in boys with pure attention-deficit/hyperactivity disorder compared to boys with pure conduct disorder during cognitive flexibility. *Human Brain Mapping, 31*(12), 1823–1833. doi: 10.1002/hbm.20975.

Rubia, K., Halari, R., Smith, A. B., Mohammed, M., Scott, S., Giampietro, V., … Brammer, M. J. (2008). Dissociated functional brain abnormalities of inhibition in boys with pure conduct disorder and in boys with pure attention deficit hyperactivity disorder. *American Journal of Psychiatry, 165*(7), 889–897. doi: 10.1176/appi.ajp.2008.07071084.

Rubia, K., Smith, A. B., Halari, R., Matsukura, F., Mohammad, M., Taylor, E., & Brammer, M. J. (2009). Disorder-specific dissociation of orbitofrontal dysfunction in boys with pure conduct disorder during reward and ventrolateral prefrontal dysfunction in boys with pure ADHD during sustained attention. *American Journal of Psychiatry, 166*(1), 83–94. doi: 10.1176/appi.ajp.2008.08020212.

Sanders, M. R. (1999). Triple P-Positive Parenting Program: Towards an empirically validated multilevel parenting and family support strategy for the prevention of behavior and emotional problems in children. *Clinical Child & Family Psychology Review, 2*(2), 71–90. doi: 10.1023/A:1021843613840.

Schepman, K., Taylor, E., Collishaw, S., & Fombonne, E. (2012). Face emotion processing in depressed children and adolescents with and without comorbid conduct disorder. *Journal of Abnormal Child Psychology, 40*(4), 583–593. doi: 10.1007/s10802-011-9587-2.

Steiner, H., & Remsing, L. (2007). Practice parameter for the assessment and treatment of children and adolescents with oppositional defiant disorder. *Journal of the American Academy of Child & Adolescent Psychiatry, 46*(1), 126–141. doi: 10.1097/01.chi.0000246060.62706.af.

Stevens, M. C., & Haney-Caron, E. (2012). Comparison of brain volume abnormalities between ADHD and conduct disorder in adolescence. *Journal of Psychiatry & Neuroscience, 37*(6), 389–398. doi: 10.1503/jpn.110148.

Stringaris, A., Maughan, B., & Goodman, R. (2010). What's in a disruptive disorder? Temperamental antecedents of oppositional defiant disorder: Findings from the Avon Longitudinal Study. *Journal of the American Academy of Child & Adolescent Psychiatry, 49*(5), 474–483. doi: 10.1016/j.jaac.2010.01.021.

Szapocznik, J., Hervis, O., & Schwartz, S. (2003). *Brief Strategic Family Therapy for Adolescent Drug Abuse*. Bethesda, MD: National Institute on Drug Abuse.

Toupin, J., Déry, M., Pauzé, R., Mercier, H., & Fortin, L. (2000). Cognitive and familial contributions to conduct disorder in children. *Journal of Child Psychology & Psychiatry & Allied Disciplines, 41*(3), 333–344. doi: 10.1017/S0021963099005296.

Tuvblad, C., & Beaver, K. M. (2013). Genetic and environmental influences on antisocial behavior. *Journal of Criminal Justice, 41*(5), 273–276. doi: 10.1016/j.jcrimjus.2013.07.007.

Van Der Meer, D. J., & Van Der Meere, J. (2004). Response inhibition in children with conduct disorder and borderline intellectual functioning. *Child Neuropsychology, 10*(3), 189–194. doi: 10.1080/09297040490911005.

Wagner, D.V., Borduin, C. M., Sawyer, A. M., & Dopp, A. R. (2014). Long-term prevention of criminality in siblings of serious and violent juvenile offenders: A 25-year follow-up to a randomized clinical trial of multisystemic therapy. *Journal of Consulting & Clinical Psychology, 82*(3), 492–499. doi: 10.1037/a0035624.

Waller, R., Gardner, F., & Hyde, L. W. (2013). What are the associations between parenting, callous–unemotional traits, and antisocial behavior in youth? A systematic review of evidence. *Clinical Psychology Review, 33*(4), 593–608. doi: http://dx.doi.org/10.1016/j.cpr.2013.03.001.

White, S. F., Brislin, S., Sinclair, S., Fowler, K. A., Pope, K., & Blair, R. J. R. (2013). The relationship between large cavum septum pellucidum and antisocial behavior, callous-unemotional traits and psychopathy in adolescents. *Journal of Child Psychology & Psychiatry & Allied Disciplines, 54*(5), 575–581. doi: 10.1111/j.1469-7610.2012.02603.x.

Wu, T., Howells, N., Burger, J., Lopez, P., Lundeen, R., & Sikkenga, A. V. (2015). *Conduct Disorder. Treating Disruptive Disorders: A Guide to Psychological, Pharmacological, and Combined Therapies.* Hoboken, NJ: Taylor and Francis. Retrieved from http://MONASH.eblib.com.au/patron/FullRecord.aspx?p=1982470, 30/5/2015.

10
DEPRESSION

Daphne Voineskos and Zafiris J. Daskalakis

Introduction

Major Depressive Disorder (MDD, depression) and associated mood syndromes are among the most common psychiatric disorders in specialist and general medical practice. These syndromes span the life cycle and present with varying symptoms. While depressive symptoms can be part of normal human behaviour, MDD can be severe and even life threatening. As with many psychiatric disorders, both nature and nurture have strong neurodevelopmental contributions vis à vis treatment response and comorbidities. Although depression can present at any age, there are striking similarities with other neurodevelopmental disorders. Across the lifespan, differences in epidemiology, risk factors, symptomatic presentation and comorbidities come to light.

In this chapter, we will attempt to elucidate recurring characteristics of depression, including those shared with other psychiatric disorders, comorbidity with other conditions, neuropsychological aspects and changes associated with symptomatology. We will define the complex neurochemical picture involving serotonergic, dopaminergic, noradrenergic, glutamatergic and GABAergic systems. We will briefly cover the role of the stress-diathesis model, early life trauma and temperament in mediating depression and mood changes.

While much has been written about depressive disorders as a whole, there continue to be questions regarding treatment algorithms, adjunctive therapies, treatment modalities and their combinations. We will cover these and more recent advances in treatment, including developments in brain stimulation therapies. In this chapter, we will attempt to address all of the above and present a cohesive approach to depression.

Preliminary considerations

The notion of depression, or melancholia, has numerous permutations throughout written history, both scientific and artistic in nature. Hippocrates wrote about an excess of "black bile", resulting in melancholia, which comprises the root of the word (melan – black, cholē – bile). This may be one of the first known writings attributing depressed mood to an internal process, as opposed to supernatural forces. Interestingly, Hippocrates' melancholia is similar to current symptomatology, including "prolonged fear or depression, irritability, restlessness, sleeplessness, aversion to food and despondency."

Modern psychiatry continues to evolve with the DSM-5 (2013). There are important changes in the realm of depression, and we will adhere to these alterations in terminology. Specifically, Premenstrual Dysphoric Disorder was moved from the "Criteria sets and axes provided for further study" to the main Depressive Disorders chapters, based on strong scientific evidence. Dysthymia has been reclassified under "Persistent Depressive Disorders", which includes both chronic MDD and dysthymic disorder, as it was previously known. The qualifier of bereavement as an exclusion criterion from depression has also been removed. It is recognized that bereavement may last much longer than the previously ascribed 2 months, and can precipitate depression with added risks for the individual. These episodes appear to occur in individuals with a personal or family history of mood disorders, and respond to the same pharmacological and psychosocial treatments as depression. DSM-5 acknowledges the close link between depressive and anxious symptoms by adding the specifier "with anxious distress". This may assist clinicians in making crucial treatment decisions and evidence demonstrates its relevance with regard to prognosis.

Returning briefly to the ancient Greeks, Aristotle astutely separated depressed states from mood alterations and responses in everyday life. An important distinction must be made between clinical mood state and emotional response to upsetting occurrences. *Mood* is defined as a pervasive and sustained emotional or psychological state. *Feelings* become entangled in this overlap, defined as the subjective experience, which, like mood, may be positive or negative. Biologically, these terms are intertwined in limbic circuits, and are highly associated with memory storage and retrieval. Moreover, the distinction between observable affect and internal mood is relevant to clinical examination. *Affect* is defined as a complex state of emotional arousal involving several feelings, which may vary over time, outwardly expressed by gesture, tone or expression. Distinguishing between these terms is helpful in clinical examination and diagnosis.

Onset and prevalence

MDD is said to have the highest lifetime prevalence of psychiatric disorders. Up to 15% of adults will suffer from depression in their lifetime. Depressive symptoms typically develop over days to weeks. Depression may appear at any age, but the likelihood of onset increases markedly with puberty and average age at onset is late 20s. There are differing reports about age of onset, with some worldwide studies showing an average first episode between ages 30–40, and a second, smaller peak of incidence between ages 50–60. There is a clear difference in prevalence between sexes. Some studies estimate lifetime prevalence to be as high as 26% for women and 12% for men.

Numerous environmental, psychosocial and biological factors place individuals at increased risk of developing depression. However, there does not appear to be a relationship to race or socioeconomic status throughout the world. There are further risk factors associated with developing a depressive episode, detailed below:

1. *Life stressors* – Frequently, depression follows psychosocial stressors, particularly death of a relative, marital separation, ending of an important relationship or job difficulties (DSM-5). Adverse childhood experiences, particularly multiple and diverse stressors during childhood, can exponentially contribute risk to the development of depression. The death of a parent increases the risk of depression for children, teens and young adults, as demonstrated by a study from the University of Pittsburgh on bereaved individuals aged 7–25 (Brent, Melhem, Donohoe, & Walker, 2009). In adults, depression appears to be more common in separated or divorced individuals, as well as those with few or no interpersonal supports.
2. *Sex* – There is a consistent 2-fold greater prevalence of depressive disorders in women over men. This has been hypothesized to be due to hormonal differences (see PMDD), the effects of childbirth and differing psychosocial stressors.
3. *Genetic and physiological* – First-degree family members of individuals with depression have a 2–4 fold higher risk for major depressive disorder than the general population, lending weight to genetic heritability of depression. Heritability is the extent a trait is genetically determined and is calculated by measuring how much of the variance in a trait is accounted for by genetic variance. Heritability can be estimated by comparing monozygotic and dizygotic twins. Since monozygotic twins share virtually 100% DNA, and dizygotic twins have shared genes similar to siblings, but identical womb environments, greater phenotype similarity in monozygotic twins suggests a heritable, genetic contribution. Stressful life events are also recognized as precipitants of depression; these events induce the HPA axis, which links cortisol with the hippocampus, a brain region involved in memory and emotion.
4. *Temperamental* – Neuroticism (negative affectivity) is a well-established risk factor for the onset of depression; high levels render individuals more likely to develop depressive episodes in response to stressful life events. Of approximately 40% heritability, neuroticism appears to account for a substantial portion of genetic liability.

Other significant risk factors such as risk genes, dementia, cognitive correlates, comorbidities and neuroanatomical aspects will be covered in a later section.

Clinical symptomatology

A depressive episode encapsulates at least 2 weeks with decrease in mood, anhedonia and at least four other symptoms, defined by DSM-5 (See table 10.1).

TABLE 10.1 DSM-5 criteria and specifiers for Major Depressive Episode (MDE)

DIAGNOSTIC CRITERIA

A. 5 (or more) of the following symptoms nearly every day during the same 2-week period, representing a change from previous functioning.
   - At least one of the symptoms must be:
     i. Depressed mood
     ii. Loss of interest or pleasure
   - Excludes symptoms clearly attributable to another medical condition

   1. Depressed mood most of the day, demonstrated through subjective report or observation from others (or irritable mood in children/adolescents).
   2. Markedly diminished interest or pleasure in almost all activities most of the day (demonstrated through subjective report or observation).
   3. Change in > 5% body weight/month (without dieting or weight gain), or decrease/increase in appetite nearly every day.
   4. Insomnia/hypersomnia.
   5. Psychomotor agitation/retardation –observable by others as opposed to subjective feelings only.
   6. Fatigue or loss of energy.
   7. Feelings of worthlessness or excessive/inappropriate guilt. These may be delusional and guilt not just regarding being unwell.
   8. Diminished ability to think/concentrate, indecisiveness (by subjective account or observed).
   9. Recurrent thoughts of death, recurrent suicidal ideation without plan or a suicide attempt or specific plan for committing suicide.

B. Symptoms cause clinically significant distress or impairment in social, occupational or other areas of functioning.

C. Not attributable to physiological effects of a substance or GMC.

D. The occurrence of the MDE is not better explained by schizoaffective disorder, schizophrenia, schizophreniform disorder, delusional disorder or other specified and unspecified psychotic disorders.

E. There has never been a manic/hypomanic episode.

Adapted from DSM-5.

Specify:

With anxious distress, mixed features, melancholic features, atypical features, mood-congruent/incongruent psychotic features, catatonia, peripartum onset or seasonal pattern (recurrent episode only).

Once a second depressive episode has occurred, the diagnosis becomes MDD, recurrent. It is important to differentiate the level and length of symptom resolution, and return to previous functioning, if present. Specifiers define each episode, and apply to the current or most recent episode of depression. We elaborate on these below:

1. With anxious distress – a new addition to the DSM-5, reflecting the frequent combination of depression with anxious symptoms. It refers specifically to restlessness, difficulty concentrating due to worry, feeling keyed up, muscle tension, ruminative worry that "something bad may happen" or fear of losing control. Individuals with anxious depression may be at risk for more disability, suicidality and diminished response to treatment.
2. With mixed features – may contribute to an individual's diagnosis of bipolar disorder, and includes some symptoms from the depressive criteria and three or more from the manic/hypomanic episode criteria, excluding distractibility.
3. With atypical features – may be a distinct biological subtype, and includes mood reactivity with ≥2 of: hypersomnia, leaden limb paralysis, interpersonal rejection sensitivity (affecting social or work life) and significant appetite/weight increase, with cravings for carbohydrate-based foods. There is some evidence for a preferential response to Monoamine Oxidase Inhibitors (MAOI) medications; overall these patients respond well to antidepressant pharmacotherapy.
4. With melancholic features – must include absolute anhedonia or no mood reactivity. It includes ≥3 of: worse mood in the mornings, early morning wakening (2 hours earlier), psychomotor retardation/agitation, decrease in appetite/weight and excessive guilt. There is a distinctive quality to the mood, seeming worse than previous episodes.
5. With psychotic features (mood-congruent or incongruent) – these include delusions and/or hallucinations. They may be mood congruent (i.e., delusions of guilt, nihilistic delusions, negative auditory hallucinations) or incongruent (i.e., delusions of grandeur, positive auditory hallucinations). The congruency qualifier should be stated explicitly.
6. With catatonia – catatonia is a group of symptoms crossing diagnostic boundaries, thus symptoms as part of depression should be explicitly stated. At least three symptoms must be observed, including mutism, negativism, catalepsy, stupor, posturing, odd mannerisms, stereotypy, agitation, echolalia, echopraxia or grimacing.
7. With peripartum onset – this specifier has been changed to include 4 weeks after delivery and the 9 months of pregnancy.

8. With seasonal pattern – a specific pattern of relapse and remission over the year, with ≥ 2 seasonal episodes of depression over the past 2 years. There should not have been any non-seasonal episodes during this period. Overall, there should be more seasonal episodes than non-seasonal. Seasonal stressors may discount this specifier (i.e., individuals who work seasonally, and become depressed with unemployment).

Comorbidity

The risk of depression increases with comorbid physical and psychiatric medical conditions. A WHO World Health Survey in the Lancet (Moussavi et al., 2007) surveyed over 200,000 patients from 60 countries. An average of 9.3–23% participants were found to have depression with ≥ 1 comorbid physical illness. Depression was significantly more likely in the presence of ≥ 1 major physical illness. Nearly a quarter (23%) of those surveyed with ≥ 2 physical conditions also suffered from depression. See Table 10.2 for more information.

1. *Physical comorbidities* – Neurological conditions including multiple sclerosis, traumatic brain injury, stroke, Parkinson's disease, and dementia of Alzheimer's type, are correlated with a higher risk of depression. There is also an increased risk for a major depressive episode after a serious cardiac event. Furthermore, chronic, disabling medical conditions like diabetes or morbid obesity may go hand in hand with major depressive episodes.

19.8% of patients with acute coronary syndrome experience depression during hospitalization (Thombs et al., 2006). Several trials examined efficacy of pharmacotherapy (Glassman et al., 2002) or psychotherapy (Berkman et al., 2003) to treat depression in cardiac patients (see Berkman et al., 2003 for more information). Oncological studies have also shown increased prevalence of depressive symptoms and disorders in oncological patients. Rates of depression are increased in stroke survivors, Multiple Sclerosis (MS) and Parkinson's Disease. Specifically, in MS, suicidal ideation is common, with up to 7.5 times the proportion of deaths due to suicide as in the age-matched general population (Sadovnick, Eisen, Ebers, & Paty, 1991). MS medications, steroids and disease-modifying drugs interacting with the immune system may have deleterious effects on mood and suicidal ideation.

In Australia, the national depression initiative "Beyondblue" has been developing partnerships with groups including Heart Foundation and Cancer Australia to sponsor research that integrates care for people with depression and physical illness. Effective chronic disease management models may help prevent the progress and secondary morbidity of chronic disease.

TABLE 10.2 General Medical Conditions commonly associated with Depression

Cardiac	Coronary Artery Disease
	Congestive Heart Failure
Pulmonary	Chronic Obstructive Pulmonary Disease
	Asthma
	Sarcoidosis
Endocrine/Metabolic	Hyperthyroidism
	Hypothyroidism
	Hyperparathyroidism
	Addison's Disease (ACTH deficiency)
	Cushing's Disease
	Hyperprolactinemia
	Porphyrias
Neurological	Stroke/Cerebrovascular Event
	Multiple Sclerosis
	Parkinson's Disease
	Dementia (of any type, i.e. Alzheimer's type, Vascular)
Vitamin Deficiencies	B12 Deficiency
	Niacin Deficiency (Pellagra)
	Folate Deficiency
	Thiamine Deficiency
	Cobalamin Deficiency
Renal	End Stage Renal Disease
Infectious Disease	HIV
	Variant Creutzfeld-Jakub Disease
Rheumatologic	Systemic Lupus Eythematosus
	Rheumatoid Arthritis
	Scleroderma
Oncological	Cancer (any site, commonly hepatic, pancreatic)
Trauma	Burn Trauma
	Brain Injury
Toxins	Mercury, Lead, Manganese, Arsenic

2. *Psychiatric comorbidities* – Depression in conjunction with another psychiatric disorder often follows a more refractory course. Psychiatric comorbidities include, but are not limited to, substance-related disorders, panic, obsessive-compulsive disorder, anorexia nervosa, bulimia nervosa and borderline personality disorder. Those with persistent depressive disorder are at higher risk for comorbid anxiety and substance use disorders. Early-onset persistent depressive disorder is strongly associated with Cluster B and C personality disorders. Men with depression frequently present with substance use disorders, whereas women present with anxiety and eating disorders. In general, comorbid substance use disorders and anxiety disorders worsen prognosis and the risk of suicide.

Rating scales

There are both self-rating and clinician-rated scales widely available in the literature. These can be used as efficacy measures for depression treatment, in clinical trials, or benchmarks in structured psychotherapy treatments. The scales below are "gold-standard" rating scales accepted throughout the field of mood disorders, and have high test-retest reliability, validity and a relatively simple scoring key.

1. Self rating scales:
   Beck Depression Inventory (BDI: Beck, Ward, Mendelson, Mock, & Erbaugh, 1961).
   Mood Assessment Scale (Geriatric Depression Scale: Yesavage et al., 1982).
   Zung Self-rating Depression Scale (Zung, 1965).
   Quick Inventory of Depressive Symptomatology (QIDS: Rush et al., 2003).
2. Clinician-rated scales:
   Hamilton Depression Rating Scale (HRSD: Hamilton, 1960).
   Montgomery-Asberg Depression Rating Scale (MADRS: Montgomery & Asberg, 1979).

Clinical vignette

A 33 year old mother of 2 children aged 4 and 6, attends an appointment and is tearful throughout the assessment. She is trained as a nurse, but has taken a sick leave over the past 2 months as she has not been able to attend work. She endorses low mood, anhedonia, low energy, disturbed concentration and attention, 20lbs of weight loss without a change in her diet habits. She denies suicidal ideation. She endorses guilt that she is unable to help her patients and care for her family, as well as worthlessness and hopelessness that she will ever be able to return to work. She has had one previous episode of depression during university, which was treated to remission with fluoxetine. She stopped the fluoxetine 8 years ago, when she began to try to have children with her husband, who is supportive and attends the appointment with her.

Genetics and epigenetics

Initially, depression was placed in the same realm as cystic fibrosis and other illnesses with monogenic heritability. This was inferred due to high heritability in twin (heritability of 40–50%), family (2–3 fold increase in lifetime risk in first degree relatives) and adoption studies. More recent studies have determined we cannot attribute all the risk of developing depression to one gene, and each gene/locus of interest may contribute part of the total genetic risk. Linkage and Genome Wide Association Studies (GWAS) show varying rates of associations. However, results from GWAS work have averaged out to less significant than previously hoped.

These results lend weight to the growing body of evidence that depression is a complex disorder with numerous genetic and environmental factors, each with differing levels of penetrance.

Given response rates to psychopharmacology (i.e., Selective Serotonin Reuptake Inhibitors [SSRIs]), there are specific neurotransmitter systems with associated genes that have been specifically explored. The serotonin transporter gene and genes involved in the serotonergic system are candidate genes for susceptibility to depression, as antidepressant medications act on these systems. This has been validated by numerous candidate gene studies.

Cognitive correlates of depression

Cognitive symptoms, acknowledged in the diagnostic criteria, include deficits in episodic memory and learning (Goodwin, 1997 for a review), whereas autobiographical memory is largely intact. Post-mortem, structural and functional imaging investigations reinforce observed cognitive dysfunction in depression. Fronto-striatal-thalamic and limbic-frontal networks and the overlap of cognitive and emotional regulation symptoms have been delineated in depression. There is also well-documented evidence of decreased hippocampal volumes and consistent executive dysfunction. It is important to understand that these cognitive deficits are not entirely due to low motivation or anhedonia, as these symptoms can remain unresolved even in remission. Cognitive deficits have also been reported in healthy first-degree relatives of patients with unipolar depression.

Depression frequently coexists with dementia or heralds its development (Jorm, 2001 for meta analysis). The proximity of the antecedent depressive episode to the onset of dementia continues to be an important, if unclear, factor. Depression has been posed in the literature both as a prodromal feature of impending dementia, and a risk factor for its later development.

Neuropathology

As mentioned, frontostriatal circuitry partly represents the macro-anatomical basis of depression. Frontal structural and functional abnormalities are reported in imaging and neurophysiological investigations. The prefrontal cortex is responsible for executive functioning, necessary to mediate heightened or conflicting emotional and behavioural responses. The "emotion and reward centres", namely striatum, amygdala and hippocampus, demonstrate reduced volumes in depression. Emotional learning is coded in hippocampal and amygdalar circuits, with the amygdala acting as a vital relay/control station, processing emotionally significant signals and orchestrating subsequent cognitive/behavioural responses through the cortex. The anterior cingulate may contribute to this limbic circuit, combining executive signals from the frontal cortex with processed amygdalar signals. The processed stimuli, with their significance and now embedded responses, are then stored in the hippocampus for future retrieval. Consistent alterations of these interconnected striatal, limbic and frontal regions in depression reinforces the brain's functioning as highly connected networks, as opposed to specified regions working in isolated silos.

Neurochemistry

The majority of early research in the neurochemistry of depression followed from the discovery of the efficacy of MAOIs and tricyclic medications, which pointed to serotonin as the neurotransmitter of depressive pathophysiology. In this section, we will cover the neurochemistry involved in the monoamine hypothesis of depression (i.e. serotonin) as well as other neurotransmitter systems, including dopamine, norepinephrine, glutamate and GABA.

Serotonin – The majority of serotonergic neuronal cell bodies are in the rostral brainstem, specifically the raphe nuclei. These project throughout the cerebral cortex, hypothalamus and limbic system. Serotonin has been the main target of neurochemical exploration, given the efficacy of serotonin reuptake inhibitors (SRIs) in treating depressive symptoms. Studies attempting to deplete serotonin have demonstrated the induction of depressive symptoms. Tryptophan hydroxylase is the rate-limiting enzyme in brain serotonin synthesis. The discovery of a new brain-specific isoform of the tryptophan hydroxylase (TPH2) has generated new interest in the connection between serotonergic systems and depression (Walther & Bader, 2003).

Dopamine – There are three important dopaminergic tracts in the brain: the nigrostriatal, mesolimbic/mesocortical and tuberoinfundibular tracts. The role of dopamine in reward mechanisms suggests a role in depression, although dopamine receptor antagonists are the treatment of choice in psychotic, not mood disorders. There are associations between depression and aberrant activity in several dopaminergic circuits, including the nigrostriatal and mesolimbic tracts.

Norepinephrine – Several antidepressant medications (e.g., venlafaxine) have specific noradrenergic activity and directed exploratory investigations of the catecholamines (norepinephrine, epinephrine and dopamine). Noradrenergic cell bodies are found in the locus ceruleus and rostral pons, and project to numerous brain areas, including the limbic system and cerebral cortex. These receptors have been implicated in both anxiety and depressive disorders.

Glutamate – Is the major excitatory neurotransmitter of the cortex and hippocampus. Glutamate binds to N-methyl-D-aspartate (NMDA) receptor sites and studies have found evidence that N-methyl-D-aspartate receptor (NMDAR) antagonists may have antidepressant effects. This evidence has lead to the "glutamatergic theory of depression".

GABA – Gamma aminobutyric acid (GABA) is a major inhibitory neurotransmitter acting throughout the brain, specifically on interneurons in the cortex.

As such, GABA has an upstream effect that modulates excitatory neurotransmitters such as norepinephrine, dopamine and serotonin. The process by which GABAergic interneurons modulate the activity of other cortical neurons is termed cortical inhibition. Dysfunctional cortical inhibition has been implicated in the pathophysiology of depression through post-mortem and imaging studies (specifically Magnetic Resonance Spectroscopy [MRS]) (Rajkowska, O'Dwyer, Teleki, Stockmeier, & Miguel-Hidalgo, 2007; Sanacora et al., 1999). GABA levels are also increased in medicated depression subjects in remission (Sanacora et al., 2004). (For review, Croarkin, Levinson, & Daskalakis, 2011).

Treatment

There are three main modalities of treatment, which can be used separately or in combination: pharmacotherapy, psychotherapy and brain stimulation. As depression is episodic, with partial to full inter-episodic recovery, physicians must also be aware of strategies to maintain wellness and prevent relapse. After a single episode, the recommendation is to remain on the same medication that was effective in acute treatment for up to 6–24 months after remission. If the patient has had two or more depressive episodes, the consensus is to remain on the antidepressant therapy for up to 5 years or for the patient's lifetime. See Table 10.3 for a simplified treatment guideline table.

1. *Pharmacotherapy*

Pharmacotherapy is a treatment of choice for depression, especially in moderate to severe episodes. Current recommendations place selective serotonin reuptake inhibitors (SSRIs), serotonin and noradrenaline reuptake inhibitors (SNRIs) and similar medications as first line options due to better safety and tolerability profiles

TABLE 10.3 Treatment of Major Depressive Episode. Adapted from combination of international guidelines (APA; CANMAT; NICE)

Episode Severity	*Treatment modality*	*Recurrent illness resistant to medication/therapy*
Mild	IPT/CBT or SSRI	
Moderate	IPT/CBT or SSRI/SNRI, Augment if partial response, TCAs vs. MAOIs if no response to two SSRI/SNRI trials.	rTMS vs. TCAs or MAOIs if no response to two SSRI/SNRI trials.
Severe	Combination therapies, consider ECT if Suicidal Ideation present	rTMS or ECT if Suicidal Ideation present
Severe with psychotic features	Antidepressant+antipsychotic or ECT	ECT

over previously preferred classes of medications (tricyclic anti-depressants [TCAs] and monoamine oxidase [MAO] inhibitors). However, TCAs and MAOIs remain good options for treatment. The first line choice of medication should be individualized, accounting for patient preference, previous response and tolerability/side effect profile. Several years ago there was concern regarding emergent suicidality with the initiation of SSRI medications. Current research does not confirm this in the adult population, although in adolescents the risk is increased 4 fold with SRIs.

Augmentation and adjunctive therapies are common in depression. Antipsychotics, benzodiazepines, mood stabilizers, thyroid medications, stimulants, sleeping aids, light therapy and others have evidence as augmentation/adjunctive agents. Furthermore, there are combination strategies that have been shown to be effective (see APA; CANMAT; NICE).

2. *Psychotherapy*

   a. Cognitive behavioural therapy (CBT) is a manualized, time-limited psychotherapy conducted in 14–20 sessions. It centres on an individual's distorted beliefs about self, the world and the future, which are theorized to contribute to depressive symptoms. Patients identify maladaptive thinking patterns and subsequently learn more helpful methods. More information can be found at the Academy of Cognitive Therapy's website (www.academyofct.org).
   b. Interpersonal Psychotherapy (IPT) is a second time-limited, manualized psychotherapy focused on interpersonal relationships and their immediate social context. It is delivered over 16 weekly sessions, divided into three phases, focusing on one or more primary areas: interpersonal role disputes, role transitions, interpersonal deficits or grief. For more information, visit the International Society for Interpersonal Psychotherapy website (www.interpersonalpsychotherapy.org).

There is substantial evidence for both CBT and IPT in acute treatment of mild to moderate depressive episodes, alone or in combination with pharmacotherapy. Further psychotherapy options with less concrete evidence are beyond the scope of this textbook, and include: supportive therapy, psychodynamic psychotherapy, behavioural activation, motivational interviewing, acceptance and commitment therapy (ACT), emotion focused therapy (EFT), bibliotherapy and cognitive-behavioural analysis system of psychotherapy (CBASP), among others.

3. *Brain Stimulation*

   a. Electroconvulsive Therapy (ECT) is the gold-standard for treatment resistant depression. An electrical current is applied to the brain via the scalp to induce a generalized seizure under anaesthesia. Patients undergo

ECT 2–3 times per week during an acute course, with significant response within 6–12 treatments. Bitemporal Standard pulse ECT has a response rate of up to 75%. While the response rate for Right Unilateral Ultrabrief ECT is slightly lower, it remains highly effective.

b. Repetitive transcranial magnetic stimulation (rTMS) is a recently developed form of brain stimulation targeting treatment resistant depression. Focused pulses of an electromagnetic coil are repetitively discharged over the scalp to stimulate cortical neurons and alter neural excitability without a seizure. High frequency rTMS applied to the left dorsolateral prefrontal cortex for 45 min, 5 days a week, for up to 30 treatments is the current standard of treatment. Briefer forms of rTMS and other brain area targets are being developed and tested for equivalent efficacy.

4. *Newer developments*

   a. DBS – Deep Brain Stimulation. A permanent neurosurgical implant is placed in the brain, with a specific target (the subgenual cingulate cortex in depression). This is connected to a pulse generator in the chest wall that is externally controlled to repetitively stimulate the target area (see Lozano et al., 2008).
   b. MST – Magnetic Seizure Therapy. A powerful repetitively discharged magnet induces a generalized seizure in a similar procedure to ECT. It is focally discharged over the prefrontal cortex and evidence shows significantly fewer cognitive side effects with MST. Trials are underway to compare efficacy with ECT (see Hoy & Fitzgerald, 2011).
   c. FEAST – Focal Electrically Administered Seizure Therapy is transcranial electrical stimulation through an anode-cathode arrangement that initiates seizures in the prefrontal cortex (see Nahas et al., 2013).
   d. Ketamine – may act as an NMDA receptor antagonist, affecting the glutamatergic system and inducing effects evident long after the "high" or intoxication has worn off. Ketamine is available orally and intranasally, but appears to have the best bioavailability when delivered through an IV. Clinical trials are currently ongoing (see Kirby, 2015).

Summary

In summary, depression is a common and disabling illness. Individuals in all age groups can be affected, and the illness can have full inter-episodic recovery or complete remission with appropriate treatment. Our understanding of the neurochemistry of depression continues to develop, and extensive work is underway in research centres across the world to develop true biomarkers and clinical measures to improve diagnosis and treatment response.

Abbreviations

BDI: Beck Depression Inventory. A gold standard rating scale used to assess symptoms of depression, developed by Aaron Beck in 1961.

CBT: Cognitive Behavioural Therapy. A time-limited, manualized psychotherapy focusing on the connection between thoughts, feelings and actions/behaviours.

DBS: Deep Brain Stimulation. A neurosurgical procedure implanting electrodes with specific brain targets, initially developed to treat movement disorders, currently being applied in depression.

DSM-5: The Diagnostic and Statistical Manual of Mental Disorders, fifth edition. Published by the American Psychiatric Association in 2013 as an update to the fourth edition (TR).

ECT: Electroconvulsive Therapy. The gold standard therapy for treatment resistant depression. Involves an electric stimulus being applied to a patient's scalp under general anaesthetic, resulting in a generalized seizure.

FEAST: Focal Electrically Administered Seizure Therapy. Transcranial electrical stimulation applied on the scalp with an anode-cathode arrangement. A new type of localized seizure therapy, with seizures occurring in the prefrontal cortex.

GABA: Gamma Aminobutyric Acid. The primary inhibitory neurotransmitter in the brain.

GABAergic: A term used to refer to something (i.e. a chemical or neuron) that primarily utilizes or modulates GABA or the GABA system.

GMC: General Medical Condition, for example a physical illness not classified as a psychiatric disorder.

GWAS: Genome Wide Association Study. Used to examine numerous common genetic variants in different individuals to look for associations with specific traits.

HPA Axis: The Hypotahlamic-Pituitary-Adrenal Axis. A complex part of the neuroendocrine system with interactions between the hypothalamus, pituitary gland and adrenal gland. It plays a part in the regulation of stress and body processes including hormones, the immune system, mood and emotions, digestion and others.

HRSD: The Hamilton Rating Scale for Depression. Also abbreviated as HAM-D. A gold standard scale to evaluate depressive symptoms, developed by Max Hamilton in 1960 and subsequently revised.

IPT: Interpersonal psychotherapy. A time-limited, manualized psychotherapy focusing on relationships.

MADRS: Montgomery-Åsberg Depression Rating Scale. A gold standard scale to evaluate depressive symptoms, developed in 1979 by Montgomery and Åsberg. There is a high degree of correlation between MADRS scores and HRSD scores.

MAOI: Monoamine Oxidase Inhibitors. One of the first classes of medications used to treat depression. These medications inhibit monamine oxidase and block the breakdown of monoamine neurotransmitters. They require a specific diet, with numerous restrictions, including abstaining from foods containing tyramine (specific cheeses, red wine, chocolate and others). The efficacy of these medications led to the development of the monoamine hypothesis.

MDD: Major Depressive Disorder.

MDE: Major Depressive Episode. A single occurrence of a clinically depressed period lasting at least 2 weeks with low mood most of the day, each day.

MS: Multiple Sclerosis.

MST: Magnetic Seizure Therapy. A developing seizure therapy for depression. A powerful magnet is focally discharged over the scalp covering the prefrontal cortex to induce a seizure under general anaesthesia.

NMDA: N-methyl-D-aspartate. A derivative of an amino acid acting as an agonist mimicking glutamate action at the NMDA receptor.

NMDAR: The NMDA receptor, see above.

PMDD: Pre-Menstrual Dysphoric Disorder. A mood disordered condition with severe psychological symptoms beginning 7–10 days prior to menstruation and decreasing within a few days of the beginning of menstruation.

QIDS: Quick Inventory of Depressive Symptomatology. A gold standard rating scale to evaluate depressive symptoms. There are both self-rating and clinician-rated versions.

rTMS: repetitive Transcranial Magnetic Stimulation. A non-convulsive brain stimulation therapy for treatment resistant depression. A figure of 8 coil is applied to a specific area of the scalp and a magnetic field generated by brief current pulses are discharged, to induce brief activity of the neurons underlying the treatment coil.

SNRI: Serotonin-Norepinephrine Reuptake Inhibitor. A class of SRI medications used to treat depressive disorders and anxiety disorders. They can also be used to treat some chronic pain disorders. Their actions are on the serotonin transporter and norepinephrine transporter proteins.

SRI: Serotonin Reuptake Inhibitor. A type of medication acting mainly to block the reuptake of serotonin by inhibiting the action of the serotonin transporter protein. This can result in increased extracellular concentrations of serotonin and thus an increase in serotonergic transmission.

SSRI: Selective Serotonin Reuptake Inhibitor. A class of SRI medications used largely to treat depressive and anxiety disorders.

TCA: Tricyclic Antidepressant. A class of compounds used as antidepressant medications, one of the earlier classes of antidepressant medications developed. These medications have good efficacy but are fatal in overdose and may have cardiac side effects.

TPH2: Tryptophan hydroxylase 2. An isozyme of trypophan hydroxylase found in humans. Expressed mainly in the serotonergic neurons.

WHO: World Health Organization.

Further readings

APA. Practice Guideline for the Treatment of Patients with Major Depressive Disorder. from https://psychiatryonline.org/pb/assets/raw/sitewide/practice_guidelines/guidelines/mdd.pdf.

CANMAT. Canadian Network for Mood and Anxiety Disorders. from http://www.canmat.org.

Croarkin, P. E., Levinson, A. J., & Daskalakis, Z. J. (2011). Evidence for GABAergic inhibitory deficits in major depressive disorder. *Neurosci Biobehav Rev, 35*(3), 818–825. doi: 10.1016/j.neubiorev.2010.10.002.

Goodwin, G. M. (1997). Neuropsychological and neuroimaging evidence for the involvement of the frontal lobes in depression. *J Psychopharmacol, 11*(2), 115–122.

Hoy, K. E., & Fitzgerald, P. B. (2011). Magnetic seizure therapy for treatment-resistant depression. *Expert Rev Med Devices, 8*(6), 723–732. doi: 10.1586/erd.11.55.

Jorm, A. F. (2001). History of depression as a risk factor for dementia: an updated review. *Aust N Z J Psychiatry, 35*(6), 776–781.

Kirby, T. (2015). Ketamine for depression: the highs and lows. *Lancet Psychiatry, 2*(9), 783–784. doi: 10.1016/S2215-0366(15)00392-2.

Lozano, A. M., Mayberg, H. S., Giacobbe, P., Hamani, C., Craddock, R. C., & Kennedy, S. H. (2008). Subcallosal cingulate gyrus deep brain stimulation for treatment-resistant depression. *Biol Psychiatry, 64*(6), 461–467. doi: 10.1016/j.biopsych.2008.05.034.

Nahas, Z., Short, B., Burns, C., Archer, M., Schmidt, M., Prudic, J., … Sackeim, H. A. (2013). A feasibility study of a new method for electrically producing seizures in man: focal electrically administered seizure therapy [FEAST]. *Brain Stimul, 6*(3), 403–408. doi: 10.1016/j.brs.2013.03.004.

NICE. Depression in adults: The treatment and management of depresison in adults. from http://www.nice.org.uk/guidance/cg90.

References

American Psychiatric Association. (2013). *Diagnostic and Statistical Manual of Mental Disorders (DSM-5)* (5th Edition ed.). Washington, DC and London: American Psychiatric Publishing.

Beck, A. T., Ward, C. H., Mendelson, M., Mock, J., & Erbaugh, J. (1961). An inventory for measuring depression. *Arch Gen Psychiatry, 4*, 561–571.

Berkman, L. F., Blumenthal, J., Burg, M., Carney, R. M., Catellier, D., Cowan, M. J., … Enhancing Recovery in Coronary Heart Disease Patients, I. (2003). Effects of treating depression and low perceived social support on clinical events after myocardial infarction: The Enhancing Recovery in Coronary Heart Disease Patients (ENRICHD) randomized trial. *JAMA, 289*(23), 3106–3116. doi: 10.1001/jama.289.23.3106.

Brent, D., Melhem, N., Donohoe, M. B., & Walker, M. (2009). The incidence and course of depression in bereaved youth 21 months after the loss of a parent to suicide, accident, or sudden natural death. *Am J Psychiatry, 166*(7), 786–794. doi: 10.1176/appi.ajp.2009.08081244.

Glassman, A. H., O'Connor, C. M., Califf, R. M., Swedberg, K., Schwartz, P., Bigger, J. T., Jr., … Sertraline Antidepressant Heart Attack Randomized Trial, G. (2002). Sertraline treatment of major depression in patients with acute MI or unstable angina. *JAMA, 288*(6), 701–709.

Hamilton, M. (1960). A rating scale for depression. *J Neurol Neurosurg Psychiatry, 23*, 56–62.

Montgomery, S. A., & Asberg, M. (1979). A new depression scale designed to be sensitive to change. *Br J Psychiatry, 134*, 382–389.

Moussavi, S., Chatterji, S., Verdes, E., Tandon, A., Patel, V., & Ustun, B. (2007). Depression, chronic diseases, and decrements in health: Results from the World Health Surveys. *Lancet, 370*(9590), 851–858. doi: 10.1016/S0140-6736(07)61415-9.

Rajkowska, G., O'Dwyer, G., Teleki, Z., Stockmeier, C. A., & Miguel-Hidalgo, J. J. (2007). GABAergic neurons immunoreactive for calcium binding proteins are reduced in the prefrontal cortex in major depression. *Neuropsychopharmacology, 32*(2), 471–482. doi: 10.1038/sj.npp.1301234.

Rush, A. J., Trivedi, M. H., Ibrahim, H. M., Carmody, T. J., Arnow, B., Klein, D. N., ... Keller, M. B. (2003). The 16-Item Quick Inventory of Depressive Symptomatology (QIDS), clinician rating (QIDS-C), and self-report (QIDS-SR): A psychometric evaluation in patients with chronic major depression. *Biol Psychiatry, 54*(5), 573–583.

Sadovnick, A. D., Eisen, K., Ebers, G. C., & Paty, D. W. (1991). Cause of death in patients attending multiple sclerosis clinics. *Neurology, 41*(8), 1193–1196.

Sanacora, G., Gueorguieva, R., Epperson, C. N., Wu, Y. T., Appel, M., Rothman, D. L., ... Mason, G. F. (2004). Subtype-specific alterations of gamma-aminobutyric acid and glutamate in patients with major depression. *Arch Gen Psychiatry, 61*(7), 705–713. doi: 10.1001/archpsyc.61.7.705.

Sanacora, G., Mason, G. F., Rothman, D. L., Behar, K. L., Hyder, F., Petroff, O. A., ... Krystal, J. H. (1999). Reduced cortical gamma-aminobutyric acid levels in depressed patients determined by proton magnetic resonance spectroscopy. *Arch Gen Psychiatry, 56*(11), 1043–1047.

Thombs, B. D., Bass, E. B., Ford, D. E., Stewart, K. J., Tsilidis, K. K., Patel, U., ... Ziegelstein, R. C. (2006). Prevalence of depression in survivors of acute myocardial infarction. *J Gen Intern Med, 21*(1), 30–38. doi: 10.1111/j.1525-1497.2005.00269.x.

Walther, D. J., & Bader, M. (2003). A unique central tryptophan hydroxylase isoform. *Biochem Pharmacol, 66*(9), 1673–1680.

Yesavage, J. A., Brink, T. L., Rose, T. L., Lum, O., Huang, V., Adey, M., & Leirer, V. O. (1982). Development and validation of a geriatric depression screening scale: A preliminary report. *J Psychiatr Res, 17*(1), 37–49.

Zung, W. W. (1965). A self-rating depression scale. *Arch Gen Psychiatry, 12*, 63–70.

11
OBSESSIVE COMPULSIVE DISORDER

Richard Moulding, Matthew. E. Hughes, Linda Byrne, Michael Do and Maja Nedeljkovic

Introduction

Within the latest version of the Diagnostic and Statistical Manual (American Psychiatric Association, 2013), Obsessive Compulsive Disorder (OCD) has been moved into a separate category of OCD-Related Disorders alongside other disorders that share its phenomenology or clinical features, including the presence of obsessions and compulsions (e.g., Body Dysmorphic Disorder; BDD), or those with difficulties with self-regulation of behaviour (e.g., Trichotillomania). In this chapter, we will discuss the phenomenology of OCD and neurodevelopmental findings, before briefly discussing treatment options for the disorder.

Preliminary considerations

Obsessive and Compulsive behaviours have been observed throughout written human history, with OCD-like behaviours noted in Buddhist texts as early as 2500 years ago (de Silva, 2006). Indeed, it has been suggested that Shakespeare's Lady Macbeth, who washed to remove feelings of guilt, reflected the author's observance of people with OCD (Moulding, Nedeljkovic, & Kyrios, 2011). OCD is characterised by the presence of obsessions and/or compulsions (APA, 2013). Obsessions are unwanted, intrusive and unpleasant images, urges or thoughts, and the compulsions are aimed at removing the distress associated with the obsessions, or preventing the harm implied by the intrusion (APA, 2013). The person must recognise the thoughts as being a product of their own mind, and at some point have insight, although insight typically wavers throughout the disorder. Obsessions are experienced as ego-dystonic – or inconsistent with the individual's sense of self. Doubt is key within the disorder, for example, an early case study noting that "... she fears that by handling money, she shall retain *something of value in her fingers* … she replies, 'my disquietude is absurd and ridiculous, but I cannot prevent it …'" (Esquirol, 1845, p. 348–350). While both intrusions/obsessions and compulsions occur in the non-clinical population with no clear boundary between clinical and non-clinical presentations (Clark et al., 2014; Olatunji, Williams, Haslam, Abramowitz, & Tolin, 2008), OCD is diagnosable when there is significant distress and/or impairment.

Onset and prevalence

Cross-national findings have consistently reported OCD prevalence rates at around 1–2% (Nedeljkovic, Moulding, Foroughi, Kyrios, & Doron, 2012). The National Epidemiological Catchment Area (ECA) Survey in the United States in 1984 using DSM-III criteria placed OCD as the 4th most common psychiatric disorder after phobias, substance use disorders and major depression, with a six-month point prevalence of 1.6% and a lifetime prevalence of 2.5% (Karno, Golding, Sorenson, & Burnam, 1988). There is no evidence that OCD is higher in particular communities, but the presentation seems to skew towards religious concerns and washing related rituals in areas where religiosity is greater, such as the Middle East, with washing rituals seemingly related to concerns about religious observance and moral cleanliness (Nedeljkovic et al., 2012).

OCD typically begins during late-adolescence to early-adulthood (Attiullah, Eisen, & Rasmussen, 2000). For example, Lensi et al. (1996) reported a mean age-of-onset of 21.1 for men and 24.3 for women, while Rasmussen and Eisen (1992) found that 65% of their sample developed their illness before 25, and less than 15% after 35 years of age. Most participants noted having subclinical symptoms prior to the onset of the disorder. OCD is typically associated with a chronic and lifelong course, with some fluctuations in symptom severity (Attiullah et al., 2000). In the longest follow-up study, the original interviewers re-examined 122 former in-patients approximately 47 years after the onset of their symptoms. Of those, 83% had improved, but only 20% had shown a full recovery, with the majority of patients having a chronic (44%) or intermittent (31%) course. Finally, 58% of the patients were reported to show qualitative changes in their symptoms (Skoog, G., & Skoog, I., 1999).

There is a slight predominance of women experiencing OCD. For example, in the ECA survey in the United States, estimates of female-male ratios varied from 1.2 to 3.1 (Bebbington et al., 1998). Some gender differences exist with regard to the presentation of OCD, and in particular, males have consistently been found to have an earlier age-of-onset (see Lochner et al., 2004). One study in 263 Italian OCD patients found males had an earlier age-of-onset, were less likely to have been married, and were more likely to have experienced sexual, exactness and symmetry obsessions, whereas women had a higher frequency of aggressive intrusions and associated panic attacks after OCD (Lensi et al., 1996). Other studies have found higher incidences of cleaning obsessions in women (Bogetto, Venturello, Albert, Maina, & Ravizza, 1999). Childhood-onset OCD has been associated with greater levels of comorbid tic disorders such as Tourette's Syndrome (Geller et al., 1998), and an increased frequency of first degree relatives with OCD or tics (Grados et al., 2001).

Obsessions and compulsions

While OCD is heterogeneous, there are highly characteristic symptom themes. Typical presentations include: individuals with contamination fears and washing/cleaning concerns (e.g., germs, dirt, asbestos, AIDS and hepatitis); individuals with obsessive doubts and checking compulsions and compulsive slowness, who often also persistently seek reassurance; individuals with unacceptable thoughts or impulses and mainly "covert" compulsions – including unwanted sexual, aggressive or blasphemous thoughts – and who respond by suppressing thoughts, compulsive praying, self-criticism, etc.; and individuals with a need for symmetry and order – for example, a need for "perfect" rooms, cupboards, picture hanging, etc., and counting or numerical thoughts. Similar presentations are seen in children, although insight may be lower (APA, 2013).

While modern attempts at finding explicit "subtypes" of OCD have generally failed, with the exception of a tic-related subtype (Leckman et al., 2010; Mansueto & Keuler, 2005), attempts at finding underlying OCD-symptom dimensions through factor analysis have been more successful. In the largest review to date – a meta-analysis of 21 studies using the gold-standard Yale-Brown Obsessive Compulsive Scale (YBOCS; Goodman et al., 1989), with the studies comprising 5124 individuals with OCD – Bloch, Landeros-Weisenberger, Rosario, Pittenger, and Leckman (2008) found evidence for a four factor structure – with dimensions of (1) "forbidden thoughts" including harm, aggressive, religious, somatic and sexual obsessions, along with checking compulsions; (2) hoarding, (3) cleaning and (4) symmetry obsessions and compulsions; although it should be noted that hoarding is now considered a distinct disorder, it appeared as a symptom dimension due to its inclusion in the symptom measure. In children, a similar structure was found, albeit with the checking compulsions shifting from the obsessions to the symmetry factor. The authors suggested that this was because "checking was … heterogeneous and associated with multiple symptom factors, normally with the most commonly held symptom factor within each age group (i.e., symmetry in children and forbidden thoughts in adults)" (Bloch et al., 2008 p. 1539).

Rating scales of severity

The gold-standard OCD measure is the clinician-rated YBOCS (Goodman et al., 1989), which has recently been updated (Y-BOCS-II; Storch et al., 2010) and is available in a child and adolescent version (CY-BOCS; Scahill et al., 1997).

The YBOCS consists of a symptom checklist in addition to a 5-item obsession and 5-item compulsion scale. Self-report OCD scales are many and varied, but most commonly include the 18-item Obsessive Compulsive Inventory-Revised (OCI-R; Foa et al., 2002); while the Dimensional Obsessive Compulsive Scale (DOCS; Abramowitz et al., 2010) is increasing in popularity. Self-report versions of the Y-BOCS are also available. All self-report measures are multidimensional, albeit with varying subscales.

Obsessive Compulsive Personality

OCD is not to be confused with the similarly-named Obsessive Compulsive *Personality* Disorder (OCPD). OCPD is a personality disorder characterised by perfectionism that interferes with task completion, dedication to work to the exclusion of leisure, rigidity and stubbornness, hypermorality and scrupulosity, over-attention to detail, miserliness, an inability to discard worn or useless items and an inability to delegate tasks (APA, 2013). While in early psychoanalytic theories, these two disorders were placed at either ends of a continuum, there is now a clear consensus that there is a distinction between the two disorders (Eisen et al., 2006). However, while there is not a specific relationship between OCPD and OCD, they share some similarities in their associated characteristics, particularly in the domains of perfectionism and the need for control. Empirically, Eisen et al. (2006) found that preoccupation with details, hoarding and perfectionism (i.e., three of the eight OCPD criteria) were significantly more common in individuals with OCD than those without OCD. Calvo et al. (2009) found that OCPD was more common in parents of children with OCD, with the same three criteria being more frequent. There is some suggestion that OCPD may be more common in early-onset OCD (Maina, Albert, Salvi, Pessina, & Bogetto, 2008) and it has been found that early-onset OCD is associated with later OCPD whether or not the OCD remits (Wewetzer et al., 2001); as such, it may be that the perfectionism and need for control prominent in OCD rituals lead to the characteristic traits of OCPD developing (Maina et al., 2008).

A neurodevelopmental disorder

A number of factors suggest that OCD may be partly a neurodevelopmental disorder. The existence of obsessive symptoms in childhood, with the presence of an early-onset group with greater tic-related comorbidities, along with evidence that some cases of OCD follow organic insult or infection, and evidence for neurological and neuropsychiatric involvement, suggest that neurodevelopmental involvement may be important at least for a proportion of OCD patients. Further symptoms that may point to such involvement are the presence in some patients of "magical" symptoms (e.g., counting in threes) and ritualised, tic-like behavioural compulsions.

The involvement of frontal circuitry within theories of OCD, which also develops rapidly during such childhood and adolescent years when OCD typically begins, is also consistent with such a viewpoint. The following case study illustrates some of the phenomenological, comorbidity and neurochemical markers that can assist in diagnosis and treatment of OCD.

Clinical vignette

A 33-year old male presented with irrational contamination fears about infecting others with a flu-like virus, despite an absence of infection and reassurance and psychoeducation from health professionals. The onset followed an outbreak of flu at the patient's workplace five years earlier and increased over time, leading to his increased isolation, cessation of work and social activities, and avoidance of crowded or busy places and of close contact with others, with the exception of his partner and health professionals. The poor insight into the irrational nature of the fears led to an initial diagnosis of delusional disorder and a resulting treatment with antipsychotic medications, which did not alleviate the symptoms. A revised diagnosis of OCD with poor insight was given following further assessment revealing a family history of anxiety and Tourette's Syndrome; more generalized contamination obsessions (e.g., contracting unspecified disease and "something bad" happening to him or partner) and ritualistic/compulsive behaviours (e.g., washing in particular order); and some limited insight during periods of lowered anxiety (e.g., during a weekend away), along with low educational background and poor understanding of biology and disease. A combined cognitive behavioural therapy and SSRI pharmacotherapy resulted in a decrease in symptoms and avoidance behaviours.

Comorbidity

Rates of comorbidity in OCD are high. Despite OCD being reclassified in DSM-5 from being an anxiety disorder, 75.8% of OCD cases identified in a community US survey had comorbid DSM-IV anxiety disorders, with Social Phobia (43.5%), Specific Phobia (42.7%), Separation Anxiety Disorder (37.1%), Panic Disorder (20.0%), and Post Traumatic Syndrome Disorder (19.1%) most common (Ruscio, Stein, Chiu, & Kessler, 2010). Comorbid anxiety disorders usually precede OCD, while depression typically follows it (Ruscio et al., 2010). Comorbidity with depression is high, with lifetime rates of 63.3% DSM-IV mood disorders found in the same survey, with Major Depressive Disorder most common (40.7%). Longer duration of OCD symptoms has been related to greater rates of depression (Diniz et al., 2004). Relative to those without OCD, individuals with OCD are more likely to have another OCD-Related disorder (APA, 2013). Specifically, hoarding symptoms have been noted in 38% of OCD patients (Samuels et al., 2007), while BDD, Trichotillomania (Hair-Pulling Disorder) and Skin-picking Disorder have been reported in 8.75%, 5.1% and 16.3% of OCD patients, respectively (Lochner et al., 2014; Lovato et al., 2012).

The relationship between OCD and several neuropsychiatric and organic movement disorders, most notably Tourette's Syndrome (TS), has been well documented (O'Connor, 2001). While earlier studies suggested that the incidence of tic disorders is fairly low in patients with OCD (e.g., 6.5% Grados et al., 2001), other studies have reported rates of up to 30% (see Leckman et al., 2010). For example, Nestadt et al. (2009) found that 26.2% of their sample had comorbid tic disorder, albeit that their sample - which was for a family-study of OCD - required diagnosis prior to 18 years of age and at least two family members with OCD, perhaps leading to greater representation of OCD with a genetic loading. As noted previously, comorbid tic disorder is associated with early-onset OCD and more common in males. Such evidence has led to the inclusion of a tic-related specifier in the DSM-5 (APA, 2013). Indeed, the differentiation of complex tics from compulsions is not a simple one; it is usually pointed out that sensory urges precede tics, whereas obsessions precede compulsions (APA, 2013). However, both tics and compulsions can be performed until there are "just-right" feelings and to relieve generalized distress (Palumbo & Kurlan, 2007).

Genetics

Generally, genetic studies on the expression of OCD fall broadly under two research streams; studies that have focused primarily on twin pairs and studies that have examined inter-familial transmission of OCD (Pauls, 2008). van Grootheest, Cath, Beekman, and Boomsma (2005) summarised findings from 13 twin studies since 1969, finding that concordance rates for monozygotic twins varied from 0% to 87%. It has been estimated that the heritability (a statistical estimation of the phenotypic variation due to genotypic variation within populations) of OCD ranges between 27% to 65% in children, and between 27% to 47% for adults (van Grootheest et al., 2005). The inter-familial risk of OCD is perhaps more accurately conceptualised as a risk factor for developing the illness. This suggestion is supported by a meta-analysis conducted by Hettema, Neale, and Kendler (2001), which showed that first degree relatives of patients with OCD evince an 8.2% aggregated risk of developing the disorder compared to 2.0% in control groups.

Neuropsychology of Obsessive Compulsive Disorder

Recently Abramovitch and colleagues (2013; in press; 2012) conducted a series of systematic reviews of the literature with regard to neuropsychological functioning in OCD. With respect to youth and children, the meta-analysis examined six areas of cognitive functioning - including Attention, Executive Functioning, Memory, Processing Speed, Visuospatial Abilities and Working Memory (Abramovitch et al., in press). Specific sub-domains of Executive Functioning were also explored including Planning, Response Inhibition and Set-shifting/Cognitive Flexibility, and verbal versus nonverbal Memory and Working Memory were also examined. All included studies utilised established methodologies, with cognitive tests used including the subtests from the Wechsler intelligence and memory batteries, the continuous performance test (CPT), Stroop task, Tower of London/Hanoi (TOL/TOH), Rey-Osterreich Complex Figure Test (ROCF), verbal fluency and the Trail making test. Overall, there was no cognitive domain where children diagnosed with OCD performed significantly worse than did healthy comparison groups (Abramovitch et al., in press). While there were no significant differences between the groups across the studies, an examination of the effect sizes for some of the sub-domains did reveal that, on average, OCD participants had disproportional difficulty in some areas. Not unexpectedly, the greatest negative effect sizes were found in the area of Executive Functioning, particularly in the sub-domain of planning. Visuospatial abilities also showed a large, negative effect size for the OCD group.

In contrast, a meta-analysis of studies in adults suggests that those with OCD appear to have more pervasive and measurable neuropsychological deficits, although the authors caution that it is unclear if the effect size differences are clinically meaningful, and that future studies should examine specific clinical presentations of OCD (Abramovitch, Abramowitz, & Mittelman, 2013). In the analysis, the OCD groups performed significantly worse than did the healthy control groups across the six major cognitive domains and their sub-domains (Abramovitch et al., 2013). Similar to the pediatric literature, a broad range of standardized tests had been used to assess the neuropsychological functioning in adults with OCD, with assessments including subtests of the adult versions of the Wechsler intelligence and memory batteries, the CPT, the Stroop task, TOL/TOH, ROCF and subtests from the Cambridge Automated Neuropsychological Test Battery (CANTAB). Memory was the domain most affected, although verbal memory was less impacted than nonverbal memory, which had the largest effect size of $d = -0.76$, indicating that, on average, the OCD group performed at three quarters of a standard deviation worse than did healthy controls in this area. Performance on tasks assessing Processing Speed, Executive Function and Attention were all in the range of around half a standard deviation worse than for the healthy controls. Age-of-onset of OCD was found to be negatively associated with effect size for Executive Functioning and its sub-domain of Set-shifting/Cognitive flexibility, indicating that *later* onset of symptoms was associated with poorer performance in these areas.

Neuropathology of Obsessive Compulsive Disorder

The neuropathology of OCD is unclear, however there is evidence that serotonergic dysfunction within the *affective cortico-basal ganglia-thalamo-cortical pathways* that are critical for regulating affective, emotional, motivational, behavioral and reward processes have a role in mediating OCD symptoms (Abramowitz, Taylor, & McKay, 2009; Menzies et al., 2008). One controversial hypothesis is that OCD derives from an autoimmune reaction to *type A β-haemolytic streptococcal* bacteria that inflame the striatum, resulting in a rapid onset of OCD symptoms in some patients who are consequently diagnosed with a Paediatric Autoimmune Neuropsychiatric Disorder Associated with Streptococcus (PANDAS) (Leonard & Swedo, 2001).

The potential role of the striatum and other basal ganglia nuclei in OCD was first suggested by Paul MacLean in the 1970s as the basal ganglia mediate ritualised, habitual and stereotyped behaviors in animals with these structures (Baxter Jr, 2003). Subsequently, OCD symptoms have been observed in patients with lesions (Laplane et al., 1989) and other disorders (e.g., TS; Stein, 2002) of the basal ganglia. Neuroimaging studies have corroborated this evidence but afforded a more detailed picture of neuropathology. Initially, positron emission tomography (PET) revealed elevated metabolic activity in the orbital frontal cortex (OFC) and the striatum of resting patients (Baxter et al., 1987; Swedo et al., 1989) that was exacerbated by symptom provocation (Rauch et al., 1994). Later work showed that selective serotonin reuptake inhibitor (SSRI) administration (Baxter, Jr, Schwartz, Bergman, & et al., 1992; Saxena et al., 2002) and cognitive-behavioral therapy (CBT; Brody et al., 1998; Schwartz, Stoessel, Baxter, Martin, & Phelps, 1996) could ameliorate anomalous activity and symptoms, and that baseline activity could predict treatment response (Rauch et al., 2002). However, other work suggested that symptoms are mediated by the thalamus and anterior cingulate cortex (ACC) (Perani et al., 1995; Saxena et al., 2009).

A meta-analysis of functional magnetic resonance imaging (fMRI) studies reported consistent abnormalities in the OFC and striatum of patients, but also in the inferior frontal, ACC, middle occipital, and parietal and cerebellar cortices, suggesting OCD pathological disturbance in both the affective and prefrontal cortico-striatal-thalamo-cortical pathways (Menzies et al., 2008). Interestingly, a recent functional connectivity study found that affective network structures exhibited hyper-connectivity, while prefrontal network structures exhibited hypo-connectivity (Harrison et al., 2009). Notably however, increased connectivity between affective structures (ventral striatum and OFC) predicted greater symptom severity (Y-BOCS), indicating symptom mediation by the affective network (Harrison et al., 2009).

Neurochemistry of Obsessive Compulsive Disorder

Serotonergic dysfunction in OCD is well established. Early work demonstrated anti-obsessional effects of the tricyclic antidepressant clomipramine (Rack & Chir, 1970) that acts by selectively blocking the reuptake of serotonin. Subsequent work showed that SSRIs and not other monoamine reuptake inhibitors provided therapeutic benefits to OCD patients (Zohar & Insel, 1987). SSRIs are now a first-line treatment for OCD, as are psychological treatments involving CBT, although up to half of patients remain unresponsive (Greist, Jefferson, Kobak, Katzelnick, & Serlin, 1995).

The dominant view of serotonergic dysfunction in OCD is that it arises from hypersensitivity of postsynaptic serotonin receptors, perhaps stemming from serotonin transporter and receptor genetic abnormalities (Greenberg et al., 1998). SSRIs act by inhibiting presynaptic reuptake of serotonin from the synaptic cleft; the consequent increase in extracellular serotonin facilitates postsynaptic serotonin binding which leads to desensitization (down-regulation) of serotonergic autoreceptors in OFC over a similar period (~8 weeks) to the psychotherapeutic effects of SSRIs (Bergqvist, Bouchard, & Blier, 1999; El Mansari, Bouchard, & Blier, 1995). Also, PET studies suggest that after an 8–12 week SSRI intervention, metabolic activity is reduced in OFC and striatum (Saxena et al., 2002; Saxena et al., 1999), and that lower baseline metabolic activity within OFC predicts response to SSRI treatment (Saxena et al., 1999).

Several researchers have explored the role of dopamine in OCD (Westenberg, Fineberg, & Denys, 2007) since dopamine agonists (Creese & Iversen, 1974) and lesions to the basal ganglia (high dopaminergic innervation: Laplane et al., 1989) can induce OCD symptoms. This work indicated that treatment-refractory patients can benefit from a combination of antipsychotic (dopamine antagonists) and SSRIs (Fineberg et al., 2006; McDougle et al., 1994), and that antipsychotics can reduce tic frequency in the OCD-related disorder TS (McDougle et al., 1994). While the role of dopamine in OCD is unclear, some work suggests that patients exhibit abnormal levels of dopamine transporters (van der Wee et al., 2014) and receptor densities (Denys, van der Wee, Janssen, De Geus, & Westenberg, 2004).

Frontostriatal circuitry and Obsessive Compulsive Disorder

The frontal lobes, located at the front of the brain, are the largest area of our brains and are considered the centre of "what makes us human". These lobes, and in particular the prefrontal and orbitofrontal areas, mediate our executive functions and our emotional functioning. Executive functions are higher-level abilities that include planning, shifting between different ideas (thinking flexibly), generating new responses (fluency), problem solving, holding and shifting attention, and abstraction. They also include the ability to inhibit inappropriate responses. The frontal lobes, and the circuits within them, continue to grow and mature throughout the individual's lifetime. As discussed previously, there is wide acceptance that the pathophysiology of OCD is associated with abnormal patterns of activity within cortico-striato-thalamo-cortical circuits (CSTC). At least five functionally and structurally segregated neural circuits or 'loops' have been identified where projections initiate from, and project back to, cortical areas including the supplementary motor area (SMA), the frontal eye fields, the dorsolateral prefrontal cortex

(DPFC), the lateral OFC and the ACC (Marsh, Maia, & Peterson, 2009). All then pass through various areas of the striatum and thalamus before looping back to the same cortical regions. The loops originating in the SMA, frontal eye fields and DPFC pass through the dorsal striatum, an area associated with habit and/or stimulus-response learning. The ventral striatum mediates reward, drive and motivation (Wise, 2004) and the latter two loops initiated in the OFC and ACC pass through this region. In OCD, there are findings that suggest abnormalities in the CSTC circuits including the OFC, ACC and the striatum, and that these anomalies may lead to the development of the disorder (Marsh et al., 2009). Within each of the five circuits there are two sub-loops that exert opposing influences on thalamocortical output at the Ventral Pallidum/Substantia Nigra (VP/SN): glutamatergic efferents from the cortex activate distinct populations of GABAergic or glutamatergic STR neurons that project to the VP/SN, forming the *direct* (activating) and *indirect* (inhibiting) pathways, respectively (Alexander, DeLong, & Strick, 1986). OCD is believed to be associated with hyperactivity of the direct pathway. For further discussion of the neurocircuitry of OCD, see Graybiel and Rauch (2000).

Treatment

As noted above, the neurochemical pathways that have been implicated in OCD include the serotonergic (Markarian et al., 2010), adrenergic (Hollander et al., 1991), and dopaminergic pathways (Husted, Shapira, & Goodman, 2005). As SSRIs have been shown to be the most effective in ameliorating the symptoms of OCD, they are generally recommended as the first line pharmacological treatment (Fineberg & Gale, 2005).

Although pharmacological treatments have been shown to alleviate the symptoms of OCD, they do not seem to resolve the underlying cause. Further, despite empirical evidence showing SSRIs to be one of the most effective pharmacological interventions for treating OCD, approximately 40% to 60% of patients fail to respond (Fineberg & Gale, 2005; Pallanti et al., 2002). Other drugs have been trialled with varying levels of success, including antipsychotics, benzodiazepines, mood stabilisers, anxiolytics, antiglutamatergics and morphine (Math & Reddy, 2007).

Finally, psychological therapy, specifically CBT, is an efficacious treatment for OCD – so much so that prominent foundations such as the National Institute for Health and Clinical Excellence (NICE, 2005) recommend it as the frontline treatment for OCD (see Kyrios, Moulding, & Bhar, 2014). Recent meta-analyses support its efficacy in group and individual formats and in children and adults (Jónsson & Hougaard, 2009; Olatunji, Davis, Powers, & Smits, 2013; Watson & Rees, 2008), although there are similar problems with respect to treatment refusal, drop-out and relapse as there are for medication approaches. These treatments are based around exposure and response prevention along with cognitive restructuring; however, as mentioned earlier, there is some evidence that they result in the normalization of functional neurological patterns as evidenced pre-and-post treatment by functional imaging. Interestingly, given the previous discussion of early-versus late onset OCD, when reviewing the literature, Leckman et al. (2010) reported that while comorbid tic disorder was a negative prognostic sign for SSRIs in childhood OCD, it did not interfere with CBT for OCD.

Summary

OCD is a highly disabling and common disorder, characterised by obsessions and compulsions, such as unwanted doubts, sexual or aggressive thoughts, concerns regarding symmetry, or contamination concerns. Neurodevelopmentally, frontal-striatal regions have been strongly implicated, with evidence to suggest the involvement of specific neurological circuitry, and robust evidence of resulting neuropsychological changes, albeit of a moderate magnitude. In particular, there appears evidence of an early onset group, who tend to be more likely male, have more OCPD features, and neurological signs such as greater tics (Taylor, 2011). However, it should also be acknowledged that cultural influences on the presentation and nature of OCD, alongside evidence of environmental influence on the formation of OCD and the utility of both pharmacological and non-pharmacological treatments, suggest that a biopsychosocial model may be of utility. For example, real memory deficits combined with high levels of responsibility may lead to a behavioral exaggeration of such deficits (i.e., "my memory is poor and I have to be absolutely sure"; Nedeljkovic, Moulding, Kyrios, & Doron, 2009), exacerbating rituals. Regardless, the evidence reviewed suggests that there are moderately effective treatments that lead to normalization of neurological alterations, but further development is required given high levels of non-response, drop-out, treatment refusal and relapse.

Abbreviations

ACC: Anterior Cingulate Cortex
BDD: Body Dysmorphic Disorder
BOLD: Blood-Oxygen Level Dependent
CANTAB: Cambridge Automated Neuropsychological Test Battery
CBT: Cognitive Behavioral Therapy
CPT: Continuous Performance Test
CSTC: Cortico-Striato-Thalamo-Cortical Circuits
DOCS: Dimensional Obsessive Compulsive Inventory
DPFC: Dorsolateral Prefrontal Cortex
ECA: National Epidemiological Catchment Area Survey
fMRI: functional Magnetic Resonance Imaging

OCD: Obsessive Compulsive Disorder
OCI-R: Obsessive Compulsive Inventory – Revised
OCPD: Obsessive Compulsive Personality Disorder
OFC: Orbital Frontal Cortext
PANDAS: Paediatric Autoimmune Neuropsychiatric Disorder Associated with Streptococcus
PET: Positron Emission Tomography
ROCF: Rey-Osterreich Complex Figure Test
SMA: Supplementary Motor Area
SSRI: Selective Serotonin Reuptake Inhibitor
TOL/TOH: Tower of London/Tower of Hanoi
TS: Tourette's Syndrome
VP/SN: Ventral Pallidum/Substantia Nigra
Y-BOCS: Yale-Brown Obsessive Compulsive Scale

Further readings

Abramovitch, A., Abramowitz, J. S., & Mittelman, A. (2013). The neuropsychology of adult obsessive-compulsive disorder: A meta-analysis. *Clinical Psychology Review, 33*(8), 1163–1171.

Abramovitch, A., Abramowitz, J. S., Mittelman, A., Stark, A., Ramsey, K., & Geller, D. A. (in press). Research Review: Neuropsychological test performance in pediatric obsessive-compulsive disorder–a meta-analysis. *Journal of Child Psychology and Psychiatry.*

Abramovitch, A., Mittelman, A., Henin, A., & Geller, D. (2012). Neuroimaging and neuropsychological findings in pediatric obsessive-compulsive disorder: a review and developmental considerations. *Neuropsychiatry, 2*(4), 313–329.

Graybiel, A. M., & Rauch, S. L. (2000). Toward a neurobiology of obsessive-compulsive disorder. *Neuron, 28*(2), 343–347.

Menzies, L., Chamberlain, S. R., Laird, A. R., Thelen, S. M., Sahakian, B. J., & Bullmore, E. T. (2008). Integrating evidence from neuroimaging and neuropsychological studies of obsessive-compulsive disorder: The orbitofronto-striatal model revisited. *Neuroscience & Biobehavioral Reviews, 32*(3), 525–549. doi: http://dx.doi.org/10.1016/j.neubiorev.2007.09.005.

National Institute of Health and Clinical Excellence. (2005). *Obsessive-Compulsive Disorder: Core Interventions in the Treatment of Obsessive-Compulsive Disorder and Body Dysmorphic Disorder.* Leicester, UK: National Collaborating Centre for Mental Health (UK).

References

Abramovitch, A., Abramowitz, J. S., & Mittelman, A. (2013). The neuropsychology of adult obsessive-compulsive disorder: A meta-analysis. *Clinical Psychology Review, 33*(8), 1163–1171.

Abramovitch, A., Abramowitz, J. S., Mittelman, A., Stark, A., Ramsey, K., & Geller, D. A. (in press). Research review: Neuropsychological test performance in pediatric obsessive-compulsive disorder – a meta-analysis. *Journal of Child Psychology and Psychiatry.*

Abramovitch, A., Mittelman, A., Henin, A., & Geller, D. (2012). Neuroimaging and neuropsychological findings in pediatric obsessive-compulsive disorder: A review and developmental considerations. *Neuropsychiatry, 2*(4), 313–329.

Abramowitz, J. S., Deacon, B. J., Olatunji, B. O., Wheaton, M. G., Berman, N. C., Losardo, D., ... Adams, T. (2010). Assessment of obsessive-compulsive symptom dimensions: Development and evaluation of the Dimensional Obsessive-Compulsive Scale. *Psychological Assessment, 22*(1), 180.

Abramowitz, J. S., Taylor, S., & McKay, D. (2009). Obsessive-compulsive disorder. *The Lancet, 374*(9688), 491–499.

Alexander, G. E., DeLong, M. R., & Strick, P. L. (1986). Parallel organization of functionally segregated circuits linking basal ganglia and cortex. *Annual Review of Neuroscience, 9*(1), 357–381.

American Psychiatric Association. (2013). *Diagnostic and Statistical Manual of Mental Disorders, (DSM-5®)*. Washington, DC: American Psychiatric Publishing.

Attiullah, N., Eisen, J. L., & Rasmussen, S. A. (2000). Clinical features of obsessive-compulsive disorder. *Psychiatric Clinics of North America, 23*(3), 469–491.

Baxter Jr, L. R. (2003). Basal ganglia systems in ritualistic social displays: Reptiles and humans; function and illness. *Physiology & Behavior, 79*(3), 451–460. doi: http://dx.doi.org/10.1016/S0031-9384(03)00164-1.

Baxter, L. R., Jr, Phelps, M. E., Mazziotta, J. C., Guze, B. H., Schwartz, J. M., & Selin, C. E. (1987). Local cerebral glucose metabolic rates in obsessive-compulsive disorder: A comparison with rates in unipolar depression and in normal controls. *Archives of General Psychiatry, 44*(3), 211–218. doi: 10.1001/archpsyc.1987.01800150017003.

Baxter, L. R., Jr, Schwartz, J. M., Bergman, K. S., & et al. (1992). Caudate glucose metabolic rate changes with both drug and behavior therapy for obsessive-compulsive disorder. *Archives of General Psychiatry, 49*(9), 681–689. doi: 10.1001/archpsyc.1992.01820090009002.

Bebbington, P. E., Dunn, G., Jenkins, R., Lewis, G., Brugha, T., Farrell, M., & Meltzer, H. (1998). The influence of age and sex on the prevalence of depressive conditions: Report from the National Survey of Psychiatric Morbidity. *Psychological Medicine, 28*(01), 9–19.

Bergqvist, P. B., Bouchard, C., & Blier, P. (1999). Effect of long-term administration of antidepressant treatments on serotonin release in brain regions involved in obsessive-compulsive disorder. *Biological Psychiatry, 45*(2), 164–174.

Bloch, M. H., Landeros-Weisenberger, A., Rosario, M. C., Pittenger, C., & Leckman, J. F. (2008). Meta-analysis of the symptom structure of obsessive-compulsive disorder. *The American Journal of Psychiatry, 165*(12), 1532–1542.

Bogetto, F., Venturello, S., Albert, U., Maina, G., & Ravizza, L. (1999). Gender-related clinical differences in obsessive-compulsive disorder. *European Psychiatry, 14*(8), 434–441.

Brody, A. L., Saxena, S., Schwartz, J. M., Stoessel, P. W., Maidment, K., Phelps, M. E., & Baxter, L. R. (1998). FDG-PET predictors of response to behavioral therapy and pharmacotherapy in obsessive compulsive disorder. *Psychiatry Research: Neuroimaging, 84*(1), 1–6.

Calvo, R., Lázaro, L., Castro-Fornieles, J., Font, E., Moreno, E., & Toro, J. (2009). Obsessive-compulsive personality disorder traits and personality dimensions in parents of children with obsessive-compulsive disorder. *European Psychiatry, 24*(3), 201–206.

Clark, D. A., Abramowitz, J., Alcolado, G. M., Alonso, P., Belloch, A., Bouvard, M., Coles, M. E., Doron, G., Fernández-Álvarez, H., & Garcia-Soriano, G. (2014). Part 3. A question of perspective: The association between intrusive thoughts and obsessionality in 11 countries. *Journal of Obsessive-Compulsive and Related Disorders, 3*(3), 292–299.

Creese, I., & Iversen, S. D. (1974). The role of forebrain dopamine systems in amphetamine induced stereotyped behavior in the rat. *Psychopharmacologia, 39*(4), 345–357.

de Silva, P. (2006). Culture and obsessive-compulsive disorder. *Psychiatry, 5*(11), 402–404.

Denys, D., van der Wee, N., Janssen, J., De Geus, F., & Westenberg, H. G. M. (2004). Low level of dopaminergic D2 receptor binding in obsessive-compulsive disorder. *Biological Psychiatry, 55*(10), 1041–1045. doi: http://dx.doi.org/10.1016/j.biopsych.2004.01.023.

Diniz, J. B., Rosario-Campos, M. C., Shavitt, R. G., Curi, M., Hounie, A. G., Brotto, S. A., & Miguel, E. C. (2004). Impact of age at onset and duration of illness on the expression of comorbidities in obsessive-compulsive disorder. *Journal of Clinical Psychiatry, 65*(1), 22–27.

Eisen, J. L., Coles, M. E., Shea, M. T., Pagano, M. E., Stout, R. L., Yen, S., … Rasmussen, S. A. (2006). Clarifying the convergence between obsessive compulsive personality disorder criteria and obsessive compulsive disorder. *Journal of Personality Disorders, 20*(3), 294–305.

El Mansari, M., Bouchard, C., & Blier, P. (1995). Alteration of serotonin release in the guinea pig orbito-frontal cortex by selective serotonin reuptake inhibitors: Relevance to treatment of obsessive-compulsive disorder. *Neuropsychopharmacology, 13*(2), 117–127.

Esquirol, E. (1845). *Mental Maladies: A Treatise on Insanity*. Lea and Blanchard.

Fineberg, N. A., & Gale, T. M. (2005). Evidence-based pharmacotherapy of obsessive-compulsive disorder. *The International Journal of Neuropsychopharmacology, 8*(01), 107–129.

Fineberg, N. A., Stein, D. J., Premkumar, P., Carey, P., Sivakumaran, T., Vythilingum, B., … Denys, D. (2006). Adjunctive quetiapine for serotonin reuptake inhibitor-resistant obsessive-compulsive disorder: A meta-analysis of randomized controlled treatment trials. *International Clinical Psychopharmacology, 21*(6), 337–343.

Foa, E. B., Huppert, J. D., Leiberg, S., Langner, R., Kichic, R., Hajcak, G., & Salkovskis, P. M. (2002). The obsessive-compulsive inventory: Development and validation of a short version. *Psychological Assessment, 14*(4), 485.

Geller, D., Biederman, J., Jones, J., Park, K., Schwartz, S., Shapiro, S., & Coffey, B. (1998). Is juvenile obsessive-compulsive disorder a developmental subtype of the disorder? A review of the pediatric literature. *Journal of the American Academy of Child & Adolescent Psychiatry, 37*(4), 420–427.

Goodman, W. K., Price, L. H., Rasmussen, S. A., Mazure, C., Fleischmann, R. L., Hill, C. L., … Charney, D. S. (1989). The Yale-Brown obsessive compulsive scale: I. Development, use, and reliability. *Archives of General Psychiatry, 46*(11), 1006–1011.

Grados, M. A., Riddle, M. A., Samuels, J. F., Liang, K.-Y., Hoehn-Saric, R., Bienvenu, O. J., … Nestadt, G. (2001). The familial phenotype of obsessive-compulsive disorder in relation to tic disorders: The Hopkins OCD family study. *Biological Psychiatry, 50*(8), 559–565.

Graybiel, A. M., & Rauch, S. L. (2000). Toward a neurobiology of obsessive-compulsive disorder. *Neuron, 28*(2), 343–347.

Greenberg, B. D., Benjamin, J., Martin, J. D., Keuler, D., Huang, S. J., Altemus, M., & Murphy, D. L. (1998). Delayed obsessive-compulsive disorder symptom exacerbation after a single dose of a serotonin antagonist in fluoxetine-treated but not untreated patients. *Psychopharmacology, 140*(4), 434.

Greist, J., Jefferson, J. W., Kobak, K. A., Katzelnick, D. J., & Serlin, R. C. (1995). Efficacy and tolerability of serotonin transport inhibitors in obsessive-compulsive disorder: A meta-analysis. *Archives of General Psychiatry, 52*(1), 53–60. doi: 10.1001/archpsyc.1995.03950130053006.

Harrison, B. J., Soriano-Mas, C., Pujol, J., Ortiz, H., López-Solà, M., Hernández-Ribas, R., … Pantelis, C. (2009). Altered corticostriatal functional connectivity in obsessive-compulsive disorder. *Archives of General Psychiatry, 66*(11), 1189–1200.

Hettema, J. M., Neale, M. C., & Kendler, K. S. (2001). A review and meta-analysis of the genetic epidemiology of anxiety disorders. *American Journal of Psychiatry, 158*(10), 1568–1578.

Hollander, E., DeCaria, C., Nitescu, A., Cooper, T., Stover, B., Gully, R., … Liebowitz, M. R. (1991). Noradrenergic function in obsessive-compulsive disorder: Behavioral and neuroendocrine responses to clonidine and comparison to healthy controls. *Psychiatry Research, 37*(2), 161–177.

Husted, D. S., Shapira, N. A., & Goodman, W. K. (2005). *Obsessive-Compulsive Disorder Neurological and Psychiatric Disorders* (pp. 171–188). Springer.

Jónsson, H., & Hougaard, E. (2009). Group cognitive behavioural therapy for obsessive-compulsive disorder: A systematic review and meta-analysis. *Acta Psychiatrica Scandinavica, 119*(2), 98–106.

Karno, M., Golding, J. M., Sorenson, S. B., & Burnam, M. A. (1988). The epidemiology of obsessive-compulsive disorder in five US communities. *Archives of General Psychiatry, 45*(12), 1094–1099.

Kyrios, M., Moulding, R., & Bhar, S. (2014). A clinician's quick guide of evidence-based approaches: Obsessive-compulsive disorder. *Clinical Psychologist, 18*(2), 96–97.

Laplane, D., Levasseur, M., Pillon, B., Dubois, B., Baulac, M., Mazoyer, B., … Baron, J. (1989). Obsessive-compulsive and other behavioural changes with bilateral basal ganglia lesions. *Brain, 112*(3), 699–725.

Leckman, J. F., Denys, D., Simpson, H. B., Mataix-Cols, D., Hollander, E., Saxena, S., Phillips, K. A. (2010). Obsessive-compulsive disorder: A review of the diagnostic criteria and possible subtypes and dimensional specifiers for DSM-V. *Depression and Anxiety, 27*(6), 507–527.

Lensi, P., Cassano, G. B., Correddu, G., Ravagli, S., Kunovac, J., & Akiskal, H. (1996). Obsessive-compulsive disorder. Familial-developmental history, symptomatology, comorbidity and course with special reference to gender-related differences. *The British Journal of Psychiatry, 169*(1), 101–107.

Leonard, H. L., & Swedo, S. E. (2001). Paediatric autoimmune neuropsychiatric disorders associated with streptococcal infection (PANDAS). *The International Journal of Neuropsychopharmacology, 4*(2), 191–198. doi: doi:10.1017/S1461145701002371.

Lochner, C., Fineberg, N. A., Zohar, J., van Ameringen, M., Juven-Wetzler, A., Altamura, A. C., … Nicolini, H. (2014). Comorbidity in obsessive-compulsive disorder (OCD): A report from the International College of Obsessive-Compulsive Spectrum Disorders (ICOCS). *Comprehensive Psychiatry, 55*(7), 1513–1519.

Lochner, C., Hemmings, S. M., Kinnear, C. J., Moolman-Smook, J. C., Corfield, V. A., Knowles, J. A., Niehaus, D. J., & Stein, D. J. (2004). Gender in obsessive-compulsive disorder: Clinical and genetic findings. *European Neuropsychopharmacology, 14*(2), 105–113.

Lovato, L., Ferrão, Y. A., Stein, D. J., Shavitt, R. G., Fontenelle, L. F., Vivan, A., … Cordioli, A. V. (2012). Skin picking and trichotillomania in adults with obsessive-compulsive disorder. *Comprehensive Psychiatry, 53*(5), 562–568.

Maina, G., Albert, U., Salvi, V., Pessina, E., & Bogetto, F. (2008). Early-onset obsessive-compulsive disorder and personality disorders in adulthood. *Psychiatry Research, 158*(2), 217–225.

Mansueto, C. S., & Keuler, D. J. (2005). Tic or compulsion? It's Tourettic OCD. *Behavior Modification, 29*(5), 784–799.

Markarian, Y., Larson, M. J., Aldea, M. A., Baldwin, S. A., Good, D., Berkeljon, A., … McKay, D. (2010). Multiple pathways to functional impairment in obsessive-compulsive disorder. *Clinical Psychology Review, 30*(1), 78–88.

Marsh, R., Maia, T.V., & Peterson, B. S. (2009). Functional disturbances within frontostriatal circuits across multiple childhood psychopathologies. *The American Journal of Psychiatry, 166*(6), 664–674.

Math, S., & Reddy, J. Y. (2007). Issues in the pharmacological treatment of obsessive-compulsive disorder. *International Journal of Clinical Practice, 61*(7), 1188–1197.

McDougle, C. J., Goodman, W. K., Leckman, J. F., Lee, N. C., Heninger, G. R., & Price, L. H. (1994). Haloperidol addition in fluvoxamine-refractory obsessive-compulsive disorder: A double-blind, placebo-controlled study in patients with and without tics. *Archives of General Psychiatry, 51*(4), 302–308.

Menzies, L., Chamberlain, S. R., Laird, A. R., Thelen, S. M., Sahakian, B. J., & Bullmore, E. T. (2008). Integrating evidence from neuroimaging and neuropsychological studies of obsessive-compulsive disorder: The orbitofronto-striatal model revisited. *Neuroscience & Biobehavioral Reviews, 32*(3), 525–549. doi: http://dx.doi.org/10.1016/j.neubiorev.2007.09.005.

Moulding, R., Nedeljkovic, M., & Kyrios, M. (2011). Obsessive compulsive disorder in the DSM. In G. Murray (Ed.), *A Critical Introduction to DSM* (pp. 151–166). New York: Nova.

National Institute of Health and Clinical Excellence. (2005). *Obsessive-Compulsive Disorder: Core Interventions in the Treatment of Obsessive-Compulsive Disorder and Body Dysmorphic Disorder.* Leicester, UK: National Collaborating Centre for Mental Health (UK).

Nedeljkovic, M., Moulding, R., Foroughi, E., Kyrios, M., & Doron, G. (2012). *Cultural Issues in Understanding and Treating Obsessive Compulsive and Spectrum Disorders.* Oxford: Oxford University Press.

Nedeljkovic, M., Moulding, R., Kyrios, M., & Doron, G. (2009). The relationship of cognitive confidence to OCD symptoms. *Journal of Anxiety Disorders, 23*(4), 463–468.

Nestadt, G., Di, C., Riddle, M., Grados, M., Greenberg, B., Fyer, A., McCracken, J., … Rasmussen, S. (2009). Obsessive-compulsive disorder: Subclassification based on co-morbidity. *Psychological Medicine, 39*(09), 1491–1501.

O'Connor, K. P. (2001). Clinical and psychological features distinguishing obsessive-compulsive and chronic tic disorders. *Clinical Psychology Review, 21*(4), 631–660.

Olatunji, B. O., Davis, M. L., Powers, M. B., & Smits, J. A. (2013). Cognitive-behavioral therapy for obsessive-compulsive disorder: A meta-analysis of treatment outcome and moderators. *Journal of Psychiatric Research, 47*(1), 33–41.

Olatunji, B. O., Williams, B. J., Haslam, N., Abramowitz, J. S., & Tolin, D. F. (2008). The latent structure of obsessive-compulsive symptoms: A taxometric study. *Depression and Anxiety, 25*(11), 956–968.

Pallanti, S., Hollander, E., Bienstock, C., Koran, L., Leckman, J., Marazziti, D., … Zohar, J. (2002). Treatment non-response in OCD: Methodological issues and operational definitions. *The International Journal of Neuropsychopharmacology, 5*(02), 181–191.

Palumbo, D., & Kurlan, R. (2007). Complex obsessive compulsive and impulsive symptoms in Tourette's syndrome. *Neuropsychiatric Disease and Treatment, 3*(5), 687.

Pauls, D. L. (2008). *The Genetics of Obsessive Compulsive Disorder: A Review of the Evidence.* Paper presented at the American Journal of Medical Genetics Part C: Seminars in Medical Genetics.

Perani, D., Colombo, C., Bressi, S., Bonfanti, A., Grassi, F., Scarone, S., … Fazio, F. (1995). [18F] FDG PET study in obsessive-compulsive disorder. A clinical/metabolic correlation study after treatment. *The British Journal of Psychiatry, 166*(2), 244–250.

Rack, M., & Chir, D. (1970). Experience with intravenous clomipramine. *Obsessional States and Their Treatment with Anafranil.*

Rasmussen, S. A., & Eisen, J. L. (1992). The epidemiology and clinical features of obsessive compulsive disorder. *Psychiatric Clinics of North America*.

Rauch, S. L., Jenike, M. A., Alpert, N. M., Baer, L., Breiter, H. C., Savage, C. R., & Fischman, A. J. (1994). Regional cerebral blood flow measured during symptom provocation in obsessive-compulsive disorder using oxygen 15—labeled carbon dioxide and positron emission tomography. *Archives of General Psychiatry, 51*(1), 62–70.

Rauch, S. L., Shin, L. M., Dougherty, D. D., Alpert, N. M., Fischman, A. J., & Jenike, M. A. (2002). Predictors of fluvoxamine response in contamination-related obsessive compulsive disorder: A PET symptom provocation study. *Neuropsychopharmacology, 27*(5), 782–791.

Ruscio, A., Stein, D., Chiu, W., & Kessler, R. (2010). The epidemiology of obsessive-compulsive disorder in the National Comorbidity Survey Replication. *Molecular Psychiatry, 15*(1), 53–63.

Samuels, J. F., Bienvenu, O. J., Pinto, A., Fyer, A. J., McCracken, J. T., Rauch, S. L., Murphy, D. L., Grados, M. A., Greenberg, B. D., & Knowles, J. A. (2007). Hoarding in obsessive-compulsive disorder: Results from the OCD Collaborative Genetics Study. *Behaviour Research and Therapy, 45*(4), 673–686.

Saxena, S., Brody, A. L., Ho, M. L., Shervin-Alborzian, B. S., Karron, M., Maidment, R. N., ... Baxter Jr, M.D. (2002). DIfferential cerebral metabolic changes with paroxetine treatment of obsessive-compulsive disorder vs major depression. *Archives of General Psychiatry, 59*(3), 250–261. doi: 10.1001/archpsyc.59.3.250.

Saxena, S., Brody, A. L., Maidment, K. M., Dunkin, J. J., Colgan, M., Alborzian, S., ... Baxter, L. R. (1999). Localized orbitofrontal and subcortical metabolic changes and predictors of response to paroxetine treatment in obsessive-compulsive disorder. *Neuropsychopharmacology, 21*(6), 683–693.

Saxena, S., Gorbis, E., O'Neill, J., Baker, S. K., Mandelkern, M. A., Maidment, K. M., ... Schwartz, J. M. (2009). Rapid effects of brief intensive cognitive-behavioral therapy on brain glucose metabolism in obsessive-compulsive disorder. *Molecular Psychiatry, 14*(2), 197–205.

Scahill, L., Riddle, M. A., McSwiggin-Hardin, M., Ort, S. I., King, R. A., Goodman, W. K., ... Leckman, J. F. (1997). Children's Yale-Brown obsessive compulsive scale: Reliability and validity. *Journal of the American Academy of Child & Adolescent Psychiatry, 36*(6), 844–852.

Schwartz, J. M., Stoessel, P. W., Baxter, L. R., Martin, K. M., & Phelps, M. E. (1996). Systematic changes in cerebral glucose metabolic rate after successful behavior modification treatment of obsessive-compulsive disorder. *Archives of General Psychiatry, 53*(2), 109–113.

Skoog, G., & Skoog, I. (1999). A 40-year follow-up of patients with obsessive-compulsive disorder. *Archives of General Psychiatry, 56*(2), 121–127.

Stein, D. J. (2002). Obsessive-compulsive disorder. *The Lancet, 360*(9330), 397–405.

Storch, E. A., Rasmussen, S. A., Price, L. H., Larson, M. J., Murphy, T. K., & Goodman, W. K. (2010). Development and psychometric evaluation of the Yale–Brown Obsessive-Compulsive Scale—Second Edition. *Psychological Assessment, 22*(2), 223.

Swedo, S. E., Schapiro, M. B., Grady, C. L., Cheslow, D. L., Leonard, H. L., Kumar, A., ... Rapoport, J. L. (1989). Cerebral glucose metabolism in childhood-onset obsessive-compulsive disorder. *Archives of General Psychiatry, 46*(6), 518–523. doi: 10.1001/archpsyc.1989.01810060038007.

Taylor, S. (2011). Early versus late onset obsessive-compulsive disorder: Evidence for distinct subtypes. *Clinical Psychology Review, 31*(7), 1083–1100.

van der Wee, N. J., Stevens, H., Hardeman, J. A., Mandl, R. C., Denys, D. A., van Megen, H. J., ... Westenberg, H. M. (2014). Enhanced dopamine transporter density in psychotropic-naive patients with obsessive-compulsive disorder shown by [123I] β-CIT SPECT. *American Journal of Psychiatry*.

van Grootheest, D. S., Cath, D. C., Beekman, A. T., & Boomsma, D. I. (2005). Twin studies on obsessive-compulsive disorder: A review. *Twin Research and Human Genetics, 8*(5), 450–458.

Watson, H. J., & Rees, C. S. (2008). Meta-analysis of randomized, controlled treatment trials for pediatric obsessive-compulsive disorder. *Journal of Child Psychology and Psychiatry, 49*(5), 489–498.

Westenberg, H. G., Fineberg, N. A., & Denys, D. (2007). Neurobiology of obsessive-compulsive disorder: Serotonin and beyond. *CNS Spectrums, 12*(S3), 14–27.

Wewetzer, C., Jans, T., Müller, B., Neudörfl, A., Bücherl, U., Remschmidt, H., … Herpertz-Dahlmann, B. (2001). Long-term outcome and prognosis of obsessive-compulsive disorder with onset in childhood or adolescence. *European Child & Adolescent Psychiatry, 10*(1), 37–46.

Wise, R. A. (2004). Dopamine, learning and motivation. *Nature Reviews Neuroscience, 5*(6), 483–494.

Zohar, J., & Insel, T. R. (1987). Obsessive-compulsive disorder: Psychobiological approaches to diagnosis, treatment, and pathophysiology. *Biological Psychiatry, 22*(6), 667–687.

12
GILLES de la TOURETTE SYNDROME

Dianne M. Sheppard, Nicole Papadopoulos and Valsamma Eapen

Introduction

Gilles de la Tourette syndrome (TS) is a neurodevelopmental disorder characterised by multiple motor tics and at least one vocal tic that have been present for over a year and onset before 18 years, according to the Diagnostic and Statistical Manual of the American Psychiatric Association (currently DSM-5, 2013) and the International Classification of Disorders (World Health Organisation Criteria [ICD -10, 1992]). It is believed that the first description of TS was by Dr Jean Marc Itard in 1825 followed by a nine-case series in 1885 by Dr Georges Albert Edouard Brutus Gilles de la Tourette, highlighting the triad of multiple motor tics, phonic tics and coprolalia (see Robertson, 2015b). The diagnostic criteria have changed over the years since DSM 1 in 1952, but uphold the tic-related criteria (above), and that the symptoms must not be attributable to the physiological effects of a substance (e.g. cocaine) or other medical condition (e.g. Huntington's Disease, post-viral encephalitis). It has been suggested that future classification may need to conceptualise a Tic Spectrum of Disorders with pure tics/Tourette disorder, as well as "TS Plus" with associated comorbidities (see Robertson & Eapen, 2014). The characteristic features of tics include the waxing and waning course with the tics changing in site and nature over time with one type of tic being replaced by a new one. The ability to voluntarily suppress the tics (duration of suppression varies based on the severity), may be followed in some by a rebound phenomenon of increased tics following the suppression, as well as suggestibility and a premonitory urge just prior to the onset of the tic relieved by performing the tic.

Associated features in TS include copro-phenomena, echo-phenomena, palipraxia, palilalia, self-injurious behaviours and non-obscene socially inappropriate (NOSI) behaviours, etc (see Clinical Symptoms section for more information).

The "pure TS" consisting of only motor and vocal tics occurs in a minority of TS patients (Eapen & Robertson, 2015); with recent reports of lifetime prevalence of *any* psychiatric comorbidity among individuals with TS of 85.7%, with 57.7% having two or more psychiatric disorders (Hirschtritt et al., 2015). While tics are the defining feature of TS, there is evidence from neuropsychological (e.g. Channon, Gunning, Frankl, & Robertson, 2006), neuro-radiological (e.g. Peterson et al., 2003) and behavioural (e.g. Peterson, Pine, Cohen, & Brook, 2001) data that it is the presence of comorbidities, such as Attention Deficit Hyperactivity Disorder (ADHD), and the socially stigmatising behaviours such as the coprophenomena that determine the course and overall outcome, especially quality of life (Eapen & Robertson, 2015; Robertson & Eapen, 2013).

Onset and prevalence

Once considered to be a rare curiosity, recent epidemiological studies suggest that TS is not uncommon with rates ranging from 0.3% to 5.7% (Robertson, 2015b); a recent meta-analysis reported a prevalence of 0.77%, with 1.06% in boys attending mainstream education (Knight et al., 2012). However, tics and TS are much more common in the special education populations in children with behavioural and emotional problems and in children with learning disabilities (Eapen, Robertson, Zeitlin, & Kurlan, 1997), and, in particular, in children with autism (Baron-Cohen, Scahill, Izaguirre, Hornsey, & Robertson, 1999). This pattern seems to suggest the involvement of overlapping neuro-developmental pathways with distinct clinical phenotypes (Eapen & Črnčec, 2009). The onset of symptoms is usually around 6 years for motor tics and 9 years for vocal tics, with worst tic severity reported at 10–11 years. Tics usually get better with advancing age, with around half showing considerably reduced or non-existent tics in adulthood.

Clinical symptoms

The clinical hallmark of Tourette syndrome is the occurrence of multiple, obtrusive motor and phonic tics that may be simple or complex and change in frequency, nature and severity over time (Robertson, 2015b). Tics are traditionally defined as repetitive, stereotyped movements or vocalisations which are *involuntary* (Singer & Walkup, 1991); though current thinking describes the tics of TS as *unvoluntary* or even *semi-voluntary* as they are performed in response to an (involuntary) premonitory sensation in order to temporarily relieve an urge or underlying discomfort (Kwak, Dat Vuong, & Jankovic, 2003). Some can transiently suppress tics with effort and increasing internal discomfort, providing additional support for their semi-voluntary nature, and recent research has shown that the premonitory urges are related to tic severity (Kwak et al., 2003) and the presence of complex tics (Eapen & Robertson, 2015).

Tics occur multiple times a day, usually in bouts and characteristically wax and wane, and can vary enormously in content and severity over time from early childhood; typically beginning with one or two simple motor and/or vocal tics, such as repetitive eye blinking, neck movements or throat clearing, and later progressing to more complex tics and associated behaviours including gestures (sometimes obscene, copropraxia), facial grimacing and retracing steps, echopraxia (repeated actions), palipraxia (repeating the last act), self-injurious behaviours, etc. (Robertson, 2014b). Phonic tics most commonly present as inarticulate sounds, such as barking, coughing and throat clearing, as well as the more complex vocalizations (e.g. animal sounds), coprolalia (swearing), echolalia (repeated vocalizations), palilalia (repetition of words or phrases or last syllable) and the non-obscene socially inappropriate behaviours (NOSI), such as discriminative verbal insults (Robertson, 2015b; Robertson & Eapen, 2013). The prevalence of these associated features varies based on the sample studied. For example, the rate of coprolalia is around 15% and for copropraxia around 5% as per the Tourette Syndrome International Database Consortium (Freeman et al., 2000), relative to the 20–40% observed to have coprolalia in clinic populations, and the 2–4% typically found in community samples of TS families (see Robertson & Eapen, 2014). TS shows quite profound clinical heterogeneity; however, a discussion of this is beyond the scope of this brief chapter (see Robertson & Eapen, 2013; Robertson, 2014a for further detail).

Comorbidity

Familial studies have consistently shown that TS symptoms rarely occur in isolation (Freeman et al., 2000; Khalifa & Von Knorring, 2005); a recent study finding just 13% of a TS cohort (n=400) had only tics while the rest showed evidence of associated comorbidities and psychopathologies (Eapen & Robertson, 2015). In terms of the clinical course, the typical pattern is a reduction in severity of the tic symptoms, and a persistence and increased interference of comorbidities with age (Robertson, 2015b). The comorbidities can be at least partly explained by genetic commonalities between TS and other neurobehavioural disorders, such that an individual is predisposed to a range of atypical behaviours and comorbidities, particularly those of obsessive-compulsive disorder (OCD) with a prevalence of 30–50% (Storch et al., 2007); and ADHD, with reported prevalence rates of 35–90% (Roessner et al., 2007); and to a lesser extent, autism spectrum disorders (ASD), with a reported rate of 13% (Eapen, McPherson, Sneddon, & Črnčec, 2013), with gender seemingly playing a modifying role (Hirschtritt et al., 2015; Robertson, 2015a, 2015b).

Other associated behaviours and psychopathologies seen in TS children at a higher rate than the general population include sleep disturbances, anxiety, depression, personality disorders, self-injurious behaviour, aggression, and conduct and oppositional defiant behaviours (Robertson, 2015b; Robertson, Cavanna, & Eapen, 2014). Although the neurobiology of TS may predispose individuals to additional psychopathology, there is speculation around whether some psychopathological symptoms are secondary to living with a socially-isolating condition (e.g. depression, anxiety), comorbid ADHD (e.g. the mood and anxiety) and/or OCD (e.g. the self-injurious behaviour) (Robertson, 2015b).

The strongest evidence of comorbidity with TS is that of obsessive-compulsive behaviours and symptoms (see above for prevalence estimates). Behaviourally, TS and OCD have features in common, especially the repetitive/obsessional quality and the behavioural disinhibition (Hollander & Stein, 1997), and they have even been considered by some as different phenotypic expressions of a common gene (Eapen, Pauls, & Robertson, 1993; Robertson, 2015b). In addition, the premonitory urge that is relieved by the performance of the tic in TS is often compared to the heightened anxiety that accompanies an urge to perform a compulsion in OCD. There is also evidence of phenomenological differences of obsessional features for those with TS and those with OCD that can likely be explained by differential neuropathology of frontostriatal circuitry (Robertson & Eapen 2013; Robertson, 2015b).

Genome-wide Complex Trait Analysis (GCTA), providing a means to more objectively quantify the genetic correlation between phenotypically related conditions, recently revealed a genetic correlation of 0.41 (se=0.15, p=0.002) between TS and OCD; remarkably close to the heritability estimates originating from historical twin and family study data (Davis et al., 2013). Despite strong evidence of shared genetic variation for TS and OCD, recent results have highlighted the complexity of the genetic relationship between TS and OCD with evidence for genetic heterogeneity. Obsessive Compulsive Behaviours (OCB) have been suggested to be an alternate phenotypic expression of the putative TS gene(s) in a subgroup with a gender dependent difference in the expression, with males presenting more with tics and females with OCB (Eapen et al., 1993). Indeed, there is some evidence that the OCD subtype that presents with tics is behaviourally distinct with a characteristic constellation of obsessions, such as intrusive images and sounds and compulsive touching, ordering and arranging, concern for symmetry, "evening up" behaviours, "just right" compulsions, tapping, staring, etc (Eapen et al., 1997; Robertson, 2015b). In addition, there is evidence that OCD may be heterogeneous with some families predisposed to OCD without tics and others to another subtype with tics, as originally put forward by Pauls et al. (1986) (Eapen & Robertson, 2015; Yu et al., 2015).

The evidence for a genetic association between TS and ADHD (see above for prevalence estimates) is equally complex, with a subgroup suggested to be genetically associated with tics and TS (Robertson, 2015b). In this regard, a recent study observed that some comorbidities may be more biologically related to OCD and/or ADHD rather than to TS with genetic correlations between TS and mood, anxiety, and disruptive behaviour disorders accounted for by ADHD and, for mood disorders, by OCD (Hirschtritt et al., 2015), which is consistent with the multistrike model of genetic heritability (see Eapen & Robertson, 2015).

Diagnostic instruments and clinical rating scales

Some of the commonly used measures for tics and related symptoms such as premonitory urge, and health-related quality of life specific to tics, are briefly described below.

The National Hospital Interview Schedule for the assessment of tics and related behaviours (NHIS) (Robertson & Eapen, 1996). This semi-structured clinical interview schedule provides an overview of demographic information as well as an assessment of TS symptoms, comorbid symptoms and diagnoses, medication history and family history information. The psychometric properties have been previously established with good inter-rater reliability and concurrent validity against the Yale Global Tic Severity Scale and DSM criteria (Robertson & Eapen, 1996). A briefer version of NHIS, The Tic Screening Questionnaire, is also available for initial screening.

The Diagnostic Confidence Index (DCI) (Robertson et al., 1999) provides a measure of whether an individual is likely to have met diagnostic criteria for TS in the past or currently.

The Yale Global Tic Severity Rating Scale (YGTSS) (Leckman et al., 1989) is a semi-structured clinician rated scale assessing tic severity based on the presence of tics in the previous week across the following dimensions: number, frequency, intensity, complexity and interference, with a separate impairment rating assessing tic-related disability.

The Parent Tic Questionnaire (PTQ) is a parent-reported assessment of the presence, frequency and intensity of tics in children (Chang, Himle, Tucker, Woods, & Piacentini, 2009) experienced in the past week, as well as a rating of tic frequency and intensity. Psychometrics demonstrate internal consistency, excellent test-retest reliability over 1–2 weeks and concurrent validity when compared to the YGTSS subscale (Woods, Piacenti, & Himle, 2007).

The Premonitory Urge Tics Scale (PUTS) assesses premonitory urges in young people with TS (Woods, Piacenti, Himle, & Chang, 2005).

Motor tic, obsessions and compulsions, vocal tic evaluation survey (MOVES) scale (Gaffney, Sieg, & Hellings, 1994) is a self-rated assessment of motor and vocal tics as well as obsessions and compulsions.

The Gilles de la Tourette Syndrome-Quality of Life Scale (GTS-QoL: Cavanna et al., 2008) assesses health-related quality of life in young patients with Tourette syndrome, across four subscales (psychological, physical, obsessional and cognitive). It has demonstrated satisfactory scaling assumptions and acceptability, as well as internal consistency, reliability and test-retest reliability and sound validity.

The assessment of comorbid conditions requires tools specific to the respective conditions and is beyond the scope of this chapter.

Clinical vignette

John is a 15 year old adolescent male who was diagnosed with Autism Spectrum Disorder (ASD) and ADHD at the age of 4 years, also noted to have severe expressive and receptive language delay. In terms of his developmental history, there was no particular complication during pregnancy or birth. His developmental milestones, including fine motor and language development, were noticeably delayed, but his gross motor function was adequate. John's recent school reports indicate that he had been performing well below the level of his peers. Currently, he also shows symptoms of anxiety largely associated with poor coping with his workload at school, difficulties with concentration, social interaction and being bullied at school. On examination, he was found to have blinking and facial tics and on further detailed interviewing, it became evident that he has had a number of motor tics as well as vocal tics which have been present at least from the age of 5 years. History also suggested that the tics changed from one site to another with one tic being replaced by a new tic, following a waxing and waning course. He also acknowledged a premonitory urge in the form of a "tingling" sensation just prior to the occurrence of the tic with relief of the sensation when he performs the tic. He reported a number of tic related obsessive compulsive behaviours, such as concern for symmetry and "evening up", having to do things "just right" and forced touching, etc. as well as non-obscene socially inappropriate (NOSI) behaviours and remarks. Given the presence of multiple motor tics and one or more vocal tics that have been present for more than a year, a diagnosis of Tourette Syndrome was made.

Family history further indicated a mixed presentation of psychiatric disorders both on the paternal and maternal sides. The presence of Tourette Syndrome, ASD, ADHD/ADD and OCD were particularly evident within the first and second-degree relatives. It is noteworthy that sixteen out of the thirty-eight biological relatives spanning three generations were found to have been previously diagnosed to have ASD, ADHD and OCD. Moreover, upon further assessment after John's diagnosis, it was revealed that his father, paternal uncle and paternal grandfather had multiple motor and vocal tics that remained undiagnosed until his assessment.

This case illustrates that tics are often missed, especially when the patient presents with more significant comorbid conditions such as ASD, as in this case. In the case of John, it became apparent that some of the difficulties experienced at school were due to NOSI behaviours, and he was also being bullied for "pulling faces", often being called a "monkey face". Appropriate psychoeducation of family and the school community as well as the use of clonidine for tics and ADHD resulted in significant overall improvement and quality of life for the patient.

Genetics and epigenetics

The heritability of TS is genetically complex; even with the recent advances in genetic technologies we still have much to learn. Complicating things further are environmental factors that have been shown to influence the expression of TS, including prenatal and perinatal influences, with factors such as intrauterine problems, low birthweight, maternal life stress during pregnancy, severe nausea, vomiting during the first trimester, maternal smoking, infections, etc. (Leckman et al., 1990) being implicated (see Robertson, 2015a for review). In particular, beta-haemolytic streptococcal infection resulting in Paediatric Autoimmune Neuropsychiatric Disorder Associated with Streptococcal infection (PANDAS) characterised by tics, obsessive compulsive behaviours and ADHD has been described, however, it has also been suggested that Tourette syndrome and PANDAS are different entities and instead that infection may serve as a trigger in predisposed individuals (Eapen & Robertson, 2015; Robertson, 2015a).

Twin and family studies have repeatedly demonstrated that TS has one of the highest familial recurrence rates of neuropsychiatric conditions with complex inheritance; monozygotic twin concordance is around 50–70%, and first degree relatives of those affected have a 5 to 15-fold increased risk (O'Rourke, Scharf, Yu, & Pauls, 2009; Scharf et al., 2013). Linkage analysis and candidate gene studies have produced inconsistent results, with no candidate genes consistently replicated (O'Rourke et al., 2009), though evidence points toward complex, polygenic heritability with environmental influences. In this regard, a number of neurodevelopmental genes have been implicated and a pathogenetic model involving the neurexin family of genes and Neurexin Transynaptic Connexus has been proposed (Clarke, Lee, & Eapen, 2012). Prior to the emergence of new technologies that have recently advanced the discipline of genetics, at least one major TS locus was identified on chromosome 2p in a study involving multigenerational families with affected sibling pairs (Tourette Syndrome Association International Consortium for Genetics, 2007).

Recent significant advances have allowed the identification of genes of small effect for a variety of heritable neuropsychiatric conditions such as TS through Genome Wide Association Studies (GWAS). The very first GWAS of TS reported a sample size of 1285 TS cases and 4964 ancestry-matched controls of European ancestry, including two population isolates. While no marker attained genome-wide significance (Scharf et al., 2013), the authors acknowledge that this is not all that surprising given the modest cohort size. Follow-up analyses examining TS genetic architecture, however, confirmed past findings that the majority of TS heritability is driven by GWAS single-nucleotide polymorphisms (SNPs) with allele frequencies >5% (Davis et al., 2013). Findings also provided evidence of a significant contribution to the genomic architecture of TS (and not OCD) from rare variants (Davis et al., 2013; Paschou et al., 2014). Further examination of the

42 top variants of interest from the initial GWAS suggested that many of these variants are likely to be true TS susceptibility alleles (Paschou et al., 2014).

Overview neuropsychology of Tourette syndrome

Neuropsychological deficits in attention, orienting and vigilance (Georgiou, Bradshaw, J.L. Phillips, Bradshaw J.A., & Chiu, 1995; Georgiou, Bradshaw, & Phillips, 1998), fine motor coordination (e.g. poor handwriting), visuomotor integration abilities (Brookshire, Butler, Ewing-Cobbs, & Fletcher, 1994) and interference control have been reported in individuals with TS. Conversely, intact executive functioning abilities have also been observed, as well as average or above average performance on cognitive measures of intellectual functioning (Yeates & Bornstein, 1994). Several studies have also demonstrated intact interference control using Stroop and Flanker tasks in adults with TS (Channon et al., 2006; Drury et al., 2011). It appears that when neuropsychological impairments have been reported, these are most often associated with comorbid psychopathologies (e.g. ADHD), suggesting that functionally significant neuropsychological impairments exist largely in individuals with TS with comorbid disorders. Future research is needed to understand the neuropsychological differences of TS-only versus comorbid subgroups.

Overview neuropathology/neurochemistry

Abnormalities within the cortico-striato-thalamo-cortical circuits and a range of neurotransmitter systems (dopamine, serotonin, opiates) have been proposed to underlie the subtle neuropsychological symptoms (e.g. reward learning, difficulties with impulse control and response inhibition) reported in TS. In particular, reduced caudate volume and cortical thinning in the frontal, parietal, sensorimotor and orbitofrontal cortex have been consistently reported. Emerging evidence also suggests that the cerebellum may also be implicated through its converging connections to the thalamus. Based on the administration of dopaminergic antagonists (such as fluphenazine, pimozide, haloperidol, risperidone and aripiprazole) shown to suppress motor and vocal tics, a preponderance of evidence supports the involvement of dopamine in TS. Specifically, supersensitive dopamine receptors, dopamine hyperinnervation, abnormal presynaptic terminal function, or excess dopamine release at the level of the striatum or cortex have been proposed, although no consistent linkage or association to candidate genes have been reported (O'Rourke et al., 2009). Multiple animal models that focus on pharmacological manipulations of single aspects of TS (e.g. motor tics, genetic mutations, comorbid symptoms) have also been developed, however exploration of these models is beyond the scope of this chapter. For a detailed review please see Bronfeld, Israelashvili, & Bar-Gad (2013).

Neurophysiological data from a range of non-invasive imaging techniques (functional magnetic resonance imaging [fMRI], positron emitting tomography

[PET], electroencephalogram [EEG], magnetoencephalogram [MEG], and transcranial magnetic stimulation [TMS]) support abnormal brain activity preceding tics in limbic circuits such as the anterior cingulate (ACC) and insular cortices, followed by activation of the sensorimotor areas with the tic onset (Bohlhalter et al., 2006). Abnormal baseline neuronal activity (Peterson et al., 1998; Worbe et al., 2012) in motor/basal ganglia pathways, correlating with tic severity, has also been consistently reported (Baym, Corbett, Wright, & Bunge, 2008; Peterson et al., 1998; Wang et al., 2011). Deep Brain Stimulation (DBS), a technique used to treat other movement disorders such as Parkinson's disease, has been used to treat severe, treatment-resistant cases of TS (with over 100 DBS surgeries reported worldwide). In particular, DBS has been applied to different regions of the motor and limbic brain circuitry, primarily the globus pallidus internus, nucleus accumbens and thalamic nuclei and has shown some success in alleviating symptoms (for a detailed review see Schrock et al., 2015).

Evolutionary/adaptive aspects

In line with the 'selfish gene' hypothesis (Dawkins, 1978), there may be some evolutionary advantages conveyed by particular genes so that they remain in the gene pool; that is, the genes that are passed on are the ones whose consequences serve their own interest in being replicated. There are several disorders of the frontostriatal system including Tourette syndrome, all of which possess a heritable component (Bradshaw & Sheppard, 2000). Their persistence in the genome likely indicates that their clinical manifestations may be associated with some form of adaptive advantage. Leckman and Cohen (1999) were amongst the first to propose that it may actually be advantageous to have a genetic vulnerability to develop TS (or OCD).

Deficient motor inhibition is one of the main pathophysiological explanations of the tics of TS (Neuner et al., 2012); thus, logically, the underlying neuropathology may also affect voluntary movements. Indeed, there are many reported case studies and reports of individuals with TS who reach highly competitive levels in sports that benefit from fast reaction times (basketball, goal-keeping in soccer, baseball, etc.), and display disinhibited, brilliant creativity and improvisation in dance and music.

Experimentally, there have also been several reports of superior motor and cognitive performance of Tourette compared to control groups (Georgiou, Bradshaw, Phillips, Cunnington, & Rogers, 1997; Mueller, Jackson, Dhalla, Datsopoulos, & Hollis, 2006; Vicario et al., 2010). The somewhat paradoxical finding that cognitive control may be enhanced in individuals with TS relative to controls has recently been reported using different paradigms (Mueller et al., 2006; Vicario et al., 2010). Combined with recent confirmatory neuroimaging results (Jung, Jackson, Parkinson, & Jackson, 2013), these findings support the contention that more efficient cognitive control in the motor domain may arise in a compensatory fashion as a result of the need to suppress tics in certain contexts (Jung et al., 2013; Vicario et al., 2010).

The neuropathological and neurochemical uniqueness of the brains of those with TS result in both the classic symptoms of TS as well as a predisposition to adaptive advantages, such as those highlighted above. The writings of patients with TS, such as Dr Lance Turtle, a UK physician (Turtle & Robertson, 2008), provide further anecdotal evidence of how these individuals perceive TS to be part of their persona; some refusing to take medication in certain contexts so as not to suppress their brilliance in sport, music or dance.

Treatment, including psychopharmacology

With regards to the use of pharmacological agents in the management of TS, Seignot (1961) was the first to describe the beneficial effects of haloperidol. While pharmacological intervention is beneficial for moderate to severe cases, for mild cases the first strategy following a diagnosis of Tourette Syndrome involves psycho-education, including explanation of the condition and available support to the patient, the family and school/workplace, etc. as appropriate. Psychological interventions found to be beneficial in TS include Habit Reversal Therapy (HRT) as well as the Comprehensive Behavioural Intervention for Tics (CBIT) (see McGuire et al., 2014). Pharmacological intervention (see Roessner & Rothenberger, 2013) is usually recommended based on a balance between what is evidence based or empirical, versus what is rational, realistic and feasible. Commonly used medications for tics other than haloperidol include antipsychotics such as pimozide (no longer used due to the cardiac side effects), risperidone, and aripiprazole. When there are co-existent tics and ADHD, noradrenergic agents such as clonidine or guanfacine (depending on availability) are used. Other less commonly used agents include topiramate, pergolide, and tetrabenazine. Other novel agents that are being trialled include selective dopamine D1 receptor antagonists and antihistaminergics. Some studies have suggested that cannabinoids may have a beneficial effect on reducing tics (Muller-Vahl, 2009) but a Cochrane review concluded that there was not sufficient evidence (Curtis, Clarke, & Rickards, 2009). Other medications used in the context of TS include Atomoxetine or stimulants for ADHD and SSRIs for OCD symptoms. It has been suggested that the site and extent of the involvement of the cortico–striatal–thalamo-cortical circuitry determine the type and severity of clinical features with a number of distinct, yet overlapping neuronal circuitry and neurotransmitters being implicated in TS (Robertson & Eapen, 2013). For example, striatal/basal ganglia area and dopamine pathways may be primarily involved in tics, the frontal cortical end of the circuitry may result in more socially inappropriate behaviours, while the dorsolateral prefrontal cortex, with both dopamine and norepinephrine, involved in ADHD. Similarly, the presence of other comorbidities such as OCD may suggest additional circuitry being involved including the basal ganglia–limbic circuitry with both serotoninergic and dopaminergic systems being involved. Thus, the management of Tourette Syndrome would need to take into account not only the tics but also associated comorbidities. In this regard, when tics and ADHD are present, the first line pharmacological agent of choice may be clonidine (Pringsheim & Steeves, 2011). In the case of tics and OCB/OCD, augmentation with a dopamine blocking agent may be needed in addition to treatment with SSRI. And in patients where tics co-occur with ASD symptoms and behavioural problems, risperidone may be a preferred first line agent.

Some of the commonly encountered co-existent psychopathology that would benefit from pharmacological treatment in its own right (independent of the treatment of tics) includes depression, anxiety (GAD, separation anxiety - sometimes secondary to treatment e.g. use of haloperidol), rage attacks and other extreme impulse dyscontrol. Other co-existent psychopathology that does not easily lend itself to pharmacological intervention includes Personality Disorder, Learning Disorder, Conduct Disorder, etc. Other treatment methods include local intramuscular injections of botulinum toxin, especially for vocal tics, and the use of Deep Brain Stimulation in refractory and severe cases (Schrock et al., 2015).

Summary

With the prevalence rate of around 1% in school aged children, Tourette syndrome is no longer considered to be rare or a bizarre curiosity. Further, there is debate as to whether it is a unitary condition but rather a Tic Spectrum Disorder with at least two subtypes identified as "Pure TS" with only tic symptoms, and "TS-Plus" with associated comorbidities and co-existent psychopathologies. With recent advances, we are one large step closer to the discovery of common TS susceptibility variants. The results of the first TS GWAS study and follow-up analyses highlight the genetic complexity of TS, and provide an essential foundation for next generation genome sequencing with additional samples that should see the identification of larger effect genes or rare gene variants, and the definitive identification of TS susceptibility genes. Clinical heterogeneity is linked to genetic heterogeneity and vice versa, and future research is indicated to delineate the aetiopathogenesis that leads to the development of different phenotypes that will need to incorporate genetics, neuroimmunology, neuroimaging, neurophysiology, neurochemistry and neuropathology, including post-mortem investigations, as well as epigenetic and environmental influences. Longitudinal studies involving detailed characterisation of phenotypes and associated features and comorbid conditions are also indicated to further understand the course, treatment response and outcomes.

Abbreviations

ACC: Anterior Cingulate Cortex
ADHD: Attention Deficit Hyperactivity Disorder
ASD: Autism Spectrum Disorders
CBIT: Comprehensive Behavioural Intervention for Tics
DBS: Deep Brain Stimulation
DCI: Diagnostic Confidence Index
DSM-1: Diagnostic and Statistical Manual of Mental Disorders – First edition
DSM-5: Diagnostic and Statistical Manual of Mental Disorders – Fifth edition
EEG: Electroencephalogram
fMRI: functional Magnetic Resonance Imaging
GAD: Generalised anxiety disorder
GCTA: Genome-wide complex train analysis
GTS-QoL: Gilles de la Tourette Syndrome – Quality of Life Scale
GWAS: Genome Wide Association Studies
HRT: Habit Reversal therapy
ICD-10: International Classifications of Disorders – 10th edition
MEG: Magnetoencephalogram
MOVES: Motor tic, obsessions and compulsions, vocal tic evaluation survey
NHIS: The National Hospital Interview Schedule for the assessment of tics and related behaviours
NOSI: non-obscene socially inappropriate behaviours
OCB: Obsessive Compulsive Behaviours
OCD: Obsessive Compulsive Disorder
PANDAS: Paediatric Autoimmune Neuropsychiatric Disorder Associated with Streptococcal infection
PTQ: Parent Tic Questionnaire
PET: Positron emitting tomography
PUTS: The Premonitory Urge Tics Scale
SSRI: Selective serotonin reuptake inhibitor
TMS: Transcranial magnetic stimulation
TS: Tourette's Syndrome
YGTSS: Yale Global Tic Severity Rating Scale

Further readings

Bradshaw, J. L., & Sheppard, D. M. (2000). The neurodevelopmental frontostriatal disorders: Evolutionary adaptiveness and anomalous lateralization. *Brain Language, 73*(2), 297–320. doi: 10.1006/brln.2000.2308.

Bronfeld, M., Israellashvili, M., & Bar-Gad, I. (2013). Pharmacological animal models of Tourette syndrome. *Neuroscience and Biobehavioural Reviews, 37*, 1101–1119.

Cavanna, A. E., & Rickards, H. (2013). The psychopathological spectrum of Gilles de la Tourette syndrome. *Neuroscience and Biobehavioural Reviews, 37*, 1008–1015.

Eapen, V., & Robertson, M. M. (2015). Are there distinct subtypes in Tourette syndrome? Pure-Tourette syndrome versus Tourette syndrome-plus, and simple versus complex tics. *Neuropsychiatric Disease and Treatment, 11*, 1431–1436. doi: 10.2147/NDT.S72284.

Ganos, C., Roessner, V., & Munchau, A. (2013). The functional anatomy of Gilles de la Tourette syndrome. *Neuroscience and Biobehavioural Reviews, 36*(6), 1050–1062.

Israelashvili, M., Loewenstern, Y., & Bar-Gad, I. (2015). Abnormal neuronal activity in Tourette syndrome and its modulation using deep brain stimulation. *Journal of Neurophysiology, 114*(1), 6–20.

Robertson, M. M. (2015a). A personal 35 year perspective on Gilles de la Tourette syndrome: Assessment, investigations, and management. *The Lancet Psychiatry, 2*(1), 88–104. doi: http://dx.doi.org/10.1016/S2215-0366(14)00133-3.

Robertson, M. M. (2015b). A personal 35 year perspective on Gilles de la Tourette syndrome: Prevalence, phenomenology, comorbidities, and coexistent psychopathologies. *The Lancet Psychiatry, 2*(1), 68–87. doi: http://dx.doi.org/10.1016/S2215-0366(14)00132-1.

Robertson, M. M., & Eapen, V. (2014). Tourette's: Syndrome, disorder or spectrum? Classificatory challenges and an appraisal of the DSM criteria. *Asian Journal of Psychiatry, 11*, 106–113.

Turtle, L., & Robertson, M. M. (2008). Tics, twitches, tales: The experiences of Gilles de la Tourette's syndrome. *American Journal of Orthopsychiatry, 78*(4), 449–455. doi: http://dx.doi.org/10.1037/a0014329.

References

American Psychiatric Association (APA). (2013). *Diagnostic and Statistical Manual of Mental Disorders (DSM-5)*. American Psychiatric Publishing.

Baron-Cohen, S., Scahill, V., Izaguirre, J., Hornsey, H., & Robertson, M. M. (1999). The prevalence of Gilles de la Tourette syndrome in children and adolescents with autism: A large scale study. *Psychological Medicine, 29*(5), 1151–1159.

Baym, C. L., Corbett, B.A., Wright, S. B., Bunge, S. A. (2008). Neural correlates of tic severity and cognitive control in children with Tourette syndrome. *Brain, 131*(pt 1), 165–179.

Bohlhalter, S., Goldfine, A., Matteson, S., Garraux, G., Hanakawa, T., Kansaku, K., Wurzman, R., & Hallett, M. (2006). Neural correlates of tic generation in Tourette syndrome: An event-related functional MRI study. *Brain, 129*(pt 8), 2029–2037.

Bradshaw, J. L., & Sheppard, D. M. (2000). The neurodevelopmental frontostriatal disorders: Evolutionary adaptiveness and anomalous lateralization. *Brain & Language, 73*(2), 297–320. doi: 10.1006/brln.2000.2308.

Bronfeld, M., Israelashvili, M., & Bar-Gad, I. (2013). Pharmacological animal models of Tourette syndrome. *Neuroscience & Biobehavioral Reviews, 37*(6), 1101–1119. doi: 10.1080/09297049.2011.613811.

Brookshire, B. L., Butler, I. J., Ewing-Cobbs, L., & Fletcher, J. (1994). Neuropsychological characteristics of children with Tourette syndrome: Evidence for a non-verbal learning disability. *Journal of Clinical and Experimental Neuropsychology, 16*(2), 289–302. doi: 10.1080/01688639408402639.

Cavanna, A. E. M., Schrag, A., Morley, D., Orth, M., Robertson, M. M., Joyce, E., Critchley, H. D., & Selai, C. (2008). The Gilles de la Tourette Syndrome-Quality of Life scale (GTS-QOL): Development and validation. *Neurology, 71*(18), 1410–1416. doi: 10.1212/01.wnl.0000327890.02893.61.

Chang, S., Himle, M. B., Tucker, B. T. P., Woods, D. W., & Piacentini, J. (2009). Initial psychometric properties of a brief parent-report instrument for assessing tic severity in children with Chronic Tic disorders. *Child & Family Behavior Therapy, 31*(3), 181–191.

Channon, S., Gunning, A., Frankl, J., & Robertson, M. M. (2006). Tourette's syndrome (TS): Cognitive performance in adults with uncomplicated TS. *Neuropsychology, 20*(1), 58.

Clarke, R. A., Lee, S., & Eapen, V. (2012). Pathogenetic model for Tourette syndrome delineates overlap with related neurodevelopmental disorders including autism. *Transl Psychiatry, 2*, e158. doi: 10.1038/tp.2012.75.

Curtis, A., Clarke, C. E., & Rickards, H. E. (2009). Cannabinoids for Tourette's syndrome. *Cochrane Database Systematic Reviews,* 7(4): CD006565. doi: 10.1002/14651858.CD006565.pub2.

Davis, L. K., Yu, D., Keenan, C. L., Gamazon, E. R., Konkashbaev, A. I., Derks, E. M., ... Scharf, J. M. (2013). Partitioning the heritability of Tourette syndrome and obsessive compulsive disorder reveals differences in genetic architecture. *PLoS Genetics, 9*(10), e1003864. doi: 1/journal.pgen.1003864.

Dawkins, R. (1978). *The Selfish Gene*. Oxford: Oxford University Press.

Drury, H., Channon, S., Barrett, R., Young, M. B., Stern, J. S., Simmons, H., & Crawford, S. (2011). Emotional processing and executive functioning in children and adults with Tourette's syndrome. *Child Neuropsychology, 18*(3), 281–298. doi: 10.1080/09297049.2011.613811.

Eapen, V., & Črnčec, R. (2009). Tourette syndrome in children and adolescents: Special considerations. *Journal of Psychosomatic Research, 67*(6), 525–532. doi: 10.1016/j.jpsychores.2009.08.003.

Eapen, V., & Robertson, M. M. (2015). Are there distinct subtypes in Tourette syndrome? Pure-Tourette syndrome versus Tourette syndrome-plus, and simple versus complex tics. *Neuropsychiatric Disease and Treatment, 11*, 1431–1436. doi: 10.2147/NDT.S72284.

Eapen, V., McPherson, S., Sneddon, C., & Črnčec, R. (2013). Tic disorders and learning disability: Clinical characteristics, cognitive performance and co-morbidity. *Australasian Journal of Special Education, 37*(4), 162–172.

Eapen, V., Pauls, D. L., & Robertson, M. M. (1993). Evidence for autosomal dominant transmission in Tourette's syndrome. United Kingdom cohort study. *The British Journal of Psychiatry, 162*(5), 593–596.

Eapen, V., Robertson, M. M., Zeitlin, H., & Kurlan, R. (1997). Gilles de la Tourette's syndrome in special education schools: A United Kingdom study. *Journal of Neurology, 244*(6), 378–382.

Freeman, R. D., Fast, D. K., Burd, L., Kerbeshian, J., Robertson, M. M., & Sandor, P. (2000). An international perspective on Tourette syndrome: Selected findings from 3500 individuals in 22 countries. *Developmental Medicine & Child Neurology, 42*(7), 436–447. doi: 10.1111/j.1469-8749.2000.tb00346.x.

Gaffney, G. R., Sieg, K., & Hellings, J. (1994). The MOVES: A self-rating scale for Tourette's syndrome. *Journal of Child and Adolescent Psychopharmacology*, 4(4), 269–280.

Georgiou, N., Bradshaw, J. L., Phillips, K. G., Bradshaw, J. A., & Chiu, E. (1995). The Simon effect and attention deficits in Gilles de la Tourette's syndrome and Huntington's disease. *Brain, 118*(5), 1305–1318.

Georgiou, N., Bradshaw, J., Phillips, J., Cunnington, R., & Rogers, M. (1997). Functional asymmetries in the movement kinematics of patients with Tourette's syndrome. *Journal of Neurology, Neurosurgery, and Psychiatry, 63*(2), 188–195.

Georgiou, N., Bradshaw, J. L., & Phillips, J. G. (1998). Directed attention in Gilles de la Tourette syndrome. *Behavioural Neurology, 11*(2), 85–91.

Hirschtritt, M. E., Lee, P. C., Pauls, D. L., Dion, Y., Grados, M. A., Illmann, C., King, R. A., Sandor, P., McMahon, W. M., Lyon, G. J.,Cath, D. C., Kurlan, R., Robertson, M. M., Osiecki, L., Scharf, J. M., & Mathews, C. A. (2015). Lifetime prevalence, age of risk, and genetic relationships of comorbid psychiatric disorders in tourette syndrome. *JAMA Psychiatry, 72*(4), 325–333. doi: 10.1001/jamapsychiatry.2014.2650.

Hollander, E., & Stein, D.J. (1997). *Obsessive Compulsive Disorders*. New York: Dekker.

Jung, J., Jackson, S. R., Parkinson, A., & Jackson, G. M. (2013). Cognitive control over motor output in Tourette syndrome. *Neuroscience & Biobehavioral Reviews, 37*(6), 1016–1025. doi: 10.1016/j.neubiorev.2012.08.009.

Khalifa, N., & Von Knorring, A. L. (2005). Tourette Syndrome and other tic disorders in a total population of children: Clinical assessment and background. *Acta Pædiatrica, 94*(11), 1608–1614. doi: 10.1111/j.1651-2227.2005.tb01837.x.

Knight, T., Steeves, T., Day, L., Lowerison, M., Jette, N., & Pringsheim, T. (2012). Prevalence of tic disorders: A systematic review and meta-analysis. *Pediatric Neurology, 47*(2), 77–90. doi: 10.1016/j.pediatrneurol.2012.05.002.

Kwak, C., Dat Vuong, K., & Jankovic, J. (2003). Premonitory sensory phenomenon in Tourette's syndrome. *Movement Disorders, 18*(12), 1530–1533. doi: 10.1002/mds.10618.

Leckman, J. F., & Cohen, D. J. (1999). Evolving models of pathogenesis. In J. F. Leckman & D. J. Cohen (Eds.), *Tourette's Syndrome-tics, Obsessions and Compulsions: Developmental Psychopathology and Clinical Care* (pp. 155–176). Hoboken, NJ: John Wiley & Sons Inc.

Leckman, J. F., Riddle, M. A., Hardin, M. T., Ort, S. I., Swartz, K. L., Stevenson, J. O. H. N., & Cohen, D. J. (1989). The Yale Global Tic Severity Scale: Initial testing of a clinician-rated scale of tic severity. *Journal of the American Academy of Child & Adolescent Psychiatry, 28*(4), 566–573.

McGuire, J. F., Piacentini, J., Brennan, E. A., Lewin, A. B., Murphy, T. K., Small, B. J., & Storch, E. A. (2014). A meta-analysis of behavior therapy for Tourette Syndrome. *Journal of Psychiatry Research, 50*: 106–112. doi: 10.1016/j.jpsychires.2013.12.009.

Mueller, S. C., Jackson, G. M., Dhalla, R., Datsopoulos, S., & Hollis, C. P. (2006). Enhanced cognitive control in young people with Tourette's syndrome. *Current Biology, 16*(6), 570–573. doi: 10.1016/j.cub.2006.01.064.

Müller-Vahl, K. R. (2009). Tourette's syndrome. In D. Kendall (Ed.), *Behavioral Neurobiology of the Endocannabinoid System*. (pp. 397–410). Berlin, Heidelberg: Springer.

Neuner, I., Arrubla, J., Ehlen, C., Janouschek, H., Nordt, C., Fimm, B., Schneider, F., Shah, N.J., Kawohl, W. (2012). Fine motor skills in adult Tourette patients are task-dependent. *BMC Neurology, 12*, 120. doi: 10.1186/1471-2377-12-120.

O'Rourke, J. A., Scharf, J. M., Yu, D., & Pauls, D. L. (2009). The genetics of Tourette syndrome: A review. *Journal of Psychosomatic Research, 67*(6), 533–545. doi: 10.1016/j.jpsychores.2009.06.006.

Paschou, P., Yu, D., Gerber, G., Evans, P., Tsetsos, F., Davis, L. K., … Scharf, J. M. (2014). Genetic association signal near NTN4 in Tourette syndrome. *Annals of Neurology, 76*(2), 310–315. doi: 10.1002/ana.24215.

Peterson, B. S., Skudlarski, P., Anderson, A. W., Zhang, H., Gatenby, J. C., Lacadie, C. M., Leckman, J. F., & Gore, J. C. (1998). A functional magnetic resonance imaging study of tic suppression in Tourette syndrome. *Archives of General Psychiatry, 55*(4), 326–333.

Peterson, B., Pine, D., Cohen, P., & Brook, J. (2001). Prospective, longitudinal study of tic, obsessive-compulsive, and attention-deficit/hyperactivity disorders in an epidemiological sample. *Journal of the American Academy of Child & Adolescent Psychiatry, 40*(6), 685–695.

Peterson, B., Thomas, P., Kane, M., Scahill, L., Zhang, H., Bronen, R., King, R.A., Leckman, J. F., & Staib, L. (2003). Basal ganglia volumes in patients with Gilles de la Tourette syndrome. *Archives of General Psychiatry, 60*(4), 415–424.

Pringsheim, T., & Steeves, T. (2011). Pharmacological treatment for Attention Deficit Hyperactivity Disorder (ADHD) in children with comorbid tic disorders. *Cochrane Database Systematic Reviews, 13*(4), CD007990. doi: 10.1002/14651858.CD007990.pub2.

Robertson, M. M. (2015a). A personal 35 year perspective on Gilles de la Tourette syndrome: Assessment, investigations, and management. *The Lancet Psychiatry, 2*(1), 88–104. doi: 10.1016/S2215-0366(14)00133-3.

Robertson, M. M. (2015b). A personal 35 year perspective on Gilles de la Tourette syndrome: Prevalence, phenomenology, comorbidities, and coexistent psychopathologies. *The Lancet Psychiatry, 2*(1), 68–87. doi: http://dx.doi.org/10.1016/S2215-0366(14)00132-1.

Robertson, M. M., & Eapen, V. (1996). The National Hospital Interview Schedule for the assessment of Gilles de la Tourette syndrome and related behaviours. *International Journal of Method in Psychiatric Research, 6*(4), 203–226. doi: 10.1002/(SICI)1234-988X(199612)6:4<203::AID-MPR165>3.3.CO;2-F.

Robertson, M. M., & Eapen, V. (2013). Wither the relationship between etiology and phenotype in Tourette Syndrome? In D. Martino & J. F. Leckman (Eds.), *Tourette Syndrome* (pp. 361–394). New York: Oxford University Press Inc.

Robertson, M. M., & Eapen, V. (2014). Tourette's Syndrome, disorder or spectrum? Classificatory challenges and an appraisal of the DSM criteria. *Asian Journal of Psychiatry, 11*, 106–113.

Robertson, M. M., Cavanna, A. E., & Eapen, V. (2014). Gilles de la Tourette Syndrome and disruptive behavior disorders: Prevalence, associations, and explanation of the relationships. *Journal* of *Neuropsychiatry Clinical Neurosciences, 27*(1), 33–41. doi: 10.1176/appi.neuropsych.13050112.

Robertson, M. M., & Eapen, V. (2014a). Tourette's Syndrome, disorder or spectrum? Classificatory challenges and an appraisal of the DSM criteria. *Asian Journal of Psychiatry, 11*, 106–113. doi: 10.1016/j.ajp.2014.05.010.

Robertson, M. M., Cavanna, A. E., & Eapen, V. (2014b). Gilles de la Tourette Syndrome and disruptive behavior disorders: Prevalence, associations, and explanation of the relationships. *The Journal of Neuropsychiatry & Clinical Neurosciences, 27*(1): 33–41. doi: 10.1176/appi.neuropsych.13050112.

Roessner, V. & Rothenberger, A. (2013). Pharmacological treatment of tics. In D. Martino, & J. F. Leckman (Eds.), *Tourette Syndrome*. New York: Oxford University Press Inc.

Roessner, V., Becker, A., Banaschewski, T., Freeman, R. D., Rothenberger, A., & Tourette Syndrome International Database. (2007). Developmental psychopathology of children and adolescents with Tourette syndrome--impact of ADHD. *European Child & Adolescent Psychiatry, 16 Suppl 1*, 24–35. doi: 10.1007/s00787-007-1004-6.

Scharf, J. M., Yu, D., Mathews, C. A., Neale, B. M., Stewart, S. E., Fagerness, J.A., et al. (2013). Genome-wide association study of Tourette's syndrome. *Molecular Psychiatry, 18*(6), 721–728. doi: 10.1038/mp.2012.69.

Schrock, L.E., Mink, J.W., Woods, D.W., Porta, M., Servello, D., Visser-Vandewalle, V., … Tourette Syndrome Association International Deep Brain Stimulation (DBS) Database and Registry Study Group. (2015). Tourette syndrome deep brain stimulation: A review and updated recommendations. *Movement Disorders, 30*(4), 448–471. doi: 10.1002/mds.26094.

Singer, H. S., & Walkup, J. T. (1991). Tourette syndrome and other tic disorders. Diagnosis, pathophysiology, and treatment. *Medicine, 70*(1), 15–32.

Storch, E. A., Merlo, L. J., Lack, C., Milsom, V. A., Geffken, G. R., Goodman, W. K., & Murphy, T.K. (2007). Quality of life in youth with Tourette's syndrome and chronic tic disorder. *Journal of Clinical Child and Adolescent Psychology, 36*, 217–227.

Tourette Syndrome Association International Consortium for Genetics. (2007). Genome scan for Tourette disorder in affected-sibling-pair and multigenerational families. *American Journal of Human Genetics, 80*(2), 265–272. doi: 10.1086/511052.

Turtle, L., & Robertson, M. M. (2008). Tics, twitches, tales: The experiences of Gilles de la Tourette's syndrome. *American Journal of Orthopsychiatry, 78*(4), 449–455. doi: 10.1037/a0014329.

Vicario, C. M., Martino, D., Spata, F., Defazio, G., Giacche, R., Martino, V., Rappo, G., Silvestri, P. R., & Cardona, F. (2010). Time processing in children with Tourette's syndrome. *Brain and Cognition, 73*(1), 28–34. doi: 10.1016/j.bandc.2010.01.008.

Wang, Z., Maia, T.V., Marsh, R., Colibazzi, T., Gerber, A., & Peterson, B. S. (2011). The neural circuits that generate tics in Tourette's syndrome. *American Journal of Psychiatry, 168*(12), 1326–1337. doi: 10.1176/appi.ajp.2011.09111692.

Woods, D. W., Piacentini, J. C., & Himle, M. B. (2007). Assessment of tic disorders. In D. W. Woods, J. C. Piacentini, J. T. Walkup (Eds). *Treating Tourette Syndrome and Tic Disorders: A Guide for Practitioners* (pp. 21–37). New York: Guilford Press.

Woods, D. W., Piacentini, J., Himle, M. B., & Chang, S. (2005). Premonitory Urge for Tics Scale (PUTS): Initial psychometric results and examination of the premonitory urge phenomenon in youths with tic disorders. *Journal of Developmental & Behavioral Pediatrics, 26*(6), 397–403.

Worbe, Y., Malherbe, C., Hartmann, A., Pélégrini-Issac, M., Messé, A., Vidailhet, M., Lehéricy, S., & Benali, H. (2012). Functional immaturity of cortico-basal ganglia networks in Gilles de la Tourette syndrome. *Brain, 135*(pt 6), 1937–1946. doi: 10.1093/brain/aws056.

World Health Organization. (1992). *The ICD-10 Classification of Mental and Behavioural Disorders: Clinical Descriptions and Diagnostic Guidelines*. Geneva: World Health Organization.

Yeates, K. O., & Bornstein, R. A. (1994). Attention deficit disorder and neuropsychological functioning in children with Tourette's syndrome. *Neuropsychology, 8*(1), 65–75. doi: 10.1037/0894-4105.8.1.65.

Yu, D., Mathews, C. A., Scharf, J. M., Neale, B. M., Davis, L. K., Gamazon, E. R., Derks, E. M., ... Pauls, D. L. (2015). Cross-disorder genome-wide analyses suggest a complex genetic relationship between Tourette's syndrome and OCD. *The American Journal of Psychiatry, 172*(1), 82–93. doi: 10.1176/appi.ajp.2014.13101306.

13
ADDICTION

Jodie Naim-Feil, Shalini Arunogiri, Primavera A. Spagnolo and Dan I. Lubman

General introduction

Drug dependence is a chronically relapsing disorder that is associated with significant costs to the individual, their family and society at large. While it is the physical aspects of dependence that bring many people into treatment (i.e. for management of physical withdrawal symptoms), it is the psychological component of dependence (i.e. addiction) that is more long-lasting and associated with subsequent relapse. Addiction can be characterized as a persistent state in which there is a diminished ability to regulate the compulsive desire to consume drugs, often regardless of potential adverse consequences. In this chapter, we shall describe the diagnostic criteria and main clinical features of dependence, including its prevalence, harms and associated comorbidities, as well as the underlying genetics. We shall also briefly outline the neurobiology of addiction, and discuss the involvement of frontostriatal circuitry in the persistence of drug-seeking behaviours. This will be followed by a review of neuropsychological, neuroimaging and brain stimulation studies of cognitive inhibitory deficits and alterations of the frontostriatal circuitry across specific substance-dependent populations (cocaine, nicotine and alcohol). We will then conclude the chapter by examining current treatment models.

Preliminary considerations

With regards to the definition of dependence, the World Health Organization (WHO) introduced 'drug dependence' as a description to encompass both *physiological* dependence (i.e. the presence of tolerance and withdrawal symptoms upon cessation of drug use) and *psychological* dependence (characterized by intense craving, loss of control of drug seeking behaviours and compulsive patterns of drug use). Modern diagnostic criteria for substance dependence (such as ICD-10 and DSM-5) continue to delineate between physiological and psychological symptoms, though both types of symptoms are not necessary for a diagnosis of substance dependence. In this chapter, the terms 'dependence' and 'addiction' will be used interchangeably to describe the persistent state in which there is a diminished ability to regulate the compulsive desire to consume drugs, regardless of adverse consequences. The term 'drug' will be used to include all psychoactive substances which have addictive properties.

Clinical symptoms

According to the American Psychiatric Association's DSM-5, a substance use disorder is identified by meeting at least two of the following criteria over a 12 month period. In this diagnostic system, the presence of a greater number of criteria indicates a higher level of severity of the disorder (American Psychiatric Association, 2013) (see Figure 13.1).

Psychological dependence

- Substance is often consumed in larger amounts or over longer periods than intended
- Unsuccessful attempts and/or persistent desire to reduce drug use
- Increased time seeking, using or recovering from substance use
- Presence of cravings and strong desire to engage in substance use
- Failure fulfilling major obligations (work/school/home) due to substance use
- Continued substance use despite interpersonal or social problems exacerbated by drug use
- Discontinuation of social, occupational or recreational activities due to substance use
- Recurrent substance use in physically hazardous situations
- Continued substance use despite awareness of physical or psychological problems caused or exacerbated by the substance

Physiological dependence

- Tolerance: Requiring increased amounts of substance to achieve intoxication or with continued use the same amount of substance produces a markedly reduced effect
- Withdrawal: The presence of withdrawal syndrome for the substance, or the substance is continued to relieve/avoid withdrawal symptoms

FIGURE 13.1 Diagnostic criteria for substance use disorders according to the DSM 5.

Likewise, the International Classification of Diseases and Health Problems (World Health Organization, 1992) has similar diagnostic criteria. Both of these diagnostic systems highlight the transition to dependence associated with the compulsive use of a substance and the increased salience of drug use, despite awareness of the negative consequences. A range of validated rating scales and screening instruments assist clinicians in the diagnosis of substance dependence. These include self-rating scales, such as the Severity of Dependence Scale (Gossop et al., 1995), Alcohol Use Disorders Identification Test (AUDIT) (Babor et al., 1992) and Drug Use Disorders Identification Test (DUDIT) (Berman et al., 2005); and clinician-administered scales Addiction Severity Index (ASI) (McLellan et al., 1980), World Mental Health Composite International Diagnostic Interview (WMH-CIDI) (World Health Organization, 1990), and Structured Clinical Interview for DSM-IV (SCID) (First et al., 2002).

Prevalence

Substance dependence remains one of the most globally-challenging and costly health, social and economic problems. For example, according to the 2013 National Survey on Drug Use and Health (NSDUH), in the United States alone, an estimated 21.6 million people aged 12 and older were diagnosed with a substance use disorder (Substance Abuse and Mental Health Services Administration, 2013). A national epidemiological survey of a representative sample of U.S. adults (n = 43,093) found the lifetime prevalence of alcohol dependence was 12.5%, and was more prevalent among men and associated with considerable disability. Of those diagnosed with alcohol dependence, only 24.1% received treatment. Significant associations between alcohol dependence, polysubstance use and comorbid psychiatric disorders (such as mood and anxiety disorders) were also reported (Hasin et al., 2007). Although rates of prevalence differ between drug groups, the rates of morbidity and mortality remain high across all of the various drug groups, including tobacco (Breslau et al., 2001), cannabis (Degenhardt et al., 2013), opioid use (Degenhardt et al., 2014), and psychostimulant drugs (UNODC, 2015). In addition, the use of multiple substances at the same time (i.e. polysubstance use) is a common feature of substance dependence and is associated with increased health risks and poor treatment outcomes (Brecht et al., 2008).

Psychiatric comorbidity

Substance use disorders also commonly co-occur with other psychiatric disorders, with nearly one in three individuals with past 12-month substance dependence meeting criteria for a comorbid mood disorder, and up to a quarter reporting an anxiety disorder (Grant et al., 2004). There are a number of aetiological pathways that may underpin this high rate of comorbidity. Neurochemical changes associated with substance intoxication and withdrawal can result in a range of psychiatric symptoms (e.g. anxiety, depression, mood swings, psychosis), and the development of a substance-induced disorder. In contrast, some individuals may use substance as a means of coping with symptoms of a mental health disorder (such as dysphoria, sleep disturbance, etc.). If the symptoms of mental illness continue to go untreated, they can perpetuate and amplify drug-seeking behaviours, resulting in the development of substance dependence. Alternatively, a common aetiological factor may predispose an individual to develop both substance dependence and a psychiatric disorder, such as early childhood trauma, which leads to increased risk of both a substance use disorder and a range of psychiatric issues (Brady and Sinha, 2005). Regardless of the aetiological pathway, when individuals present with comorbid issues, it can often be challenging for clinicians to ascertain whether the psychiatric disorder is primary or substance-induced, especially if there is ongoing substance use. A period of abstinence can be crucial to understanding the relationship between the two disorders, and to make a clear diagnosis. However, this approach can be challenging when drug use is ongoing or there is limited access to detoxification support.

Long-term estimates of recovery are difficult to establish due to diagnostic challenges, the episodic nature of the illness, and a protracted time-course of recovery. Recent epidemiological studies suggest that approximately 58% of substance-dependent individuals achieve sustained recovery (Sheedy and Whitter, 2009), and while these estimates may not refer to full remission, they refer to individuals transcending their symptoms and contributing to society. This is supported by an increasing number of studies which highlight the role of psychological, environmental and social factors that promote resilience and recovery (Best and Lubman, 2012). This has been paralleled by growth in the understanding of the genetic and neurobiological underpinnings of addictive disorders and potential targets for pharmacological treatments, leading to a rejuvenated era of research and discovery in this field.

Clinical vignette

John, a 45-year-old man, presents to his general practitioner with problems sleeping. He says he is drinking between one to two bottles of wine every evening. He initially enjoyed having a drink with his wife at dinner, but his drinking has increased gradually over the past year as his workload has increased. Financial pressures requiring him to dismiss a number of employees caused him much stress. He now feels that he needs to drink every day to help him sleep and relax after his stressful work days. He also describes feeling nauseated, tremulous and unwell if he tries to stop drinking. John's wife suggested that he take a break from drinking alcohol as he is very irritable, neglecting his commitments of late and has cut ties with many of his friends. She claims that alcohol is always his answer to stressful situations.

John's doctor completes the alcohol use disorders identification test (AUDIT) with him and finds that John is drinking at a level indicative of alcohol dependence. His doctor also explores the links between John's alcohol use and his mental health, suggesting that he may be developing an alcohol-induced depressive disorder. The doctor recommends that John starts by treating his alcohol dependence and prescribes John a brief course of benzodiazepines (diazepam) to manage alcohol withdrawal, advising him on how to take this medication once he stops drinking. He also prescribes naltrexone to help manage cravings and reduce John's alcohol use. The doctor then refers John to a psychologist for counselling. The psychologist thoroughly assesses his alcohol use and its impact on his mental health. He explores John's family and developmental history: John experienced a childhood where alcohol use was common, his father being often angry and verbally aggressive when intoxicated. Using a 12-week cognitive-behavioural therapeutic approach, John's psychologist explores the relationship between his workplace stress and his drinking, relating this to his difficulties in managing conflict and confrontation.

After three months of therapy, John reduces his drinking dramatically and has a period of abstinence from alcohol. His sleep and depressive symptoms improve significantly and he can function better at his workplace. However, he experiences a relapse following an argument with his wife over their finances. He returns to his psychologist, reflects on the triggers for this relapse and works on developing skills to manage this relationship conflict. His psychologist recommends that he attends a support group such as Alcoholics Anonymous (AA) to help maintain sobriety and strengthen his social support. One year later, John is attending AA meetings regularly, occasionally meets with his psychologist, and maintains abstinence from alcohol. He has insight into situations which make him vulnerable to relapse and focuses on developing coping strategies to manage future situations.

Genetics and epigenetics of addiction

Evidence from family, adoption and twin studies converge on the relevance of genetic factors in the development of addiction (Heath et al., 1997; Tsuang et al., 1996). Twin studies indicate that genes influence each stage from initiation to dependence, although the genetic determinants may differ. In addition to genetic factors, other *intrinsic* factors (e.g. sex, age, age at first use, pre-existing addictive disorder, or other mental illness), together with *extrinsic* factors (e.g. drug availability, peer influences, social support, childhood adversity, parenting style, socioeconomic status), contribute to the initiation of use, and the progression from use to dependence (Goldman et al., 2005). Therefore, addiction is an etiologically complex condition that results from multiple genetic and environmental risk factors. The relative importance of these factors varies across the lifespan and at different stages of the addictive disorder. For example, a recent twin study demonstrated that in early adolescence, the initiation and use of nicotine, alcohol and cannabis was strongly determined by familial and social factors, but these gradually declined in importance during the progression to young and middle adulthood, when genetic factors become maximal (Kendler et al., 2008).

Heritability of addictive disorders varies across different drugs, ranging on the heritability index from 0.39 for hallucinogens to 0.72 for cocaine (Goldman et al., 2005). A number of genetic factors are also substance-specific, while others are shared between different substances (Goldman and Bergen, 1998). Substance-specific genes include genes for metabolic enzymes (ALDH2, ADH1B, CYP2D6) as well as genes encoding gatekeeper molecules such as drug receptors (e.g. CHRNA5, OPRM1). On the other hand, genes influencing diverse aspects of addiction neurobiology (anxiety, impulsivity and reward), including genes such as monoamine oxidase A (MAOA), the serotonin transporter (SLC6A4), and catechol-O-methyl transferase (COMT), have been implicated in the shared genetic liability between addiction and other psychiatric diseases. For example, initial experimentation with drugs or escalation to chronic use at a young age accompanies other behavioural indices of impulsivity (i.e. conduct problems), and thus genes influencing impulsivity will likely have a general effect on addiction (Agrawal et al., 2012). Based on these observations, a strategy designed to improve gene discovery in addiction is the study of *intermediate phenotypes*. Such phenotypes result from the deconstruction of phenotypes into elements that are aetiologically less complex and that present with shared genetic factors. For example, twin studies have demonstrated that a common factor encompassing externalizing disorders, such as antisocial personality disorder (ASPD) and conduct disorder (CD), accounted for 71% of the genetic liability to alcoholism and 67% of the inheritance of vulnerability to illicit drug abuse or dependence (Goldman et al., 2005).

Such an approach, together with genome-wide methods and candidate gene studies, has facilitated the identification of several genes involved in addictive disorders. However, several obstacles are still present. Firstly, addiction is a complex trait, characterized by a great degree of variance in behavioural manifestations, and this makes it difficult to detect the effect of a single gene. Secondly, gene hunting for disorders such as addiction was considered as a low priority as the development of addiction was traditionally conceived as an individual choice rather than a disease, and moreover, as a disease highly amenable to environmental modification (Merikangas and Risch, 2003). However, as neurobiological models of addiction progress, it is apparent that addiction results from both pre-alterations (vulnerability) and/or post-alterations (drug effects) in neuro-circuitry, such as the frontostriatal system (Kravitz et al., 2015). These models have the potential to enhance the identification of the genetic determinants of addiction, thus improving our ability to characterize vulnerable individuals, develop new treatments or tailor current treatment options. For example, geneticists can use an OPRM1 variant to predict treatment response to naltrexone in alcohol dependence, with carriers of the Asp40 allele more highly likely to show clinical improvement (Anton et al., 2008).

Similarly, CHRNA5Asn398Asp (Munafò et al., 2011) and DBH (Leventhal et al., 2014) has been reported to influence smoking cessation treatment.

Neurobiology of addiction

Acute drug exposure enhances dopaminergic neurotransmission within the mesocorticolimbic 'reward' circuitry (Melis et al., 2005). The reward circuitry consists of dopaminergic neurons originating from cell bodies in the ventral tegmental area (VTA) that project to limbic structures (i.e. the mesolimbic pathway) and cortical areas (i.e. the mesocortical pathway) (Feltenstein and See, 2008). Within this reward-related circuitry, psychostimulant drugs, such as cocaine, increase extracellular dopamine levels by blocking reuptake of dopamine by the dopamine transporter (Ersche and Sahakian, 2007), while other drugs of abuse, such as alcohol and nicotine, work indirectly by acting on neurons containing γ-aminobutyric acid (GABA) or glutamate (GLU) which, in turn, increases dopaminergic neurotransmission within the mesocorticolimbic circuitry (Markou, 2008; Tambour and Quertemont, 2007). This critical circuitry mediates the evolutionary behaviours associated with natural rewards, such as food, water, sex and nurturing one's young. Drugs of abuse are rewarding and reinforcing as they also increase dopamine within this circuitry. However, repeated drug exposure induces compensatory neuroadaptations within the mesocorticolimbic circuitry, which act to oppose the effects of acute drug administration; these neuroadaptations result in the suppression of dopaminergic neurotransmission (Melis et al., 2005).

Recent addiction models have expanded the traditional mesolimbic 'reward' circuitry involved in addiction to include two separate, yet interconnected systems: the limbic system in the incentive-sensitization of drugs (Robinson and Berridge, 2001) and the prefrontal circuitry in the compulsive aspects of drug seeking (Goldstein and Volkow, 2002; Jentsch and Taylor, 1999; Lubman et al., 2004). Recent advances in neuroimaging and brain stimulation techniques have allowed researchers to directly examine the neural systems underlying regulatory control (i.e. the prefrontal cortex) and have highlighted its critical role in regulating the compulsive desire to consume drugs despite adverse consequences. Indeed, neuropsychological studies have found that individuals who are chronically exposed to addictive drugs often present with executive, inhibitory and decision-making impairments, and these cognitive deficits are accompanied by abnormalities within the frontostriatal circuitry (Verdejo-García et al., 2006).

The prefrontal cortex, cognitive control and compulsive drug-seeking

The ability to maintain cognitive inhibitory control and suppress responses to automatic yet inappropriate stimuli relies on the integrated function of neural systems within the prefrontal cortex (PFC) (Fuster, 2001). Two cortical systems within the basal ganglia are required for effective cognitive inhibitory control: one consisting of the dorsolateral prefrontal (DLPFC) and orbitofrontal (OFC) circuitry, and the second, involving the anterior cingulate (ACC) (Blasi et al., 2006).

The DLPFC functions in an executive manner and plays an essential role in response inhibition (Garavan et al., 2002). The DLPFC is critical to the updating and integrating information about projected task-related outcomes and translating this input into the selection of an appropriate behavioural response. Dysfunction of this circuitry could impact on an individuals' ability to assimilate information regarding potential outcomes and lead to the selection of ongoing risky behavioural choices.

The OFC is considered fundamental to the suppression of irrelevant or interfering impulses, behaviours or thoughts (Winstanley, 2007). Dysfunction of the OFC is related primarily to aberrant impulsive and disinhibited social behaviours and faulty decision-making. Neuroimaging studies report dysfunction of the OFC across substance dependent populations and provide evidence of a relationship between altered OFC, impaired decision-making skills and the compulsive aspects of addiction (Volkow and Fowler, 2000). Additionally, the OFC has connections with subcortical regions, including the nucleus accumbens and basolateral amygdala. The OFC integrates information relayed from these subcortical regions and generates a set of outcome expectancies (Schoenbaum et al., 2006). The inability to adequately assimilate the negative outcome expectancies into decision-making schema could explain why individuals with a compromised OFC find it difficult to abstain from continued drug seeking despite the known aversive risks.

One of the many functions of the ACC is its involvement in error detection and conflict monitoring (Kerns et al., 2004). Dysfunction of the ACC can disrupt the process of evaluating an erroneous outcome and impact on one's ability to identify the likelihood of a negative outcome. Neuroimaging studies have provided extensive evidence of ACC dysfunction in substance dependence populations, which could relate to the impaired ability to accurately assess the negative outcomes associated with chronic drug use (Yücel and Lubman, 2007). As such, substance-dependent individuals may have diminished sensitivity to the evaluation of risk associated with continued drug use.

Thus, various brain systems within the frontostriatal circuitry appear to play a critical role in the maintenance of addictive behaviours. The next section reviews neurocognitive, neuroimaging and brain stimulation studies that highlight frontally-mediated cognitive inhibitory impairments in substance-dependent populations (focusing here on cocaine, nicotine and alcohol). When combined, these studies provide consistent evidence for dysregulation of frontostriatal circuitry in compulsive drug-seeking.

Chronic cocaine use and the prefrontal cortex

Cocaine, a short-acting psychostimulant drug, is highly reinforcing and addictive. Cocaine has a direct effect on dopamine signaling, which promotes dopamine transmission by binding to the dopamine transporter, blocking the synaptic dopamine re-uptake, and resulting in the build-up of extracellular dopamine in the mesolimbic structures of the brain (Kalivas, 2007). Repetitive cocaine use generates profound addiction in humans and neurotransmitter systems such as dopamine, GLU and GABA are implicated in models of cocaine dependence.

Neuropsychological studies

Acute cocaine administration has been found to improve and possibly *normalise* cognitive function in cocaine users (Garavan et al., 2008), while chronic cocaine use is associated with cognitive impairment across the domains of inhibitory control, decision-making and performance monitoring (Fillmore and Rush, 2002). Additionally, the severity of these cognitive impairments predicts treatment compliance and therapeutic response.

Neuroimaging studies

Consistent with these findings, structural MRI studies show reductions in grey matter tissue density in the frontal cortical brain regions of cocaine (both current and abstinent) users compared to controls (Franklin et al., 2002; Matochik et al., 2003), with OFC grey matter loss correlating with increased cocaine-related compulsivity (Ersche et al., 2011). Additionally, decreases in grey matter of the frontal cortex were found to be inversely correlated with duration of cocaine abuse (Ersche et al., 2011), while diffusion tensor imaging (DTI) studies identified a relationship between altered patterns of frontal connectivity and cocaine dependence (Lim et al., 2002).

On a functional level, resting-state functional magnetic resonance imaging (fMRI) studies show that active cocaine users present with functional connectivity decreases within the mesocorticolimbic circuitry (Gu et al., 2010), while acute intravenous administration of cocaine produces activation with this downregulated system (Garavan et al., 2008). Further, reduced activation of frontal regions, such as the PFC and ACC (Li et al., 2008) of cocaine users is associated with impaired cognitive inhibition, craving (Risinger et al., 2005) and heightened levels of impulsivity (Hu et al., 2015). PET studies also show that chronic cocaine users demonstrate decreased relative prefrontal cerebral blood flow (Volkow et al., 1988) and reduced frontal cerebral glucose metabolism (Volkow et al., 1992) compared to healthy controls. Patterns of altered activation of the prefrontal cortex are also evident in abstinent cocaine users, with altered patterns of activation of the OFC during decision making tasks (Bolla et al., 2003), and the ACC and lateral PFC throughout tasks of cognitive and attentional control (Bolla et al., 2004a). Additionally, the amount of cocaine consumed prior to abstinence correlates with altered activation of these frontal regions (Bolla et al., 2004b).

Brain stimulation studies

A single session of high frequency repetitive Transcranial Magnetic Stimulation (rTMS) to the right DLPFC transiently reduced cocaine craving in cocaine-dependent patients (Camprodon et al., 2007), while ten sessions of high frequency rTMS to the left DLPFC in cocaine-dependent patients post-detoxification caused a gradual decrease in cocaine craving (Politi et al., 2008). Based on these findings, the authors suggest that up-regulating DLPFC excitability in a cocaine-dependent brain can reduce craving for cocaine.

Chronic nicotine use and the prefrontal cortex

Nicotine, a highly addictive psychostimulant, is a major psychotropic component of tobacco smoke (Dani et al., 2001). Nicotine interacts with nicotinic acetylcholine receptors, resulting in increased dopamine neurotransmission within the mesocorticolimbic circuitry via dopaminergic neurons, as well as through GABA and GLU synaptic transmission (Mansvelder et al., 2002). Discontinuation of nicotine intake can result in unpleasant somatic and affective withdrawal symptoms (De Biasi and Dani, 2011).

Neuropsychological studies

Early studies focused on the acute cognitive-enhancing effects of nicotine exposure across several domains, such as executive functioning, attention and working memory (Heishman et al., 2010; Swan and Lessov-Schlaggar, 2007). However, at the same time, nicotine abstinence was related to reduced performance in attentional control (Ernst et al., 2001), response inhibition (Dawkins et al., 2009) and decision-making (Field et al., 2006). These effects were confirmed by a recent study which found that acute nicotine administration *reversed* abstinence-related inhibitory deficits in chronic smokers (Dawkins et al., 2007). This led to the proposition that acute nicotine exposure may *normalise* cognitive deficits in chronic smokers. Over time, dependence on nicotine could exacerbate these cognitive symptoms and lead to increased difficulty regulating nicotine use, despite apparent negative consequences (Nesic et al., 2011).

Neuroimaging studies

On a structural level, recent structural MRI studies have identified that chronic smokers exhibit significantly reduced cortical grey matter volumes and densities in frontal regions and the ACC (Liao et al., 2012). Severity of smoking was also found to be related to reductions in grey matter density (Brody et al., 2004), grey matter volume (Gallinat et al., 2006) and cortical thickness (Kühn et al., 2010) within the prefrontal cortex.

On a functional level, active smokers exposed to smoking-cues show increased cerebral blood flow (CBF) in the prefrontal cortex and associated regions, as well as activation of the anterior cingulate cortex. Additionally, increased activations within subregions of the PFC were related to *smoking-expectancy*; suggesting that activation of the OFC and DLPFC is modulated by the anticipation of future nicotine-exposure (McBride et al., 2006). Indeed, increased perfusion (Franklin et al., 2007) and activation (McBride et al., 2006) of the DLPFC were found to be associated with heightened craving. PET studies examining metabolic changes induced by nicotine-cue exposure in heavy smokers found cigarette cue-exposure induced increased metabolism in the PFC, left anterior temporal lobe and the bilateral ACC (Brody et al., 2002a). Further, subjective levels of craving correlated with metabolism in the frontal regions (including the OFC, DLPFC and ACC) (Brody et al., 2002b; Rose et al., 2007).

Brain stimulation studies

Brain stimulation studies report that high frequency stimulation (rTMS and tDCS) over the frontal cortex is capable of reducing levels of craving (Amiaz et al., 2009; Fregni et al., 2008), the number of cigarettes smoked (Eichhammer et al., 2003; Johann et al., 2003) and nicotine cue-induced craving (Boggio et al., 2009; Li et al., 2013).

Chronic alcohol use and the prefrontal cortex

Ethanol, the psychoactive ingredient in alcoholic beverages, acts as a central nervous system depressant (Conte et al., 2008). Acute alcohol consumption increases extracellular dopamine levels in the mesocorticolimbic circuitry indirectly through GABA and GLU systems. Chronic exposure induces compensatory neuroadaptations to counter these acute effects, resulting in the suppression of dopaminergic neurotransmission (Kalivas et al., 2009).

Neuropsychological studies

Neuropsychological studies report that alcohol dependent individuals exhibit regulatory deficits across the domains of executive control, cognitive inhibition and decision-making (Naim-Feil et al., 2014; Noël et al., 2007). These cognitive impairments persist beyond abstinence and relate to poor treatment outcome (Bates et al., 2002).

Neuroimaging studies

Structural MRI studies report altered frontal brain morphometry (Pfefferbaum et al., 1998), as well as a relationship between volumetric reductions of these frontal regions and poor cognitive performance in alcohol-dependent individuals (Chanraud et al., 2007), with DLPFC volumetric reductions persisting beyond abstinence (Makris et al., 2008). DTI studies identify widespread reductions in frontal white matter tracts within frontostriatal systems (Fortier et al., 2014), with heavy drinking associated with microstructural white matter damage (Pfefferbaum et al.,

2014) which persists in alcohol-dependent patients who relapse (relative to those who abstained) (Shear et al., 1994).

On a functional level, fMRI studies report reduced cerebral perfusion in prefrontal and left parietal regions (Clark et al., 2007), while alcohol cue-reactivity is related to increased activation of the frontal and limbic areas (Tapert et al., 2004) in alcohol-dependent females. Other studies demonstrate a relationship between altered patterns of frontal brain activation and cognitive performance in alcohol-dependent individuals (Pfefferbaum et al., 2001). Indeed, abstinent alcohol-dependent patients exhibit impaired impulse control as reflected by decreased cortical activation of the DLPFC, as well as increased risk-taking related to reduced activation of the medial OFC, bilateral parietal cortices and rostral ACC (Li et al., 2009). PET studies report a relationship between alcohol dependence and metabolic abnormalities in frontal circuitry (Volkow et al., 2007). Left DLPFC hypometabolism (Dao-Castellana et al., 1998), alterations in regional cerebral blood flow (CBF) (Noel et al., 2001) and perfusion of the frontal regions (Demir et al., 2002) correlate with poorer performance on various cognitive tasks. With regards to craving, detoxified alcohol-dependent patients exposed to an alcoholic cue show significant increases in CBF in the ventral putamen (which receives input from the frontal cortex), DLPFC, insula and cerebellum and these increases correlate with self-reported craving (Olbrich et al., 2006).

Brain stimulation studies

A recent combined TMS-EEG study provided the first report of suppressed cortical inhibition within the *frontal cortex* of alcohol dependent patients post-detoxification. These findings support the notion that repetitive alcohol use leads to compensatory neuroadaptations, such as suppressed cortical inhibitory neurotransmission in the frontal cortex and surrounding regions, and these neural alterations persist beyond abstinence (Naim-Feil et al., IN PRESS). Brain stimulation studies have also examined the efficacy of applying techniques such as Transcranial Direct Current Stimulation (tDCS) and rTMS to the DLPFC and medial frontal cortex in attenuating alcohol-seeking behaviours. Two studies reported that application of high frequency rTMS to the right DLPFC (Mishra et al., 2010) or low frequency rTMS double-cone stimulation to the medial frontal cortex (targeting the ACC) (De Ridder et al., 2011) reduced levels of alcohol craving, while a tDCS study demonstrated that both anodal-left/cathodal-right and anodal-right/cathodal-left tDCS conditions led to decreases in alcohol craving levels (Boggio et al., 2008). Contrary to these findings, two studies reported that rTMS to the left DLPFC (Höppner et al., 2011) or the right DLPFC (Herremans et al., 2012) did not reduce alcohol craving. This discrepancy may relate to methodological factors, such as stimulation parameters, number of stimulation sessions and site of stimulation.

Brief overview

These studies provide initial evidence of frontostriatal dysfunction in substance-dependent populations. Neuropsychological studies demonstrate cognitive inhibitory deficits across cocaine, nicotine and alcohol-dependent populations, with deficits identified in cocaine and alcohol-dependent groups also relating to treatment response. Structural alterations of the frontal cortices were also observed across cocaine, nicotine and alcohol-dependent populations. In chronic smokers, these structural alterations were amplified by the severity of nicotine exposure, while in alcohol-dependent individuals these structural deficits persisted beyond abstinence and were predictive of relapse. From a functional perspective, chronic cocaine, nicotine and alcohol-dependent individuals all exhibited altered patterns of frontal brain activity. In both cocaine users and alcohol-dependent individuals, these frontal alterations were related to cognitive inhibitory impairments and craving, and persisted beyond abstinence. In chronic smokers, these frontal alterations related to smoking-expectancy, cue-exposure and heightened levels of craving. Preliminary brain stimulation studies examined the efficacy of targeting these frontal regions and demonstrated that they were able to reduce craving levels and chronic drug consumption in cocaine and nicotine-dependent individuals, although studies in alcohol dependence were mixed. Collectively, these studies provide compelling evidence for the relationship between frontostriatal dysfunction (specifically the three PFC-striatothalamic circuits – the DLPFC, OFC and ACC), regulatory deficits and persistent drug-seeking behaviours, and highlight the importance of targeting frontostriatal deficits in the treatment of addiction.

Implications for treatment

While standard clinical models of care do not directly focus on the remediation of these cognitive inhibitory deficits, most addiction services do employ therapeutic strategies that target PFC function. For example, psychological treatments, such as motivational interviewing, are designed to improve response selection (i.e. examining the positive and negative values of continued drug use). Other strategies, such as cognitive behavioural therapy, include the teaching of improved drug-refusal skills and adaptive coping skills to assist with the inhibition of compulsive drug cravings (Yücel and Lubman, 2007), while mindfulness-based relapse prevention therapies help patients increase awareness of their triggers and responses, accept uncomfortable mental states and challenge acting on 'auto-pilot' (Witkiewitz et al., 2005).

Pharmacological interventions for addiction have not classically targeted prefrontal circuitry. However, there are an increasing number of medications that target reward and craving mechanisms, including the alcohol pharmacotherapies acamprosate (Kalk and Lingford-Hughes, 2014) and naltrexone (Pettinati et al., 2006). Another novel area of interest is the development of pharmacotherapies that impact on GLU and GABA neurotransmitter systems and modulate dopaminergic transmission. Such medications may have a role in enhancing PFC function, thereby improving decision making or inhibitory control (Addolorato et al., 2012). One example is topiramate, an anti-epileptic medication, which is being trialed for its ability to reduce craving and consumption of cocaine (Johnson et al., 2013) and alcohol (Guglielmo et al., 2015). Another approach is the use of cognitive enhancing drugs (commonly used for ADHD) to counter the cognitive impairments associated with chronic drug use (Sofuoglu et al., 2013). For instance, modafinil may increase extracellular dopamine in the prefrontal cortex (Dackis et al., 2004).

Experimental approaches, such as the use of non-invasive brain stimulation techniques, (e.g. TMS and tDCS) are also being explored as potential treatment strategies for substance dependence. Preliminary studies suggest that application of brain stimulation techniques can induce transient decreases in craving levels and drug consumption (Naim-Feil and Zangen, 2013). However, further large-scale studies are required to more conclusively evaluate the clinical efficacy of these techniques.

Summary

Substance dependence is a chronic relapsing and devastating psychiatric disorder. Understanding the progression from recreational use to dependence remains a critical issue for the diagnosis and treatment of these disorders. Genetic studies suggest that addiction is an aetiologically complex disorder resulting from the influence of multiple genetic and environmental factors. Recent neurobiological models of addiction have expanded the traditional mesolimbic 'reward' circuitry to include two parallel, yet interconnected systems: the limbic system in the incentive-sensitization of drugs and the prefrontal cortex in the compulsive nature of drug-seeking. The frontal circuitry is thought to play a critical regulatory role in inhibiting the prepotent desire to consume drugs regardless of the consequences. This is supported by a growing number of studies demonstrating a relationship between frontostriatal dysfunction, regulatory deficits and the persistence of drug-seeking behaviours. An improved understanding of the multifaceted nature of addiction is critical for identifying those who are more vulnerable to the development of dependence, improving therapeutic strategies that reduce drug-seeking behaviours and enhancing treatment and recovery outcomes.

Abbreviations

ACC: anterior cingulate cortex
DLFFC: dorsolateral prefrontal cortex
GABA: γ-aminobutyric acid

GLU: glutamate
OFC: orbital frontal cortex
PFC: prefrontal cortex
tDCS: transcranial direct current stimulation
TMS: transcranial magnetic stimulation

Further readings

Daglish, M., Lingford-Hughes, A., Nutt, D. (2005). Human functional neuroimaging connectivity research in dependence. *Reviews in the Neurosciences, 16,* 151–157.

Feil, J., Zangen, A. (2010). Brain stimulation in the study and treatment of addiction. *Neuroscience & Biobehavioral Reviews, 34,* 559–574.

Feltenstein, M.W., See, R.E. (2008). The neurocircuitry of addiction: An overview. *British Journal of Pharmacology, 154,* 261–274.

Goldman, D., Oroszi, G., Ducci, F. (2005). The genetics of addictions: Uncovering the genes. *Nature Reviews Genetics, 6,* 521–532.

Hyman, S.E., Malenka, R.C. (2001). Addiction and the brain: The neurobiology of compulsion and its persistence. *Nature Reviews Neuroscience, 2,* 695–703.

Robinson, T.E., Berridge, K.C. (2001). Incentive-sensitization and addiction. *Addiction, 96,* 103–114.

Verdejo-García, A., Bechara, A., Recknor, E.C., Pérez-García, M. (2006). Executive dysfunction in substance dependent individuals during drug use and abstinence: An examination of the behavioral, cognitive and emotional correlates of addiction. *Journal of the International Neuropsychological Society, 12,* 405–415.

References

Addolorato, G., Leggio, L., Hopf, F. W., Diana, M., & Bonci, A. (2012). Novel therapeutic strategies for alcohol and drug addiction: Focus on GABA, ion channels and transcranial magnetic stimulation. *Neuropsychopharmacology, 37*(1), 163–177.

Agrawal, A., Verweij, K. J., Gillespie, N. A., Heath, A. C., Lessov-Schlaggar, C. N., Martin, N. G., … & Lynskey, M. T. (2012). The genetics of addiction—A translational perspective. *Translational Psychiatry, 17*(2), 54.

American Psychiatric Association. (2013). *Diagnostic and Statistical Manual of Mental Disorders: DSM-5* (5th ed.). Arlington, VA: American Psychiatric Publishing.

Amiaz, R., Levy, D., Vainiger, D., Grunhaus, L., & Zangen, A. (2009). Repeated high-frequency transcranial magnetic stimulation over the dorsolateral prefrontal cortex reduces cigarette craving and consumption. *Addiction, 104*(4), 653–660.

Anton, R. F., Oroszi, G., O'Malley, S., Couper, D., Swift, R., Pettinati, H., & Goldman, D. (2008). An Evaluation of μ-Opioid Receptor (OPRM1) as a predictor of naltrexone response in the treatment of alcohol dependence: Results from the Combined Pharmacotherapies and Behavioral Interventions for Alcohol Dependence (COMBINE) Study. *Archives of General Psychiatry, 65*(2), 135–144.

Babor, T. F., de la Fuente, J. R., Saunders, J., & Grant, M. (1992). *AUDIT: The Alcohol Use Disorders Identification Test. Guidelines for Use in Primary Health Care.* Geneva, Switzerland: World Health Organization.

Bates, M. E., Bowden, S. C., & Barry, D. (2002). Neurocognitive impairment associated with alcohol use disorders: Implications for treatment. *Experimental and Clinical Psychopharmacology, 10*(3), 193–212.

Berman, A. H., Bergman, H., Palmstierna, T., & Schlyter, F. (2005). Evaluation of the Drug Use Disorders Identification Test (DUDIT) in criminal justice and detoxification settings and in a Swedish population sample. *European Addiction Research, 11*(1), 22–31.

Best, D.W., & Lubman, D. I. (2012). The recovery paradigm: A model of hope and change for alcohol and drug addiction. *Australian Family Physician, 41*(8), 593.

Blasi, G., Goldberg, T. E., Weickert, T., Das, S., Kohn, P., Zoltick, B., … & Mattay, V. S. (2006). Brain regions underlying response inhibition and interference monitoring and suppression. *European Journal of Neuroscience, 23*(6), 1658–1664.

Boggio, P. S., Liguori, P., Sultani, N., Rezende, L., Fecteau, S., & Fregni, F. (2009). Cumulative priming effects of cortical stimulation on smoking cue-induced craving. *Neuroscience Letters, 463*(1), 82–86.

Boggio, P. S., Sultani, N., Fecteau, S., Merabet, L., Mecca, T., Pascual-Leone, A., … & Fregni, F. (2008). Prefrontal cortex modulation using transcranial DC stimulation reduces alcohol craving: A double-blind, sham-controlled study. *Drug & Alcohol Dependence, 92*(1–3), 55–60.

Bolla, K., Ernst, M., Kiehl, K., Mouratidis, M., Eldreth, D., Contoreggi, C., … & London, E. (2004). Prefrontal cortical dysfunction in abstinent cocaine abusers. *The Journal of Neuropsychiatry & Clinical Neurosciences, 16*(4), 456–464.

Bolla, K. I., Eldreth, D. A., London, E. D., Kiehl, K. A., Mouratidis, M., Contoreggi, C., … & Ernst, M. (2003). Orbitofrontal cortex dysfunction in abstinent cocaine abusers performing a decision-making task. *NeuroImage, 19*(3), 1085–1094.

Brady, K. T., & Sinha, R. (2005). Co-occurring mental and substance use disorders: The neurobiological effects of chronic stress. *The American Journal of Psychiatry, 162*, 1483–1493.

Brecht, M.-L., Huang, D., Evans, E., & Hser, Y.-I. (2008). Polydrug use and implications for longitudinal research: Ten-year trajectories for heroin, cocaine, and methamphetamine users. *Drug & Alcohol Dependence, 96*(3), 193–201.

Breslau, N., Johnson, E. O., Hiripi, E., & Kessler, R. (2001). Nicotine dependence in the United States: Prevalence, trends, and smoking persistence. *Archives of General Psychiatry, 58*(9), 810–816.

Brody, A. L., Mandelkern, M. A., Jarvik, M. E., Lee, G. S., Smith, E. C., Huang, J. C., … & London, E. D. (2004). Differences between smokers and nonsmokers in regional gray matter volumes and densities. *Biological Psychiatry, 55*(1), 77–84.

Brody, A. L., Mandelkern, M. A., London, E. D., Childress, A. R., Lee, G. S., Bota, R. G., … & Jarvik, M. E. (2002). Brain metabolic changes during cigarette craving. *Archives of General Psychiatry, 59*(12), 1162–1172.

Brody, A. L., Mandelkern, M. A., London, E. D., Childress, A. R., Lee, G. S., Bota, R. G., … & Jarvik, M. E. (2002). Brain metabolic changes during cigarette craving. *Archives of General Psychiatry, 59*(12), 1162–1172.

Camprodon, J. A., Martínez-Raga, J., Alonso-Alonso, M., Shih, M. C., & Pascual-Leone, A. (2007). One session of high frequency repetitive transcranial magnetic stimulation (rTMS) to the right prefrontal cortex transiently reduces cocaine craving. *Drug Alcohol Dependence, 86*(1), 91–94.

Chanraud, S., Martelli, C., Delain, F., Kostogianni, N., Douaud, G., Aubin, H. J., … & Martinot, J. L. (2007). Brain morphometry and cognitive performance in detoxified alcohol-dependents with preserved psychosocial functioning. *Neuropsychopharmacology, 32*(2), 429–438.

Clark, C. P., Brown, G. G., Eyler, L. T., Drummond, S. P., Braun, D. R., & Tapert, S. F. (2007). Decreased perfusion in young alcohol-dependent women as compared with age-matched controls. *American Journal of Drug Alcohol Abuse, 33*(1), 13–19.

Conte, A., Attilia, M. L., Gilio, F., Iacovelli, E., Frasca, V., Bettolo, C. M., ... & Inghilleri, M. (2008). Acute and chronic effects of ethanol on cortical excitability. *Clinical Neurophysiology, 119*(3), 667–674.

Dackis, C. A., Kampman, K. M., Lynch, K. G., Pettinati, H. M., & O'Brien, C. P. (2004). A double-blind, placebo-controlled trial of Modafinil for cocaine dependence. *Neuropsychopharmacology, 30*(1), 205–211.

Dani, J. A., Ji, D., & Zhou, F. M. (2001). Synaptic plasticity and nicotine addiction. *Neuron, 31*(3), 349–352.

Dao-Castellana, M. H., Samson, Y., Legault, F., Martinot, J. L., Aubin, H. J., Crouzel, C., ... & Syrota, A. (1998). Frontal dysfunction in neurologically normal chronic alcoholic subjects: Metabolic and neuropsychological findings. *Psychological Medicine, 28*(5), 1039–1048.

Dawkins, L., Powell, J., West, R., Powell, J., & Pickering, A. (2007). A double-blind placebo-controlled experimental study of nicotine: II—Effects on response inhibition and executive functioning. *Psychopharmacology, 190*(4), 457–467.

Dawkins, L., Powell, J. H., Pickering, A., Powell, J., & West, R. (2009). Patterns of change in withdrawal symptoms, desire to smoke, reward motivation and response inhibition across 3 months of smoking abstinence. *Addiction, 104*(5), 850–858.

De Biasi, M., & Dani, J. A. (2011). Reward, addiction, withdrawal to nicotine. *Annual Review of Neuroscience, 34*, 105–130.

De Ridder, D., Vanneste, S., Kovacs, S., Sunaert, S., & Dom, G. (2011). Transient alcohol craving suppression by rTMS of dorsal anterior cingulate: An fMRI and LORETA EEG study. *Neuroscience Letters, 496*(1), 5–10.

Degenhardt, L., Charlson, F., Mathers, B., Hall, W. D., Flaxman, A. D., Johns, N., & Vos, T. (2014). The global epidemiology and burden of opioid dependence: Results from the global burden of disease 2010 study. *Addiction, 109*(8), 1320–1333.

Degenhardt, L., Ferrari, A. J., Calabria, B., Hall, W. D., Norman, R. E., McGrath, J., ... & Whiteford, H. A. (2013). The global epidemiology and contribution of cannabis use and dependence to the global burden of disease: Results from the GBD 2010 study.

Demir, B., Uluq, B. D., Erqun, E. L., & Erbas, B. (2002). Regional cerebral blood flow and neuropsychological functioning in early and late onset alcoholism. *115*(3), 115–125.

Eichhammer, P., Johann, M., Kharraz, A., Binder, H., Pittrow, D., Wodarz, N., & Hajak, G. (2003). High-frequency repetitive transcranial magnetic stimulation decreases cigarette smoking. *Journal of Clinical Psychiatry, 64*(8), 951–953.

Ernst, M., Heishman, S. J., Spurgeon, L., & London, E. D. (2001). Smoking history and nicotine effects on cognitive performance. *Neuropsychopharmacology, 25*(3), 313–319.

Ersche, K., & Sahakian, B. (2007). The neuropsychology of amphetamine and opiate dependence: Implications for treatment. *Neuropsychology Review, 17*(3), 317–336.

Ersche, K. D., Barnes, A., Jones, P. S., Morein-Zamir, S., Robbins, T. W., & Bullmore, E. T. (2011). Abnormal structure of frontostriatal brain systems is associated with aspects of impulsivity and compulsivity in cocaine dependence. *Brain, 134*(pt 7), 2013–2024.

Feltenstein, M. W., & See, R. E. (2008). The neurocircuitry of addiction: An overview. *British Journal of Pharmacology, 154*(2), 261–274.

Field, M., Santarcangelo, M., Sumnall, H., Goudie, A., & Cole, J. (2006). Delay discounting and the behavioural economics of cigarette purchases in smokers: The effects of nicotine deprivation. *Psychopharmacology, 186*(2), 255–263.

Fillmore, M. T., & Rush, C. R. (2002). Impaired inhibitory control of behavior in chronic cocaine users. *Drug & Alcohol Dependence, 66*(3), 265–273.

First, M. B., Spitzer, R. L., Gibbon, M., & Williams, J. B. W. (2002). *Structured Clinical Interview for DSM-IV-TR Axis I Disorders, Research Version, Patient Edition. (SCID- I/P).* New York: Biometrics Research, New York Psychiatric Institute.

Fortier, C. B., Leritz, E. C., Salat, D. H., Lindemer, E., Maksimovskiy, A. L., Shepel, J., … & McGlinchey, R. E. (2014). Widespread effects of alcohol on white matter microstructure. *Alcoholism: Clinical & Experimental Research, 38*(12), 2925–2933.

Franklin, T. R., Acton, P. D., Maldjian, J. A., Gray, J. D., Croft, J. R., Dackis, C. A., … & Childress, A. R. (2002). Decreased gray matter concentration in the insular, orbitofrontal, cingulate, and temporal cortices of cocaine patients. *Biological Psychiatry, 51*(2), 134–142.

Franklin, T. R., Wang, Z., Wang, J., Sciortino, N., Harper, D., Li, Y., … & Childress, A. R. (2007). Limbic activation to cigarette smoking cues independent of nicotine withdrawal: A perfusion fMRI study. *Neuropsychopharmacology, 32*(11), 2301–2309.

Fregni, F., Liguori, P., Fecteau, S., Nitsche, M. A., Pascual-Leone, A., & Boggio, P. S. (2008). Cortical stimulation of the prefrontal cortex with transcranial direct current stimulation reduces cue-provoked smoking craving: A randomized, sham-controlled study. *Journal of Clinical Psychiatry, 69*, 32–40.

Fuster, J. M. (2001). The prefrontal cortex - An update: Time is of the essence. *Neuron, 30*(2), 319–333.

Gallinat, J., Meisenzahl, E., Jacobsen, L. K., Kalus, P., Bierbrauer, J., Kienast, T., … & Staedtgen, M. (2006). Smoking and structural brain deficits: A volumetric MR investigation. *European Journal of Neuroscience, 24*(6), 1744–1750.

Garavan, H., Kaufman, J. N., & Hester, R. (2008). Acute effects of cocaine on the neurobiology of cognitive control. *Philosophical Transactions of the Royal Society B: Biological Sciences, 363*(1507), 3267–3276.

Garavan, H., Ross, T. J., Murphy, K., Roche, R. A. P., & Stein, E. A. (2002). Dissociable executive functions in the dynamic control of behavior: Inhibition, error detection, and correction. *NeuroImage, 17*(4), 1820–1829.

Goldman, D., & Bergen, A. (1998). General and specific inheritance of substance abuse and alcoholism. *Archives of General Psychiatry, 55*(11), 964–965.

Goldman, D., Oroszi, G., & Ducci, F. (2005). The genetics of addictions: Uncovering the genes. *Nature Reviews Genetics, 6*(7), 521–532.

Goldstein, R. Z., & Volkow, N. D. (2002). Drug addiction and its underlying neurobiological basis: Neuroimaging evidence for the involvement of the frontal cortex. *American Journal of Psychiatry, 159*(10), 1642–1652.

Gossop, M., Darke, S., Griffiths, P., Hando, J., Powis, B., Hall, W., & Strang, J. (1995). The Severity of Dependence Scale (SDS): Psychometric properties of the SDS in English and Australian samples of heroin, cocaine and amphetamine users. *Addiction, 90*(5), 607–614.

Grant, B. F., Stinson, F. S., Dawson, D. A., Chou, S. P., Dufour, M. C., Compton, W., … & Kaplan, K. (2004). Prevalence and co-occurrence of substance use disorders and independent mood and anxiety disorders: Results from the national epidemiologic survey on alcohol and related conditions. *Archives of General Psychiatry, 61*(8), 807–816.

Gu, H., Salmeron, B. J., Ross, T. J., Geng, X., Zhan, W., Stein, E. A., & Yang, Y. (2010). Mesocorticolimbic circuits are impaired in chronic cocaine users as demonstrated by resting-state functional connectivity. *NeuroImage, 53*(2), 593–601.

Guglielmo, R., Martinotti, G., Quatrale, M., Ioime, L., Kadilli, I., Di Nicola, M., & Janiri, L. (2015). Topiramate in alcohol use disorders: Review and update. *CNS Drugs, 29*(5), 383–395.

Hasin, D. S., Stinson, F. S., Ogburn, E., & Grant, B. F. (2007). Prevalence, correlates, disability, and comorbidity of DSM-IV alcohol abuse and dependence in the United States: Results from the National Epidemiologic Survey on alcohol and related conditions. *Archives of General Psychiatry, 64*(7), 830–842.

Heath, A. C., Bucholz, K. K., Madden, P. A. F., Dinwiddie, S. H., Slutske, W. S., Bierut, L. J., … & Martin, N. G. (1997). Genetic and environmental contributions to alcohol dependence risk in a national twin sample: Consistency of findings in women and men. *Psychological Medicine, 27*(6), 1381–1396.

Heishman, S., Kleykamp, B., & Singleton, E. (2010). Meta-analysis of the acute effects of nicotine and smoking on human performance. *Psychopharmacology, 210*(4), 453–469.

Herremans, S. C., Baeken, C., Vanderbruggen, N., Vanderhasselt, M. A., Zeeuws, D., Santermans, L., & De Raedt, R. (2012). No influence of one right-sided prefrontal HF-rTMS session on alcohol craving in recently detoxified alcohol-dependent patients: Results of a naturalistic study. *Drug & Alcohol Dependence, 120*(1–3), 209–213.

Höppner, J., Broese, T., Wendler, L., Berger, C., & Thome, J. (2011). Repetitive transcranial magnetic stimulation (rTMS) for treatment of alcohol dependence. *World Journal of Biological Psychiatry, 12*(SUPPL. 1), 57–62.

Hu, Y., Salmeron, B., Gu, H., Stein, E. A., & Yang, Y. (2015). Impaired functional connectivity within and between frontostriatal circuits and its association with compulsive drug use and trait impulsivity in cocaine addiction. *JAMA Psychiatry, 72*(6), 584–592.

Jentsch, J. D., & Taylor, J. R. (1999). Impulsivity resulting from frontostriatal dysfunction in drug abuse: Implications for the control of behavior by reward-related stimuli. *Psychopharmacology, 146*(4), 373–390.

Johann, M., Wiegand, R., Kharraz, A., Bobbe, G., Sommer, G., Hajak, G., … & Eichhammer, P. (2003). Transcranial magnetic stimulation for nicotine dependence. *Psychiatrische Praxis, 30*(Supp 2), S129–131.

Johnson, B. A., Ait-Daoud, N., Wang, X. Q., Penberthy, J. K., Javors, M. A., Seneviratne, C., & Liu, L. (2013). Topiramate for the treatment of cocaine addiction: A randomized clinical trial. *JAMA Psychiatry, 70*(12), 1338–1346.

Kalivas, P. W. (2007). Neurobiology of cocaine addiction: Implications for new pharmacotherapy. *American Journal on Addictions, 16*(2), 71–78.

Kalivas, P. W., LaLumiere, R. T., Knackstedt, L., & Shen, H. (2009). Glutamate transmission in addiction. *Neuropharmacology, 56*(Supplement 1), 169–173.

Kalk, N. J., & Lingford-Hughes, A. R. (2014). The clinical pharmacology of acamprosate. *British Journal of Clinical Pharmacology,* 77(2), 315–323.

Kendler, K. S., Schmitt, E., Aggen, S. H., & Prescott, C. A. (2008). Genetic and environmental influences on alcohol, caffeine, cannabis, and nicotine use from early adolescence to middle adulthood. *Archives of General Psychiatry, 65*(6), 674–682.

Kerns, J. G., Cohen, J. D., MacDonald Iii, A. W., Cho, R. Y., Stenger, V. A., & Carter, C. S. (2004). Anterior cingulate conflict monitoring and adjustments in control. *Science, 303*(5660), 1023–1026.

Kravitz, A. V., Tomasi, D., LeBlanc, K. H., Baler, R., Volkow, N. D., Bonci, A., & Ferré, S. (2015). Cortico-striatal circuits: Novel therapeutic targets for substance use disorders. *Brain Research*. Doi 10.1016/j.brainres.2015.03.048.

Kühn, S., Schubert, F., & Gallinat, J. (2010). Reduced thickness of medial orbitofrontal cortex in smokers. *Biological Psychiatry, 68*(11), 1061–1065.

Leventhal, A. M., Lee, W., Bergen, A. W., Swan, G. E., Tyndale, R. F., Lerman, C., & Conti, D.V. (2014). Nicotine dependence as a moderator of genetic influences on smoking cessation treatment outcome. *Drug and Alcohol Dependence, 138*(1), 109–117.

Li, C. R., Luo, X., Yan, P., Bergquist, K., & Sinha, R. (2009). Altered impulse control in alcohol dependence: Neural measures of stop signal performance. *Alcoholism: Clinical & Experimental Research, 33*(4), 740–750.

Li, C. S. R., Huang, C., Yan, P., Bhagwagar, Z., Milivojevic, V., & Sinha, R. (2008). Neural correlates of impulse control during stop signal inhibition in cocaine-dependent men. *Neuropsychopharmacology, 33*(8), 1798–1806.

Li, X., Hartwell, K. J., Owens, M., LeMatty, T., Borckardt, J. J., Hanlon, C. A., … & George, M. S. (2013). Repetitive transcranial magnetic stimulation of the dorsolateral prefrontal cortex reduces nicotine cue craving. *Biological Psychiatry, 73*(8), 714–720.

Liao, Y., Tang, J., Liu, T., Chen, X., & Hao, W. (2012). Differences between smokers and non-smokers in regional gray matter volumes: A voxel-based morphometry study. *Addiction Biology, 17*(6), 977–980.

Lim, K. O., Choi, S. J., Pomara, N., Wolkin, A., & Rotrosen, J. P. (2002). Reduced frontal white matter integrity in cocaine dependence: A controlled diffusion tensor imaging study. *Biological Psychiatry, 51*(11), 890–895.

Lubman, D. I., Yücel, M., & Pantelis, C. (2004). Addiction, a condition of compulsive behaviour? Neuroimaging and neuropsychological evidence of inhibitory dysregulation. *Addiction, 99*(12), 1491–1502.

Makris, N., Oscar-Berman, M., Kim, S., Hodge, S. M., Kennedy, D. N., Caviness, V. S., … & Harris, G. J. (2008). Decreased volume of the brain reward system in alcoholism. *Biological Psychiatry, 64*(3), 192–202.

Mansvelder, H. D., Keath, J. R., & McGehee, D. S. (2002). Synaptic mechanisms underlie nicotine-induced excitability of brain reward areas. *Neuron, 33*(6), 905–919.

Markou, A. (2008). Review. Neurobiology of nicotine dependence. *Philosophical Transactions of the Royal Society B: Biological Sciences, 363*(1507), 3159–3168.

Matochik, J. A., London, E. D., Eldreth, D. A., Cadet, J. L., & Bolla, K. I. (2003). Frontal cortical tissue composition in abstinent cocaine abusers: A magnetic resonance imaging study. *NeuroImage, 19*(3), 1095–1102.

McBride, D., Barrett, S. P., Kelly, J. T., Aw, A., & Dagher, A. (2006). Effects of expectancy and abstinence on the neural response to smoking cues in cigarette smokers: An fMRI study. *Neuropsychopharmacology, 31*(12), 2728–2738.

McLellan, A. T., Luborsky, L., Woody, G. E., & O'Brien, C. P. (1980). An improved diagnostic evaluation instrument for substance abuse patients: The Addiction severity index. *The Journal of Nervous & Mental Disease, 168*(1), 26–33.

Melis, M., Spiga, S., & Diana, M. (2005). The dopamine hypothesis of drug addiction: Hypodopaminergic state. *International Review of Neurobiology* (Vol. 63, pp. 101–154): Academic Press.

Merikangas, K. R., & Risch, N. (2003). Genomic priorities and public health. *Science, 302*(5645), 599–601.

Mishra, B. R., Nizamie, S. H., Das, B., & Praharaj, S. K. (2010). Efficacy of repetitive transcranial magnetic stimulation in alcohol dependence: A sham-controlled study. *Addiction, 105*(1), 49–55.

Munafò, M. R., Johnstone, E. C., Walther, D., Uhl, G. R., Murphy, M. F. G., & Aveyard, P. (2011). CHRNA3 rs1051730 genotype and short-term smoking cessation. *Nicotine & Tobacco Research, 13*(10), 982–988.

Naim-Feil, J., Bradshaw, J., Rogasch, N., Daskalakis, Z., Sheppard, D., Lubman, D., & Fitzgerald, P. (IN PRESS). Cortical inhibition within motor and frontal regions in alcohol dependence post-detoxification: A pilot TMS-EEG study. *The World Journal of Biological Psychiatry*.

Naim-Feil, J., Fitzgerald, P. B., Bradshaw, J. L., Lubman, D. I., & Sheppard, D. (2014). Neurocognitive deficits, craving, and abstinence among alcohol-dependent individuals following detoxification. *Archives of Clinical Neuropsychology, 29*(1), 26–37.

Naim-Feil, J., & Zangen, A. (2013) Addiction. *Vol. 116. Handbook of Clinical Neurology 116,* 613–30. doi: 10.1016/B978-0-444-53497-2.00049-8.

Nesic, J., Rusted, J., Duka, T., & Jackson, A. (2011). Degree of dependence influences the effect of smoking on cognitive flexibility. *Pharmacology Biochemistry & Behavior, 98*(3), 376–384.

Noel, X., Paternot, J., Van der Linden, M., Sferrazza, R., Verhas, M., Hanak, C., ... & Verbanck, P. (2001). Correlation between inhibition, working memory and delimited frontal area blood flow measured by 99mTc-BICISATE SPECT in alcohol-dependent patients. *Alcohol Alcohol., 36*(6), 556–563.

Noël, X., Van der Linden, M., d'Acremont, M., Bechara, A., Dan, B., Hanak, C., & Verbanck, P. (2007). Alcohol cues increase cognitive impulsivity in individuals with alcoholism. *Psychopharmacology, 192*(2), 291–298.

Olbrich, H. M., Valerius, G., Paris, C., Hagenbuch, F., Ebert, D., & Juengling, F. D. (2006). Brain activation during craving for alcohol measured by positron emission tomography. *Australian & New Zealand Journal of Psychiatry, 40*(2), 171–178.

Pettinati, H. M., O'Brien, C. P., Rabinowitz, A. R., Wortman, S. P., Oslin, D. W., Kampman, K. M., & Dackis, C. A. (2006). The status of naltrexone in the treatment of alcohol dependence: Specific effects on heavy drinking. *Journal of Clinical Psychopharmacology, 26*(6), 610–625.

Pfefferbaum, A., Desmond, J. E., Galloway, C., Menon, V., Glover, G. H., & Sullivan, E. V. (2001). Reorganization of frontal systems used by alcoholics for spatial working memory: An fMRI study. *NeuroImage, 14*(1), 7–20.

Pfefferbaum, A., Rosenbloom, M. J., Chu, W., Sassoon, S. A., Rohlfing, T., Pohl, K. M., ... & Sullivan, E. V. (2014). White matter microstructural recovery with abstinence and decline with relapse in alcohol dependence interacts with normal ageing: A controlled longitudinal DTI study. *The Lancet Psychiatry, 1*(3), 202–212.

Pfefferbaum, A., Sullivan, E. V., Rosenbloom, M. J., Mathalon, D. H., & Lim, K. O. (1998). A controlled study of cortical gray matter and ventricular changes in alcoholic men over a 5-year interval. *Archives of General Psychiatry, 55*(10), 905–912.

Politi, E., Fauci, E., Santoro, A., & Smeraldi, E. (2008). Daily sessions of transcranial magnetic stimulation to the left prefrontal cortex gradually reduce cocaine craving. *American Journal on Addictions: The Official Journal of the American Academy of Addiction Psychiatry, 17*(4), 345–346.

Risinger, R. C., Salmeron, B. J., Ross, T. J., Amen, S. L., Sanfilipo, M., Hoffmann, R. G., ... & Stein, E. A. (2005). Neural correlates of high and craving during cocaine self-administration using BOLD fMRI. *NeuroImage, 26*(4), 1097–1108.

Robinson, T. E., & Berridge, K. C. (2001). Incentive-sensitization and addiction. *Addiction, 96*(1), 103–114.

Rose, J. E., Behm, F. M., Salley, A. N., Bates, J. E., Coleman, R. E., Hawk, T. C., & Turkington, T. G. (2007). Regional brain activity correlates of nicotine dependence. *Neuropsychopharmacology, 32*(12), 2441–2452.

Schoenbaum, G., Roesch, M. R., & Stalnaker, T. A. (2006). Orbitofrontal cortex, decision-making and drug addiction. *Trends in Neurosciences, 29*(2), 116–124.

Shear, P. K., Jernigan, T. L., & Butters, N. (1994). Volumetric magnetic resonance imaging quantification of longitudinal brain changes in abstinent alcoholics. *Alcoholism: Clinical & Experimental Research, 18*(1), 172–176.

Sheedy, C. K., & Whitter, M. (2009). *Guiding Principles and Elements of Recovery-Oriented Systems of Care: What Do We Know from the Research?* HHS Publication No. (SMA) 09–4439. Rockville, MD: Center for Substance Abuse Treatment, Substance Abuse and Mental Health Services Administration.

Sofuoglu, M., DeVito, E. E., Waters, A. J., & Carroll, K. M. (2013). Cognitive enhancement as a treatment for drug addictions. *Neuropharmacology, 64*, 452–463.

Substance Abuse and Mental Health Services Administration. (2013). *Results from the 2012 National Survey on Drug Use and Health: Summary of National Findings,* NSDUH Series H-48, HHS Publication No. (SMA) 14–4863. Rockville, MD: Substance Abuse and Mental Health Services Administration.

Swan, G., & Lessov-Schlaggar, C. (2007). The effects of tobacco smoke and nicotine on cognition and the brain. *Neuropsychology Review, 17*(3), 259–273.

Tambour, S., & Quertemont, E. (2007). Preclinical and clinical pharmacology of alcohol dependence. *Fundamental & Clinical Pharmacology, 21*(1), 9–28.

Tapert, S. F., Brown, G. G., Baratta, M.V., & Brown, S. A. (2004). fMRI BOLD response to alcohol stimuli in alcohol-dependent young women. *Addictive Behaviours, 29*(1), 33–50.

Tsuang, M. T., Lyons, M. J., Eisen, S. A., Goldberg, J., True, W., Lin, N., … & Eaves, L. (1996). Genetic influences on DSM-III-R drug abuse and dependence: A study of 3,372 twin pairs. *American Journal of Medical Genetics—Seminars in Medical Genetics, 67*(5), 473–477.

UNODC. (2015). *United Nations Office on Drugs and Crime.* World Drug Report 2015.

Verdejo-García, A., Bechara, A., Recknor, E. C., & Pérez-García, M. (2006). Executive dysfunction in substance dependent individuals during drug use and abstinence: An examination of the behavioral, cognitive and emotional correlates of addiction. *Journal of the International Neuropsychological Society, 12*(3), 405–415.

Volkow, N. D., & Fowler, J. S. (2000). Addiction, a disease of compulsion and drive: Involvement of the orbitofrontal cortex. *Cerebral Cortex, 10*(3), 318–325.

Volkow, N. D., Hitzemann, R., Wang, G. J., Fowler, J. S., Wolf, A. P., Dewey, S. L., & Handlesman, L. (1992). Long-term frontal brain metabolic changes in cocaine abusers. *Synapse, 11*(3), 184–190.

Volkow, N. D., Mullani, N., Gould, K. L., Adler, S., & Krajewski, K. (1988). Cerebral blood flow in chronic cocaine users: A study with positron emission tomography. *The British Journal of Psychiatry 152*, 641–648.

Volkow, N. D., Wang, G. J., Telang, F., Fowler, J. S., Logan, J., Jayne, M., … & Wong, C. (2007). Profound decreases in dopamine release in striatum in detoxified alcoholics: Possible orbitofrontal involvement. *Journal of Neuroscience, 27*(46), 12700–12706.

Winstanley, C. A. (2007). The orbitofrontal cortex, impulsivity, and addiction: Probing orbitofrontal dysfunction at the neural, neurochemical, and molecular level. *Annals of the New York Academy of Sciences,* (1121), 639–655.

Witkiewitz, K., Marlatt, G. A., & Walker, D. (2005). Mindfulness-based relapse prevention for alcohol and substance use disorders. *Journal of Cognitive Psychotherapy, 19*(3), 211–228.

World Health Organization. (1990). *The World Health Organization World Mental Health Composite International Diagnostic Interview (WHO WMH-CIDI)*. Geneva, Switzerland: World Health Organization.

World Health Organization. (1992). *The ICD-10 Classification of Mental and Behavioural Disorders: Clinical Descriptions and Diagnostic Guidelines.* Geneva, Switzerland: World Health Organization.

Yücel, M., & Lubman, D. I. (2007). Neurocognitive and neuroimaging evidence of behavioural dysregulation in human drug addiction: Implications for diagnosis, treatment and prevention. *Drug & Alcohol Review, 26*(1), 33–39.

14
GAMBLING DISORDER

Felicity K. Lorains, Julie C. Stout, Peter G. Enticott and John L. Bradshaw

Introduction

Gambling is a pastime for many people; however, it can become a serious problem for a small proportion of people. Gambling disorder (GD) shares features with many other disorders including substance use disorders, impulse control disorders and obsessive compulsive disorder (OCD). Initially GD was considered an impulse control disorder, and listed in the Diagnostic and Statistic Manual of Mental Health Disorders-4 (DSM-4) alongside kleptomania and pyromania (American Psychiatric Association, 2000). However, the latest revision of the DSM (DSM-5) has reclassified GD into the renamed 'Substance-Related and Addictive Disorders' category and GD is the first 'behavioural addiction' included in this category (APA, 2013). The reclassification of GD reflects an evolving understanding of the similarities between GD and substance-based addictions in clinical characteristics, genetic origins and neuropsychological and neurobiological underpinnings (e.g., Brewer & Potenza, 2008; van Holst, van den Brink, Veltman, & Goudriaan, 2010). Therefore, GD presents a unique opportunity to examine the effects of an addictive behaviour without the influence of an exogenous drug. In this chapter we discuss the symptomatology, onset, prevalence, comorbid disorders and treatment options for GD. Furthermore, we review the evidence of genetic, neuropsychological and neurochemical contributions to GD and examine the evidence for fronto-striatal dysfunction in this disorder.

Preliminary considerations

A variety of different terms are used in the literature to refer to people with gambling problems including: 'problem gambling', 'pathological gambling', 'compulsive gambling' and 'at-risk gambling'. Given the recent reclassification and renaming as Gambling Disorder, we will use this term throughout this chapter. However, like many disorders, gambling problems are proposed to lie on a continuum, and although some individuals may not meet diagnostic criteria, negative impacts are still likely to be present.

Emerging evidence indicates that GD is heterogeneous in both cause and clinical presentation. For example, gamblers who prefer certain gambling forms or who have comorbidities may also have different underlying cognitive or neurobiological characteristics. Theoretical models of GD have now incorporated this notion of heterogeneity and acknowledged that GD is likely to be associated with multiple different pathways (Blaszczynski & Nower, 2002; Sharpe, 2002). However, there is currently no consensus regarding exact subtypes of gamblers, consequently, in this chapter we will not differentiate between subtypes of gamblers, although this is an important future direction.

Onset and prevalence

The 12-month prevalence rate of adult GD is estimated to be 2.3% (Williams, Volberg, & Stevens, 2012), whereas the lifetime prevalence of adult GD is between 0.4–0.6% according to DSM-IV criteria (Kessler et al., 2008; Petry, Stinson, & Grant, 2005). However, the prevalence of GD is higher among certain groups including adolescents, substance abusers, incarcerated individuals and ethnic minorities (e.g., Gerstein et al., 1999; Welte, Barnes, Tidwell, & Hoffman, 2008). Furthermore, an additional 2.3% of the population endorse at least one DSM-IV gambling criterion, suggesting they may be at-risk for developing GD (Kessler et al., 2008).

People with GD generally begin gambling at an earlier age (average 18 years) than gamblers without GD (average 21 years) and onset of symptoms generally occurs in early adulthood (Kessler et al., 2008). However, GD is most commonly diagnosed in adults aged 30–50 years old (Kessler et al., 2008; Petry et al., 2005). Younger age of onset has been associated with greater GD severity, whilst older age of onset has been linked with greater general (non-gambling) psychopathology (Jiménez-Murcia et al., 2010). Like substance use disorders, GD follows a fluctuating course of improving, relapsing and remission (Ledgerwood & Petry, 2006). On average, people with GD report 9.4 years of the disorder (Kessler et al., 2008), however, there are likely to be periods within this that are free from gambling with a period of problematic gambling lasting on average one year (Slutske, 2006).

Men are 4.5 times more likely to develop GD than women (Kessler et al., 2008). However, the prevalence of female GD has increased over time, and this has been linked to the increased availability of electronic gaming machines (EGM) (Dowling, 2013), which are more popular among women and linked to faster development of GD (Tavares et al., 2003). Males typically begin gambling at an earlier age and develop the disorder earlier than females, whereas women generally begin gambling later in life, but progress more quickly to GD (Ibáñez, Blanco, Moreryra, & Sáiz-Ruiz, 2003).

Clinical symptoms

GD is characterised by difficulty limiting time or money gambling, which results in adverse effects on personal, financial, familial or vocational pursuits. The clinical symptoms of GD include preoccupation with gambling, tolerance and withdrawal symptoms, inability to control gambling, and negative effects which impact daily functioning. GD cannot occur in the context of a manic episode.

Preoccupation includes frequently thinking about gambling, ways to continue gambling or re-living gambling experiences. Craving and urges to gamble also commonly occur. People with GD frequently develop a tolerance to gambling and gamble with increasing amounts of money over time. Tolerance has been attributed to an increased need for excitement and cognitive distortions (e.g., a belief that gambling with larger amounts of money will increase the chance of winning [Blaszczynski, Walker, Sharpe, & Nower, 2008]). Withdrawal symptoms can occur when quitting or reducing gambling frequency and commonly include irritability and restlessness, although they can include depression, anxiety, anger, guilt, racing heart, sweating, sleeping problems and headaches (Blaszczynski et al., 2008). Loss of control over gambling and an inability to stop gambling are other key features, as well as the presence of "chasing losses" whereby disordered gamblers will continue to gamble in an attempt to win back previous losses.

Negative consequences of GD include increased psychological distress and affective symptoms, difficulties with interpersonal relationships, poor quality of life and negative impacts on employment (e.g., Dickerson, Baron, Hong, & Cottrell, 1996; Petry et al., 2005). People with GD commonly lie to family members and friends about their gambling and require financial assistance (Kalischuk, Nowatzki, Cardwell, Klein, & Solowoniuk, 2006). Furthermore, approximately 20% of people with GD have committed illegal actions and 11% report being arrested or incarcerated secondary to gambling problems (Potenza, Steinberg, McLaughlin, Rounsaville, & O'Malley, 2000).

Although not a diagnostic criterion, cognitive distortions and erroneous thoughts are common in GD (Myrseth, Brunborg, & Eidem, 2010). Cognitive distortions can include: an exaggerated belief of the ability to win, superstitious beliefs, attributional biases (i.e., wins are associated with skill and losses are ignored), selective memory for wins, the illusion of control and the gamblers' fallacy where a win is perceived to be 'due' (Joukhador, Maccallum, & Blaszczynski, 2003).

Comorbidity

Between 79.1 and 96.3% of people with GD meet criteria for at least one comorbid mental health disorder during their lifetime (Kessler et al., 2008; Park et al., 2010). In community GD samples, nicotine dependence is most common (60.1%), followed by alcohol/substance use disorder (57.5%), any mood disorder (37.9%) and any anxiety disorder (37.4%) (Lorains, Cowlishaw, & Thomas, 2011). However, in treatment-seeking samples, mood disorders are most common (23.1%), followed by alcohol use disorders (21.2%), anxiety disorders (17.6%), substance (non-alcohol) use disorder (7.0%), Attention Deficit Hyperactivity Disorder (9.3%) and psychotic disorders (4.7%) (Dowling et al., 2015). In addition, nearly half of treatment-seeking people with GD meet the criteria for a personality disorder (Dowling et al., 2014). Lastly, people with GD frequently meet the criteria for more than one comorbid disorder simultaneously (multi-morbidity), further complicating this heterogeneous disorder (Kessler et al., 2008).

Whether comorbid disorders develop before or after GD is likely to vary individually. There is evidence of mood disorders developing after GD as a result of financial and psychological distress (Kim, Grant, Eckert, Faris, & Hartman, 2006), however, there is also evidence that anxiety disorders (except PTSD), major depressive disorder and alcohol/drug abuse are more likely to occur before GD (Kessler et al., 2008).

Diagnostic instruments and clinical rating scales

The diagnostic and measurement scales for GD include:

- Diagnostic and Statistical Manual (DSM) for Mental Disorders (Version 5) (APA, 2013).
- International Classification of Diseases (ICD-10) criteria (World Health Organization, 2004).
- The South Oaks Gambling Screen (SOGS) (Lesieur & Blume, 1987).
- The Problem Gambling Severity Index (PGSI) from the Canadian Problem Gambling Index (Ferris & Wynne, 2001).
- DSM criteria-based measurement tools, such as the Diagnostic Interview Schedule and the National Opinion Research Centre DSM Screen for Gambling Problems (NODS) (Winters, Specker, & Stinchfield, 2002).
- Diagnostic Interview for Gambling Severity (DIGS) (Winters et al., 2002).
- Structured Clinical Interview for Pathological Gambling (Grant, Steinberg, Kim, Rounsaville, & Potenza, 2004).

Clinical vignette

Sue is a 55 year old woman with a 20 year history of uncontrollable gambling on EGMs. Below she describes her experience of living with GD:

> "Like many others, I experienced a big win during one of my first EGM games, and I believe this was connected to developing a GD. Initially, I found EGMs were an enjoyable way to spend spare time with family and friends.

However, they slowly grew on me, and over time, I viewed EGMs as a distraction from everyday life. Over 10 years, I spent more and more money and time gambling. Gambling seemed like an ideal way of escaping from difficult personal issues. I found comfort in the anonymous environment gambling provided. I had a chosen machine and believed this machine was lucky. I would insist on being left alone, usually for hours. I didn't want to gamble with friends or try different games. When my family was away I would spend the night there. It was all about me and the machine. I felt helpless in controlling my gambling urges and experienced depressive episodes. I felt too ashamed to tell anyone about my problem. Over time, gambling meant I was unable to pay bills and eventually resulted in losing my job. However, if you'd met me you may not have known I had a gambling problem. I appeared like any other ordinary person but I felt like two different people. After experiencing a particularly bad depressive episode, I sought help. I tried different counsellors and treatment programs. Sometimes this worked and I abstained from gambling for months, however, I have relapsed many times".

Genetics and molecular genetics of gambling disorder

GD is more common among people who perceive a parent to have a GD (Gupta & Derevensky, 1998) and among first-degree relatives of people with GD (Black, Monahan, Temkit, & Shaw, 2006). Heritability of GD is estimated to be 50–60% (Lobo & Kennedy, 2009), however, environmental factors, such as availability of and access to gambling, are also requisites. Additionally, there appears to be a shared genetic vulnerability between GD and antisocial behaviours (Slutske et al., 2001), alcohol dependence (Slutske et al., 2000) and major depressive disorder (Potenza, Xian, Shah, Scherrer, & Eisen, 2005).

Evidence exists of alterations to genes associated with dopamine, serotonin and norepinephrine systems in GD. People with GD demonstrate alterations in a D2 receptor gene (Comings et al., 1996), a variant allele of the D4 receptor gene (Comings et al., 1999), polymorphisms of the DRD1 gene (Lobo et al., 2007) and have lower dopamine concentration but an increase in dopamine metabolites in cerebrospinal fluid (CSF) (Bergh, Eklund, Sodersten, & Nordin, 1997). GD has also been associated with a variant of the serotonin transporter gene in males (Pérez de Castro, Ibánez, Saiz-Ruiz, & Fernández-Piqueras, 1999) and increased noradrenaline and its metabolite in the CSF (Bergh et al., 1997). In addition, there is evidence of lower platelet monoamine-oxidase in GD, (Blanco, Orensanz-Munoz, Blanco-Jerez, & Saiz-Ruiz, 1996) and an association between allele distribution on the monoamine oxidase A gene and severe gambling in males (Ibanez, Perez De Castro, Fernandez-Piqueras, Blanco, & Saiz-Ruiz, 2000). Finally, Comings et al. (2001) provided evidence that dopamine, serotonin and norepinephrine genes all contribute to the risk of GD.

Overview of the neuropsychology of gambling disorder

There is evidence of complex executive functioning impairments in GD, whereas basic processing speed, attention, and learning and memory are likely to be preserved (Goudriaan, Oosterlaan, de Beurs, & van den Brink, 2006a). Research, to date, has focused on inhibitory control, attentional bias and decision making.

There is some evidence that people with GD demonstrate *poor* inhibitory control on the Go/No-Go task and the Stop Signal Task (e.g., Goudriaan, Oosterlaan, de Beurs, & van den Brink, 2005; Kertzman et al., 2008; Odlaug, Chamberlain, Kim, Schreiber, & Grant, 2011). People with GD also demonstrate poor interference control on the Stroop task (e.g., Kalechstein et al., 2007; Kertzman, Lidogoster, Aizer, Kotler, & Dannon, 2011). Mixed evidence exists for whether gambling severity is associated with response inhibition (Leiserson & Pihl, 2007; Odlaug et al., 2011). Despite these findings, there is also evidence for *intact* inhibitory control on response inhibition (Ledgerwood et al., 2012; Lorains, Stout, Bradshaw, Dowling, & Enticott, 2014b) and interference control tasks (Brand et al., 2005; Ledgerwood et al., 2012). Thus, there are findings from well-designed studies of both *poor* and *intact* inhibitory control in GD. These discrepancies do not seem to be explained by the tasks, samples, gambling severity or comorbid mental health disorders.

Mixed evidence also exists as to whether GD is associated with an attentional bias towards gambling cues. Molde et al. (2010) found that people with GD demonstrate an attentional bias to win-related gambling stimuli on a pictorial emotional Stroop task, and Brevers et al. (2011a) found that people with GD demonstrated an attentional bias towards gambling cues in a flicker paradigm. However, no group differences were seen in an attentional blink paradigm (Brevers et al., 2011b) or an emotional Stroop task (Lorains et al., 2014a).

Strong evidence indicates impaired decision making among people with GD. GD is consistently associated with poor decision making under risk and ambiguity on the Iowa Gambling Task (IGT) (Goudriaan et al., 2005; Kertzman et al., 2011). Mixed evidence exists for whether gambling severity is associated with IGT performance (Lakey, Goodie, & Campbell, 2007; Roca et al., 2008); however, the presence of comorbid disorders suggests poorer IGT performance (e.g.,Petry, 2001). In addition, people with GD demonstrate similar IGT performance to alcohol abusers (Goudriaan et al., 2005), further supporting the links between these disorders. Two studies investigated underlying factors contributing to poor IGT performance in GD. Goudriaan, Oosterlaan, de Beurs, and van den Brink (2006b) found that abnormal physiological responses underlie IGT decision making, thus providing support for somatic marker hypothesis in GD (Bechara & Damasio, 2005). Using cognitive modelling, however, Lorains et al. (2014a) demonstrated that IGT performance in GD is associated with a greater attention to the magnitude of gains and less choice consistency.

GD is also associated with poor decision making on other risky, ambiguous tasks (e.g., Lawrence, Luty, Bogdan, Sahakian, & Clark, 2009). Furthermore, people with

GD display an impulsive decision making style characterised by rapid responses without appropriate consideration of options, with poor performances on delay discounting tasks (e.g., Ledgerwood, Alessi, Phoenix, & Petry, 2009) and other impulsive decision making tasks (Lawrence et al., 2009; Ledgerwood et al., 2009). However, two delay discounting studies yielded conflicting results (Holt, Green, & Myerson, 2003; Madden, Petry, & Johnson, 2009). Furthermore, people with GD have demonstrated poor decision making even with explicit risks (Brand et al., 2005), are more willing to sacrifice smaller certain rewards for a larger uncertain reward (Madden et al., 2009) and are less sensitive to losses during decision making (Lorains et al., 2014a).

Preliminary evidence also indicates impairments in cognitive flexibility, idea generation and planning in GD. People with GD have demonstrated poor cognitive flexibility on the Wisconsin Card Sorting Test (Rugle & Melamed, 1993) and the Trail Making Test (Part B) (Kalechstein et al., 2007). Recently, Boog et al. (2014) reported impaired reward-based cognitive flexibility in GD, with intact non-reward based cognitive flexibility, suggesting reward-based learning may be central to cognitive inflexibility in GD. Furthermore, people with GD demonstrate reduced idea generation on a verbal fluency task (Goudriaan et al., 2006a; Roca et al., 2008); however, one contradictory finding exists (Marazziti et al., 2008). Lastly, preliminary evidence indicates poor planning in GD on the Tower of London task (Goudriaan et al., 2006a; Ledgerwood et al., 2012). However, de Ruiter et al. (2009) found no differences between GD, smokers and controls, although a smaller sample size was used.

Overview of the neuropathology of gambling disorder

Fronto-striatal circuitry and gambling disorder

A small but growing neuroimaging field has focused on cue reactivity, inhibitory control, decision making, and reward and punishment tasks in GD. Unlike substance-based addictive disorders, there is currently no evidence of alterations in grey matter volumes or morphological brain abnormalities in GD (van Holst, de Ruiter, van den Brink, Veltman, & Goudriaan, 2012). However, research has demonstrated differential brain activation patterns in the fronto-striatal circuitry and mesolimbic reward pathways of people with GD.

In cue reactivity studies, some evidence indicates *reduced* functional magnetic resonance imaging (fMRI) activation when people with GD view gambling scenarios (frontal and orbitofrontal cortex, caudate/basal ganglia and thalamus) or evaluate pictures for high personal relevance (bilateral nucleus accumbens, left putamen) (de Greck et al., 2010; Potenza et al., 2003b). However, more commonly, when people with GD view gambling-related stimuli, *increased* fMRI activation has been reported in dorsolateral prefrontal cortex (DLPFC), medial prefrontal cortex, anterior cingulate cortex, ventral striatum, parahippocampal gyrus, middle temporal gyrus and amygdala (Balodis, Lacadie, & Potenza, 2012a; Goudriaan, de Ruiter, van den Brink, Oosterlaan, & Veltman, 2010; van Holst, van Holstein, van den Brink, Veltman, & Goudriaan, 2012). People with GD have also demonstrated greater cue reactivity to gambling stimuli than controls using electroencephalography (EEG) (Wölfling et al., 2011). In contrast, during the presence of interference stimuli and inhibition tasks, people with GD have displayed reduced activation in the left ventromedial prefrontal cortex (VMPFC), superior aspect of the OFC, right dorsomedial prefrontal cortex and dorsal anterior cingulate cortex (de Ruiter, Oosterlaan, Veltman, van den Brink, & Goudriaan, 2011; Potenza et al., 2003a).

During decision making tasks, aberrant reward processing has been demonstrated in GD. On the IGT, Tanabe et al. (2007) reported that participants with comorbid GD and substance-dependence displayed reduced VMPFC activity, whilst Power, Goodyear, and Crockford (2011) found that people with GD demonstrated increased orbitofrontal cortex (OFC), caudate and amygdala activation during high-risk IGT decisions. Similarly, EEG evidence suggests increased sensitivity to IGT outcomes in the medial frontal region of people with GD (Oberg, Christie, & Tata, 2011). People with GD also display enhanced neural value correlations in reward areas (ventral striatum, VMPFC, substantia nigra/ventral tegmental area) during delay discounting (Miedl, Peters, & Büchel, 2012). Studies examining decision making during gambling games have demonstrated *increased* neural activation in people with GD. For example, Miedl, Fehr, Meyer, & Herrmann (2010) found that during blackjack, people with GD displayed increased activation in the superior temporal gyrus, right inferior frontal/orbitofrontal gyrus and right medial pulvinar during high-risk choices and decreased activation during low-risk choices. The opposite pattern was found in controls.

On reward and punishment tasks, people with GD have demonstrated reduced VLPFC activation during monetary gain and loss of the Probabilistic Response Learning Task (de Ruiter et al., 2009), and reduced ventral striatum activation during reward anticipation, reduced VMPFC activation during reward outcome and reduced insula activation during loss outcomes of the Monetary Incentive Delay Task (Balodis et al., 2012b). Furthermore, during a simple guessing game, people with GD displayed reduced right ventral striatum and VMPFC activation compared to controls, and gambling severity was negatively correlated with activation in these areas (de Greck et al., 2010; Reuter et al., 2005). In contrast, on a simple guessing game examining reward expectation, van Holst, Veltman, Büchel, van den Brink, and Goudriaan (2012) found that people with GD demonstrated greater activation in the bilateral dorsal striatum during large monetary amounts, and greater activation in the dorsal striatum and left OFC during gain related expectations. Additionally, Worhunsky, Malison, Rogers, and Potenza (2014) found that people with GD displayed increased anticipatory reward activation in the ventral striatum, insula and medial prefrontal cortex during a slot-machine task. The differences in neural activation patterns may be associated with differences in study design, decision phase, level of risk/reward and personal relevance of the task. Finally, people with GD activate regions associated with "win" conditions (uncus, right anterior medial temporal lobe and right inferior occipital gyrus) during a near miss (i.e., outcomes proximal to a win), indicating that they may view near misses more as wins (Habib & Dixon, 2010).

Providing further support of the role of the fronto-striatal networks, GD has been reported in patients with damage to the VMPFC (Floris, Cannas, Melis, Solla, & Marrosu, 2008), during the early stages of the frontal variant of fronto-temporal dementia (Nakaaki et al., 2007), and during bilateral subthalamic stimulation in Parkinson's disease (Smeding et al., 2007). In addition, a recent fMRI meta-analysis reported that collectively people with GD demonstrate increased activation in right lentiform nucleus and left middle occipital gyrus during cognitive tasks, and that gambling severity is associated with increased right lentiform nucleus and bilateral parahippocampus activation but reduced right middle frontal gyrus activation (Meng et al., 2014).

Neurochemistry of Gambling Disorder

Given the links between dopamine and the mesolimbic reward circuitry and its involvement in substance-based addictive disorders, dopamine has primarily been investigated in the neurochemistry of GD. To date, no group difference has been found between people with GD and controls in striatal D2/D3 receptor availability and dopamine release (Boileau et al., 2012; Clark et al., 2012). However, individual GD traits (impulsivity and gambling severity) may be associated with dopamine receptor binding (Boileau et al., 2012; Clark et al., 2012). Furthermore, altered dopamine release influences decision making differently in people with GD and controls, and increased dopamine release is associated with poorer decision making, increased risk-taking and excitement in GD (Linnet, Møller, Peterson, Gjedde, & Doudet, 2010a, 2010b; Linnet, Peterson, Doudet, Gjedde, & Moller, 2010c). Finally, dopamine agonist treatment for Parkinson's disease has been associated with GD (Pirritano et al., 2014).

Treatment

Several psychological and pharmacological treatments have been trialled in GD. Psychological studies have focused on cognitive behavioural therapy (CBT), motivational interviewing (MI) or motivational enhancement therapy; however, psychoanalytical, psychodynamic, Gamblers Anonymous and self-help treatments also exist (Cowlishaw et al., 2012; Pallesen, Mitsem, Kvale, Johnsen, & Molde, 2005). A Cochrane review found evidence for the short term (0–3 months) efficacy of CBT in reducing gambling behaviour and other GD symptoms, and preliminary evidence for MI in reducing gambling behaviour (Cowlishaw et al., 2012). However, the long term effectiveness of psychological treatments is not well known and results were based on limited research (Cowlishaw et al., 2012).

In the pharmacological literature, antidepressants (e.g., Black et al., 2007; Saiz-Ruiz et al., 2005) and mood stabilisers (lithium and topiramate) (Berlin et al., 2013; Hollander, Pallanti, Allen, Sood, & Baldini Rossi, 2005) have demonstrated mixed results in GD, whilst atypical antipsychotics have not been effective (e.g., McElroy, Nelson, Welge, Kaehler, & Keck Jr, 2008). In contrast, opioid antagonists have demonstrated promising results, with naltrexone and nalmefene reducing gambling symptoms (Grant, Kim, & Hartman, 2008; Grant, Odlaug, Potenza, Hollander, & Kim, 2010). However, a further naltrexone study (with a lower dose) was not effective (Toneatto, Brands, & Selby, 2009). Recently, preliminary evidence supports the use of glutamatergic agents (Grant, Chamberlain, Odlaug, Potenza, & Kim, 2010; Grant, Kim, & Odlaug, 2007).

Regardless of treatment, relapse rates remain high, with only 8% of people with GD abstinent 12 months post quitting (Hodgins & el-Guebaly, 2004). In addition, most people with GD do not seek treatment, with only 7–12% of people with GD ever presenting formally for treatment; therefore there is a high rate of natural recovery in GD (Slutske, 2006).

Summary

GD is a complex psychiatric disorder which shares similarities with many other disorders including OCD, impulse control disorders and Attention Deficit Hyperactivity Disorder, although it is most closely aligned with substance-based addictive disorders. GD is primarily associated with a loss of self-regulation and control which manifests as urges/cravings, withdrawal symptoms, preoccupation and tolerance, which leads to dysfunction in everyday life.

GD symptoms manifest in early adulthood, although symptoms develop gradually, and diagnosis is often not for many years. Similar to other disorders, men are more likely to develop GD earlier than women, although the prevalence of GD in women is increasing. High rates of comorbid psychiatric disorders are common in GD. Similar to other disorders associated with impaired control, GD is associated with a fluctuating course of relapsing, recovery and remission. There is evidence of a genetic link in GD, and a genetic association between GD and substance-based addictive disorders, depression and personality traits (e.g., antisocial behaviour). However, no candidate genes have been identified to date. Dopamine, serotonin and norepinephrine systems are all reportedly involved, although similar to substance-based addictive disorders, dopamine appears to be most strongly associated with GD.

Neuropsychological evidence suggests that GD is associated with impairments in certain higher-level executive functions. There is robust evidence of impaired decision making in GD. People with GD make poor decisions under risk and ambiguity and demonstrate an impulsive decision making style despite explicit risk/reward information, and this appears to be associated with abnormal reward processing.

There is partial support for poor inhibitory control and greater attentional bias towards gambling cues. It is likely that poor inhibitory control and attentional bias may occur under certain conditions and may vary individually. Furthermore, preliminary evidence suggests poor cognitive flexibility, idea generation and planning in GD.

Neurobiologically, strong evidence implicates the fronto-striatal circuitry and mesolimbic reward pathways in GD. In the presence of gambling stimuli or during gambling, people with GD generally demonstrate increased activation in regions associated with the reward pathways and fronto-striatal networks (i.e., DLPFC, OFC, parahippocampal gyrus and amygdala). In contrast, people with GD appear to demonstrate reduced fronto-striatal activation during inhibitory control tasks, and aberrant reward processing occurs during decision making and reward and punishment paradigms. Collectively, these findings provide support for altered fronto-striatal functioning and mesolimbic reward pathways in people with GD, and activation likely differs situationally.

In regards to treatment, CBT, MI and opioid antagonists have demonstrated efficacy in reducing gambling symptoms, particularly over the short term and there is promising recent evidence for glutamatergic agents. However, the long term benefits of these treatments are not well known and further research is required, as most studies were of limited duration and used small heterogeneous sample sizes. Akin to many disorders associated with the fronto-striatal networks, GD is heterogeneous in its nature and manifestation. Heterogeneity is present in the clinical symptoms, onset, genetics, neuropsychology, neurobiology and neurochemistry, and growing evidence indicates subtypes of GD may exist.

Research in GD is still in its infancy and the neuropsychological and neurobiological underpinnings of this complex disorder are only beginning to emerge. However, there is clear evidence that dysfunction occurs within the fronto-striatal circuitry and mesolimbic reward systems of people with GD, and this dysfunction likely relates to difficulties in higher-level executive functions. In this regard, GD may pave the way for understanding of other potential "behavioural addictions".

Abbreviations

APA: American Psychological Association
CBT: Cognitive Behaviour Therapy
DSM: Diagnostic and Statistical Manual of Mental Health Disorders
EEG: Electroencephalography
EGM: Electronic Gaming Machine
fMRI: functional Magnetic Resonance Imaging
GD: Gambling Disorder
IGT: Iowa Gambling Task
MI: Motivational Interviewing

OFC: Orbitofrontal Cortex
VLPFC: Ventrolateral Prefrontal Cortex
VMPFC: Ventromedial Prefrontal Cortex

Further readings

Blaszczynski, A., & Nower, L. (2002). A pathways model of problem and pathological gambling. *Addiction, 97,* 487–499.

Brewer, J. A., & Potenza, M. N. (2008). The neurobiology and genetics of impulse control disorders: Relationships to drug addictions. *Biochemical Pharmacology, 75,* 63–75.

Cowlishaw, S., Merkouris, S., Dowling, N., Anderson, C., Jackson, A., & Thomas, S. (2012). Psychological therapies for pathological and problem gambling. *Cochrane Database Systematic Reviews, 11,* CD008937.

Grant, J. E., Odlaug, B. L., & Schreiber, L. R. N. (2014). Pharmacological treatments in pathological gambling. *British Journal of Clinical Pharmacology, 77,* 375–381.

van Holst, R. J., van den Brink, W., Veltman, D. J., & Goudriaan, A. E. (2010). Why gamblers fail to win: A review of cognitive and neuroimaging findings in pathological gambling. *Neuroscience and Biobehavioral Reviews, 34,* 87–107.

Verdejo-García, A., Lawrence, A. J., & Clark, L. (2008). Impulsivity as a vulnerability marker for substance-use disorders: Review of findings from high-risk research, problem gamblers and genetic association studies. *Neuroscience & Biobehavioral Reviews, 32,* 777–810.

References

American Psychiatric Association (APA). (2000). *Diagnostic and Statistical Manual of Mental Disorders (DSM-IV-TR).* Washington, DC: APA.

American Psychiatric Association (APA). (2013). *Diagnostic and Statistical Manual of Mental Disorders (DSM-5).* American Psychiatric Publishing.

Balodis, I., Lacadie, C., & Potenza, M. (2012a). A preliminary study of the neural correlates of the intensities of self-reported gambling urges and emotions in men with pathological gambling. *Journal of Gambling Studies, 28*(3), 493–513. doi: 10.1007/s10899-011-9259-8.

Balodis, I. M., Kober, H., Worhunsky, P. D., Stevens, M. C., Pearlson, G. D., & Potenza, M.N. (2012b). Diminished frontostriatal activity during processing of monetary rewards and losses in pathological gambling. *Biological Psychiatry, 71*(8), 749–757. doi: 10.1016/j.biopsych.2012.01.006.

Bechara, A., & Damasio, A. R. (2005). The somatic marker hypothesis: A neural theory of economic decision. *Games and Economic Behavior, 52*(2), 336–372. doi:10.1016/j.geb.2004.06.010.

Bergh, C., Eklund, T., Sodersten, P., & Nordin, C. (1997). Altered dopamine function in pathological gambling. *Psychological Medicine, 27*(2), 473–475.

Berlin, H. A., Braun, A., Simeon, D., Koran, L. M., Potenza, M. N., McElroy, S. L., … & Hollander, E. (2013). A double-blind, placebo-controlled trial of topiramate for pathological gambling. *The World Journal of Biological Psychiatry, 14*(2), 121–128. doi: 10.3109/15622975.2011.560964.

Black, D. W., Arndt, S., Coryell, W. H., Argo, T., Forbush, K. T., Shaw, M. C., … & Allen, J. (2007). Bupropion in the treatment of pathological gambling: A randomized, double-blind, placebo-controlled, flexible-dose study. *Journal of Clinical Psychopharmacology, 27*(2), 143–150.

Black, D.W., Monahan, P. O., Temkit, M. H., & Shaw, M. (2006). A family study of pathological gambling. *Psychiatry Research, 141*, 295–303.

Blanco, C., Orensanz-Munoz, L., Blanco-Jerez, C., & Saiz-Ruiz, J. (1996). Pathological gambling and platelet MAO activity: A psychobiological study. *American Journal of Psychiatry, 153*(1), 119–121.

Blaszczynski, A., & Nower, L. (2002). A pathways model of problem and pathological gambling. *Addiction, 97*(5), 487–499.

Blaszczynski, A., Walker, M., Sharpe, L., & Nower, L. (2008). Withdrawal and tolerance phenomenon in problem gambling. *International Gambling Studies, 8*, 179–192.

Boileau, I., Payer, D., Chugani, B., Lobo, D., Behzadi, A., Rusjan, P.M., ... & Zack, M. (2012). The D2/3 dopamine receptor in pathological gambling: A position emission tomography study with [11C]-(+)-propyl-hexahydro-naphtho-oxazin and [11C]raclopride. *Addiction, 108*(5), 953–63. doi: 10.1111/add.12066.

Boog, M., Hoppener, P., V. D. Wetering, B. J., Goudriaan, A. E., Boog, M. C., & Franken, I. H. (2014). Cognitive inflexibility in gamblers is primarily present in reward-related decision making. *Frontiers in Human Neuroscience, 8*, 569. doi: 10.3389/fnhum.2014.00569.

Brand, M., Kalbe, E., Labudda, K., Fujiwara, E., Kessler, J., & Markowitsch, H. J. (2005). Decision-making impairments in patients with pathological gambling. *Psychiatry Research, 133*(1), 91–99.

Brevers, D., Cleeremans, A., Bechara, A., Laloyaux, C., Kornreich, C., Verbanck, P., & Noel, X. (2011a). Time course of attentional bias for gambling information in problem gambling. *Psychology of Addictive Behaviors, 25*(4), 675–82. doi: 10.1037/a0024201.

Brevers, D., Cleeremans, A., Tibboel, H., Bechara, A., Kornreich, C., Verbanck, P., & Noel, X. (2011b). Reduced attentional blink for gambling-related stimuli in problem gamblers. *Journal of Behavior Therapy and Experimental Psychiatry, 42*(3), 265–269. doi: 10.1016/j.jbtep.2011.01.005.

Brewer, J. A., & Potenza, M. N. (2008). The neurobiology and genetics of impulse control disorders: Relationships to drug addictions. *Biochemical Pharmacology, 75*(1), 63–75.

Clark, L., Stokes, P. R., Wu, K., Michalczuk, R., Benecke, A., Watson, B. J., ... & Lingford-Hughes, A.R. (2012). Striatal dopamine D2/D3 receptor binding in pathological gambling is correlated with mood-related impulsivity. *Neuroimage, 63*(1), 40–46. doi: 10.1016/j.neuroimage.2012.06.067.

Cognat, E., Lagarde, J., Decaix, C., Hainque, E., Azizi, L., Gaura-Schmidt, V., ... & Levy, R. (2010). "Habit" gambling behaviour caused by ischemic lesions affecting the cognitive territories of the basal ganglia. *Journal of Neurology, 257*(10), 1628–1632. doi: 10.1007/s00415-010-5579-3.

Comings, D. E., Gade-Andavolu, R., Gonzalez, N., Wu, S., Muhleman, D., Chen, C., ... & Rosenthal, R.J. (2001). The additive effect of neurotransmitter genes in pathological gambling. *Clinical Genetics, 60*(2), 107–116.

Comings, D. E., Gonzalez, N., Wu, S., Gade, R., Muhleman, D., Saucier, G., ... & MacMurray, J.P. (1999). Studies of the 48 bp repeat polymorphism of the DRD4 gene in impulsive, compulsive, addictive behaviors: Tourette syndrome, ADHD, pathological gambling, and substance abuse. *American Journal of Medical Genetics-Neuropsychiatric Genetics, 88*(4), 358–368.

Comings, D. E., Rosenthal, R. J., Lesieur, H. R., Rugle, L. J., Muhleman, D., Chiu, C., ... & Gade, R. (1996). A study of the dopamine D2 receptor gene in pathological gambling. *Pharmacogenetics and Genomics, 63*, 223–234.

Cowlishaw, S., Merkouris, S., Dowling, N., Anderson, C., Jackson, A., & Thomas, S. (2012). Psychological therapies for pathological and problem gambling. *The Cochrane Database of Systematic Reviews, 11*, CD008937. doi: 10.1002/14651858.CD008937.pub2.

de Greck, M., Enzi, B., Prorsch, U., Gantman, A., Tempelmann, C., & Northoff, G. (2010). Decreased neuronal activity in reward circuitry of pathological gamblers during processing of personal relevant stimuli. *Human Brain Mapping, 31*(11), 1802–1812. doi: 10.1002/hbm.20981.

de Ruiter, M. B., Oosterlaan, J., Veltman, D. J., van den Brink, W., & Goudriaan, A. E. (2011). Similar hyporesponsiveness of the dorsomedial prefrontal cortex in problem gamblers and heavy smokers during an inhibitory control task. *Drug and Alcohol Dependence, 121*(1–2), 81–89. doi: 10.1016/j.drugalcdep.2011.08.010.

de Ruiter, M. B., Veltman, D. J., Goudriaan, A. E., Oosterlaan, J., Sjoerds, Z., & van den Brink, W. (2009). Response perseveration and ventral prefrontal sensitivity to reward and punishment in male problem gamblers and smokers. *Neuropsychopharmacology, 34*(4), 1027–1038. doi: 10.1038/npp.2008.

Dickerson, M., Baron, E., Hong, S. M., & Cottrell, D. (1996). Estimating the extent and degree of gambling related problems in the Australian population: A national survey. *Journal of Gambling Studies, 12*(2), 161–178. doi: 10.1007/BF01539172.

Dowling, N. (2013). The cognitive-behavioural treatment of female problem gambling. In D. C. Richard, A. Blaszczynski & L. Nower (Eds.), *Wiley-Blackwell Handbook of Disordered Gambling* (pp. 225–250). Chichester, England: Wiley-Blackwell.

Dowling, N. A., Cowlishaw, S., Jackson, A. C., Merkouris, S. S., Francis, K. L., & Christensen, D.R. (2014). Systematic review and meta-analysis of the prevalence of comorbid personality disorders in treatment-seeking problem and pathological gambling. *Journal of Personality Disorders, 23*, 1–20.

Dowling, N. A., Cowlishaw, S., Jackson, A. C., Merkouris, S. S., Francis, K. L., & Christensen, D. R. (2015). Prevalence of psychiatric co-morbidity in treatment-seeking problem gamblers: A systematic review and meta-analysis. *Australian and New Zealand Journal of Psychiatry, 46*(6), 519–39. doi: 10.1177/0004867415575774.

Fagundo, A. B., Fernandez-Aranda, F., de la Torre, R., Verdejo-Garcia, A., Granero, R., Penelo, E., ... & Jimenez-Murcia, S. (2014). Dopamine DRD2/ANKK1 Taq1a and DAT1VNTR polymorphisms are associated with a cognitive flexibility profile in pathological gamblers. *Journal of Psychopharmacology, 28*(12), 1170–1177. doi: 10.1177/0269881114551079.

Ferris, J., & Wynne, H. (2001). *The Canadian Problem Gambling Index: Final Report.* Ottawa, ON: Canadian Centre on Substance Abuse (CCSA).

Floris, G., Cannas, A., Melis, M., Solla, P., & Marrosu, M.G. (2008). Pathological gambling, delusional parasitosis and adipsia as a post-haemorrhagic syndrome: A case report. *Neurocase, 14(5)* 385–389. doi: 10.1080/13554790802385418.

Gerstein, D., Hoffmann, J., Larison, C., Laszlo, E., Murphy, S., Palmer, A., ... & Sinclair, S. (1999). *Gambling Impact and Behavior Study: Report to the National Gambling Impact Study Commission.* Chicago: National Opinion Research Center at the University of Chicago.

Goudriaan, A. E., de Ruiter, M. B., van den Brink, W., Oosterlaan, J., & Veltman, D.J. (2010). Brain activation patterns associated with cue reactivity and craving in abstinent problem gamblers, heavy smokers and healthy controls: An fMRI study. *Addiction Biology, 15*(4), 491–503. doi: 10.1111/j.1369-1600.2010.00242.x.

Goudriaan, A. E., Oosterlaan, J., de Beurs, E., & van den Brink, W. (2005). Decision making in pathological gambling: A comparison between pathological gamblers, alcohol dependents, persons with Tourette syndrome, and normal controls. *Cognitive Brain Research, 23*(1), 137–151.

Goudriaan, A. E., Oosterlaan, J., de Beurs, E., & van den Brink, W. (2006a). Neurocognitive functions in pathological gambling: A comparison with alcohol dependence, Tourette syndrome and normal controls. *Addiction, 101*(1), 534–547.

Goudriaan, A. E., Oosterlaan, J., de Beurs, E., & van den Brink, W. (2006b). Psychophysiological determinants and concomitants of deficient decision making in pathological gamblers. *Drug and Alcohol Dependence, 84*(3), 231–239.

Grant, J. E., Chamberlain, S. R., Odlaug, B. L., Potenza, M. N., & Kim, S. W. (2010). Memantine shows promise in reducing gambling severity and cognitive inflexibility in pathological gambling: A pilot study. *Psychopharmacology, 212*(4), 603–612. doi: 10.1007/s00213-010-1994-5.

Grant, J. E., Kim, S.W., & Hartman, B. K. (2008). A double-blind, placebo-controlled study of the opiate antagonist naltrexone in the treatment of pathological gambling urges. *Journal of Clinical Psychiatry, 69*(5), 783–789.

Grant, J. E., Kim, S. W., & Odlaug, B. L. (2007). N-acetyl cysteine, a glutamate-modulating agent, in the treatment of pathological gambling: A pilot study. *Biological Psychiatry, 62*(5), 652–657.

Grant, J. E., Odlaug, B. L., Potenza, M. N., Hollander, E., & Kim, S. W. (2010). Nalmefene in the treatment of pathological gambling: Multicentre, double-blind, placebo-controlled study. *The British Journal of Psychiatry, 197*(4), 330–331. doi: 10.1192/bjp.bp.110.078105.

Grant, J. E., Steinberg, M. A., Kim, S. W., Rounsaville, B. J., & Potenza, M. N. (2004). Preliminary validity and reliability testing of a structured clinical interview for pathological gambling. *Psychiatry Research, 128*(1), 79–88.

Gupta, R., & Derevensky, J. (1998). Adolescent gambling behavior: A prevalence study and examination of the correlates associated with problem gambling. *Journal of Gambling Studies, 14*(4), 319–345.

Habib, R., & Dixon, M. R. (2010). Neurobehavioral evidence for the "near-miss" effect in pathological gamblers. *Journal of the Experimental Analysis of Behavior, 93*(3), 313–328. doi: 10.1901/jeab.2010.93-313.

Hewig, J., Kretschmer, N., Trippe, R. H., Hecht, H., Coles, M. G., Holroyd, C. B., & Miltner, W. H. (2010). Hypersensitivity to reward in problem gamblers. *Biological Psychiatry, 67*(8), 781–783.

Hodgins, D. C., & el-Guebaly, N. (2004). Retrospective and prospective reports of precipitants to relapse in pathological gambling. *Journal of Consulting and Clinical Psychology, 72*(1), 72–80.

Hollander, E., Pallanti, S., Allen, A., Sood, E., & Baldini Rossi, N. (2005). Does sustained-release lithium reduce impulsive gambling and affective instability versus placebo in pathological gamblers with bipolar spectrum disorders? *The American Journal of Psychiatry, 162*(1), 137–145.

Holt, D. D., Green, L., & Myerson, J. (2003). Is discounting impulsive? Evidence from temporal and probability discounting in gambling and non-gambling college students. *Behavioural Processes, 64*(3), 355–367.

Ibáñez, A., Blanco, C., Moreryra, P., & Sáiz-Ruiz, J. (2003). Gender differences in pathological gambling. *The Journal of Clinical Psychiatry, 64*(3), 295–301.

Ibanez, A., Perez De Castro, I., Fernandez-Piqueras, J., Blanco, C., & Saiz-Ruiz, J. (2000). Pathological gambling and DNA polymorphic markers at MAO-A and MAO-B genes. *Molecular Psychiatry, 5*(1), 105–109.

Jiménez-Murcia, S., Álvarez-Moya, E. M., Stinchfield, R., Fernández-Aranda, F., Granero, R., Aymamí, N., … & Menchón, J. (2010). Age of onset in pathological gambling: Clinical, therapeutic and personality correlates. *Journal of Gambling Studies, 26*(2), 235–248. doi: 10.1007/s10899-009-9175-3.

Joukhador, J., Maccallum, F., & Blaszczynski, A. (2003). Differences in cognitive distortions between problem and social gamblers. *Psychological Reports, 92*(3 pt 2), 1203–1214.

Kalechstein, A. D., Fong, T., Rosenthal, R. J., Davis, A., Vanyo, H., & Newton, T. F. (2007). Pathological gamblers demonstrate frontal lobe impairment consistent with that of methamphetamine-dependent individuals. *Journal of Neuropsychiatry and Clinical Neurosciences, 19*(3), 298–303.

Kalischuk, R. G., Nowatzki, N., Cardwell, K., Klein, K., & Solowoniuk, J. (2006). Problem gambling and its impact on families: A literature review. *International Gambling Studies, 6(1)* 31–60. 10.1080/14459790600644176.

Kertzman, S., Lidogoster, H., Aizer, A., Kotler, M., & Dannon, P. N. (2011). Risk-taking decisions in pathological gamblers is not a result of their impaired inhibition ability. *Psychiatry Research, 188*(1), 71–77. doi: 10.1016/j.psychres.2011.02.021.

Kertzman, S., Lowengrub, K., Aizer, A., Vainder, M., Kotler, M., & Dannon, P. N. (2008). Go-no-go performance in pathological gamblers. *Psychiatry Research, 161*(1), 1–10. doi: 10.1016/j.psychres.2007.06.026.

Kessler, R. C., Hwang, I., LaBrie, R., Petukhova, M., Sampson, N. A., Winters, K. C., & Shaffer, H.J. (2008). DSM-IV pathological gambling in the national comorbidity survey replication. *Psychological Medicine, 38*(9), 1351–1360. doi: 10.1017/S0033291708002900.

Kim, S. W., Grant, J. E., Eckert, E. D., Faris, P. L., & Hartman, B. K. (2006). Pathological gambling and mood disorders: Clinical associations and treatment implications. *Journal of Affective Disorders, 92*(1), 109–116.

Lakey, C. E., Goodie, A. S., & Campbell, W. (2007). Frequent card playing and pathological gambling: The utility of the Georgia Gambling Task and Iowa Gambling Task for predicting pathology. *Journal of Gambling Studies, 23*(3), 285–297.

Lawrence, A. J., Luty, J., Bogdan, N. A., Sahakian, B. J., & Clark, L. (2009). Problem gamblers share deficits in impulsive decision-making with alcohol-dependent individuals. *Addiction, 104*(6), 1006–1015. doi: 10.1111/j.1360-0443.2009.02533.x.

Ledgerwood, D., Orr, E., Kaploun, K., Milosevic, A., Frisch, G., Rupcich, N., & Lundahl, L. (2012). Executive function in pathological gamblers and healthy controls. *Journal of Gambling Studies, 28*(1), 89–103. doi: 10.1007/s10899-010-9237-6.

Ledgerwood, D. M., Alessi, S. M., Phoenix, N., & Petry, N. M. (2009). Behavioral assessment of impulsivity in pathological gamblers with and without substance use disorder histories versus healthy controls. *Drug and Alcohol Dependence, 105*(1–2), 89–96. doi: 10.1016/j.drugalcdep.2009.06.011.

Ledgerwood, D. M., & Petry, N. M. (2006). What do we know about relapse in pathological gambling? *Clinical Psychology Review, 26*(2), 216–228.

Leiserson, V., & Pihl, R. O. (2007). Reward-sensitivity, inhibition of reward-seeking, and dorsolateral prefrontal working memory function in problem gamblers not in treatment. *Journal of Gambling Studies, 23*(4), 435–455.

Lesieur, H. R., & Blume, S. B. (1987). The South Oaks Gambling Screen (SOGS)—A new instrument for the identification of pathological gamblers. *American Journal of Psychiatry, 144*(9), 1184–1188.

Linnet, J., Møller, A., Peterson, E., Gjedde, A., & Doudet, D. (2010a). Dopamine release in ventral striatum during Iowa Gambling Task performance is associated with increased excitement levels in pathological gambling. *Addiction, 106*(2), 383–390. doi: 10.1111/j.1360-0443.2010.03126.x.

Linnet, J., Møller, A., Peterson, E., Gjedde, A., & Doudet, D. (2010b). Inverse association between dopaminergic neurotransmission and Iowa Gambling Task performance in pathological gamblers and healthy controls. *Scandinavian Journal of Psychology, 52*(1), 28–34. doi: 10.1111/j.1467-9450.2010.00837.x.

Linnet, J., Peterson, E., Doudet, D., Gjedde, A., & Moller, A. (2010c). Dopamine release in ventral striatum of pathological gamblers losing money. *Acta Psychiatrica Scandinavica, 122i(4)*, 326–333. doi: 10.1111/j.1600-0447.2010.01591.x.

Lobo, D. S., Vallada, H. P., Knight, J., Martins, S. S., Tavares, H., Gentil, V., & Kennedy, J.L. (2007). Dopamine genes and pathological gambling in discordant sib-pairs. *Journal of Gambling Studies, 23*(4), 421–433.

Lobo, D. S. S., & Kennedy, J. L. (2009). Genetic aspects of pathological gambling: A complex disorder with shared genetic vulnerabilities. *Addiction, 104*(9), 1454–1465. doi: 10.1111/j.1360-0443.2009.02671.x.

Lorains, F. K., Cowlishaw, S., & Thomas, S. A. (2011). Prevalence of comorbid disorders in problem and pathological gambling: Systematic review and meta-analysis of population surveys. *Addiction, 106*(3), 490–498. doi: 10.1111/j.1360-0443.2010.03300.x.

Lorains, F. K., Dowling, N. A., Enticott, P. G., Bradshaw, J. L., Trueblood, J. S., & Stout, J. C. (2014a). Strategic and non-strategic problem gamblers differ on decision-making under risk and ambiguity. *Addiction, 109*(7), 1128–1137. doi: 10.1111/add.12494.

Lorains, F. K., Stout, J. C., Bradshaw, J. L., Dowling, N. A., & Enticott, P. G. (2014b). Self-reported impulsivity and inhibitory control in problem gamblers. *Journal of Clinical and Experimental Neuropsychology, 36*(2), 144–157. doi: 10.1080/13803395.2013.873773.

Madden, G. J., Petry, N. M., & Johnson, P. S. (2009). Pathological gamblers discount probabilistic rewards less steeply than matched controls. *Experimental and Clinical Psychopharmacology, 17*(5), 283–290. doi: 10.1037/a0016806.

Marazziti, D., Dell'Osso, M. C., Conversano, C., Consoli, G., Vivarelli, L., Mungai, F., … & Golia, F. (2008). Executive function abnormalities in pathological gamblers. *Clinical Practice & Epidemiology in Mental Health, 4*, 7. doi: 10.1186/1745-0179-4-7.

McElroy, S. L., Nelson, E. B., Welge, J. A., Kaehler, L., & Keck Jr, P. E. (2008). Olanzapine in the treatment of pathological gambling: A negative randomized placebo-controlled trial. *Journal of Clinical Psychiatry, 69*(3), 433–440.

Meng, Y. J., Deng, W., Wang, H. Y., Guo, W. J., Li, T., Lam, C., & Lin, X. (2014). Reward pathway dysfunction in gambling disorder: A meta-analysis of functional magnetic resonance imaging studies. *Behavioural Brain Research, 275*, 243–251. doi: 10.1016/j.bbr.2014.08.057.

Miedl, S. F., Fehr, T., Meyer, G., & Herrmann, M. (2010). Neurobiological correlates of problem gambling in a quasi-realistic blackjack scenario as revealed by fMRI. *Psychiatry Research, 181*(3), 165–173. doi: 10.1016/j.pscychresns.2009.11.008.

Miedl, S. F., Peters, J., & Büchel, C. (2012). Altered neural reward representations in pathological gamblers revealed by delay and probability discounting. *Archives of General Psychiatry, 69*(2), 177–186. doi: 10.1001/archgenpsychiatry.2011.1552.

Molde, H., Pallesen, S., Sætrevik, B., Hammerborg, D. K., Laberg, J. C., & Johnsen, B. H. (2010). Attentional biases among pathological gamblers. *International Gambling Studies, 10*, 45–59.

Myrseth, H., Brunborg, G., & Eidem, M. (2010). Differences in cognitive distortions between pathological and non-pathological gamblers with preferences for chance or skill games. *Journal of Gambling Studies, 26*, 561–569.

Nakaaki, S., Murata, Y., Sato, J., Shinagawa, Y., Hongo, J., Tatsumi, H., … & Furukawa, T.A. (2007). Impairment of decision-making cognition in a case of frontotemporal lobar degeneration (FTLD) presenting with pathologic gambling and hoarding as the initial symptoms. *Cognitive and Behavioral Neurology, 20*, 121–125.

Oberg, S. A. K., Christie, G. J., & Tata, M. S. (2011). Problem gamblers exhibit reward hypersensitivity in medial frontal cortex during gambling. *Neuropsychologia, 49*, 3768–3775.

Odlaug, B. L., Chamberlain, S. R., Kim, S. W., Schreiber, L. R. N., & Grant, J. E. (2011). A neurocognitive comparison of cognitive flexibility and response inhibition in gamblers with varying degrees of clinical severity. *Psychological Medicine, 41*, 2111–2119.

Pallesen, S., Mitsem, M., Kvale, G., Johnsen, B. H., & Molde, H. (2005). Outcome of psychological treatments of pathological gambling: A review and meta-analysis. *Addiction, 100*, 1412–1422.

Park, S., Cho, M., Jeon, H., Lee, H., Bae, J., Park, J., … & Hong, J. (2010). Prevalence, clinical correlations, comorbidities, and suicidal tendencies in pathological Korean gamblers: Results from the Korean epidemiologic catchment area study. *Social Psychiatry and Psychiatric Epidemiology, 45*, 621–629.

Pérez de Castro, I., Ibánez, A., Saiz-Ruiz, J., & Fernández-Piqueras, J. (1999). Genetic contribution to pathological gambling: Possible association between a functional DNA polymorphism at the serotonin transporter gene (5-HTT) and affected men. *Pharmacogenetics and Genomics, 9*, 397–400.

Petry, N. M. (2001). Substance abuse, pathological gambling, and impulsiveness. *Drug & Alcohol Dependence, 63*, 29–38.

Petry, N. M., Stinson, F. S., & Grant, B. F. (2005). Comorbidity of DSM-IV pathological gambling and other psychiatric disorders: Results from the National Epidemiologic Survey on Alcohol and related conditions. *Journal of Clinical Psychiatry, 66*, 564–574.

Pirritano, D., Plastino, M., Bosco, D., Gallelli, L., Siniscalchi, A., & De Sarro, G. (2014). Gambling disorder during dopamine replacement treatment in Parkinson's disease: A comprehensive review. *Biomed Research International, 2014*, 728038. doi: 10.1155/2014/728038.

Potenza, M., N, Leung, H. C., Blumberg, H., P, Peterson, B., S, Fulbright, R. K., Lacadie, C.M., Skudlarski, P., & Gore, J.C. (2003a). An FMRI Stroop task study of ventromedial prefrontal cortical function in pathological gamblers. *American Journal of Psychiatry, 160*, 1990.

Potenza, M., Steinberg, M., McLaughlin, S., Rounsaville, B., & O'Malley, S. (2000). Illegal behaviors in problem gambling: Analysis of data from a gambling helpline. *Journal of the American Academy of Psychiatry and the Law Online, 28*, 389–403.

Potenza, M. N., Steinberg, M. A., Skudlarski, P., Fulbright, R. K., Lacadie, C. M., Wilber, … & Wexler, B. E. (2003b). Gambling urges in pathological gambling: A functional magnetic resonance imaging study. *Archives of General Psychiatry, 60*, 828–836.

Potenza, M. N., Xian, H., Shah, K., Scherrer, J. F., & Eisen, S.A. (2005). Shared genetic contributions to pathological gambling and major depression in men. *Archives of General Psychiatry, 62*, 1015–1021.

Power, Y., Goodyear, B., & Crockford, D. (2011). Neural correlates of pathological gamblers preference for immediate rewards during the Iowa Gambling Task: An fMRI study. *Journal of Gambling Studies, 28*, 623–636.

Reuter, J., Raedler, T., Rose, M., Hand, I., Glascher, J., & Buchel, C. (2005). Pathological gambling is linked to reduced activation of the mesolimbic reward system. *Nature Neuroscience, 8*, 147–148.

Roca, M., Torralva, T., Lopez, P., Cetkovich, M., Clark, L., & Manes, F. (2008). Executive functions in pathologic gamblers selected in an ecologic setting. *Cognitive and Behavioral Neurology, 21*, 1–4.

Rugle, L., & Melamed, L. (1993). Neuropsychological assessment of attention problems in pathological gamblers. *Journal of Nervous and Mental Disease, 181*, 107–112.

Saiz-Ruiz, J., Blanco, C., Ibáñez, A., Masramon, X., Gómez, M. M., Madrigal, M., & Diez, T. (2005). Sertraline treatment of pathological gambling: A pilot study. *The Journal of Clinical Psychiatry, 66*, 28–33.

Sharpe, L. (2002). A reformulated cognitive-behavioral model of problem gambling: A biopsychosocial perspective. *Clinical Psychology Review, 22*, 1–25.

Slutske, W. S. (2006). Natural recovery and treatment-seeking in pathological gambling: Results of two U.S. national surveys. *The American Journal of Psychiatry, 163*(2), 297–302.

Slutske, W. S., Eisen, S., True, W. R., Lyons, M. J., Goldberg, J., & Tsuang, M. (2000). Common genetic vulnerability for pathological gambling and alcohol dependence in men. *Archives of General Psychiatry, 57*, 666–673.

Slutske, W.S., Eisen, S., Xian, H., True, W.R., Lyons, M.J., Goldberg, J., & Tsuang, M. (2001). A twin study of the association between pathological gambling and antisocial personality disorder. *Journal of Abnormal Psychology, 110*, 297–308.

Smeding, H., Goudriaan, A., Foncke, E., Schuurman, P., Speelman, J., & Schmand, B. (2007). Pathological gambling after bilateral subthalamic nucleus stimulation in Parkinson disease. *Journal of Neurology, Neurosurgery & Psychiatry, 78*, 517–519.

Tanabe, J., Thompson, L., Claus, E., Dalwani, M., Hutchison, K., & Banish, M.T. (2007). Prefrontal cortex activity is reduced in gambling and nongambling substance users during decision-making. *Human Brain Mapping, 28*, 1276–1286.

Tavares, H., Martins, S. S., Lobo, D. S., Silveira, C. M., Gentil, V., & Hodgins, D. C. (2003). Factors at play in faster progression for female pathological gamblers: An exploratory analysis. *The Journal of Clinical Psychiatry, 64*(4), 433–438.

Toneatto, T., Brands, B., & Selby, P. (2009). A randomized, double-blind, placebo-controlled trial of naltrexone in the treatment of concurrent alcohol use disorder and pathological gambling. *Am J Addict, 18*, 219–225.

van Holst, R. J., de Ruiter, M. B., van den Brink, W., Veltman, D. J., & Goudriaan, A. E. (2012). A voxel-based morphometry study comparing problem gamblers, alcohol abusers, and healthy controls. *Drug and Alcohol Dependence, 124*, 142–148.

van Holst, R. J., van den Brink, W., Veltman, D. J., & Goudriaan, A. E. (2010). Why gamblers fail to win: A review of cognitive and neuroimaging findings in pathological gambling. *Neuroscience and Biobehavioral Reviews, 34*, 87–107.

van Holst, R. J., van Holstein, M., van den Brink, W., Veltman, D. J., & Goudriaan, A. (2012). Response inhibition during cue reactivity in problem gamblers: An fMRI study. *Plos One*, 7(3).e30909. doi: 10.1371/journal.pone.0030909.

van Holst, R. J., Veltman, D. J., Büchel, C., van den Brink, W., & Goudriaan, A. E. (2012). Distorted expectancy coding in problem gambling: Is the addictive in the anticipation? *Biological Psychiatry, 71*, 741–748.

Welte, J., Barnes, G., Tidwell, M. C., & Hoffman, J. (2008). The prevalence of problem gambling among U.S. adolescents and young adults: Results from a national survey. *Journal of Gambling Studies, 24*, 119–133.

Williams, R. J., Volberg, R., & Stevens, R. M. G. (2012). *The Population Prevalence of Problem Gambling: Methodological Influences, Standardized Rates, Jurisdictional Differences, and*

Worldwide Trends. Report prepared for the Ontario Problem Gambling Research Centre and the Ontario Ministry of Health and Long Term Care. Retrieved from http://hdl.handle.net/10133/3068.

Winters, K. C., Specker, S., & Stinchfield, R. S. (2002). Measuring pathological gambling with the diagnostic interview for gambling severity (DIGS). In J. J. Marotta, J. A. Cornelius & W. R. Eadington (Eds.), *The Downside: Problem and Pathological Gambling* (pp. 143–148). Reno, NV: University of Nevada.

Wölfling, K., Mörsen, C. P., Duven, E., Albrecht, U., Grüsser, S. M., & Flor, H. (2011). To gamble or not to gamble: At risk for craving and relapse—Learned motivated attention in pathological gambling. *Biological Psychology, 87*, 275–281.

Worhunsky, P. D., Malison, R. T., Rogers, R. D., & Potenza, M. N. (2014). Altered neural correlates of reward and loss processing during simulated slot-machine fMRI in pathological gambling and cocaine dependence. *Drug Alcohol Depend, 145*, 77–86.

World Health Organization. (2004). *The International Classification of Diseases (ICD-10)*. Geneva: World Health Organization.

15
SCHIZOPHRENIA

Tamara May and Paul B. Fitzgerald

Introduction

Schizophrenia is a complex disorder, the aetiology of which remains uncertain despite decades of dedicated research. Numerous studies have uncovered a diverse range of changes in the brains of persons with schizophrenia. These lines of research have included genetic analyses, the study of the post-mortem brains of patients with schizophrenia, the study of the living brain with structural and functional neuroimaging and investigations of neurochemical markers of brain function. These studies have progressively enhanced our knowledge as to the brain processes implicated in this disorder, but as yet we do not have a universally accepted comprehensive hypothesis or theory. Most of the traditional theories, which have focused on individual neurotransmitter systems, fail to adequately represent the complexity and inconsistencies seen in the research literature. Regardless, this is a disorder that is common and produces great disability and suffering. It warrants an ongoing committed approach to uncover its secrets in a manner that leads to improved clinical outcomes. In this chapter we will provide an overview of the disorder and describe the emerging understanding of its cause(s) and how these relate to neurodevelopment and fronto-striatal systems.

Clinical symptoms

According to the Diagnostic and Statistical Manual of Mental Disorders 5th Edition (DSM-5; APA, 2013), Schizophrenia Spectrum disorders lie on a gradient of severity and include Schizotypal Personality Disorder, Delusional Disorder, Brief Psychotic Disorder, Schizophreniform Disorder, Schizophrenia and Schizoaffective disorder. Five domains of abnormalities define the schizophrenia spectrum:

delusions, hallucinations, disorganised thinking, grossly disorganised or abnormal motor behaviour and negative symptoms. An individual may have one or several of these symptoms, resulting in a heterogeneous clinical picture. The symptoms are clustered into relatively independent categories which may point to distinct neural substrates (Bradshaw, 2001).

Delusions are set beliefs which will not change despite conflicting evidence (APA, 2013). They can involve a variety of themes including persecutory, referential, somatic, religious and grandiose, and can be classified further into bizarre or non-bizarre. Bizarre delusions are implausible and not derived from ordinary life experiences, whereas non-bizarre delusions are plausible. Delusions are typically socially oriented, occurring in the context of contemporary social interactions, based on making mistakes in logic and having false premises (Bradshaw, 2001).

Hallucinations are alterations in perceptions that occur without external stimuli (APA, 2013). These appear vivid and clear to the individual, like normal perceptions and not under voluntary control, and are misattributed to real or external sources. Auditory hallucinations are most common in schizophrenia but hallucinations can occur in any sensory modality. Auditory hallucinations are usually experienced as voices which are perceived as distinct from one's own thoughts. Hallucinations and delusions are sometimes referred to as positive symptoms, given an increase or distortion of normal functioning.

Disorganised or incoherent thinking (formal thought disorder) relates to aspects of speech where responses are tangential and conversation may switch from one topic to another (derailment or loose associations) (APA, 2013). Speech may be so severely disorganised as to be incoherent and similar to receptive aphasia, being muddled with words that have no relationship to each other or no apparent meaning.

Grossly disorganised or abnormal motor behaviour can be varied in presentation, from childlike silliness to agitation, which impacts on the performance of daily living activities (APA, 2013). Catatonia involves a significant decrease in reactivity to one's environment and is at the extreme end of disorganised behaviour. Repetitive stereotyped movements, mutism and echoing speech are also part of grossly disorganised behaviour, but may occur in other conditions such as autism spectrum disorder.

Negative symptoms include diminished emotional expression or blunted affect, alogia, anhedonia, social withdrawal and avolition - the decrease in motivated self-initiated purposeful activities (APA, 2013). Negative symptoms may be one of the most disabling aspects of the condition, responding more poorly to treatment than positive symptoms and persisting over time with impacts on social and occupational functioning.

A diagnosis of DSM-5 Schizophrenia requires two of the above five domains of symptoms to have been present for the majority of a one month period, refer to Table 15.1. One of the domains must be delusions, hallucinations or disorganised speech. In addition, the individual's functioning must have become significantly impaired since the onset of the symptoms. The disturbance must have persisted for at least 6 months, which may include prodromal or residual symptoms. In addition,

TABLE 15.1 DSM-5 Diagnostic Criteria for Schizophrenia

A. Two (or more) of the following, each present for a significant portion of time during a 1-month period (or less if successfully treated). At least one of these must be (1), (2), or (3):

1. Delusions.
2. Hallucinations.
3. Disorganized speech (e.g, frequent derailment or incoherence)
4. Grossly disorganized or catatonic behaviour.
5. Negative symptoms (i.e. diminished emotional expression or avolition).

B. For a significant portion of the time since the onset of the disturbance, level of functioning in one or more major areas, such as work, interpersonal relationships or self-care, is markedly below the level achieved prior to the onset (or when the onset is in childhood or adolescence, there is failure to achieve expected level of interpersonal, academic or occupational functioning).

C. Continuous signs of the disturbance persist for at least 6 months. This 6-month period must include at least 1 month of symptoms (or less, if successfully treated) that meet Criterion A (i.e. active phase symptoms) and may include periods of prodomal or residual symptoms. During these prodromal or residual periods, the signs of the disturbances may be manifested by only negative symptoms or by two or more symptoms listed in Criterion A present in an attenuated form (e.g. odd beliefs, unusual perceptual experiences).

D. Schizoaffective disorder and depressive or bipolar disorder with psychotic features have been ruled out because either 1) no major depressive or manic episodes have occurred concurrently with the active-phase symptoms, or 2) if mood episodes have occurred during active-phase symptoms, they have been present for a minority of the total duration of the active and residual periods of the illness.

E. The disturbance is not attributable to the physiological effects of a substance (e.g. a drug of abuse, a medication) or another medical condition.

F. If there is a history of autism spectrum disorder or a communication disorder of childhood onset, the additional diagnosis of schizophrenia is made only if prominent delusions or hallucinations, in addition to the other required symptoms of schizophrenia, are also present for at least 1 month (or less if successfully treated).

there must be an exclusion of diagnoses of Schizoaffective disorder, which involves the presence of both mood (bipolar or unipolar) and schizophrenia symptoms, and bipolar disorder with psychotic features.

Clinical vignette

Matthew is a 30 year old, unemployed single male who lives alone in accommodation funded by his parents. Matthew was an average student, completed high school and commenced university. During this period, Matthew's functioning began to deteriorate after witnessing a friend die in a car accident in which he was the driver. His mood became dysthymic, he disengaged socially, failed his subjects and neglected his nutritional and hygiene needs. He gradually became paranoid he was being pursued by the police for culpable driving despite being cleared of wrongdoing. He became aggressive toward his mother. Following a short period of attempted treatment by a community outreach team, he was admitted to a psychiatric hospital and diagnosed with first onset psychosis. Matthew was treated with antipsychotic medication which reduced his paranoia, however, he later ceased his medication and symptoms returned. He was diagnosed with schizophrenia and has limited motivation to work or study and relies heavily on his parents for financial support.

Prevalence, onset, course and gender

The lifetime prevalence of schizophrenia is between 0.3–0.7% of the population (APA, 2013). Onset is typically gradual and for males is generally in the early- to mid-20s (18–25 years) and in the late-20s for females (25–35 years) (APA, 2013). Although schizophrenia may not manifest until an individual enters their twenties, longitudinal studies show subtle symptoms in childhood, including lower cognitive and motor performance (Dickson, Laurens, Cullen, & Hodgins, 2012; Erlenmeyer-Kimling et al., 2000; Rapoport, Giedd, & Gogtay, 2012). These subtle symptoms occur before the onset of the full condition, including during the prodrome, defined as the time when baseline functioning declines, up until the time the individual meets criteria for schizophrenia (White, Anjum, & Schulz, 2014; Yung et al., 2004). Prodromal symptoms are non-specific and include cognitive deficits, affective disturbances such as depression, social isolation and more broadly, school failure (Allen, Strauss, Barchard, Vertinski, Carpenter, & Buchanan, (2013); Lynall et al., 2010).

Around 20% of individuals who manifest schizophrenia have a good outcome; however, most individuals require ongoing help with tasks of daily living and continue to experience significant psychiatric symptoms; a minority will experience a progressive deterioration (APA, 2013; Lang, F., Kösters, Lang, S., Becker, & Jäger, 2013). Earlier onset of schizophrenia is associated with a poorer prognosis (Clemmensen, Vernal, & Steinhausen, 2012). The rate of completed suicide in schizophrenia was previously thought to be between 10–15%; however, more recent research indicates the rate is closer to 5%, which most often occurs around clinical onset (Palmer, Pankratz, & Bostwick, 2005). Overall, individuals with schizophrenia have a 15–25-year reduction in life expectancy, due in part to increased levels of suicide and medical comorbidity and complications (Laursen, Munk-Olsen, & Vestergaard, 2012; Laursen et al., 2013).

Comorbidity and differential diagnosis

Substantial psychiatric comorbidity exists in schizophrenia, including depression (50%), substance abuse (47%), post traumatic stress disorder (29%), obsessive compulsive disorder (23%) and panic disorder (15%) (Buckley, Miller, Lehrer, & Castle, 2009). Comorbidities are linked with poorer outcomes and commence early on in the condition, with around 30–36% of first episode psychosis patients already experiencing a comorbidity (Sim, Chua, Chan, Mahendran, & Chong, 2006; Sim et al., 2004).

Individuals with schizophrenia are also more likely than the general population to experience chronic medical conditions (Laursen et al., 2012). This includes hypothyroidism, chronic obstructive pulmonary disease, diabetes with complications, hepatitis C, fluid/electrolyte disorders and nicotine dependence which may be an act of 'self-medication', similar to that seen in Huntington's disease (Carney, Jones, & Woolson, 2006). This may, in part, relate to failing to receive medical services due to the psychiatric condition itself (Koran et al., 1989). It is estimated that physical comorbidity accounts for 60% of premature deaths not related to suicide in individuals with schizophrenia, hence detection and treatment of physical comorbidities is critical (Lambert, Velakoulis, & Pantelis, 2003).

Genetics and environment

Schizophrenia was once thought to be a neurodegenerative condition similar to Huntington's disease, but is now generally agreed to be a disorder of aberrant neurodevelopmental processes which occur well before the appearance of clinical symptoms (Erlenmeyer-Kimling et al., 2000; Rapoport et al., 2012; Woods, 2014). Degenerative processes may also be present, possibly in only a subset of patients, and relate to the same underlying pathological processes which cause abnormal development (Kobayashi et al., 2014). There are likely to be multiple pathological processes in the aetiology of schizophrenia which result in the highly heterogeneous symptom presentation. Biological abnormalities may confer vulnerability and interact with environmental stressors to produce the condition via a stress-vulnerability model.

Genetic factors

Schizophrenia is a highly heritable condition. Twin studies show that monozygotic (MZ) twins have 50–60% concordance for schizophrenia (Cardno & Gottesman, 2000). However, no single gene has been identified that causes the condition. There are a number of susceptibility genes implicated, including NRG1 (neuroregulin 1), DTNBP1 (dysbindin), DRD1–4 (dopamine receptors D1–D4), DISC1, COMT (catechol-O-methyl-transferase), GRM3 (metabotropic glutamate receptor), MHC, TCF4, NRGN and ZNF7804A (Stefansson et al., 2009; Tandon, Keshavan, & Nasrallah, 2008; Williams et al., 2011).

Further genetic and neurodevelopmental evidence comes from the multiple dysmorphic features, or minor physical abnormalities, which have been well documented in individuals with schizophrenia and more recently in their relatives (Ismail, Cantor-Graae, & McNeil, 2014; Lane et al., 1997; Scutt, Chow, Weksberg, Honer, & Bassett, 2001). These include a narrowing and elongation of the mid-face and lower face (Lane et al., 1997). Schizophrenia is associated with rare genetic conditions including 22q11 deletion syndrome, with 25% of those with this syndrome having comorbid schizophrenia and those with schizophrenia being 40–80 times more likely than the general population to have the deletion (Bassett, Chow, & Weksberg, 2000; Scutt et al., 2001). This condition is characterised by a long, narrow face, flat cheeks, narrow palpebral fissures, retruded jaw and tapered fingers.

These rare genetic conditions are associated with Copy Number Variants (CNVs), which are deletions or duplications in the genome which can result in gain or loss of expression of the genes they contain. Rare CNVs associated with schizophrenia include deletions at 1q21, 2p53, 3q29, 15p11.2, 15q11.3, 17q12, 22q11.2 and Neurexin 1 (NRXN1) and duplications at 7q36.3, 25q11–13, 16p11.2 and 16p13.1 (Kirov et al., 2009; Levinson et al., 2011; Walsh et al., 2008). The presence of CNVs is associated with a more severe phenotype including childhood-onset schizophrenia (Walsh et al., 2008). Many of these CNVs are present in other neurodevelopmental conditions such as autism spectrum disorder, Attention Deficit Hyperactivity Disorder and intellectual disability, suggesting common brain developmental pathways across disorders (Moreno-De-Luca et al., 2010). These conditions may share pathogenic mechanisms despite different behavioural manifestations (Burbach & van der Zwaag, 2009).

Environmental factors

A number of environmental factors are influential in the pathogenesis of schizophrenia. Prenatal exposure to infection (including influenza, elevated toxoplasma antibody, rubella and genital–reproductive infections) is associated with an increased risk of schizophrenia in offspring (Brown, 2011). Season of birth is also implicated, with higher incidence in those born in late winter/early spring and summer, which may relate to maternal exposure to infectious agents during pregnancy (Mortensen et al., 1999). A range of obstetric complications including placenta pathology are linked to schizophrenia, as are low birth weight and prematurity (Johnson & Marlow, 2011). Advanced paternal age is associated with increased de novo CNVs conferring increased risk (Kong et al., 2012). Complex Developmental Trauma has also been associated with an increased risk of developing psychosis (Morgan & Fisher, 2007). Growing up in an urban environment also confers heightened risk, which may be due to a general stress factor or to increased exposure to influenza (van Os, Kenis, & Rutten, 2010). Migration and being an ethnic minority both pose heightened risk of psychosis, which is linked to chronic social adversity (Bourque, Van der Ven, & Malla, 2011). Overall, the genetic and environmental factors linked with schizophrenia are generally nonspecific and associated with other disorders of neurodevelopment.

Neuropathology

Brain structure

Schizophrenia results in significant structural changes to the brain, which may commence early in development and prior to clinical onset and persist throughout childhood and into adulthood. Studies of high-risk prenatals and infants with mothers with schizophrenia spectrum disorder have revealed, in males only, larger intracranial volume, cerebrospinal fluid, total grey matter and lateral ventricle volumes compared with controls (Gilmore et al., 2010). This contrasts with the reduced grey matter found in adolescence and adulthood schizophrenia; nevertheless it parallels the increased brain volumes seen in infancy in other neurodevelopmental conditions such as autism spectrum disorder.

Longitudinal studies of childhood onset schizophrenia have revealed significant grey matter reductions localised to the frontal and temporal lobes by 20 years of age (Greenstein et al., 2006). In adults, grey matter reductions are present in the anterior cingulate, frontal (particularly medial and inferior) and temporal lobes, hippocampus/amygdala, thalamus and insula and these may be magnified over time (Shepherd, Laurens, Matheson, Carr, & Green, 2012). In addition, there is increased volume of the ventricles and cavum septum pellucidum (Shepherd et al., 2012). Changes in brain volume continue to occur with the onset of the condition, specifically a shrinking of the brain, which may be as a consequence of psychosis though it may also be in part a consequence of medication use. Medication is a confounding variable when interpreting brain volume abnormalities over time, yet even when this factor is taken into account, significant brain volume changes are present (Van Haren, Cahn, Pol, & Kahn, 2012).

Basal ganglia (BG) disorders, such as Huntington's disease and Parkinson's disease, are associated with movement and other symptoms similar to schizophrenia including involuntary movements, catatonia, psychosis and affective disturbance. However, the extent of BG disruption in schizophrenia is still being elucidated, with both increased and decreased volumes found post-mortem (Bogerts, Meertz, & Schönfeldt-Bausch, 1985; Corson, Nopoulos, Andreasen, Heckel, & Arndt, 1999). Recent studies of medication naïve patients with first episode psychosis (with and without movement disorders) and schizophrenia patients have found no differences in BG volumes compared with controls (Gur et al., 2014; Lang et al., 2014). Medication use appears to be related to extrapyramidal symptoms in schizophrenia, which may be linked to enlargement of the BG; however, the contribution of illness versus medication is still being determined (Gur et al., 2014; Lang et al., 2014).

The cerebellum has also been implicated in schizophrenia, with irregular Purkinje cell arrangement and loss described as early as 1959. Recent studies have equivocal findings in regard to volumetric comparisons; however, cerebellar asymmetry differences may be involved (Levitt et al., 2014). Left-greater-than-right hemispheric volume asymmetry has been found that may relate to particular cognitive deficits, given language processing and verbal working memory tasks both activate the right inferior cerebellar hemisphere (Levitt et al., 2014; Loeber, Cintron, & Yurgelun-Todd, 2014).

Reductions in white matter are also present in schizophrenia indicating disturbed structural connectivity in the brain (Konrad & Winterer, 2008; Lynall et al., 2010). These changes predate the first episode of psychosis and occur in medication naive patients (Yao et al., 2013). White matter abnormalities are present in many of the significant white matter pathways including the corpus callosum, insula, anterior limbs of the internal capsule, superior longitudinal fasciculus, cingulum, arcuate fasiculus and uncinate (Konrad & Winterer, 2008; Shepherd et al., 2012). Recent volumetric meta-analysis of white matter revealed that frontal, parietal and temporal lobe volumes show significant longitudinal reductions in people with schizophrenia (Olabi et al., 2011). Taken together, there is clear evidence for underlying brain abnormalities in both white and grey matter in schizophrenia, which begin early in development and confer vulnerability for the condition.

Neurotransmitters

Dopamine, glutamate, serotonin and gamma amino butyric acid (GABA) are all implicated in schizophrenia, and may act in a synergistic manner, with imbalances in one affecting some or all of the others. In particular, dopamine has been a focus, given antipsychotic medications used to treat schizophrenia primarily affect dopamine, with most blocking the D2 dopamine receptor (Kapur & Remington, 2001). Drugs which increase dopamine, such as amphetamines, generally cause positive symptoms such as delusions and hallucinations, even in otherwise healthy individuals, and drugs which act to reduce dopamine levels result in decreased or ceased positive symptoms. Thus arose the dopamine hypothesis of schizophrenia, which posits that psychotic symptoms of schizophrenia are due at least in part to increased dopamine release from the central dopamine pathway, and increased dopaminergic transmission (Crow, 1980). A recent meta-analysis has shown that presynaptic dopaminergic function is altered in schizophrenia, with no or less evidence that there are alterations in dopamine transporter and receptor availability (Howes et al., 2012). The dopamine hypothesis has been updated to highlight a more complex role involving abnormal, rather than just excess, dopamine and better explain the range of symptoms (Davis & Kahn, 1991). There may be excessive phasic dopamine release in specific regions of the basal ganglia, possibly related to the presence of positive symptoms. Recent research also suggests areas of reduced dopamine release in the frontal lobes, particularly within the dorsolateral prefrontal cortex, which may be associated with negative and cognitive symptoms including deficits in working memory (Slifstein et al., 2015) and catatonia when present.

Brain glutamatergic pathways have also been implicated, including impairments in signalling at synaptic N-methyl-D-aspartate (NMDA)-type glutamate receptors

(NMDARs). Drugs, such as ketamine, which block neurotransmission at the NMDAR, produce a range of schizophrenia symptoms including positive symptoms, negative symptoms and disorganised thought, as well as cognitive impairment (Poels et al., 2014). Thus arose the glutamate hypothesis of schizophrenia which suggests there is hypofunction of the NMDAR (Kantrowitz & Javitt, 2010).

GABA is the major inhibitory neurotransmitter in the brain, and there is substantial evidence that cortical GABA neurotransmission is also altered in schizophrenia. This includes decreased GABA synthesis and uptake, which is revealed in post-mortem studies of individuals with schizophrenia (Simpson, Slater, Deakin, Royston, & Skan, 1989; Stan & Lewis, 2012). Cognitive impairments in information processing and working memory found in schizophrenia may be associated with the deficits found in GABAergic inhibition (Daskalakis, Fitzgerald, & Christensen, 2007; Lewis & Gonzalez-Burgos, 2006; Lewis, Hashimoto, & Volk, 2005; Lewis & Moghaddam, 2006).

There have been mixed findings regarding serotonin's involvement in schizophrenia. Prior to the dopamine hypothesis, serotonin was implicated via the hallucinogenic symptoms produced from lysergic acid (LSD), which has affinity for serotonin receptors (Breier, 1995). Serotonin acts together with dopamine, with some atypical antipsychotics having dual serotonin-dopamine antagonism. Earlier studies indicated a reduced density of 5-HT2 receptors in the prefrontal cortex in schizophrenia; however, more recent studies have failed to replicate this finding (Lewis et al., 2014).

Neuropsychology

Cognitive impairment, although not part of the diagnostic criteria, is considered a core deficit in schizophrenia and occurs across most aspects of cognition, including attention, language, memory and the executive functions (Keefe & Fenton, 2007). Attention problems present in schizophrenia as deficits in vigilance, concentration and distractibility (Bradshaw, 2001; Jeste et al., 1996). Executive functioning problems include set-shifting deficits, present on tasks such as the Wisconsin Card Sorting Task, and difficulties with abstract reasoning, monitoring behaviour, inhibition and poor planning (Bradshaw, 2001; Pantelis et al., 1999). Memory problems occur at all stages of encoding, retrieval and recognition, affecting working memory and verbal memory (Conklin, Curtis, Katsanis, & Iacono, 2000; Lee & Park, 2005). These cognitive deficits overlap with other conditions and are nonspecific to schizophrenia. Impairment in cognition is not a consequence of pharmacological treatments or illness chronicity and is present in a mild form in relatives of those with schizophrenia and may reflect genetic risk for the condition. Cognitive impairments are usually moderate to severe and remain relatively stable throughout the illness, even after recovery (Harvey, Green, Keefe, & Velligan, 2004; Rajji et al., 2013).

Subtle cognitive deficits can be identified early in childhood in individuals at high risk. For example, deficits in working memory and attention have been found in children under 9 years old who have parents with schizophrenia (Erlenmeyer-Kimling et al., 2000). Language and speech impairments are also present before the onset of childhood schizophrenia (Nicolson et al., 2014). IQ deficits have been found before 13 years of age in individuals who later develop schizophrenia (Dickson et al., 2012). In the schizophrenia prodrome, cognitive deficits manifest in auditory working memory, verbal fluency/processing speed and declarative verbal memory (Mesholam-Gately, Giuliano, Goff, Faraone, & Seidman, 2009; Simon et al., 2007). The type and severity of cognitive impairment may depend on the age of onset of symptoms (Rajji, Ismail, & Mulsant, 2009). First episode schizophrenia is marked by more severe deficits in immediate verbal memory and processing speed, although there are generalised deficits compared to controls across most neurocognitive measures including attention, language, executive functioning, memory and IQ (Mesholam-Gately et al., 2009). These deficits are similar to those found in chronic, older, adult patients with schizophrenia (Heinrichs & Zakzanis, 1998). The cognitive impairments found in schizophrenia have a pervasive impact on the ability to carry out tasks of daily living, to work and socialise, making them particularly disabling (Kitchen, Rofail, Heron, & Sacco, 2012).

Treatment, including psychopharmacology

Pharmacologic treatments

Symptom specific pharmacological treatments for schizophrenia have been available since the effects of chlorpromazine were uncovered in the mid-20th century. Until the 1990s, pharmaceutical treatment for schizophrenia consisted of a range of first generation antipsychotic drugs such as haloperidol, fluphenazine, thioridazine and zuclopenthixol, which were predominantly high or low potency blockers of the dopamine D2 receptor. These medications were effective in the amelioration of positive symptoms in about 70% of patients, but had little impact on negative and cognitive symptoms (Tandon, Nasrallah, & Keshavan, 2009). Their use was complicated by high rates of extrapyramidal side effects such as parkinsonism and tardive dyskinesia (Dolder & Jeste, 2003), probably made considerably worse over time by the use of doses that were considerably in excess of those required to adequately block the D2 receptor.

We now also have a range of second-generation antipsychotics (sometimes described as atypical antipsychotics), which have been progressively developed over the last 20 years. These have a relatively broader range of actions, although it is likely that the main antipsychotic effects of all of these drugs are mediated through blockade of the dopamine D2 receptor. Drugs like risperidone and asenapine predominantly affect the dopamine D2 and serotonin 5 HT2a receptors. The degree to which serotonergic blockade influences the effects of these drugs remains unclear.

Aripiprazole is unusual as a partial agonist of the dopamine D2 receptor. Olanzapine and quetiapine have a slightly more complex effect on a range of other neurotransmitter systems, as does clozapine, a drug with a unique clinical profile (Tandon, Nasrallah, & Keshavan, 2010). The development of clozapine actually preceded that of the other second-generation medications, although it was not widely used until the 1990s due to other serious side effects. It has specific efficacy for patients with treatment-resistant schizophrenia, something that has not been shown with any other antipsychotic (Chakos, Lieberman, Hoffman, Bradford, & Sheitman, 2001). Its use is complicated by the possible development of agranulocytosis, myocarditis and seizures at high dose. Other second-generation antipsychotics have a variable range of side effects including substantial weight gain with olanzapine, sedation with quetiapine and elevated prolactin with risperidone (Crossley, Constante, McGuire, & Power, 2010; Lieberman et al., 2005; Sikich et al., 2008).

Overall, the development of second-generation antipsychotics has substantially enhanced the treatment options for patients with schizophrenia, and this development occurred with a trend towards more rational dosing of all antipsychotic medications. However, except for clozapine, none of these drugs have efficacy in treatment resistant patients and they have limited benefits for negative and cognitive symptoms (Crossley et al., 2010; Jones et al., 2006; Lieberman et al., 2005). They do have effects on the acute treatment of symptoms and in relapse prevention (Leucht et al., 2003). Over time, treatment with these medications is associated with reduced relapse rates (Cheung, 1981; Moller, 2000) and potentially with better functioning (Marshall et al., 2005).

Other psychotropic medications are used in patients with schizophrenia to target comorbid symptoms. These include antidepressants, anticonvulsants and benzodiazapines for symptoms of depression, anxiety, aggression and insomnia (Pickar, Vinik, & Bartko, 2008).

Psychological interventions

If schizophrenia is precipitated by stress in an individual with an underlying biological vulnerability, efforts to reduce stress have the potential to reduce relapse (Mueser, Deavers, Penn, & Cassisi, 2013). Along these lines, a range of different psychosocial treatments have been used in schizophrenia. These include Cognitive Behavioural Therapy (CBT), social skills training, cognitive training and family-based psychoeducational programs (Bustillo, Lauriello, Horan, & Keith, 2014; Mueser et al., 2013; Wykes et al., 2002). Meta-analyses show a number of treatment approaches to be effective in reducing the symptoms of schizophrenia and associated impairment.

CBT for psychotic symptoms significantly reduces psychotic symptoms, negative symptoms and mood symptoms (Wykes, Steel, Everitt, & Tarrier, 2008). Cognitive remediation training programs typically target attention, memory, executive function, social cognition or metacognition and have larger effects when combined with additional rehabilitation programs (Wykes, Huddy, Cellard, McGurk, & Czobor, 2014). Social skills training programs increase social skills and have additional positive impacts on daily living skills and community functioning (Kurtz & Mueser, 2008; Pfammatter, Junghan, & Brenner, 2006). Given that many individuals with schizophrenia live at home with their families of origin due to the severity of their symptoms, psychoeducation for family members is important. Without this aspect, families may have difficulty understanding and managing the symptoms of schizophrenia as well as navigating the mental health system, thus increasing family stress, resulting in an increased risk of relapse (Hooley, 2007). Family psychoeducational programs for schizophrenia reduce relapses, hospitalisations and increase treatment adherence, and may also reduce the levels of expressed emotion within families (Pharoah, Mari, Rathbone, & Wong, 2010).

Psychosocial treatments which contain multiple elements for first episode psychosis show promise in reducing symptoms, re-hospitilisations and improving function (Penn, Waldheter, Perkins, Mueser, & Lieberman, 2014). Other promising treatments include supported education and housing, social cognition training, peer support services, healthy lifestyle interventions and specific treatments for substance abuse, post traumatic stress disorder and comorbid medical conditions (Mueser et al., 2013).

Summary

Schizophrenia is clearly a complex disorder which affects a substantial number of individuals in our community and that leads to increased morbidity and substantial disability. It has a highly heterogeneous presentation and overlaps substantially with a range of other psychiatric disorders. The aetiology of schizophrenia has not yet been fully elucidated. The pattern of the emergence of the symptoms of this disorder is clearly consistent with a neurodevelopmental origin. There are a range of potential genetic, neurochemical and environmental factors that seemingly contribute to the progressive development of this disorder, as individuals progress from childhood through adolescence and into early adult life. There are widespread brain changes in individuals with schizophrenia and disruption in several neurotransmitter systems. It appears likely that there are pathological abnormalities in dopamine, glutamate and GABA, but it remains unclear whether these changes vary within or between individuals and how these varying pathophysiologies relate to different symptom presentations.

We currently have a range of drug and psychological treatments. However, even when these are applied in optimal ways, a significant proportion of patients continue to experience marked disability. Ongoing research is required to develop better symptomatic strategies and approaches to treatment that are based on a better understanding of the underlying brain and psychological processes that contribute to the development of this distressing disorder.

Glossary

Active Phase: Period where symptoms are acute
Alogia: Poverty of speech; a general lack of additional, unprompted content seen in normal speech
Anhedonia: The inability to experience pleasure from activities usually found enjoyable
Aphasia: A general impairment in linguistic ability
Avolition: The decrease in motivated self-initiated purposeful activities
CNV: Copy NumberVariants - are deletions or duplications in the genome which can result in gain or loss of expression of the genes they contain
First Episode: First manifestation of schizophrenia meeting the diagnostic symptom and time criteria
Negative Symptoms: Flattened affect, disorganised speech/alogia, avolition
Positive Symptoms: Hallucinations, delusions, disorganised or incoherent thinking (formal thought disorder), grossly disorganised behaviour including catatonia
Prodromal Phase: The time when baseline functioning declines, up until the time the individual meets criteria for schizophrenia
Residual Phase: When the symptoms have lessened in severity after an active phase

Further readings

Howes, O. D., Kambeitz, J., Kim, E., Stahl, D., Slifstein, M., Abi-Dargham, A., & Kapur, S. (2012). The nature of dopamine dysfunction in schizophrenia and what this means for treatment: Meta-analysis of imaging studies. *Archives of General Psychiatry, 69*(8), 776–786.

Olabi, B., Ellison-Wright, I., McIntosh, A. M., Wood, S. J., Bullmore, E., & Lawrie, S. M. (2011). Are there progressive brain changes in schizophrenia? A meta-analysis of structural magnetic resonance imaging studies. *Biological Psychiatry, 70*(1), 88–96.

Poels, E., Kegeles, L., Kantrowitz, J., Slifstein, M., Javitt, D., Lieberman, J., … Girgis, R. (2014). Imaging glutamate in schizophrenia: Review of findings and implications for drug discovery. *Molecular Psychiatry, 19*(1), 20–29.

Rapoport, J., Giedd, J., & Gogtay, N. (2012). Neurodevelopmental model of schizophrenia: Update 2012. *Molecular Psychiatry, 17*(12), 1228–1238.

Shepherd, A. M., Laurens, K. R., Matheson, S. L., Carr, V. J., & Green, M. J. (2012). Systematic meta-review and quality assessment of the structural brain alterations in schizophrenia. *Neuroscience & Biobehavioral Reviews, 36*(4), 1342–1356.

van Os, J., Kenis, G., & Rutten, B. P. (2010). The environment and schizophrenia. *Nature, 468*(7321), 203–212.

References

Allen, D. N., Strauss, G. P., Barchard, K. A., Vertinski, M., Carpenter, W. T., & Buchanan, R. W. (2013). Changes in academic and social premorbid adjustment across sex and developmental period in individuals with schizophrenia. *Schizophrenia Research, 146*, 132.

APA. (2013). *Diagnostic and Statistical Manual of Mental Disorders* (5th Ed). Arlington, VA: American Psychiatric Association.

Bassett, A. S., Chow, E. W., & Weksberg, R. (2000). Chromosomal abnormalities and schizophrenia. *American Journal of Medical Genetics, 97*(1), 45–51.

Bogerts, B., Meertz, E., & Schönfeldt-Bausch, R. (1985). Basal ganglia and limbic system pathology in schizophrenia: A morphometric study of brain volume and shrinkage. *Archives of General Psychiatry, 42*(8), 784–791.

Bourque, F., Van der Ven, E., & Malla, A. (2011). A meta-analysis of the risk for psychotic disorders among first-and second-generation immigrants. *Psychological Medicine, 41*(05), 897–910.

Bradshaw, J. L. (2001). Developmental disorders of the frontostriatal system. *Neuropsychological Neuropsychiatric and Evolutionary Perspectives,* Psychology Press/Taylor & Francis, Hove.

Breier, A. (1995). Serotonin, schizophrenia and antipsychotic drug action. *Schizophrenia Research, 14*(3), 187–202.

Brown, A. S. (2011). Exposure to prenatal infection and risk of schizophrenia. *Frontiers in Psychiatry, 2*, 63. doi: 10.3389/fpsyt.2011.00063.

Buckley, P. F., Miller, B. J., Lehrer, D. S., & Castle, D. J. (2009). Psychiatric comorbidities and schizophrenia. *Schizophrenia Bulletin, 35*(2), 383–402.

Burbach, J. P. H., & van der Zwaag, B. (2009). Contact in the genetics of autism and schizophrenia. *Trends in Neurosciences, 32*(2), 69–72.

Bustillo, J. R., Lauriello, J., Horan, W. P., & Keith, S. J. (2014). The psychosocial treatment of schizophrenia: An update. *American Journal of Psychiatry.*

Cardno, A. G., & Gottesman, I. I. (2000). Twin studies of schizophrenia: From bow-and-arrow concordances to star wars Mx and functional genomics. *American Journal of Medical Genetics, 97*(1), 12–17.

Carney, C. P., Jones, L., & Woolson, R. F. (2006). Medical comorbidity in women and men with schizophrenia: A population-based controlled study. *Journal of General Internal Medicine, 21*(11), 1133–1137.

Chakos, M., Lieberman, J., Hoffman, E., Bradford, D., & Sheitman, B. (2001). Effectiveness of second-generation antipsychotics in patients with treatment-resistant schizophrenia: A review and meta-analysis of randomized trials. *Am Journal of Psychiatry, 158*(4), 518–526.

Cheung, H. K. (1981). Schizophrenics fully remitted on neuroleptics for 3–5 years—To stop or continue drugs? *The British Journal of Psychiatry, 138*, 490–494.

Clemmensen, L., Vernal, D. L., & Steinhausen, H.-C. (2012). A systematic review of the long-term outcome of early onset schizophrenia. *BMC Psychiatry, 12*(1), 150.

Conklin, H. M., Curtis, C. E., Katsanis, J., & Iacono, W. G. (2000). Verbal working memory impairment in schizophrenia patients and their first-degree relatives: Evidence from the digit span task. *American Journal of Psychiatry, 157*(2), 275–277.

Corson, P. W., Nopoulos, P., Andreasen, N. C., Heckel, D., & Arndt, S. (1999). Caudate size in first-episode neuroleptic-naive schizophrenic patients measured using an artificial neural network. *Biological Psychiatry, 46*(5), 712–720.

Crossley, N. A., Constante, M., McGuire, P., & Power, P. (2010). Efficacy of atypical v. typical antipsychotics in the treatment of early psychosis: Meta-analysis. *The British Journal of Psychiatry, 196*(6), 434–439. doi: 10.1192/bjp.bp.109.066217.

Crow, T. J. (1980). Molecular pathology of schizophrenia: More than one disease process? *BMJ, 280*(6207), 66–68.

Daskalakis, Z. J., Fitzgerald, P. B., & Christensen, B. K. (2007). The role of cortical inhibition in the pathophysiology and treatment of schizophrenia. *Brain Research Reviews, 56*(2), 427–442. doi: 10.1016/j.brainresrev.2007.09.006.

Davis, K. L., & Kahn, R. S. (1991). Dopamine in schizophrenia: A review and reconceptualization. *The American Journal of Psychiatry, 148*(11), 1474.

Dickson, H., Laurens, K., Cullen, A., & Hodgins, S. (2012). Meta-analyses of cognitive and motor function in youth aged 16 years and younger who subsequently develop schizophrenia. *Psychological Medicine, 42*(04), 743–755.

Dolder, C. R., & Jeste, D.V. (2003). Incidence of tardive dyskinesia with typical versus atypical antipsychotics in very high risk patients. *Biological Psychiatry, 53*(12), 1142–1145.

Erlenmeyer-Kimling, L., Rock, D., Roberts, S. A., Janal, M., Kestenbaum, C., Cornblatt, B., ... Gottesman, I. I. (2000). Attention, memory, and motor skills as childhood predictors of schizophrenia-related psychoses: The New York High-Risk Project. *American Journal of Psychiatry, 157*(9), 1416–1422.

Gilmore, J. H., Kang, C., Evans, D. D., Wolfe, H. M., Smith, J. K., Lieberman, J. A., ... Gerig, G. (2010). Prenatal and neonatal brain structure and white matter maturation in children at high risk for schizophrenia. *American Journal of Psychiatry*.

Greenstein, D., Lerch, J., Shaw, P., Clasen, L., Giedd, J., Gochman, P., ... Gogtay, N. (2006). Childhood onset schizophrenia: Cortical brain abnormalities as young adults. *Journal of Child Psychology and Psychiatry, 47*(10), 1003–1012.

Gur, R. E., Maany, V., Mozley, P. D., Swanson, C., Bilker, W., & Gur, R. C. (1998). Subcortical MRI volumes in neuroleptic-naive and treated patients with schizophrenia. *American Journal of Psychiatry, 155*(12), 1711–1717.

Harvey, P. D., Green, M. F., Keefe, R. S., & Velligan, D. I. (2004). Cognitive functioning in schizophrenia: A consensus statement on its role in the definition and evaluation of effective treatments for the illness. *Journal of Clinical Psychiatry*.

Heinrichs, R. W., & Zakzanis, K. K. (1998). Neurocognitive deficit in schizophrenia: A quantitative review of the evidence. *Neuropsychology, 12*(3), 426.

Hooley, J. M. (2007). Expressed emotion and relapse of psychopathology. *Annual Review of Clininical Psychology, 3*, 329–352.

Howes, O. D., Kambeitz, J., Kim, E., Stahl, D., Slifstein, M., Abi-Dargham, A., & Kapur, S. (2012). The nature of dopamine dysfunction in schizophrenia and what this means for treatment: Meta-analysis of imaging studies. *Archives of General Psychiatry, 69*(8), 776–786.

Ismail, B., Cantor-Graae, E., & McNeil, T. F. (2014). Minor physical anomalies in schizophrenic patients and their siblings. *The American Journal of Psychiatry, 155*(12). 1695–1702.

Jeste, D. V., Heaton, S. C., Paulsen, J. S., Ercoli, L., Harris, M. J., & Heaton, R. K. (1996). Clinical and neuropsychological comparison of psychotic depression with nonpsychotic depression and schizophrenia. *The American Journal of Psychiatry, 153*(4), 490–496.

Johnson, S., & Marlow, N. (2011). Preterm birth and childhood psychiatric disorders. *Pediatric Research, 69*, 11R–18R.

Jones, P. B., Barnes, T. R., Davies, L., Dunn, G., Lloyd, H., Hayhurst, K. P., ... Lewis, S. W. (2006). Randomized controlled trial of the effect on Quality of Life of second- vs first-generation antipsychotic drugs in schizophrenia: Cost Utility of the Latest Antipsychotic Drugs in Schizophrenia Study (CUtLASS 1). *Archives of General Psychiatry, 63*(10), 1079–1087. doi: 10.1001/archpsyc.63.10.1079.

Kantrowitz, J. T., & Javitt, D. C. (2010). N-methyl-d-aspartate (NMDA) receptor dysfunction or dysregulation: The final common pathway on the road to schizophrenia? *Brain Research Bulletin, 83*(3), 108–121.

Kapur, S., & Remington, G. (2001). Dopamine D2 receptors and their role in atypical antipsychotic action: Still necessary and may even be sufficient. *Biological Psychiatry, 50*(11), 873–883.

Keefe, R. S., & Fenton, W. S. (2007). How should DSM-V criteria for schizophrenia include cognitive impairment? *Schizophrenia Bulletin, 33*(4), 912–920.

Kirov, G., Grozeva, D., Norton, N., Ivanov, D., Mantripragada, K. K., Holmans, P., … Consortium, I. S. (2009). Support for the involvement of large copy number variants in the pathogenesis of schizophrenia. *Human Molecular Genetics, 18*(8), 1497–1503.

Kitchen, H., Rofail, D., Heron, L., & Sacco, P. (2012). Cognitive impairment associated with schizophrenia: A review of the humanistic burden. *Advances In Therapy, 29*(2), 148–162.

Kobayashi, H., Isohanni, M., Jääskeläinen, E., Miettunen, J., Veijola, J., Haapea, M., … Murray, G. K. (2014). Linking the developmental and degenerative theories of schizophrenia: Association between infant development and adult cognitive decline. *Schizophrenia Bulletin*, sbu010.

Kong, A., Frigge, M. L., Masson, G., Besenbacher, S., Sulem, P., Magnusson, G., … Jonasdottir, A. (2012). Rate of de novo mutations and the importance of father's age to disease risk. *Nature, 488*(7412), 471–475.

Konrad, A., & Winterer, G. (2008). Disturbed structural connectivity in schizophrenia—Primary factor in pathology or epiphenomenon? *Schizophrenia Bulletin, 34*(1), 72–92.

Koran, L. M., Sox, H. C., Marton, K. I., Moltzen, S., Sox, C. H., Kraemer, H. C., … Levin, L. C. (1989). Medical evaluation of psychiatric patients: I. results in a state mental health system. *Archives of General Psychiatry, 46*(8), 733–740.

Kurtz, M. M., & Mueser, K. T. (2008). A meta-analysis of controlled research on social skills training for schizophrenia. *Journal of Consulting and Clinical Psychology, 76*(3), 491.

Lambert, T. J., Velakoulis, D., & Pantelis, C. (2003). Medical comorbidity in schizophrenia. *Medical Journal of Australia, 178*(9), S67.

Lane, A., Kinsella, A., Murphy, P., Byrne, M., Keenan, J., Colgan, K., … Waddington, J. (1997). The anthropometric assessment of dysmorphic features in schizophrenia as an index of its developmental origins. *Psychological Medicine, 27*(05), 1155–1164.

Lang, D. J., Kopala, L. C., Vandorpe, R. A., Rui, Q., Smith, G. N., Goghari, V. M., & Honer, W. G. (2014). An MRI study of basal ganglia volumes in first-episode schizophrenia patients treated with risperidone. *The American Journal of Psychiatry*.

Lang, F., Kösters, M., Lang, S., Becker, T., & Jäger, M. (2013). Psychopathological long-term outcome of schizophrenia–A review. *Acta Psychiatrica Scandinavica, 127*(3), 173–182.

Laursen, T. M., Munk-Olsen, T., & Vestergaard, M. (2012). Life expectancy and cardiovascular mortality in persons with schizophrenia. *Current Opinion in Psychiatry, 25*(2), 83–88.

Laursen, T. M., Wahlbeck, K., Hällgren, J., Westman, J., Ösby, U., Alinaghizadeh, H., … Nordentoft, M. (2013). Life expectancy and death by diseases of the circulatory system in patients with bipolar disorder or schizophrenia in the Nordic countries. *PLoS One, 8*(6), 1–7.

Lee, J., & Park, S. (2005). Working memory impairments in schizophrenia: A meta-analysis. *Journal of Abnormal Psychology, 114*(4), 599.

Leucht, S., Barnes, T. R., Kissling, W., Engel, R. R., Correll, C., & Kane, J. M. (2003). Relapse prevention in schizophrenia with new-generation antipsychotics: A systematic review and exploratory meta-analysis of randomized, controlled trials. *The American Journal of Psychiatry, 160*(7), 1209–1222.

Levinson, D. F., Duan, J., Oh, S., Wang, K., Sanders, A. R., Shi, J., … Amin, F. (2011). Copy number variants in schizophrenia: Confirmation of five previous findings and new evidence for 3q29 microdeletions and VIPR2 duplications. *The American Journal of Psychiatry*.

Levitt, J. J., McCarley, R. W., Nestor, P. G., Petrescu, C., Donnino, R., Hirayasu, Y., … Shenton, M. E. (2014). Quantitative volumetric MRI study of the cerebellum and vermis in schizophrenia: Clinical and cognitive correlates. *The American Journal of Psychiatry*.

Lewis, D. A., & Gonzalez-Burgos, G. (2006). Pathophysiologically based treatment interventions in schizophrenia. *Nature Medicine, 12*(9), 1016–1022. doi: 10.1038/nm1478.

Lewis, D. A., Hashimoto, T., & Volk, D. W. (2005). Cortical inhibitory neurons and schizophrenia. *Nature Reviews Neuroscience, 6*(4), 312–324. doi: 10.1038/nrn1648.

Lewis, D. A., & Moghaddam, B. (2006). Cognitive dysfunction in schizophrenia: Convergence of gamma-aminobutyric acid and glutamate alterations. *Archives of Neurology, 63*(10), 1372–1376. doi: 10.1001/archneur.63.10.1372.

Lewis, R., Kapur, S., Jones, C., DaSilva, J., Brown, G. M., Wilson, A. A., … & Zipursky, R. B. (1999). Serotonin 5-HT2 receptors in schizophrenia: A PET study using [18F] setoperone in neuroleptic-naive patients and normal subjects. *American Journal of Psychiatry, 156*(1), 72–78.

Lieberman, J. A., Stroup, T. S., McEvoy, J. P., Swartz, M. S., Rosenheck, R. A., Perkins, D. O., … and John K. Hsiao, M.D. for the Clinical Antipsychotic Trials of Intervention Effectiveness (CATIE) Investigators. (2005). Effectiveness of antipsychotic drugs in patients with chronic schizophrenia. *The New England Journal of Medicine, 353*(12), 1209–1223. doi: 10.1056/NEJMoa051688.

Loeber, R. T., Cintron, C. M., & Yurgelun-Todd, D. A. (2014). Morphometry of individual cerebellar lobules in schizophrenia. *The American Journal of Psychiatry*.

Lynall, M.-E., Bassett, D. S., Kerwin, R., McKenna, P. J., Kitzbichler, M., Muller, U., & Bullmore, E. (2010). Functional connectivity and brain networks in schizophrenia. *The Journal of Neuroscience, 30*(28), 9477–9487.

Marshall, M., Lewis, S., Lockwood, A., Drake, R., Jones, P., & Croudace, T. (2005). Association between duration of untreated psychosis and outcome in cohorts of first-episode patients: A systematic review. *Archives of General Psychiatry, 62*(9), 975–983. doi: 10.1001/archpsyc.62.9.975.

Mesholam-Gately, R. I., Giuliano, A. J., Goff, K. P., Faraone, S. V., & Seidman, L. J. (2009). Neurocognition in first-episode schizophrenia: A meta-analytic review. *Neuropsychology, 23*(3), 315.

Moller, H. J. (2000). State of the art of drug treatment of schizophrenia and the future position of the novel/atypical antipsychotics. *World Journal of Biological Psychiatry, 1*(4), 204–214.

Moreno-De-Luca, D., Mulle, J. G., Kaminsky, E. B., Sanders, S. J., Myers, S. M., Adam, M. P., … Weik, L. (2010). Deletion 17q12 is a recurrent copy number variant that confers high risk of autism and schizophrenia. *The American Journal of Human Genetics, 87*(5), 618–630.

Morgan, C., & Fisher, H. (2007). Environment and schizophrenia: Environmental factors in schizophrenia: Childhood trauma—A critical review. *Schizophrenia Bulletin, 33*(1), 3–10.

Mortensen, P. B., Pedersen, C. B., Westergaard, T., Wohlfahrt, J., Ewald, H., Mors, O., … Melbye, M. (1999). Effects of family history and place and season of birth on the risk of schizophrenia. *The New England Journal of Medicine, 340*(8), 603–608.

Mueser, K. T., Deavers, F., Penn, D. L., & Cassisi, J. E. (2013). Psychosocial treatments for schizophrenia. *Annual Review of Clinical Psychology, 9*, 465–497.

Nicolson, R., Lenane, M., Singaracharlu, S., Malaspina, D., Giedd, J. N., Hamburger, S. D., … Fernandez, T. (2014). Premorbid speech and language impairments in childhood-onset schizophrenia: Association with risk factors. *The American Journal of Psychiatry*.

Olabi, B., Ellison-Wright, I., McIntosh, A. M., Wood, S. J., Bullmore, E., & Lawrie, S. M. (2011). Are there progressive brain changes in schizophrenia? A meta-analysis of structural magnetic resonance imaging studies. *Biological Psychiatry, 70*(1), 88–96.

Palmer, B. A., Pankratz, V. S., & Bostwick, J. M. (2005). The lifetime risk of suicide in schizophrenia: A reexamination. *Archives of General Psychiatry, 62*(3), 247–253.

Pantelis, C., Barber, F. Z., Barnes, T. R., Nelson, H. E., Owen, A. M., & Robbins, T. W. (1999). Comparison of set-shifting ability in patients with chronic schizophrenia and frontal lobe damage. *Schizophrenia Research, 37*(3), 251–270.

Penn, D. L., Waldheter, E. J., Perkins, D. O., Mueser, K. T., & Lieberman, J. A. (2014). Psychosocial treatment for first-episode psychosis: A research update. *The American Journal of Psychiatry*.

Pfammatter, M., Junghan, U. M., & Brenner, H. D. (2006). Efficacy of psychological therapy in schizophrenia: Conclusions from meta-analyses. *Schizophrenia Bulletin, 32*(suppl 1), S64-S80.

Pharoah, F., Mari, J., Rathbone, J., & Wong, W. (2010). Family intervention for schizophrenia. *Cochrane Database of Systematic Reviews, 12*. CD000088. doi: 10.1002/14651858.

Pickar, D., Vinik, J., & Bartko, J. J. (2008). Pharmacotherapy of schizophrenic patients: Preponderance of off-label drug use. *PLoS One, 3*(9), e3150. doi: 10.1371/journal.pone.0003150.

Poels, E., Kegeles, L., Kantrowitz, J., Slifstein, M., Javitt, D., Lieberman, J., … Girgis, R. (2014). Imaging glutamate in schizophrenia: Review of findings and implications for drug discovery. *Molecular Psychiatry, 19*(1), 20–29.

Rajji, T., Ismail, Z., & Mulsant, B. (2009). Age at onset and cognition in schizophrenia: Meta-analysis. *The British Journal of Psychiatry, 195*(4), 286–293.

Rajji, T. K., Voineskos, A. N., Butters, M. A., Miranda, D., Arenovich, T., Menon, M., … Mulsant, B. H. (2013). Cognitive performance of individuals with schizophrenia across seven decades: A study using the MATRICS consensus cognitive battery. *The American Journal of Geriatric Psychiatry, 21*(2), 108–118.

Rapoport, J., Giedd, J., & Gogtay, N. (2012). Neurodevelopmental model of schizophrenia: Update 2012. *Molecular Psychiatry, 17*(12), 1228–1238.

Scutt, L., Chow, E., Weksberg, R., Honer, W., & Bassett, A. S. (2001). Patterns of dysmorphic features in schizophrenia. *American Journal of Medical Genetics, 105*(8), 713–723.

Shepherd, A. M., Laurens, K. R., Matheson, S. L., Carr, V. J., & Green, M. J. (2012). Systematic meta-review and quality assessment of the structural brain alterations in schizophrenia. *Neuroscience & Biobehavioral Reviews, 36*(4), 1342–1356.

Sikich, L., Frazier, J. A., McClellan, J., Findling, R. L., Vitiello, B., Ritz, L., … Lieberman, J. A. (2008). Double-blind comparison of first- and second-generation antipsychotics in early-onset schizophrenia and schizo-affective disorder: Findings from the treatment of early-onset schizophrenia spectrum disorders (TEOSS) study. *The American Journal of Psychiatry, 165*(11), 1420–1431. doi: 10.1176/appi.ajp.2008.08050756.

Sim, K., Chua, T. H., Chan, Y. H., Mahendran, R., & Chong, S. A. (2006). Psychiatric comorbidity in first episode schizophrenia: A 2 year, longitudinal outcome study. *Journal of Psychiatric Research, 40*(7), 656–663.

Sim, K., Swapna, V., Mythily, S., Mahendran, R., Kua, E., McGorry, P., & Chong, S. (2004). Psychiatric comorbidity in first episode psychosis: The Early Psychosis Intervention Program (EPIP) experience. *Acta Psychiatrica Scandinavica, 109*(1), 23–29.

Simon, A. E., Cattapan-Ludewig, K., Zmilacher, S., Arbach, D., Gruber, K., Dvorsky, D. N., … Umbricht, D. (2007). Cognitive functioning in the schizophrenia prodrome. *Schizophrenia Bulletin, 33*(3), 761–771.

Simpson, M., Slater, P., Deakin, J., Royston, M., & Skan, W. (1989). Reduced GABA uptake sites in the temporal lobe in schizophrenia. *Neuroscience Letters, 107*(1), 211–215.

Slifstein, M., van de Giessen, E., Van Snellenberg, J., Thompson, J. L., Narendran, R., Gil, R., … Moore, H. (2015). Deficits in prefrontal cortical and extrastriatal dopamine release in schizophrenia: A positron emission tomographic functional magnetic resonance imaging study. *JAMA Psychiatry, 72*(4), 316–324.

Stan, A., & Lewis, D. A. (2012). Altered cortical GABA neurotransmission in schizophrenia: Insights into novel therapeutic strategies. *Current Pharmaceutical Biotechnology, 13*(8), 1557.

Stefansson, H., Ophoff, R. A., Steinberg, S., Andreassen, O. A., Cichon, S., Rujescu, D., … Collier, D. A. (2009). Common variants conferring risk of schizophrenia. *Nature, 460*(7256), 744–747. doi: 10.1038/nature08186.

Tandon, R., Keshavan, M. S., & Nasrallah, H. A. (2008). Schizophrenia, "just the facts" what we know in 2008. 2. Epidemiology and etiology. *Schizophrenia Research, 102*(1–3), 1–18. doi: 10.1016/j.schres.2008.04.011.

Tandon, R., Nasrallah, H. A., & Keshavan, M. S. (2009). Schizophrenia, "just the facts" 4. Clinical features and conceptualization. *Schizophrenia Research, 110*(1-3), 1–23. doi: 10.1016/j.schres.2009.03.005.

Tandon, R., Nasrallah, H. A., & Keshavan, M. S. (2010). Schizophrenia, "just the facts" 5. Treatment and prevention. Past, present, and future. *Schizophrenia Research, 122*(1–3), 1–23. doi: 10.1016/j.schres.2010.05.025.

Van Haren, N., Cahn, W., Pol, H. H., & Kahn, R. (2012). The course of brain abnormalities in schizophrenia: Can we slow the progression? *Journal of Psychopharmacology, 26*(5 suppl), 8–14.

van Os, J., Kenis, G., & Rutten, B. P. (2010). The environment and schizophrenia. *Nature, 468*(7321), 203–212.

Walsh, T., McClellan, J. M., McCarthy, S. E., Addington, A. M., Pierce, S. B., Cooper, G. M., … Bhandari, A. (2008). Rare structural variants disrupt multiple genes in neurodevelopmental pathways in schizophrenia. *Science, 320*(5875), 539–543.

White, T., Anjum, A., & Schulz, S. C. (2014). The schizophrenia prodrome. *The American Journal of Psychiatry, 163*(3), 376–380.

Williams, H. J., Norton, N., Dwyer, S., Moskvina, V., Nikolov, I., Carroll, L., … O'Donovan, M. C. (2011). Fine mapping of ZNF804A and genome-wide significant evidence for its involvement in schizophrenia and bipolar disorder. *Molecular Psychiatry, 16*(4), 429–441. doi: 10.1038/mp.2010.36.

Woods, B. T. (2014). Is schizophrenia a progressive neurodevelopmental disorder? Toward a unitary pathogenetic mechanism. *The British Journal of Psychiatry, 181*(2), 144–152.

Wykes, T., Brammer, M., Mellers, J., Bray, P., Reeder, C., Williams, C., & Corner, J. (2002). Effects on the brain of a psychological treatment: Cognitive remediation therapy functional magnetic resonance imaging in schizophrenia. *The British Journal of Psychiatry, 181*(2), 144–152.

Wykes, T., Huddy, V., Cellard, C., McGurk, S. R., & Czobor, P. (2014). A meta-analysis of cognitive remediation for schizophrenia: Methodology and effect sizes. *The American Journal of Psychiatry*.

Wykes, T., Steel, C., Everitt, B., & Tarrier, N. (2008). Cognitive behavior therapy for schizophrenia: Effect sizes, clinical models, and methodological rigor. *Schizophrenia Bulletin, 34*(3), 523–537.

Yao, L., Lui, S., Liao, Y., Du, M.Y., Hu, N., Thomas, J. A., & Gong, Q.-Y. (2013). White matter deficits in first episode schizophrenia: An activation likelihood estimation meta-analysis. *Progress in Neuro-Psychopharmacology and Biological Psychiatry, 45*, 100–106.

Yung, A. R., McGorry, P. D., McFarlane, C. A., Jackson, H. J., Patton, G. C., & Rakkar, A. (2004). Monitoring and care of young people at incipient risk of psychosis. *Schizophrenia Bulletin, 22*(2), 283–303.

16
WILLIAMS SYNDROME

Darren R. Hocking

Introduction

Williams syndrome (WS) is a rare genetically based developmental disorder with a unique cognitive and behavioural profile. At the cognitive level, individuals with WS commonly have mild to moderate intellectual disability with relative strengths in language, short-term verbal memory and face processing accompanied by more profound weaknesses in visuospatial construction, drawing, number processing and visuomotor integration (Hocking et al., 2008; Mervis, et al., 2000). Behaviourally, individuals with WS are described as overly friendly, gregarious, empathic, with a profile of indiscriminant social drive or "hypersociability", but with difficulties in interpreting social cues and norms, alongside increased inattention, distractibility and nonsocial anxiety (Morris, 2010). At the neural level, there is increasing evidence for widespread brain abnormalities including: anomalous activation of frontostriatal regions that may relate to problems in suppression of inappropriate social behaviours (Mobbs et al., 2007); structural abnormalities in cortico-striatal-thalamo-cerebellar circuits linked to increased inattention and hyperactivity symptoms (Campbell et al., 2009) and reduced volume and connectivity in posterior parietal areas (dorsal visual stream) supporting visuospatial and visuomotor functions (Hoeft et al., 2007; Meyer-Lindenberg et al., 2004).

Despite its rarity, the intense study of WS has its roots in the theoretical debate about modularity of domain-specific abilities in developmental disorders (i.e. independence of language from cognition), which could be shown to dissociate in cases of adult neuropsychological patients. This view of uneven cognitive profiles that remain static and rely solely on the end state (nativist, modular view) has been largely challenged by the research examining developmental trajectories across several domains in WS that emphasise dynamic processes that shape the uneven profile over developmental time (Karmiloff-Smith, 2009). We shall see that this neuroconstructivist approach extends to other modules or domains previously not considered core phenotypic features (e.g. motor control), where domain-general strengths and weaknesses in cognitive processes (e.g. executive function) can have widespread and cascading effects on domain-specific behavioural outcomes.

We first review studies on clinical symptoms and comorbidities and then turn to studies of genotype-phenotype correlations using atypical/partial deletion cases as illustrative examples. We next discuss how patterns of strengths and weaknesses in the neuropsychological profile are broadly consistent with the verbal and spatial dissociation in WS, and then outline how poor planning and visuomotor integration impact on gait and motor features in WS. We will then review studies of atypical structure, neural activation and functional connectivity within and between key regions underlying the unique cognitive and behavioural phenotype in WS. In addition, we will briefly discuss the limited pharmacological and behavioural interventions.

Preliminary considerations

In the unique strengths and weaknesses in the cognitive and behavioural profile associated with WS, there is considerable heterogeneity both between and within individuals (Porter & Coltheart, 2005). There is also much genetic heterogeneity, with regard to the size of the deletion, with a subset of WS individuals showing smaller, larger or partial deletions (Borg et al., 1995; Fryssira et al., 1997; Porter et al., 2012), and inversion or duplication rather than deletion (Tassbehji, 2003; Osborne et al., 2001). This has prompted a re-examination of the common depiction of WS as demonstrating near-normal language and face processing, in the context of profound weaknesses in visuospatial and visuomotor integration (Hocking, et al., 2008). More recent studies have identified distinct subgroups in WS based on strengths and weaknesses in a broad range of neuropsychological functions (Porter & Coltheart, 2005), and genetic variability may map onto the behavioural heterogeneity. Thus, it is important to bear in mind the considerable heterogeneity in WS when interpreting the results of the studies reviewed in the next sections.

Clinical vignette

"Jenny is an 8-year-old girl who is described as overfriendly, irresistibly drawn to strangers, with extreme empathy and lack of social fear, and unusually prolonged eye contact. She has particular strengths in producing language in the most loquacious way despite her low intellectual ability (IQ = 60). Jenny has much affinity for music, especially her sense of rhythm and ability to remember lyrics, with extreme emotional reactions to music. Despite these relative strengths, she experiences specific fears especially related to loud noises, severe learning difficulties, impulsiveness and poor concentration in the classroom. Jenny has extremely poor gross and fine motor skills; she is unable to tie her own shoe laces, and has difficulty judging steps and obstacles around the house, and is unable to draw even the most simple geometric shapes. Despite her strong desire to make friends, she has difficulty making and maintaining peer relationships, often seeking out the company of adults and her younger siblings."

Prevalence, clinical symptoms and comorbidity

WS is a rare developmental disorder with estimates of prevalence usually given as 1 in 20,000 live births, although a subsequent population study reported a prevalence of 1 in 7,500 (Strømme et al., 2002). This discrepancy may reflect better diagnosis of the unique clinical features such as characteristic facial and behavioural features, alongside the gold standard diagnostic test, fluorescent in-situ hybridization (FISH), commonly indicating deletion of the elastin (*ELN*) gene. Individuals with WS have characteristic facial dysmorphology, short stature and global developmental delay, including congenital cardiovascular disease, infantile hypercalcemia and a distinctive neurological profile (Hocking et al., 2008). Both children and adults with WS commonly report sensorineural hearing loss, and an unusual sensitivity to noise (i.e. hyperacusis) (Gothelf et al., 2006; Elsabbagh et al., 2011).

The most common comorbidities in individuals with WS include Attention Deficit Hyperactivity Disorder (ADHD) and anxiety. Children with WS have a high frequency of ADHD symptoms (Rhodes et al., 2011), with many meeting DSM-IV-TR criteria for ADHD as the most common comorbid diagnosis (64.7%), compared to the low rates seen in the general population and other genetic disorders such as Down syndrome (DS) (6.1%) (Leyfer et al., 2006). Of those who met ADHD criteria, 69% were in the inattentive subtype, 27% were in the combined subtype and only 4% were within the Hyperactive/Impulsive subtype. Studies using DSM-IV interviews with parents of children with WS report that the rate of specific phobia is higher in children with WS (between 45–54%) than in developmental disabilities (DD) of mixed etiology (Dykens, 2003; Leyfer et al., 2006), with fear of loud noises being the most common (Green et al., 2012). Obsessive-compulsive symptoms and repetitive behaviours show similarly higher rates (54.8%) compared to DD (17.1%), the most common being aggressive obsessions (e.g. fear of hurting oneself or others) (Green et al., 2012). Generalised anxiety disorder is less frequently diagnosed in children with WS (rates vary from 6–24%), although their worries mainly refer to anticipation about (either positive or negative) future events that often fail to meet diagnostic criteria (Green et al., 2012; Leyfer et al., 2006). Thus, the anxiety in WS may lie at the intersection between obsessiveness and intolerance of uncertainty bearing some similarities to ASD (Wigham et al., 2015).

Indeed, elevated rates of socio-communicative and reciprocal social difficulties in WS suggest some overlap with ASD (Klein-Tasman et al., 2007; Lincoln et al., 2007). In one study, approximately half the sample of young children with

WS were classified by the Autism Diagnostic Observation Schedule (ADOS) as sharing difficulties similar to children with pervasive developmental disorder—not otherwise specified, with problems in pointing, gestures, giving, showing and eye contact (Klein-Tasman et al., 2007). Thus, although individuals with WS appear overly friendly, empathic and socially disinhibited, the significant comorbidities including anxiety, inattention, hyperactivity and reciprocal social difficulties indicate some commonalities with ASD. These social and behavioural difficulties may explain later problems in making and maintaining peer relationships, which can lead to isolation in over 70% of WS adults (Davies et al., 1998; Udwin, Yule & Martin, 1987).

Genetics and genotype-phenotype correlations

WS is caused by a hemizygous (i.e. deletion of one of the two copies) deletion of approximately 28 genes on the long arm of chromosome region 7q11.23. The deletion is usually sporadic, arising from instability at the 7q11.23 locus, leaving the region prone to chromosomal rearrangement during meiosis and is the result of unequal crossing over at misaligned repeat segments. This leads to a common deletion size in most cases, which is typically around ~1.6 mega base (Mb) pairs, and is of interest because 22 of the 28 transcripts that lie within the WS critical region (WSCR) are highly expressed in the brain. Moreover, some of the deleted genes are general transcription factors with downstream effects on the expression of many other genes. Patients with only a partial deletion of the WSCR have dramatically increased our understanding of the links between candidate genes and phenotypic cognitive, social and visuomotor features characteristic of WS.

LIM domain kinase 1

Based on two partial deletion cases involving deletion of only *ELN* and *LIMK1*, hemizygosity of *LIMK1* was the first gene implicated in core impairments in visuospatial constructive cognition in WS (Frangiskakis et al., 1996). However, patients with similar deletions, including *LIMK1*, who also displayed SVAS, did not show the characteristic visuospatial cognitive deficits when using a more in-depth range of standardised and experimental measures of visuospatial functioning (Gray et al., 2006). Thus *LIMK1* deletion alone is not sufficient to cause the impairments in the visuoconstructive phenotype in WS (Antonell et al., 2010a, 2010b).

General transcription factor II-I genes

General transcription factor II-I genes (*GTF21* & *GTF2IRD1*) belong to a family of transcription factors, appearing near the distal deletion breakpoint, and interact with multiple proteins and DNA involved in developmental pathways. Therefore, the GTF2 genes emerge as strong candidates for the main neurological features of WS. Hirota et al. (2003) suggested that *GTF21* and *GTF2IRD1* are likely to disproportionately contribute to the development of brain regions involved in visuospatial functioning in WS. However, a subsequent study in a partial deletion patient that included *GTF2IRD1,* but not *GTF21,* suggested that *GTF2IRD1* may contribute to visuospatial impairments as assessed on spatial subtests of the Wechsler Intelligence Scales for Preschool and Primary School Children (Dai et al., 2009). Thus genes at the telomeric end of WSCR make a significant contribution to the characteristic spatial cognitive deficits in WS.

Karmiloff-Smith et al. (2012), however, report a partial deletion case from *FKBP6* to *GTF2IRD1* (HR), compared to a case with only four telemetric genes deleted (JB), including *GTF21, NCF1* and *GTF21RD2.* The former displayed relatively spared visuospatial functioning on psychometric tests (not typical of WS), alongside enhanced sociability and elevated anxiety as also seen in WS, whereas the latter showed a more autistic-like profile (Karmiloff-Smith et al., 2012). Interestingly, altered expression or duplication of *GTF21* in WSCR has been linked to severe social interaction problems and repetitive behaviours associated with ASD (Malenfant et al., 2012). More recently, Hoeft et al. (2014) used an imaging genetics approach in atypical versus "classic deletion" cases with WS, and identified 1) *GTF21* and *GTF2IRD1* as candidate genes contributing to deficits in visuospatial/visuomotor integration, intraparietal sulcus as well as overall grey matter structure, 2) *LIMK1* for aberrant morphometry of 'social brain' networks (amygdala, orbitofrontal cortex, fusiform gyrus) and social approach behaviour, and 3) STX1A, and/or CYLN2 in overall white matter structure.

These findings raise interesting questions about the role of genes at the more telemetric end of WSCR in severity of cognitive impairment. Indeed, individuals with slightly larger deletions including *GTF2IRD2* (approximately 1.8 Mb), present with more severe impairments in executive function (cognitive flexibility), social and spatial functioning than those within the "classic deletion" WS range (Porter et al., 2012).

It is therefore likely that more than one candidate gene, as well as neighboring genes outside the WSCR, gene-gene interactions, and environmental and stochastic processes, contribute in varying degrees to the characteristic WS phenotype. It should be noted that contributions of genes expressed on the non-deleted chromosome may also influence the WS cognitive and behavioural phenotype. This may arise from DNA sequence variations and epigenetic effects such as DNA methylation (i.e. molecular factors that influence genetic activity or expression without alterations to the primary DNA sequence).

Overview neuropsychology of Williams syndrome

Individuals with WS have been characterised as possessing mild to moderate intellectual disability (IQ between 50 and 60, range 40–100), although debate continues about the importance of IQ test selection and limitations of using average IQ scores given the uneven cognitive profiles both between and within individuals (Porter & Coltheart, 2005). The largest discrepancy is most evident in the relative strengths in verbal skills, with verbal IQ typically higher than nonverbal or performance IQ (Martens et al., 2008). Perhaps the most striking feature to arise from this uneven profile is the modality-specific effects on attention, executive function, memory and planning that tap into the visuospatial domain, an area of profound weakness in WS, and suggestive of disruption to frontoparietal circuits as reviewed in Chapter 19.

Visuospatial, language and face processing

Similar to autism, individuals with WS show a bias toward local feature processing at the expense of processing the global properties of stimuli. For example, early studies employing Navon-type stimuli revealed a superiority at processing the small, constituent numbers (local level) than the larger figures constituted by smaller characters (global level) in both WS and ASD (Bellugi et al., 1988; Birhle et al., 1989; Rinehart et al., 2000). However, a closer inspection of performance by Porter and Coltheart (2006) reveals that individuals with WS show a local bias in *attention* that does not extend to *perception* tasks such as drawing, and is apparent on naming tasks without a constructional component. Hoffman et al. (2003) examined eye fixations when solving block construction tasks, and showed that deficits in global processing may reflect impaired spatial representations (i.e. spatial structure of blocks and their location) that interact with executive processes, such as planning, when puzzles increase in complexity. Thus, theoretical perspectives may need to be revised to account for interactions across attention, executive processes and spatial cognition, and it is perhaps an over simplification to describe individuals with WS as 'local processors'.

Aside from these findings, the debate about modularity of mind has its roots in early reports of individuals with WS scoring in the normal range on language and some face-processing tasks using the Benton Facial Recognition Test (Bellugi et al., 1999). Although expressive (concrete) language and verbal (phonological) short-term memory are relative strengths in WS, the onset of language is significantly delayed, with considerable weaknesses in relational/conceptual vocabulary and pragmatic aspects of language (Mervis & John, 2010). Indeed, toddlers with WS are impaired in triadic joint interaction (Laing et al., 2002), comprehension of communicative intent behind pointing gestures and eye gaze (John & Mervis, 2010) and their use of referential word production occurs well before the ability to produce pointing gestures, contrary to that seen in typical development (Mervis et al., 2003).

The notion of an 'intact' face processing module has similarly been challenged, as people with WS appear to achieve normal scores using atypical cognitive strategies. These processing strategies are characterised by less reliance on configural processing of second-order relational information (i.e. sensitivity to spatial relationships between individual features), and greater dependence on featural processing (i.e. ability to identify the face based on individual features) (Karmiloff-Smith et al., 2004). Although holistic first-order processing (i.e. processing of the face gestalt, or the face as a whole image) may seem intact in WS (Tager et al., 2003), holistic face processing shows developmental delay even though performance is in the 'normal' range later in development (Annaz et al., 2009; Karmiloff-Smith et al., 2004). Moreover, neural responses when processing faces in WS have been shown to be atypical on electroencephalogram (EEG), event-related potentials (ERPs) and magnetoencephalography (MEG) (Grice et al., 2001; Nakamura et al., 2006). As Karmiloff-Smith et al. (2004) suggest, the previous inconsistencies in face processing in WS may relate to seemingly typical face processing being driven by atypical neural processing and underlying cognitive strategies, and the often erroneous assumption that performance in the 'normal range' reflects typical rather than deviant developmental trajectories beginning early in development.

Attention, memory and executive functions

Visual search performance and control of attention in children with WS seem to resemble those described for adult patients with lesions of frontal and parietal lobes. Early difficulties in the selection of targets for visual attention (i.e. selective attention deficits reflected in erroneous responses to distractors) have been described in children with WS (Cornish et al., 2007; Scerif et al., 2004); although abnormalities in attention disengagement associated with impaired saccadic eye movements may underlie some of the visual search deficits (Brown et al., 2003; van der Geest et al., 2004). Atkinson et al. (2003) propose that atypical development of frontoparietal circuits may underpin many of the factors involved in impairments on a range of executive function and inhibition tasks in WS. The phenomenon of 'sticky fixation' was described by Atkinson et al., (2003; Atkinson & Braddick, 2011), with some children with WS incapable of disengaging their attention from a particularly salient target (see also, Brown et al., 2003). Indeed, impairments may only become discernible when inhibition tasks require spatially-directed responses (e.g. on a counterpointing task analogous to an antisaccade task) compared to that on Stroop-like naming tasks requiring suppression of a verbal response (Atkinson et al., 2003). Therefore, the use of verbal strategies to scaffold relative weaknesses in other areas (i.e. visuospatial domain) may represent an adaptive approach to overcome impairments on tasks that require frontoparietal function.

On standardised neuropsychological tests, the executive function profile is one of fractionation in WS, although the profile is not sufficiently different to distinguish from the impairments seen across other genetic syndromes such as DS (Hocking et al., 2014). Although individuals with WS evidence significantly better verbal short-term memory than spatial memory (Jarrold et al., 1999), their impairments on verbal and spatial working memory tasks which require a high level of mental manipulation are comparable to chronological age (CA)- and IQ-matched individuals with DS (Edgin et al., 2010; Devenny et al., 2004). Importantly, individuals with WS perform more poorly on planning tasks such as the Tower of London test than those with DS, where participants are required to reproduce a sequence of movements of balls on pegs to match a goal arrangement (Constanzo et al., 2013). We have similarly found that adults with WS show particularly poor planning during increased demands for accuracy on a computerised Fitts' reciprocal aiming task compared to CA- and IQ-matched individuals with DS (Hocking et al., 2011a). Thus, poor planning may interact dynamically with a range of impairments in WS, from visuospatial abilities associated with block construction to drawing the global features of stimuli, even extending to motor and gait features, reviewed in the next section.

Motor planning, visuomotor integration and gait features

Abnormalities of gait, impairments in stair and surface stepping and poor visuomotor integration are common in WS (Cowie et al., 2012; Hocking et al., 2008). Initial reports suggested that basic gait characteristics resembled a basal ganglia-Parkinsonian pattern manifested as reduced gait speed and stride length (i.e. deficiencies in internal regulation of stride length) with a widened step width as a compensatory strategy for postural instability (Hocking et al., 2009). However, a subsequent study suggested that the primary deficit is not one of internal regulation of stride length, as external visual cues, which normally improve gait in Parkinson disease, by circumventing the faulty internal generation of movement by the basal ganglia-supplementary loop, failed to improve spatiotemporal gait patterns in adults with WS (Hocking et al., 2010). Rather, the well-known visuomotor integration and executive attention deficits may underlie the greater deterioration in gait during both external (visual cues) and internal (attentional strategy to increase stride length) cueing in WS. Indeed, difficulties with stair descent are common in children with WS, which could arise from impairments in executive attention, planning, visuospatial processing of depth cues and visuomotor integration. In general, in children and adolescents with WS, during step descent the overall stepping speed is slowed irrespective of changes in step height, and scaling of movement kinematics does not show the same relation to visually determined step height as seen in typically developing 3-year-olds (Cowie et al., 2012). In a study involving gait adaptation during obstacle crossing (Hocking et al., 2011b), we found late adjustments to foot placement in the final steps prior to stepping over an obstacle in WS when compared to CA- and IQ-matched individuals with DS and TD controls. Therefore, the lack of anticipatory gait adjustments in WS may reflect poor planning and flexibility within the visuomotor system required to transform sensorimotor information during gait adaptation.

The areas involved in gait and posture heavily interact with higher-level cognitive processes such as executive control in WS (Hocking et al., 2013, 2014). Indeed, our recent work on cognitive-motor interference in WS has revealed significant dual-task costs in choice stepping reaction times while performing a concurrent verbal fluency task (Hocking et al., 2013); progressive slowing and more variable step initiation times during a Go/NoGo stepping task which was associated with ADHD-related inattention (Hocking et al., 2013) and greater dual-task gait costs when performing a secondary verbal fluency task that correlated with everyday executive functioning (Hocking et al., 2014). Together these findings suggest widespread effects of fronto-striato-parietal dysfunction on cognitive control of movement and everyday Executive Function (EF) and ADHD-related characteristics in WS.

Overview neuropathology/neurochemistry

Frontostriatal and frontoparietal circuitry in Williams syndrome

Several cognitive and behavioural features, including increased rates of ADHD and poor inhibition described above, hint toward aberrant development of frontostriatal circuits in WS. Moreover, the compulsion to engage and approach both familiar and unfamiliar people may originate in core impairments in response inhibition (Porter et al., 2007). In a functional magnetic resonance imaging (fMRI) study, individuals with WS showed comparable behavioural accuracy (albeit slower reaction time) on a Go/NoGo task to that seen among age-matched typically developing (TD) controls (Mobbs et al., 2007). The between group comparisons for functional activation relative to controls, however, revealed reduced activation in the dorsolateral prefrontal cortex and dorsal anterior cingulate cortex (regions involved in executive control), and in the striatum (especially the putamen, which is involved in motor planning) in the WS group. There was also *increased* activation in the medial precuneus and posterior cingulate cortex in WS relative to controls (Mobbs et al., 2006), and intriguingly these same areas show *reduced* activation during Go/NoGo performance in children with ADHD (Rubia et al., 2005). These findings highlight the plasticity of the WS brain whereby behavioural functioning is maintained by compensatory pathways and neural restructuring to overcome frontostriatal dysfunction.

Although volumes of frontal brain regions are relatively more preserved than posterior brain regions in WS (Chiang et al., 2007; Eckert et al., 2005), neuroimaging studies consistently report structural abnormalities in fronto-striatal-thalamic regions. Of the very few studies using voxel-based morphometry (VBM) in children with WS, Campbell et al. (2009) showed reduced grey matter volume in the left parieto-occipital regions, right posterior cingulate gyrus and the basal ganglia.

By contrast, there were significant grey matter increases in the frontal lobes, anterior cingulate gyrus and left frontal lobe, alongside increases in white matter in the anterior cingulate. In the WS group, increased rates of ADHD-related inattention were positively correlated with reduced frontal and increased cerebellum and caudate nucleus grey matter volumes. Interestingly, alterations in cortico-striatal-thalamic loops have been suggested to reflect maturation of cognitive control and planning of actions across childhood and adolescence (Haber & Calzavara, 2009), and these cortico-striatal-thalamic as well as cerebellar abnormalities have been linked to the symptoms in ADHD (Krain & Castellanos, 2006).

In addition to commonalities and differences in the neural basis of inhibition and ADHD-like deficits, the broad range of impairments in visual attention, spatial cognition, planning and visuomotor integration also implicate dysfunction of the frontoparietal circuits. The most consistently reported finding is reduced grey matter volume in the posterior parietal areas, which has been suggested to underlie the most characteristic visuomotor features of WS (Hocking et al., 2008). Additionally, the corpus callosum is more elongated, with an abnormal thickness profile (Chiang et al., 2007; Sampaio et al., 2010). Importantly, studies have also identified bilaterally reduced grey matter volume in the intraparietal sulcus (Boddaert et al., 2006; Eckert et al., 2006), increased cortical folding in parieto-occipital regions (Schmitt et al., 2002; Gaser et al., 2006) and bilaterally reduced sulcal depths in these same regions in WS (Eisenberg et al., 2010; Van Essen et al., 2006). The functional correlates of these structural abnormalities in the parieto-occipital/intraparietal sulcus regions were identified using path analysis and VBM showing less connectivity with later dorsal stream regions in high functioning (IQs within the normal range) individuals with WS (Meyer-Lindenberg et al., 2004). In the same WS group, the directly adjacent dorsal stream areas showed significant bilateral hypoactivation during performance on spatial localisation and visuospatial construction tasks.

Although these findings may indicate relatively normal ventral stream functioning in WS, there appear to be abnormalities in functional connectivity between ventral visual areas, and key dorsal stream and social processing regions in the same high functioning WS group (Sarpal et al., 2008). Specifically, ventral stream areas such as the fusiform face area (FFA: involved in face processing), and the parahippocampal place area (PPA: crucial for spatial navigation), showed reduced functional connectivity with the intraparietal sulcus, while the FFA showed reduced connections to the amygdala and parts of the frontal cortex (Sarpal et al., 2008). These latter regions, especially the amygdala and orbitofrontal cortex, show reduced connectivity during presentation of threatening faces (Meyer-Lindenberg et al., 2005), which may underlie the lack of social fear, nonsocial anxieties and uninhibited social approach behaviour in WS.

Cerebellum and Williams syndrome

Although not typically regarded as a cerebellar disorder, the previously described impairments in reaching, balance and locomotion, alongside deficits in attention, executive function and visuospatial skills, as well as disinhibited social behaviour in WS, suggest some overlap with *cerebellar cognitive affective syndrome* (Schmahmann & Sherman, 1998) (described in detail in Chapter 3). Despite the overall reduced brain volume in individuals with WS (typically only reaching 80% of TD adult brains; Chiang et al., 2007; Jernigan & Bellugi, 1994), structural imaging studies of the cerebellum are inconsistent. Some studies report relatively enlarged volumes of the cerebellar vermis (Osório et al., 2014; Schmitt et al., 2001); others report preserved cerebellar volumes (Chiang et al., 2007; Reiss et al., 2000). These inconsistencies are likely related to the unique size and shape of the WS brain that may introduce bias during the pre-processing stage when using automated methods such as VBM (Eckert et al., 2006).

More recent VBM studies that overcome these limitations in WS have revealed associations between right cerebellar GM density and performance on linguistic measures (morpho-syntactic and praxis), and between right superior frontal gyrus, left inferior parietal lobule and cerebellum, and performance on visuospatial tasks (Block Design) (Menghini et al., 2011). Furthermore, there is unequal distribution of white matter with much less reduction in cerebellar white matter compared to that observed in the cerebrum (Osório et al., 2014; Reiss et al., 2000). An earlier study showed anomalous neural density in the cerebellum (abnormal ratio of choline and creatine to N-aceylaspartate), which correlated with performance on language, visuospatial and processing speed tasks in WS (Rae et al., 1998). Further evidence for the cerebellar role in cognition comes from Menghini et al. (2013), who showed that a larger volume of the posterior cerebellar vermis lobules VI-VII correlated with lower scores on serial reaction time (implicit learning), phonological fluency and verbal short-term memory tasks in individuals with WS.

Together, these findings emphasise the developmental vulnerability of the cerebellum in WS, and the potential effects of anomalous cerebellar functioning on other affected regions that are reciprocally connected via cerebello-cortical networks.

Functional and structural connectivity in Williams syndrome

The previous functional neuroimaging findings point to anomalous functional connectivity within and between dorsal/ventral visual stream regions, suggesting that alterations to white matter connectivity might account for the link between the WS hemideletion and visuospatial abnormalities in WS. Indeed, Diffusion Tensor Imaging (DTI) studies indicate greater fractional anisotropy (FA: an index of microstructural integrity) in the right superior longitudinal fasciculus in high functioning WS (Marenco et al., 2007), and when comparing 'typical' WS to developmentally delayed individuals (Hoeft et al., 2007). Importantly, impairments in visuospatial construction (Wechsler Object Assembly) have been linked to this anomalous inter-regional network connectivity in WS (Hoeft et al., 2007). Moreover, major white matter tracts do not show the normal asymmetry (left > right) in degree of coherence in fibre orientation, with preferential right hemisphere involvement that may contribute to impairments in visuospatial construction and social cognition (Marenco et al., 2007). Similarly, reduced FA in corticospinal and corticocerebellar tracts may contribute to the neurological abnormalities, such as abnormal gait, balance and muscle weakness (Arlinghaus et al., 2011), which we have previously reported in adults with WS (Hocking et al., 2009).

Treatment/including psychopharmacology

Although considerable progress has been made toward a more nuanced approach to characterising the WS behavioural and neural phenotype, the development and evaluation of interventions is still in its infancy. There are only a few case reports or studies with small samples that report the use of methylphenidate in the treatment of ADHD in children with WS with mixed efficacy (Bawden et al., 1997; Zwaigenbaum et al., 2006). More recently, a larger study of children and adolescents with WS found that 72.2% using methylphenidate showed significant improvements using the clinical global impression scale (Green et al., 2012). However, in two WS cases, methylphenidate was no more effective than placebo in treatment of ADHD symptoms measured by the Conners Parent Rating Scale (Zwaigenbaum et al., 2006).

Given that other developmental disorders such as ASD share characteristics in common with WS (weaknesses in relational/conceptual language and pragmatics), language interventions designed for ASD may also be appropriate, with some modification, in children with WS. Moreover, the assessment, formulation and treatment strategies for anxiety in WS should be mindful of enhanced vulnerability to experiencing generalised anxiety and specific phobias, which may not overlap with ASD (Rodgers et al., 2012). Given that most current interventions are designed to address phenotypic features, rather than etiology, many of the treatment programs designed for ASD may also be suitable for children with WS. For example, variants of Applied Behaviour Analysis (ABA) combined with a strong emphasis on social skills training may reduce undesirable behaviours, while promoting key social behaviours (e.g. Early Start Denver Model) necessary for successful peer relationships in children with WS.

Summary

Despite the initial portrayals of WS as characterised by an uneven profile of peaks and troughs associated with its phenotypic outcome, there is now a more nuanced view of the considerable heterogeneity across and within domains in WS. The genetic heterogeneity and inconsistencies across genetic studies of WS mirror the overall variability within the cognitive and behavioural phenotype. The pattern of strengths and weaknesses in verbal and spatial cognition is often consistent across domains, while in other contexts (e.g. when higher level mental manipulation is required) they appear not to fully mirror the verbal and spatial dissociations commonly depicted in WS.

Even domains considered to be relative strengths in WS, such as face processing and language, may rely on atypical cognitive processes (e.g. analysis of individual facial features), and there exists a number of abnormalities in the use of relational or conceptual vocabulary and pragmatics, which share some overlap with ASD. In the domains of visual search and attention, the early difficulties in attention disengagement may well explain a range of difficulties in selective attention and face processing. Moreover, the profound deficits in planning and visuomotor integration in WS may partially explain their poor performance in visually-guided locomotion and stair descent, and their relation to specific aspects of executive control suggests that cognitive processes outside the domain of interest may have considerable impact on behavioural outcomes.

Seemingly near-normal performance may be supported by atypical neural activation, maintained by compensatory neural restructuring within frontostriatal and frontoparietal circuits. Even in areas of the brain that show relatively normal structure and function such as the ventral stream, there exists abnormal functional connectivity with other regions subserving visuospatial and face processing, possibly indicative of compensatory functional reorganisation. Similarly, despite a relatively normal or enlarged cerebellum, changes in neuronal density and relation of cerebellar volume to individual differences in various cognitive tasks suggest anomalous connectivity within cerebellar-cortico networks.

In conclusion, the considerable overlap with the autism spectrum including difficulties with social reciprocity, anxiety, communication and initiating joint attention challenges the common lay characterisation of WS as the "opposite" of ASD. It will be critical to consider how deficits in one or more domain general processes can influence and interact with phenotypic outcomes from infancy onward. Such an approach should inform syndrome-specific interventions that target domain general processes that can influence cross-domain interactions later in life, thereby providing the essential building blocks to help children with WS reach their full potential.

Abbreviations

ADHD: Attention Deficit Hyperactivity Disorder
ADOS: Autism Diagnostic Observation Schedule
ASD: Autism Spectrum Disorder
CA: Chronological age
CCAS: Cerebellar Cognitive Affective Syndrome
DS: Down syndrome
DTI: Diffusion Tensor Imaging
EEG: Electroencephalogram

EF: Executive function
ERPs: Event Related Potentials
FA: Fractional anisotropy
FFA: Fusiform Face Area
FISH: Fluorescent in-situ hybridization
fMRI: Functional magnetic resonance imaging
MA: Mental age
Mb: Mega base pairs
MEG: Magnetoencephalography
PPA: Parahippocampal Place Area
SVAS: Supravalvular Aortic Stenosis
TD: Typically developing
VBM: Voxel-based morphometry
WS: Williams syndrome

Further readings

Eckert, M. A., Galaburda, A. M., Mills, D. L., Bellugi, U., Korenberg, J. R., & Reiss, A. L. (2006). The neurobiology of Williams syndrome: Cascading influences of visual system impairment? *Cellular and Molecular Life Sciences, 63*(16), 1867–75.

Haas, B. W, Reiss, A. L. (2012). Social brain development in Williams syndrome: The current status and directions for future research. *Frontiers in Psychology, 3*, 186.

Järvinen, A., Korenberg, J. R., & Bellugi, U. (2013). The social phenotype of Williams syndrome. *Current Opinion in Neurobiology, 23*(3), 414–22.

Karmiloff-Smith, A. (2012). Perspectives on the dynamic development of cognitive capacities: Insights from Williams syndrome. *Current Opinion in Neurology, 25*(2), 106–11.

Martens, M. A., Wilson, S. J., & Reutens, D. C. (2008). Research Review: Williams syndrome: A critical review of the cognitive, behavioral, and neuroanatomical phenotype. *Journal of Child Psychology and Psychiatry, 49*(6), 576–608.

Meyer-Lindenberg, A., Mervis, C. B., & Berman, K. F. (2006). Neural mechanisms in Williams syndrome: A unique window to genetic influences on cognition and behaviour. *Nature Reviews Neuroscience,* 7(5), 380–93.

Morris, C. A. (2010). The behavioral phenotype of Williams syndrome: A recognizable pattern of neurodevelopment. *American Journal of Medical Genetics. Part C. Seminars in Medical Genetics, 154C*(4), 427–31.

Van Herwegen, J. (2015). Williams syndrome and its cognitive profile: The importance of eye movements. *Psychology Research and Behavior Management, 8*, 143–51.

References

Annaz D, Karmiloff-Smith A, Johnson, M. H., & Thomas, M. S. (2009). A cross-syndrome study of the development of holistic face recognition in children with autism, Down syndrome, and Williams syndrome. *Journal of Experimental Child Psychology, 102*(4), 456–86.

Antonell, A., Del Campo, M., Magano, L. F., Kaufmann, L., de la Iglesia, J.M., Gallastegui, F... Pérez-Jurado, L.A. (2010a). Partial 7q11.23 deletions further implicate GTF2I and GTF2IRD1 as the main genes responsible for the Williams-Beuren syndrome neurocognitive profile. *Journal of Medical Genetics, 47*(5), 312–20.

Antonell, A., Vilardell, M., & Pérez Jurado, L. A. (2010b). Transcriptome profile in Williams-Beuren syndrome lymphoblast cells reveals gene pathways implicated in glucose intolerance and visuospatial construction deficits. *Human Genetics, 128(1)*, 27–37.

Arlinghaus, L. R., Thornton-Wells, T. A., Dykens, E. M., & Anderson, A. W. (2011). Alterations in diffusion properties of white matter in Williams syndrome. *Magnetic Resonance Imaging, 29*(9), 1165–74.

Atkinson, J., Braddick, O. (2011). From genes to brain development to phenotypic behavior: "Dorsal-stream vulnerability" in relation to spatial cognition, attention, and planning of actions in Williams syndrome (WS) and other developmental disorders. *Progress in Brain Research, 189*, 261–83.

Atkinson, J., Braddick, O., Anker, S., Curran, W., Andrew, R., Wattam-Bell, J., et al. (2003). Neurobiological models of visuospatial cognition in children with Williams syndrome: Measures of dorsal-stream and frontal function. *Developmental Neuropsychology, 23*(1&2), 139–172.

Bawden, H. N., MacDonald, G. W., & Shea, S. (1997). Treatment of children with Williams syndrome with methylphenidate. *Journal of Child Neurology, 12*(4), 248–52.

Bellugi, U., Lichtenberger, L., Mills, D., Galaburda, A., & Korenberg, J.R. (1999). Bridging cognition, the brain and molecular genetics: Evidence from Williams syndrome. *Trends in Neuroscience, 22*(5), 197–207.

Bellugi, U., Marks, S., Bihrle, A., & Sabo, H. (1988). Dissociation between language and cognitive functions in Williams syndrome. In D. Bishop & K. Mogford (Eds), *Language Development in Exceptional Circumstances* (pp. 177–89). Hove: Psychology Press.

Bihrle, A. M., Bellugi, U., Delis, D., Marks, S. (1989). Seeing either the forest or the trees: Dissociation in visuospatial processing. *Brain and Cognition, 11*(1), 37–49.

Borg, I., Delhanty, J. D., & Baraitserer, M. (1995). Detection of hemizygosity at the elastin locus by FISH analysis as a diagnostic test in both classical and atypical cases of Williams syndrome. *Journal of Medical Genetics, 32*, 692–696.

Boddaert, N., Mochel, F., Meresse, I., Seidenwurm, D., Cachia, A., Brunelle, F., … Zilbovicius, M. (2006). Parieto-occipital grey matter abnormalities in children with Williams syndrome. *Neuroimage, 30*(3), 721–5.

Brown, J. H., Johnson, M. H., Paterson, S. J., Gilmore, R., Longhi, E., & Karmiloff-Smith, A. (2003). Spatial representation and attention in toddlers with Williams syndrome and Down syndrome. *Neuropsychologia, 41*(8), 1037–46.

Campbell, L. E., Daly, E., Toal, F., Stevens, A., Azuma, R., Karmiloff-Smith, A., … Murphy, K. C. (2009). Brain structural differences associated with the behavioural phenotype in children with Williams syndrome. *Brain Research, 1258*, 96–107.

Chiang, M. C., Reiss, A. L., Lee, A. D., Bellugi, U., Galaburda, A. M., Korenberg, J. R., … Thompson, P. M. (2007). 3D pattern of brain abnormalities in Williams syndrome visualized using tensor-based morphometry. *Neuroimage, 36*(4), 1096–109.

Costanzo, F., Varuzza, C., Menghini, D., Addona, F., Gianesini, T., & Vicari, S. (2013). Executive functions in intellectual disabilities: A comparison between Williams syndrome and Down syndrome. *Research in Developmental Disabilities, 34*(5), 1770–80.

Cornish, K., Scerif, G., & Karmiloff-Smith, A. (2007). Tracing syndrome-specific trajectories of attention across the lifespan. *Cortex, 43*, 672–685.

Cowie, D., Braddick, O., & Atkinson, J. (2012). Visually guided step descent in children with Williams Syndrome. *Developmental Science, 15*(1), 74–86.

Dai, L., Bellugi, U., Chen, X. N., Pulst-Korenberg, A. M., Järvinen-Pasley, A., Tirosh-Wagner, … Korenberg J. R. (2009). Is it Williams syndrome? GTF2IRD1 implicated in visual-spatial construction and GTF2I in sociability revealed by high resolution arrays. *American Journal of Medical Genetics. Part A, 149A*(3), 302–14.

Davies, M., Udwin, O., & Howlin, P. (1998). Adults with Williams syndrome. Preliminary study of social, emotional and behavioural difficulties. *British Journal of Psychiatry, 172,* 273–6.

Devenny, D. A., Krinsky-McHale, S. J., Kittler, P. M., Flory, M., Jenkins, E., Brown, W. T. (2004). Age-associated memory changes in adults with Williams syndrome. *Developmental Neuropsychology, 26*(3), 691–706.

Dykens, E. M. (2003). Anxiety, fears, and phobias in persons with Williams syndrome. *Developmental Neuropsychology, 23*(1–2), 291–316.

Eckert, M. A., Hu, D., Eliez, S., Bellugi, U., Galaburda, A., Korenberg, J., … Reiss, A. L. (2005). Evidence for superior parietal impairment in Williams syndrome. *Neurology, 64,* 152–153.

Eckert, M. A., Tenforde, A., Galaburda, A. M., Bellugi, U., Korenberg, J. R., Mills, D., & Reiss, A. L. (2006). To modulate or not to modulate: Differing results in uniquely shaped Williams syndrome brains. *Neuroimage, 32*(3), 1001–7.

Edgin, J. O., Pennington, B. F., & Mervis, C. B. (2010). Neuropsychological components of intellectual disability: The contributions of immediate, working, and associative memory. *Journal of Intellectual Disability Research, 54*(5), 406–417.

Eisenberg, D. P., Jabbi, M., & Berman, K. F. (2010). Bridging the gene-behavior divide through neuroimaging deletion syndromes: Velocardiofacial (22q11.2 Deletion) and Williams (7q11.23 Deletion) syndromes. *Neuroimage, 53*(3), 857–69.

Elsabbagh, M., Cohen, H., Cohen, M., Rosen, S., & Karmiloff-Smith, A. (2011). Severity of hyperacusis predicts individual differences in speech perception in Williams syndrome. *Journal of Intellectual Disability Research, 55*(6), 563–71.

Fryssira, H., Palmer, R., Hallidie-Smith, K. A., Taylor, J, Donnai, D, & Reardon, W. (1997). Flourescent in situ hybridisation (FISH) for hemizygous deletion at the elastin locus in patients with isolated supravalvar aortic stenosis. *Journal of Medical Genetics, 34,* 306–308.

Gaser, C., Luders, E., Thompson, P. M., Lee, A. D., Dutton, R. A., Geaga, J, A., Reiss, A. L. (2006). Increased local gyrification mapped in Williams syndrome. *Neuroimage, 33*(1), 46–54.

Gothelf, D., Farber, N., Raveh, E., Apter, A., & Attias, J. (2006). Hyperacusis in Williams syndrome: Characteristics and associated neuroaudiologic abnormalities. *Neurology, 66*(3), 390–5.

Gray, V., Karmiloff-Smith, A., Funnell, E., & Tassabehji, M. (2006). In-depth analysis of spatial cognition in Williams syndrome: A critical assessment of the role of the LIMK1 gene. *Neuropsychologia, 44*(5), 679–85.

Green, T., Avda, S., Dotan, I., Zarchi, O., Basel-Vanagaite, L., Zalsman, G., … Gothelf, D. (2012). Phenotypic psychiatric characterization of children with Williams syndrome and response of those with ADHD to methylphenidate treatment. *American Journal of Medical Genetics, 159B*(1), 13–20.

Grice, S. J., Spratling, M. W., Karmiloff-Smith, A., Halit, H., Csibra, G., de Haan, M., & Johnson, M. H. (2001). Disordered visual processing and oscillatory brain activity in autism and Williams syndrome. *Neuroreport, 12*(12), 2697–700.

Haber, S. N., Calzavara, R. (2009). The cortico-basal ganglia integrative network: The role of the thalamus. *Brain Research Bulletin, 78*(2–3), 69–74.

Hirota, H., Matsuoka, R., Chen, X. N., Salandanan, L. S., Lincoln, A., Rose, F. E., … Korenberg, J. R. (2003). Williams syndrome deficits in visual spatial processing linked to GTF2IRD1 and GTF2I on chromosome 7q11.23. *Genetic Medicine, 5*(4), 311–21.

Hocking, D. R., Bradshaw, J. L., & Rinehart, N. J. (2008). Fronto-parietal and cerebellar contributions to motor dysfunction in Williams syndrome: A review and future directions. *Neuroscience and Biobehavioral Reviews, 32*(3), 497–507.

Hocking, D. R., McGinley, J. L., Moss, S. A., Bradshaw, J. L., & Rinehart, N. J. (2010). Effects of external and internal cues on gait function in Williams syndrome. *Journal of the Neurological Sciences, 291*, 57–63.

Hocking, D. R., Menant, J. C., Kirk, H. E., Lord, S., & Porter, M. A. (2014). Gait profiles as indicators of domain-specific impairments in executive control across neurodevelopmental disorders. *Research in Developmental Disabilities, 35*(1), 203–14.

Hocking, D. R., Rinehart, N. J., McGinley, J. L., & Bradshaw, J. L. (2009). Gait function in adults with Williams syndrome. *Experimental Brain Research, 192*(4), 695–702.

Hocking, D., Rinehart, N., McGinley, J., Moss, S., & Bradshaw, J. (2011a). A kinematic analysis of visually-guided movement in Williams syndrome. *Journal of the Neurological Sciences, 301*(1–2), 51–58.

Hocking, D. R., Rinehart, N. J., McGinley, J. L., Galna, B., Moss, S. A., & Bradshaw, J. L. (2011b). Gait adaptation during obstacle crossing reveals impairments in the visual control of locomotion in Williams syndrome. *Neuroscience, 197*, 320–329.

Hocking, D. R., Thomas, D., Menant, J., Porter, M. A., Smith, S., Lord, S., & Cornish, K. M. (2013). The interplay between executive control and motor functioning in Williams syndrome. *Developmental Science, 16*(3), 428–42.

Hoeft, F., Barnea-Goraly, N., Haas, B. W., Golarai, G., Ng, D., Mills, D., … Reiss, A. L. (2007). More is not always better: Increased fractional anisotropy of superior longitudinal fasciculus associated with poor visuospatial abilities in Williams syndrome. *Journal of Neuroscience, 27*(44), 11960–5.

Hoeft, F., Dai, L., Haas, B. W., Sheau, K., Mimura, M., Mills, D., … Reiss, A. L. (2014). Mapping genetically controlled neural circuits to social behaviour and visuo-motor integration by a preliminary examination of atypical deletions with Williams syndrome. *PLoS One, 9*(8), e104088.

Hoffman, J. E., Landau, B., & Pagani, B. (2003). Spatial breakdown in spatial construction: Evidence from eye fixations in children with Williams syndrome. *Cognitive Psychology, 46*(3), 260–301.

Jarrold, C., Baddeley, A. D., & Hewes, A. K. (1999). Genetically dissociated components of working memory: Evidence from Down's and Williams syndrome. *Neuropsychologia, 37*(6), 637–51.

Jernigan, T. L., & Bellugi, U. (1994). Neuroanatomical distinctions between Williams and Down syndromes. In S. Broman & J. Grafnab (Eds), *Atypical Cognitive Deficits in Developmental Disorders: Implications in Brain Function* (pp. 57–66). Hillsdale, NJ: Lawrence Erlbaum.

Karmiloff-Smith, A. (2009). Nativism versus neuroconstructivism: Rethinking the study of developmental disorders. *Developmental Psychology, 45*(1), 56–63.

Karmiloff-Smith, A., Broadbent, H., Farran, E. K., Longhi, E., D'Souza, D., Metcalfe, K., … Sansbury, F. (2012). Social cognition in Williams syndrome: Genotype/phenotype insights from partial deletion patients. *Frontiers in Psychology, 3*, 168.

Karmiloff-Smith, A., Thomas, M., Annaz, D., Humphreys, K., Ewing, S., Brace, N., … Campbell, R. (2004). Exploring the Williams syndrome face-processing debate: The importance of building developmental trajectories. *Journal of Child Psychology and Psychiatry, 45*(7), 1258–74.

Klein-Tasman, B. P., Mervis, C. B., Lord, C., & Phillips, K. D. (2007). Socio-communicative deficits in young children with Williams syndrome: Performance on the Autism Diagnostic Observation Schedule. *Child Neuropsychology, 13*(5), 444–67.

Krain, A. L., & Castellanos, F. X. (2006). Brain development and ADHD. *Clinical Psychology Review, 26*(4), 433–44.

Laing, E., Butterworth, G., Ansari, D., Gsodl, M., Longhi, E., Panagiotaki, G., Paterson, S., & Karmiloff-Smith, A. (2002). Atypical development of language and social communication in toddlers with Williams syndrome. *Developmental Science, 5*, 233–246.

Leyfer, O. T., Woodruff-Borden, J., Klein-Tasman, B. P., Fricke, J. S., & Mervis, C. B. (2006). Prevalence of psychiatric disorders in 4 to 16-year-olds with Williams syndrome. *American Journal of Medical Genetics: Neuropsychiatric Genetics, 141B*(6), 615–22.

Lincoln, A. J., Searcy, Y. M., Jones, W., & Lord, C. (2007). Social interaction behaviors discriminate young children with autism and Williams syndrome. *Journal of the American Academy of Child and Adolescent Psychiatry, 46*(3), 323–31.

Marenco, S., Siuta, M. A., Kippenhan, J. S., Grodofsky, S., Chang, W. L., Kohn, P., … Berman, K. F. (2007). Genetic contributions to white matter architecture revealed by diffusion tensor imaging in Williams syndrome. *Proceedings of the National Academy of Sciences USA, 104*(38), 15117–22.

Martens, M.A., Wilson, S.J., & Reutens, D.C. (2008). Research review: Williams syndrome: A critical review of the cognitive, behavioral, and neuroanatomical phenotype. *Journal of Child Psychology and Psychiatry, 49*(6), 576–608.

Melenfant, P., Liu, X., Hudson, M. L., et al. (2012). Association of GTF2i in the Williams-Beuren syndrome critical region with autism spectrum disorders. *Journal of Autism and Developmental Disorders, 42*(7), 1459–69.

Menghini, D., Di Paola, M., Federico, F., Vicari, S., Petrosini, L., Caltagirone, C., Bozzali, M. (2011). Relationship between brain abnormalities and cognitive profile in Williams syndrome. *Behavior Genetics, 41*(3), 394–402.

Menghini, D., Di Paola, M., Murri, R., Costanzo, F., Caltagirone, C., Vicari, S., Petrosini, L. (2013). Cerebellar vermis abnormalities and cognitive functions in individuals with Williams syndrome. *Research in Developmental Disabilities, 34*(7), 2118–26.

Meyer-Lindenberg, A., Hariri, A. R., Munoz, K. E., Mervis, C. B., Mattay, V. S., Morris, C. A., & Berman, K. F. (2005). Neural correlates of genetically abnormal social cognition in Williams syndrome. *Nature Neuroscience, 8*(8), 991–3.

Meyer-Lindenberg, A., Kohn, P., Mervis, C. B., Kippenhan, J. S., Olsen, R. K., Morris, C.A., & Berman, K.F. (2004). Neural basis of genetically determined visuospatial construction deficit in Williams syndrome. *Neuron, 43*, 623–631.

Mervis, C. B., & John, A. E. (2010). Comprehension of the communicative intent behind pointing and gazing gestures by young children with Williams syndrome or Down syndrome. *Journal of Speech, Language and Hearing Research, 53*(4), 950–60.

Mervis, C. B., Robinson, B. F., Bertrand, J., Morris, C. A., Klein-Tasman, B. P., & Armstrong, S. C. (2000). The Williams syndrome cognitive profile. *Brain and Cognition, 44*, 604–628.

Mervis, C. B., Robinson, B. F., Rowe, M. L., Becerra, A. M., & Klein-Tasman, B. P. (2003). Language abilities of individuals who have Williams syndrome. In: L. Abbeduto (Ed). *International Review of Research in Mental Retardation*. (pp. 35–81). Orlando, FL: Academic Press.

Mobbs, D., Eckert, M. A., Mills, D., Korenberg, J., Bellugi, U., Galaburda, A. M., & Reiss A. L. (2007). Frontostriatal dysfunction during response inhibition in Williams syndrome. *Biological Psychiatry, 62*(3), 256–61.

Morris, CA. (2010). The behavioral phenotype of Williams syndrome: A recognizable pattern of neurodevelopment. *American Journal of Medical Genetics. Part C, Seminar in Medical Genetics, 154C*(4), 427–31.

Nakamura, M., Watanabe, S., Gunji, A., & Kakigi, R. (2006). The magnetoencephalographic response to upright and inverted face stimuli in a patient with Williams syndrome. *Pediatric Neurology, 34*(5), 412–414.

Osborne, L. R., Li, M., Pober, B., Chitayat, D., Bodurtha, J. Mandel, A., … Scherer, S. W. (2001). A 1.5 million-base pair inversion polymorphism in families with Williams-Beuren syndrome. *Nature Genetics, 29,* 321–325.

Osório, A., Soares, J. M., Prieto, M. F., Vasconcelos, C., Fernandes, C., Sousa, S., … Sampaio, A. (2014). Cerebral and cerebellar MRI volumes in Williams syndrome. *Research in Developmental Disabilities, 35*(4), 922–8.

Porter, M. A., & Coltheart, M. (2005). Cognitive heterogeneity in Williams syndrome. *Developmental Neuropsychology, 27*(2), 275–306.

Porter, M. A., & Coltheart, M. (2006). Global and local processing in Williams syndrome, autism, and Down syndrome: Attention, perception and construction. *Developmental Neuropsychology, 30*(3), 771–789.

Porter, M. A., Coltheart, M., & Langdon, R. (2007). The neuropsychological basis of hypersociability in Williams and Downs syndrome. *Neuropsychologia, 45,* 2839–2849.

Porter, M. A., Dobson-Stone, C., Kwok, J. B. J., Schofield, P. R., Beckett, W., & Tassabehji, M. (2012). A role for transcription factor GTF2IRD2 in executive function in Williams-Beuren syndrome. *PLoS One,* 7(10), e47457.

Rae, C., Karmiloff-Smith, A., Lee, M. A., Dixon, R. M., Grant, J., Blamire, A. M., … Radda, G. K. (1998). Brain biochemistry in Williams syndrome: Evidence for a role of the cerebellum in cognition? *Neurology, 51*(1), 33–40.

Reiss, A. L., Eliez, S., Schmitt, J. E., Straus, E., Lai, Z., Jones, W., & Bellugi, U. (2000). Neuroanatomy of Williams syndrome: A high-resolution MRI study. *Journal of Cognitive Neuroscience, 12 (Suppl 1*), 65–73.

Rhodes, S. M., Riby, D., Matthews, K., & Coghill, D. R. (2011). Attention-deficit/hyperactivity disorder and Williams syndrome: Shared behavioral and neuropsychological profiles. *Journal of Clinical and Experimental Neuropsychology, 33*(1), 147–156.

Rinehart, N. J., Bradshaw, J. L., Moss, S.A., Brereton, A. V., & Tonge, B. J. (2000). Atypical interference of local detail on global processing in high-functioning autism and Asperger's disorder. *Journal of Child Psychology and Psychiatry, and Allied Disciplines, 41*(6), 769–78.

Rodgers, J., Riby, D. M., Janes, E, Connolly B., & McConachie, H. (2012). Anxiety and repetitive behaviours in autism spectrum disorders and Williams syndrome: A cross-syndrome comparison. *Journal of Autism and Developmental Disorders, 42*(2), 175–80.

Rubia, K., Smith, A. B., Brammer, M. J., Toone, B., & Taylor, E. (2005). Abnormal brain activation during inhibition and error detection in medication-naive adolescents with ADHD. *American Journal of Psychiatry, 162*(6), 1067–75.

Sampaio, A., Bouix, S., Sousa, N., Vasconcelos, C., Férnandez, M., Shenton, M. E., & Gonçalves, Ó.F. (2010). Morphometry of corpus callosum in Williams syndrome: Shape as an index of neural development. *Brain Structure and Function, 218*(3), 711–20.

Sarpal, D., Buchsbaum, B. R., Kohn, P. D., Kippenhan, J. S., Mervis, C. B., Morris, C. A., … Berman, K. F. (2008). A genetic model for understanding higher order visual processing:

Functional interactions of the ventral visual stream in Williams syndrome. *Cerebral Cortex, 18*(10), 2402–9.

Scerif, G., Cornish, K., Wilding, J., Driver, J., & Karmiloff-Smith, A. (2004). Visual search in typically developing toddlers and toddlers with Fragile X or Williams syndrome. *Developmental Science,* 7(1), 116–30.

Schmahmann, J. D., & Sherman, J. C. (1998). The cerebellar cognitive affective syndrome. *Brain, 121*(Pt 4), 561–79.

Schmitt, J. E., Eliez, S., Warsofsky, I. S., Bellugi, U., & Reiss, A. L. (2001). Enlarged cerebellar vermis in Williams syndrome. *Journal of Psychiatry Research, 35*(4), 225–9.

Schmitt, J. E., Watts, K., Eliez, S., Bellugi, U., Galaburda, A. M., & Reiss, A. L. (2002). Increased gyrification in Williams syndrome: Evidence using 3D MRI methods. *Developmental Medicine and Child Neurology, 44*(5), 292–5.

StrØmme, P., BjØrnstad, P. G., & Ramstad, K. (2002). Prevalence estimation of Williams syndrome. *Journal of Child Neurology, 17*, 269–271.

Tager-Flusberg, H., Plesa-Skwerer, D., Faja, S., & Joseph, R. M. (2003). People with Williams syndrome process faces holistically. *Cognition, 89*(1), 11–24.

Tassabehji, M. (2003). Williams-Beuren syndrome: A challenge for genotype-phenotype correlations. *Human Molecular Genetics, 12*(2), R229-R237.

Udwin, Yule, W., & Martin, N. (1987). Cognitive abilities and behavioral characteristics of children with idiopathic hypercalcemia. *Journal of Child Psychology and Psychiatry and Allied Disciplines, 28*, 297–309.

van der Geest, J. N., Lagers-van Haselen, G. C., van Hagen, J. M., Govaerts, L. C., de Coo, I. F., de Zeeuw, C. I., & Frens, M. A. (2004). Saccade dysmetria in Williams-Beuren syndrome. *Neuropsychologia, 42*(5), 569–76.

Van Essen, D. C., Dierker, D., Snyder, A. Z., Raichle, M. E., Reiss, A. L., & Korenberg, J. (2006). Symmetry of cortical folding abnormalities in Williams syndrome revealed by surface-based analyses. *Journal of Neuroscience, 26*(20), 5470–83.

Wigham, S., Rodgers, J., South, M., McConachie, H., & Freeston, M. (2015). The interplay between sensory processing abnormalities, intolerance of uncertainty, anxiety and restricted and repetitive behaviours in autism spectrum disorder. *Journal of Autism and Developmental Disorders, 45*(4), 943–52.

Zwaigenbaum, L., Dick, P., Handley-Derry, M., Malone, M., & Jacobson, S. (2006). "N of 1" trials of methylphenidate in two children with William syndrome and attention deficit hyperactivity disorder. *Journal of Developmental and Physical Disabilities, 18*(1), 45–58.

17
FRIEDREICH ATAXIA

Louise A. Corben, Eppie M. Yiu, Marguerite V. Evans-Galea and Martin B. Delatycki

Introduction

Friedreich ataxia (FRDA), the most common inherited ataxia, was first described as a distinct clinical syndrome in 1863 by Nicholaus Friedreich, Professor of Medicine in Heidelberg, Germany (Friedreich, 1863, 1876, 1877). The well documented clinical features of FRDA include progressive ataxia, spasticity, absent lower limb reflexes, impaired vibration sense and proprioception, scoliosis, foot deformity and cardiomyopathy (Delatycki, Williamson, & Forrest, 2000; Harding, 1981). In 1996, the discovery by Campuzano and colleagues of the mutations in the *FXN* gene that underlie FRDA enabled molecular diagnosis of affected individuals (Campuzano et al., 1996). Despite the extraordinary progress in our understanding of FRDA in the last 150 years, there is still no proven treatment that can slow the progression or eventual outcome of this life-shortening condition.

Prevalence, onset and progression

With an incidence of approximately 1 in 29,000 and a carrier rate of 1:85, FRDA occurs predominantly in Caucasians and affects both sexes equally (Cossee et al., 1997). Inheritance is autosomal recessive and it is not uncommon for more than one child in a family to be affected by FRDA. The onset of symptoms in typical FRDA is on average in the mid teen years, however, variable age of onset is apparent even between siblings (Delatycki et al., 1999; Dürr et al., 1996). About 25% of individuals presenting with FRDA fall outside the diagnostic criteria as described by Harding (Delatycki & Corben, 2012). These individuals include those with Late Onset Friedreich Ataxia (LOFA), defined as onset between 25 and 39 years, and Very Late Onset Friedreich Ataxia (VLOFA), defined as onset ≥ 40 years

(Bidichandani, Garcia, Patel, & Dimachkie, 2000). Typically FRDA is progressive, with the average time from symptom onset to wheelchair dependency being about 10 to 15 years (Delatycki & Corben, 2012; Dürr et al., 1996). The mean age at death in typical FRDA is reported to be late in the third decade (De Michele et al., 1996; Harding, 1981; Tsou et al., 2011) with 59% of deaths attributed to cardiac dysfunction (Tsou et al., 2011).

Clinical symptoms

Neurological symptoms

In rare cases, cardiac, diabetes or orthopaedic manifestation may precede neurological signs (Chakraborty et al., 2015; Quercia et al., 2010; Reetz et al., 2015), however, in the majority of individuals the heralding symptoms of FRDA are gait instability and/or generalised clumsiness due to a combination of cerebellar and spinocerebellar degeneration, sensory and vestibular neuropathy (Delatycki & Corben, 2012; Reetz et al., 2015). The blend of cerebellar and afferent ataxia results in a wide-based ataxic gait associated with frequent falls. As the disease progresses, the individual requires increased external support to walk until they are eventually unable to mobilise and become wheelchair dependent (Delatycki & Corben, 2012; Harding, 1981; Pandolfo, 2009). Progressive limb weakness occurring in tandem with ataxia and spasticity further compromises trunk control and upper and lower limb function (Milne, Campagna, Delatycki, & Corben, 2013; Parkinson, Boesch, Nachbauer, Mariotti, & Giunti, 2013; Schulz et al., 2009). A mixed picture of upper and lower motor neuron findings is typical, with areflexia, extensor plantar responses, and abnormal vibration sensation and proprioception on neurologic examination (Delatycki et al., 2000; Parkinson et al., 2013).

The impact of FRDA on motor control is multimodal, appearing as dysmetria, dysdiadochokinesis, weakness and spasticity in both upper and lower limbs (Parkinson et al., 2013). In speech it is apparent as dysarthria, generally noticeable early in the disease trajectory and invariably progressive (Delatycki & Corben, 2012; Folker et al., 2010). Likewise in swallowing, dysphagia, initially thought to be associated with more advanced FRDA, is now reported relatively early in the disease course (Vogel, Brown, Folker, Corben, & Delatycki, 2014). Oculomotor findings associated with FRDA include prolonged saccadic latency, square wave jerks and difficulty with fixation including ocular flutter (Fahey et al., 2008). Some individuals with FRDA develop clinically apparent optic atrophy, whilst many others have subclinical retinal nerve fibre thinning (Noval, Contreras, Sanz-Gallego, Manrique, & Arpa, 2012; Seyer et al., 2013).

A reduction in hearing had been previously reported in only 8–13% of individuals with FRDA (Dürr et al., 1996; Harding, 1981). However, in the setting of typically normal or near-normal sound detection, almost all individuals with FRDA will progress to display abnormal neural conduction in the central auditory pathways and associated distorted perception of speech (Rance et al., 2010; Rance et al., 2008). Functionally, this impairment is apparent as reduced auditory processing in a noisy environment. The severity of the auditory impairment in FRDA, reported to be a result of an axonopathy in the cochlear nerve, mirrors disease progression (Rance, Corben, & Delatycki, 2012).

Non-neurological symptoms

The most common cause of death in FRDA is cardiac dysfunction, apparent as changes in both left ventricular (LV) structure and function (Tsou et al., 2011). Most individuals with FRDA, particularly those with an earlier age of disease onset, demonstrate abnormalities in LV wall thickness and mass index, as measured by echocardiography, however only some progress to dilated cardiomyopathy and cardiac failure (Mottram et al., 2011; Regner et al., 2012; Weidemann et al., 2013). Whilst occasionally present early in the disease process, supraventricular arrhythmias are more common in advanced disease (Tsou et al., 2011; Weidemann et al., 2013). The variable cardiac phenotype associated with FRDA does not always parallel the neurological phenotype (Dutka, Donnelly, Nihoyannopoulos, Oakley, & Nunez, 1999).

Scoliosis occurs in most individuals with FRDA (Shapiro & Specht, 1993), and is usually more severe in individuals with symptom onset prior to 10 years of age (Labelle, Tohme, Duhaime, & Allard, 1986; Milbrandt, Kunes, & Karol, 2008). Further skeletal changes occurring frequently in individuals with FRDA are pes cavus and foot and ankle equinovarus deformity, the latter having the greater impact on mobility (Delatycki & Corben, 2012; Delatycki et al., 2005).

Diabetes mellitus occurs in about 12% of individuals with FRDA (Cnop, Mulder, & Igoillo-Esteve, 2013). Low bone density and reduced vitamin D levels have also been recently demonstrated in individuals with FRDA (Eigentler et al., 2014). A recent study reported a greater incidence of sleep related breathing disorders, in particular obstructive and central sleep apnoea in individuals with FRDA (Corben, Ho, Copland, Tai, & Delatycki, 2013).

Clinical vignette

Ten year old Sam, who was previously healthy, was noticed by his parents to be falling over more than usual. Although initially the GP reassured Sam's parents that there was nothing to be concerned about and he is "just a bit of clumsy kid growing into his body", Sam was ultimately referred to see a neurologist. The neurologist found that Sam had a wide-based gait, absent lower limb reflexes, bilateral pes cavus and scoliosis. He ordered molecular testing for Friedreich ataxia and the diagnosis was confirmed with Sam being homozygous for two intron 1 *FXN* GAA expansions of 800 and 1150 repeats. Sam's parents were informed about the autosomal recessive inheritance of Friedreich ataxia. They were fearful that their younger daughter, Stella who was aged 8, had also inherited the double dose of the faulty gene. Sam's parents understood there were no treatments proven to slow the progression of Friedreich ataxia, yet, despite this knowledge, were determined to ensure that Friedreich ataxia did not define Sam, nor what he aspired to achieve. Their determination ensured the implementation of interventions at school, home and through therapy to maximise Sam's function.

Genetics

The most common disease-causing mutation in FRDA is a Guanine-Adenine-Adenine (GAA) trinucleotide repeat expansion in the first intron of *FXN* (Campuzano et al., 1996; Pandolfo, 2009). In unaffected individuals, *FXN* typically contains 6–36 GAA repeats while individuals with FRDA have anywhere from 56 to >1,000 GAA repeats (Pandolfo, 2009). Approximately 96% of affected individuals are homozygous for expanded intron 1 GAA repeats. This results in reduced *FXN* transcript and the encoded mitochondrial protein frataxin is generally expressed at less than one third of the normal levels (Campuzano et al., 1996). This reduction in frataxin levels is considered the main driver of pathogenesis, however, repeat-associated pathologies may also play a role (Evans-Galea, Lockhart, Galea, Hannan, & Delatycki, 2014). About 4% of individuals with FRDA are compound heterozygous for an expanded allele and a second detrimental mutation in *FXN*, such as a missense, nonsense, splice-site, or insertion/deletion mutation (Cossée et al., 1999). These mutations may result in an atypical FRDA phenotype (De Castro et al., 2000).

Frataxin is a ubiquitously expressed protein that is essential for life, playing a role in iron-sulphur cluster assembly, heme biosynthesis and intracellular iron homeostasis (Pandolfo & Pastore, 2009; Pastore & Puccio, 2013). Absence of frataxin in homozygous knock-out mice results in embryonic lethality (Cossee et al., 2000). Expression of frataxin is highest in mitochondria-rich tissues such as the heart and the spinal cord, with the dorsal root ganglion (DRG) sensory neurons and the granular layer of the cerebellum also being major sites of expression (Santos et al., 2010). In FRDA, dysregulated iron metabolism results in the loss of iron-sulfur clusters and mitochondrial iron accumulation (Pandolfo & Pastore, 2009; Pastore & Puccio, 2013). These impact mitochondrial function and lead to defects in energy production and increased oxidative stress (Calabrese et al., 2005).

Despite the diverse phenotype associated with FRDA, consistent correlations have been found between the number of GAA repeats on the smaller allele (GAA1) and age at onset (De Michele et al., 1998; Delatycki et al., 2000; Ribaï et al., 2007), swift disease progression (Mateo et al., 2004), time to wheelchair use, cardiomyopathy, presence of scoliosis, impaired vibration sense and presence of foot deformity (Delatycki et al., 1999). Individuals with LOFA or VLOFA have smaller GAA repeat size, slower disease progression and fewer related symptoms such as pes cavus and scoliosis (De Michele et al., 1994). However, the heterogeneous FRDA phenotype is not all explained by GAA repeat length as corroborated by the size of the GAA1 allele only accounting for approximately 47% of age of onset (Montermini, Andermann, et al., 1997; Montermini, Richter, et al., 1997; Santos et al., 2010). Other genetic and environmental modifiers may alter the expression of the disease (Bidichandani et al., 2000; Kelly et al., 2011). A recent study postulated that variance in pathology onset may also point to factors such as somatic GAA expansions occurring throughout development and beyond, thus influencing *FXN* transcription and subsequent frataxin expression (Koeppen & Mazurkiewicz, 2013).

A number of epigenetic changes are associated with FRDA, including differential DNA methylation and altered histone modifications. In the blood and buccal cells of individuals with FRDA, there is increased DNA methylation at CpG dinucleotides in *FXN* upstream of the expanded GAA repeat and decreased methylation downstream compared with unaffected individuals (Castaldo et al., 2008; Evans-Galea et al., 2012). Similar changes in methylation have been observed in post-mortem heart and brain samples from individuals with FRDA compared to unaffected individuals (Al-Mahdawi et al., 2008).

Cognitive and behavioural implications of FRDA

The cognitive and behavioural implications of FRDA have been the focus of research for nearly three decades (Corben et al., 2012). Early studies reported a specific finding of slowed information processing in individuals with FRDA (Botez-Marquard & Botez, 1993; Corben et al., 2006; Hart, Henry, Kwentus, & Leshner, 1986; Hart, Kwentus, Leshner, & Frazier, 1985; White, Lalonde, & Botez-Marquard, 2000). The few early studies exploring the neurobehavioural profile associated with FRDA exemplify the contemporaneous view that the role of the cerebellum was confined to coordinating voluntary movement. It was not until more recent studies unequivocally demonstrated the role of the cerebellum in cognitive, language and affective regulation (Manto & Lorivel, 2011; Schmahmann, 2004; Timmann et al., 2010) that there was an associated interest in examining the effect of FRDA on cognitive development and function.

Neuropsychological assessments have been widely used to measure neurobehavioural impairment in FRDA (Ciancarelli, Cofini, & Carolei, 2010; Manto & Lorivel, 2011; Mantovan et al., 2006; Wollmann, Barroso, Monton, & Nieto, 2002). Mantovan and colleagues identified that individuals with FRDA were impaired in specific neuropsychological tasks compared to control participants, as evidenced by reduced abstract thinking, concept formation and visuospatial reasoning (Mantovan et al., 2006). de Nóbrega and colleagues utilised phonemic, semantic and action verbal fluency tasks to evaluate executive function in individuals with FRDA compared to matched controls (de Nóbrega, Nieto, Barrosso, & Montón, 2007). Individuals with FRDA were significantly more impaired in performance on the phonemic and action fluency tests when compared to control participants (de Nóbrega et al., 2007). To dissect the FRDA-associated speech motor impairment from cognitive performance, de Nóbrega and colleagues investigated the relationship between language and reaction time (RT) tasks and noted the source of the group difference lay not with dysarthria associated with FRDA, but rather with impairment in the neural circuitry associated with executive function. This seminal study highlighted the importance of separating the motor and non-motor aspects of FRDA in order to examine cognitive function (de Nóbrega et al., 2007). Neito and colleagues completed neuropsychological assessment of 36 individuals with FRDA noting impairments in conceptual thinking, verbal fluency and acquisition of verbal information, visuoperceptive and visuoconstructive functions and processing speed (Nieto et al., 2012). A later study by this team used a similar paradigm, however they stratified the cohort of individuals with FRDA into typical onset (n=29) and LOFA (n=7)(Nieto, Correia, de Nobrega, Monton, & Barroso, 2013). Both groups exhibited impairment in motor processing speed, conceptual thinking and verbal fluency, however only the typical onset group demonstrated slowed cognition and impairment in visuoperceptive and visuoconstructive capacity. Neito and colleagues concluded that individuals with later disease onset may sustain less cognitive impairment, supporting the contention that FRDA-associated cognitive impairment may be as a consequence of disrupted neurodevelopmental processes (Nieto et al., 2013). Nauchbauer and colleagues also utilised neuropsychological assessments to explore attention, memory, executive function and visual perception in 29 individuals with FRDA and 28 matched control participants (Nachbauer et al., 2014). Correlation of the assessment results with clinical parameters indicated that a higher age of onset predicted better neuropsychological performance, further supporting the notion that cognitive impairment in FRDA is at least partly a neurodevelopmental phenomenon. Critically, a higher age of onset may predict more favourable cognitive capacity in individuals with FRDA (Nachbauer et al., 2014).

Whilst the use of neuropsychological assessments to evaluate cognition in people with FRDA has persisted, it is difficult to extrapolate these findings to individuals capacity to manage daily activities that demand flexible and comprehensive cognitive abilities. Individuals with FRDA have proven themselves capable of achieving high levels of education and participating in intelligent and relevant discourse, despite their age at disease onset (Gibilisco & Vogel, 2013). It may be postulated that individuals with an earlier age of onset become increasingly physically impaired at a critical time of their neural development and education. Poor performance on specific intelligence tests may well reflect compromised educational opportunities (Bürk, 2007; Ciancarelli et al., 2010). Alternatively, the neuropsychological changes in individuals with FRDA may reflect direct impact of the condition on the cerebral cortex and/or primary cerebellar pathology which subsequently disrupts the cerebello-thalamo-cortical loops critical to neurobehavioural performance (Doron, Funk, & Glickstein, 2010; Timmann et al., 2010).

Historically, an effective avenue to explore cognitive function has been through the use of paradigms that measure RT (Salthouse & Heddon, 2002). Whilst utilising RT paradigms to characterise cognitive function in FRDA is tantalising, careful consideration is warranted regarding the confound associated with motor impairment. To address this issue and explore neurobehavioural function using non-neuropsychological assessment paradigms, Corben and colleagues conducted a number of studies using RT; however they used a subtractive analytic methodology to determine the effect of the underlying cognitive load on performance in FRDA (Corben, Akhlaghi, et al., 2011; Corben, Delatycki, Bradshaw, Churchyard, & Georgiou-Karistianis, 2011; Corben et al., 2010; Corben, Georgiou-Karistianis, et al., 2011). These studies examined the psychomotor capacity of individuals with FRDA to respond to unexpected change in requisite movement, to utilise advance information to plan movement, to generate a motoric response to incongruent stimuli and to accommodate changes in moving to targets differing in size and distance apart. Successful completion of these motor tasks requires preplanning of movement and online error detection and correction. The cerebellum and its connections to the frontal cortex via cerebro-ponto-cerebello-thalamo-cerebral loops are fundamental to both processes. Performance on these tasks was correlated with clinical parameters including age at disease onset and compared to matched control participants. These studies confirmed individuals with FRDA had difficulty with tasks requiring initiation and preparation of complex motor tasks, and ongoing planning including error detection and correction. These results support the contention of likely impairment in neural connectivity between the cerebellum and cortical structures usually implicated in complex cognitive function. Importantly, in most of these studies there was a significant relationship between worse performance and an earlier age of disease onset, again indicating the impact of reduced frataxin on the developing neural system underlying motor cognition in individuals with FRDA (Corben, Akhlaghi, et al., 2011; Corben et al., 2011; Corben et al., 2010; Corben, Georgiou-Karistianis, et al., 2011).

The ocular motor system is increasingly viewed as a model motor system, with a growing number of studies using saccadic eye movements as an experimental tool to gain insights into the cognitive processes that govern motor control and goal directed behaviour (White & Fielding, 2012). Examination of the cognitive control of eye movements provides an ideal method to further understand the cognitive impairment associated with FRDA. Fielding and colleagues examined antisaccade and memory-guided saccade characteristics in 13 individuals with FRDA and matched control participants (Fielding et al., 2010). Compared to control participants, individuals with FRDA demonstrated impaired inhibitory control and spatial working memory as evidenced by disproportionally greater and significantly different antisaccade and memory-guided saccades. Importantly, the difference lay in the inhibitory control of reflexive saccades, rather than being a generalised slowing of eye movement. Unsurprisingly, given a reduction in inhibitory control, individuals with FRDA made significantly more directional errors than control participants (Fielding et al., 2010). Hocking and colleagues further examined inhibitory control in eye movements by employing a gap overlap task to evaluate attentional engagement and disengagement of eye movements in FRDA (Hocking et al., 2014). The requirement to disengage attention from fixation to a target in the presence of a distractor proved challenging for individuals with FRDA compared to matched control participants. Consistent with previous studies by Corben and colleagues, significant correlations were found between impaired ocular motor control and clinical parameters including FARS score and disease duration. A fundamental component of task success lies in the capacity to successfully inhibit a pre-potent response (disengage from fixation) and move to subsequently engage in generating a suitable response. Cortical areas responsible for exogenous shifts of attention and response selection include the posterior and superior parietal areas, dorsolateral prefrontal cortex (DLPFC) and the anterior cingulate cortex (ACC) (Braver, Barch, Gray, Molfese, & Snyder, 2001; Loose, Kaufmann, Tucha, Auer, & Lange, 2006). Successful completion of these ocular motor tasks requires robust cerebellar access to these cortical areas (Fielding et al., 2010; White & Fielding, 2012).

The issue of potential attentional and memory impairment in individuals with FRDA was further explored by Klopper and colleagues utilising The Test of Everyday Attention (Klopper et al., 2011). Significant impairment in sustained volitional attention and working memory was noted in individuals with FRDA again indicating disruption to cerebello-thalamo-cortical pathways governing attention (Klopper et al., 2011). Impairment in working memory correlated significantly with some clinical parameters, in particular the length of the smaller GAA repeat expansion, implicating again the effect of reduced frataxin on developing brain function.

Neuropathology associated with FRDA

Beyond the initial descriptions by Friedreich regarding the neuropathology associated with FRDA, the extensive work of Koeppen and colleagues has been critical in understanding the extent and breadth of the neuropathology related to FRDA (Koeppen, 2011; Koeppen, Davis, & Morral, 2011; Koeppen et al., 2013; Koeppen & Mazurkiewicz, 2013; Koeppen et al., 2009; Koeppen, Morral, McComb, & Feustel, 2011; Koeppen, Ramirez, Becker, Feustel, & Mazurkiewicz, 2015; Morral, Davis, Qian, Gelman, & Koeppen, 2010). Reflecting the selective vulnerability of tissues to reduced frataxin, Koeppen and colleagues have confirmed that the major sites of neuropathology in FRDA are the DRG and posterior columns of the spinal cord, spinocerebellar tracts, corticospinal tracts and DN of the cerebellum (Koeppen & Mazurkiewicz, 2013). The main developmental and degenerative changes in DRG relate to the reduction in large axons and thick myelinated fibres which occurs early in the course of the disease (Koeppen et al., 2009). The loss of DRG neurons has a domino effect on related structures resulting in the significant reduction of dorsal column fibres and afferent connections to the dorsal nuclei of Clarke (Koeppen & Mazurkiewicz, 2013). The disabling peripheral neuropathy associated with FRDA is likely secondary to the loss of axons and disturbed Schwann cell function (Morral et al., 2010).

In terms of morphology and volume, the cerebellar cortex is essentially unaffected in FRDA (Koeppen, 2011; Mascalchi, 2013; Stefanescu et al., 2015). In comparison, atrophy of the DN and its efferent myelinated fibres is apparent with severe loss of large neurons believed to be the major cause of the dysmetria, dysarthria and dysphagia that characterises FRDA (Koeppen, Davis, et al., 2011; Stefanescu et al., 2015).

Neuroimaging in FRDA

In recent years, multiple neuroimaging studies have used transcranial magnetic stimulation (Brighina et al., 2005), structural magnetic resonance imaging (MRI) (Akhlaghi et al., 2011; Della Nave, Ginestroni, Giannelli, et al., 2008; Stefanescu et al., 2015), tractography (Akhlaghi et al., 2014; Clemm von Hohenberg et al., 2013; Corben, Kashuk, et al., 2014; Della Nave, Ginestroni, Tessa, et al., 2008; Egger et al., 2014; Mascalchi, 2013; Pagani et al., 2010; Vieira Karuta et al., 2015; Zalesky et al., 2014), transcranial sonography (Synofzik, Godau, Lindig, Schols, & Berg, 2011), whole brain voxel-based morphometry (VBM) (Franca et al., 2009; Santner, Schocke, Boesch, Nachbauer, & Egger, 2014; Silva et al., 2013) and functional MRI (Akhlaghi et al., 2012; Georgiou-Karistianis et al., 2012; Ginestroni et al., 2012) to elucidate the specific cortical and cerebellar regions affected in FRDA.

VBM has demonstrated volume loss in the DN as well as dorsal medulla, rostral vermis and infero-medial portions of the cerebellar hemispheres in individuals with FRDA compared to control participants (Della Nave et al., 2008). In addition, atrophy of the superior cerebellar peduncles (SCP), containing efferent fibres projecting from the DN to the motor, premotor, oculomotor and prefrontal regions, has been demonstrated in individuals with FRDA (Akhlaghi et al., 2011; Della Nave et al., 2008). Diffusion tensor imaging (DTI) has demonstrated white matter (WM) changes in individuals with FRDA, including disruption to WM tracts that link the cerebellum to the cerebrum via the thalamus (Akhlaghi et al., 2014; Clemm von Hohenberg et al., 2013; Egger et al., 2014; Pagani et al., 2010; Vieira Karuta et al., 2015; Zalesky et al., 2014). Indeed, Akhlaghi and colleagues demonstrated the compromised integrity of the dentato-thalamo-cortical and dentato-rubral tracts was significantly correlated with reduced cognitive performance in individuals with FRDA indicating a role of disturbed cerebello-thalamo-cortical connectivity beyond the well documented WM changes, in the cognitive impairment associated with FRDA (Akhlaghi et al., 2014). Zalesky and colleagues utilised connectomic mapping and super resolution track imaging techniques to elegantly demonstrate connectivity disruptions in FRDA (Zalesky et al., 2014). Connectomic mapping identified a 16% dimunition of stream lines connecting the cerebellum to distant regions such as the supplementary motor area, the cingulate cortex, frontal cortices, putamen and pallidum (Zalesky et al., 2014). Not surprisingly, these cortical and subcortical areas are critical regions for motor planning and inhibitory control. Functional MRI confirms changes in activation due to disrupted cerebello-thalamo-cortical connectivity (Akhlaghi et al., 2012; Ginestroni et al., 2012; Mantovan et al., 2006). Georgiou-Karistianis and colleagues demonstrated changes in functional activation in cortical and subcortical regions in individuals with FRDA compared to control participants in response to a conflict resolution task. Of particular note in individuals with FRDA was comparable reduced activation in the prefrontal and parietal regions underlying attention; and in the posterior processing areas such as the superior temporal gyrus, inferior parietal lobule and the cingulate gyrus, all implicated in response selection (Georgiou-Karistianis et al., 2012).

Diagnostic instruments and clinical ratings scales

Given there are currently no treatments available that are proven to halt the inexorable decline seen in individuals with FRDA, the challenge facing clinicians in evaluating the efficacy of interventions is the accurate and efficient measurement of disease progression (Delatycki, 2009). The difficulty relates to both the gradual nature of disease progression and its phenotypic variability. The effect of FRDA on the individual can be determined by general neurological measures and/or measures of more specific areas of neurological decline such as gait, oculomotor, upper limb, speech, audiologic and cognitive function. Non-neurological areas such as cardiac involvement and quality of life may also be measured (Delatycki, 2009). The three main rating scales currently used to measure clinical severity of FRDA include: the International Cooperative Rating Scale (ICARS) (Metz et al., 2013; Trouillas et al., 1997), the Friedreich Ataxia Rating Scale (FARS) (Subramony et al., 2005) and the Scale for Assessment and Rating of Ataxia (SARA) (Schmitz-Hübsch et al., 2006).

Treatment

There are currently no proven disease-modifying therapies for FRDA, and management focuses on monitoring for, and the symptomatic treatment of, the neurologic and extra-neurologic complications of FRDA, as well as provision of psychosocial support for individuals and their families. This is best achieved in a multidisciplinary setting. Consensus-based guidelines for the management of FRDA have recently been published and serve as an excellent resource internationally for clinicians and families (Corben, Lynch, et al., 2014).

Allied health therapy aims to optimise strength, mobility, transfers (e.g. to/from wheelchair), balance, joint range of motion, speech and communication, and bulbar function. The provision of customised wheelchairs, seating and equipment can enhance function and independence. Intensive rehabilitation programs are effective in achieving sustained improvements in functional independence in those with a recent deterioration in function, for example after an acute medical event (Milne et al., 2012).

Neurogenic bladder dysfunction may be symptomatically improved by the use of anticholinergic agents (Corben, Lynch, et al., 2014; Schulz et al., 2009). Bone health management includes adequate calcium and vitamin D intake, and consideration of bone densitometry assessment for those at high risk of osteoporosis, e.g. wheelchair dependent individuals (Eigentler et al., 2014). Sleep studies should be performed on those with symptoms of sleep-disordered breathing, and treatment for obstructive sleep apnoea instituted when appropriate (Corben, et al., 2013).

The clinician should screen for mood disorders and social isolation, not only in individuals with FRDA, but also their families. Psychological support and the use of antidepressants should be instituted where necessary, and additional psychosocial support encompassing school/work issues and financial assistance is often welcomed. Genetic counselling should be offered to all families and individuals with FRDA. Presymptomatic testing of minors (e.g. siblings of children with FRDA) is a current area of controversy that requires further research (Lowe, Corben, Duncan, Yoon, & Delatycki, 2015).

The search for disease-modifying therapies for FRDA remains active, with the three main therapeutic approaches including antioxidants and enhancers of mitochondrial function, iron chelators and agents that increase frataxin expression. A number of drugs have reached the human clinical trial phase, however, to date none have proven beneficial nor been approved for use in FRDA.

Summary

Pathology associated with FRDA targets multiple organ systems and sites in the central and peripheral nervous system resulting in numerous symptoms. There is now well established evidence that there are specific neurobehavioural deficits associated with FRDA and these are likely to reflect reduced cerebello-thalamo-cortico connectivity. The neuropathology associated with FRDA and most often preceding the first symptoms is a consequence of neuronal death secondary to frataxin deficiency. The temporal relationship between the onset of neuropathology and subsequent symptoms remains ambiguous, however the relationship between age at disease onset and neurobehavioural changes indicates the developing neural system is particularly sensitive to reduced frataxin. Yet the deficits described thus far are quite specific and generally do not preclude a person with FRDA from participating in school and university, gaining meaningful employment and partnering and raising a family. It may be postulated that despite well-documented neurobehavioural changes associated with FRDA, compensatory measures such as reorganisation of the cerebellar-cortical network during neural maturation and beyond may contribute to the apparent aptitude of individuals with FRDA. Understanding the heterogeneous nature of FRDA-related cognitive changes and their underpinning mechanisms as well as the capacity for reorganisation warrants ongoing research to ensure the impairments associated with FRDA do not influence an individual's capacity to participate in all aspects of life.

Abbreviations

DN: Dentate Nucleus
DRG: Dorsal Root Ganglion
DTI: Diffusion tensor imaging
FARS: Friedreich Ataxia Rating Scale
FRDA: Friedreich Ataxia
FXN: Frataxin
GAA: Guanine-Adenine-Adenine
HDAC: Histone Deacetylase
ICARS: International Cooperative Ataxia Rating Scale
LOFA: Late Onset Friedreich Ataxia
LV: Left ventricular
MRI: Magnetic Resonance Imaging
MRS: Magnetic Resonance Spectroscopy
OCT: Optical Coherence Tomography
OSA: Obstructive Sleep Apnea
QOL: Quality of Life
RT: Reaction Time
SARA: The scale for the assessment and rating of ataxia
SCP: Superior cerebellar peduncle
SDB: Sleep Disordered Breathing
UMN: Upper Motor Neuron
VBM: Voxel-based morphometry
VLOFA: Very Late Onset Friedreich Ataxia
WHO: World Health Organization
WM: White Matter

Further readings

Corben, L. A., Georgiou-Karistianis, N., Bradshaw, J. L., Evans-Galea, M. V., Churchyard, A. J., & Delatycki, M.B. *Characterising the Neuropathology and Neurobehavioural Phenotype in Friedreich Ataxia in Tandem Repeat Polymorphisms: Genetic Plasticity, Neural Diversity and Disease* (Ed: A Hannan). Landes Bioscience and Springer Science+Business Media. 2012.

Corben, L. A., Lynch, D. R., Pandolfo, M., Schulz, J., & Delatycki, M. B. (2014)/ Consensus clinical management guidelines for Friedreich ataxia. Orphanet *Journal of Rare Diseases 9*,184. http://www.curefa.org/clinical-care-guidelines.

Evans-Galea, M.V., Carrodus, N., Rowley, S. M., Corben, L.A., Tai, G., Saffery, R., … Sarsero, J. P. (2012). FXN Methylation Predicts Expression and Clinical Outcome in Friedreich Ataxia. *Annals of Neurology, 71*(4), 487–97.

Evans-Galea, M. V., Pebay, A., Dottori, M., Corben, L. A., Ong, S. H., Lockhart, P. J., & Delatycki, M. B. (2014). Cell and Gene Therapy for Friedreich ataxia – progress to date. *Human Gene Therapy, 25*(8), 684–693.

Gomes, C. M. & Santos, R. (2013). Neurodegeneration in Friedreich's Ataxia: From defective frataxin to oxidative stress. *Oxidative Medicine and Cellular Longevity* 2013,487534 doi.org/10.1155/2013/487534.

Milne, S., Campagna, E., Delatycki, M. B., & Corben, L. A. (2013). *Rehabilitation for Individuals with Friedreich Ataxia: A Model of Comprehensive Care* in *Rehabilitation in Movement Disorders* (Eds: M Morris & R Iansek). Cambridge: University Press.

Tai, G., Corben, L. A., Gurrin, L., Yiu, E. M., Churchyard, A., Fahey, M., Hoare, B., ... Delatycki, M. B. (2015) A study of up to twelve years follow-up of Friedreich ataxia utilising four measurement tools. *Journal of Neurology, Neurosurgery and Psychiatry,* 86(6), 660–6.

References

Akhlaghi, H., Corben, L., Georgiou-Karistianis, N., Bradshaw, J., Delatycki, M. B., Storey, E., & Egan, G. F. (2012). A functional MRI study of motor dysfunction in Friedreich's ataxia. *Brain Research, 1471*, 138–154. doi: 10.1016/j.brainres.2012.06.035.

Akhlaghi, H., Corben, L., Georgiou-Karistianis, N., Bradshaw, J., Storey, E., Delatycki, M. B., & Egan, G. F. (2011). Superior cerebellar peduncle atrophy in Friedreich's ataxia correlates with disease symptoms. *Cerebellum, 10*(1), 81–87. doi: 10.1007/s12311-010-0232-3.

Akhlaghi, H., Yu, J., Corben, L., Georgiou-Karistianis, N., Bradshaw, J. L., Storey, E., ... Egan, G. F. (2014). Cognitive deficits in Friedreich ataxia correlate with micro-structural changes in dentatorubral tract. *Cerebellum, 13*(2), 187–198. doi: 10.1007/s12311-013-0525-4.

Al-Mahdawi, S., Pinto, R. M., Ismail, O., Vashney, D., Lymperi, S., Sandi, C., ... Pook, M. (2008). The Friedreich ataxia GAA repeat expansion mutation induces comparable epigenetic changes in human and transgenic mouse brain and heart tissues. *Human Molecular Genetics, 17*(5), 735–746.

Bidichandani, S. I., Garcia, C. A., Patel, P. I., & Dimachkie, M. M. (2000). Very late-onset Friedreich ataxia despite large GAA triplet repeat expansions. *Archives of Neurology, 57*(2), 246–251.

Botez-Marquard, T., & Botez, M. I. (1993). Cognitive behavior in heredodegenerative ataxias. *European Neurology, 33*(5), 351–357.

Braver, T., Barch, D., Gray, J., Molfese, D., & Snyder, A. (2001). Anterior cingulate cortex and response conflict: Effects of frequency, inhibition and errors. *Cerebral Cortex, 11*(September), 825–836.

Brighina, F., Scalia, S., Gennuso, M., Lupo, I., Matta, F., Piccoli, T., & Fierro, B. (2005). Hypo-excitability of cortical areas in patients affected by Friedreich ataxia: A TMS study. *Journal of the Neurological Sciences, 235*(1–2), 19–22.

Bürk, K. (2007). Cognition in hereditary ataxia. *Cerebellum, 6*(3), 280–286.

Calabrese, V., Lodi, R., Tonon, C., D'Agata, V., Sapienza, M., Scapagnini, G., ...Butterfield, D. A. (2005). Oxidative stress, mitochondrial dysfunction and cellular stress response in Friedreich's ataxia. *Journal of Neurological Sciences, 233*(1–2), 145–162.

Campuzano, V., Montermini, L., Molto, M. D., Pianese, L., Cossee, M., Cavalcanti, F., ... Monticelli, A. (1996). Friedreich's ataxia: Autosomal recessive disease caused by an intronic GAA triplet repeat expansion. *Science, 271*(5254), 1423–1427.

Castaldo, I., Pinelli, M., Monticelli, A., Acquaviva, F., Giacchetti, M., Filla, A., ... Cocozza, S. (2008). DNA methylation in intron 1 of the frataxin gene is related to GAA repeat length and age of onset in Friedreich ataxia patients. *Journal of Medical Genetics, 45*(12), 808–812. doi: 10.1136/jmg.2008.058594.

Chakraborty, P. P., Ray, S., Bhattacharjee, R., Ghosh, S., Mukhopadhyay, P., Mukhopadhyay, S., & Chowdhury, S. (2015). First presentation of diabetes as diabetic ketoacidosis in a case of Friedreich's ataxia. *Clinical Diabetes, 33*(2), 84–86. doi: 10.2337/diaclin.33.2.84.

Ciancarelli, I., Cofini, V., & Carolei, A. (2010). Evaluation of neuropsychological functions in patients with Friedreich ataxia before and after cognitive therapy. *Functional Neurology, 25*(2), 81–85.

Clemm von Hohenberg, C., Schocke, M. F., Wigand, M. C., Nachbauer, W., Guttmann, C. R., Kubicki, M., … Egger, K. (2013). Radial diffusivity in the cerebellar peduncles correlates with clinical severity in Friedreich ataxia. *Neurological Sciences, 34*(8), 1459–1462. doi: 10.1007/s10072-013-1402-0.

Cnop, M., Mulder, H., & Igoillo-Esteve, M. (2013). Diabetes in Friedreich ataxia. *Journal of Neurochemistry, 126 Suppl 1*, 94–102. doi: 10.1111/jnc.12216.

Corben, L. A., Akhlaghi, H., Georgiou-Karistianis, N., Bradshaw, J. L., Egan, G. F., Storey, E., … Delatycki, M. B. (2011). Impaired inhibition of prepotent motor tendencies in Friedreich ataxia demonstrated by the Simon interference task. *Brain Cognition, 76*(1), 140–145. doi: doi:10.1016/j.bandc.2011.02.002.

Corben, L. A., Delatycki, M. B., Bradshaw, J. L., Churchyard, A. J., & Georgiou-Karistianis, N. (2011). Utilization of advance motor information is impaired in Friedreich ataxia. *Cerebellum, 10*(4), 793–803.

Corben, L. A., Delatycki, M. B., Bradshaw, J. L., Horne, M. K., Fahey, M. C., Churchyard, A. C., & Georgiou-Karistanis, N. (2010). Impairment in motor reprogramming in Friedreich ataxia reflecting possible cerebellar dysfunction. *Journal of Neurology, 257*(5), 782–791.

Corben, L. A., Georgiou-Karistianis, N., Bradshaw, J. L., Evans-Galea, M.V., Churchyard, A. J., & Delatycki, M. B. (2012). Characterising the Neuropathology and Neurobehavioural Phenotype in Friedreich Ataxia. In A. Hannan (Ed.), *Tandem Repeat Polymorphisms: Genetic Plasticity, Neural Diversity and Disease.* (pp. 169–184) Texas: Landes Bioscience and Springer Science and Business Media.

Corben, L. A., Georgiou-Karistianis, N., Bradshaw, J. L., Hocking, D. R., Churchyard, A. J., & Delatycki, M. B. (2011). The Fitts task reveals impairments in planning and online control of movement in Friedreich ataxia: Reduced cerebellar-cortico connectivity? *Neuroscience, 192*, 382–390. doi: 10.1016/j.neuroscience.2011.06.057.

Corben, L. A., Georgiou-Karistianis, N., Fahey, M. C., Storey, E., Churchyard, A., Horne, M. K., … Delatycki, M. B. (2006). Towards an understanding of cognitive function in Friedreich ataxia. *Brain Research Bulletin, 70*, 197–202.

Corben, L. A., Ho, M., Copland, J., Tai, G., & Delatycki, M. B. (2013). Increased prevalence of sleep-disordered breathing in Friedreich ataxia. *Neurology, 81*(1), 46–51. doi: 10.1212/WNL.0b013e318297ef18.

Corben, L. A., Kashuk, S. R., Akhlaghi, H., Jamadar, S., Delatycki, M. B., Fielding, J., … Egan, G. F. (2014). Myelin paucity of the superior cerebellar peduncle in individuals with Friedreich ataxia: An MRI magnetization transfer imaging study. *Journal of the Neurological Sciences, 343*(1–2), 138–143. doi: 10.1016/j.jns.2014.05.057.

Corben, L. A., Lynch, D., Pandolfo, M., Schulz, J. B., & Delatycki, M. B. (2014). Consensus clinical management guidelines for Friedreich ataxia. *Orphanet Journal of Rare Diseases, 9*, 184. doi: 10.1186/s13023-014-0184-7.

Cossée, M., Dürr, A., Schmitt, M., Dahl, N., Trouillas, P., Allinson, P., … Pandolfo, M. (1999). Friedreich's ataxia: Point mutations and clinical presentation of compound heterozygotes. *Annals of Neurology, 45*(2), 200–206.

Cossée, M., Puccio, H., Gansmuller, A., Koutnikova, H., Dierich, A., LeMeur, M., … Koenig, M. (2000). Inactivation of the Friedreich ataxia mouse gene leads to early embryonic lethality without iron accumulation. *Human Molecular Genetics, 9*(8), 1219–1226.

Cossée, M., Schmitt, M., Campuzano, V., Reutenauer, L., Moutou, C., Mandel, J. L., & Koenig, M. (1997). Evolution of the Friedreich's ataxia trinucleotide repeat expansion: Founder effect and premutations. *Proceedings of the National Academy of Sciences of the United States of America, 94*(14), 7452–7457.

De Castro, M., Garcia-Planells, J., Monros, E., Canizares, J., Vazquez-Manrique, R., Vilchez, J. J., … Palau, F. (2000). Genotype and phenotype analysis of Friedreich's ataxia compound heterozygous patients. *Human Genetics, 106*(1), 86–92.

De Michele, G., Filla, A., Cavalcanti, F., Di Maio, L., Pianese, L., Castaldo, I., … Campanella, G. (1994). Late onset Friedreich's disease: Clinical features and mapping of mutation to the FRDA locus. *Journal of Neurology, Neurosurgery & Psychiatry, 57*(8), 977–979.

De Michele, G., Filla, A., Criscuolo, C., Scarano, V., Cavalcanti, F., Pianese, L., … Cocozza, S. (1998). Determinants of onset age in Friedreich's ataxia. *Journal of Neurology, 245*(3), 166–168.

De Michele, G., Perrone, F., Filla, A., Mirante, E., Giordano, M., De Placido, S., & Campanella, G. (1996). Age of onset, sex, and cardiomyopathy as predictors of disability and survival in Friedreich's disease: A retrospective study on 119 patients. *Neurology, 47*(5), 1260–1264.

de Nóbrega, E., Nieto, A., Barrosso, J., & Montón, F. (2007). Differential impairment in semantic, phonemic, and action fluency performance in Friedreich's ataxia: Possible evidence of prefrontal dysfunction. *Journal of International Neuropsychology Society, 13*(6), 944–952.

Delatycki, M. B. (2009). Evaluating the progression of Friedreich ataxia and its treatment. *Journal of Neurology, 256*, 36–41. doi: 10.1007/s00415-009-1007-y.

Delatycki, M. B., & Corben, L. A. (2012). Clinical features of Friedreich ataxia. *Journal of Child Neurology, 27*(9), 1133–1137. doi: 10.1177/0883073812448230.

Delatycki, M. B., Holian, A., Corben, L., Rawicki, H. B., Blackburn, C., Hoare, B., … Churchyard, A. (2005). Surgery for equinovarus deformity in Friedreich's ataxia improves mobility and independence. *Clinical Orthopaedics & Related Research,* (430), 138–141.

Delatycki, M. B., Paris, D. B., Gardner, R. J., Nicholson, G. A., Nassif, N., Storey, E., … Forrest, S. M. (1999). Clinical and genetic study of Friedreich ataxia in an Australian population. *American Journal of Medical Genetics, 87*(2), 168–174.

Delatycki, M. B., Williamson, R., & Forrest, S. M. (2000). Friedreich ataxia: An overview. *Journal of Medical Genetics, 37*(1), 1–8.

Della Nave, R., Ginestroni, A., Giannelli, M., Tessa, C., Salvatore, E., Salvi, F., …. Mascalchi, M. (2008). Brain structural damage in Friedreich's ataxia. *Journal of Neurology, Neurosurgery & Psychiatry, 79*, 82–85.

Della Nave, R., Ginestroni, A., Tessa, C., Salvatore, E., Bartolomei, I., Salvi, F., … Mascalchi, M. (2008). Brain white matter tracts degeneration in Friedreich ataxia. An in vivo MRI study using tract-based spatial statistics and voxel-based morphometry. *Neuroimage, 40*(1), 19–25. doi: 10.1016/j.neuroimage.2007.11.050.

Doron, K. W., Funk, C. M., & Glickstein, M. (2010). Fronto-cerebellar circuits and eye movement control: A diffusion imaging tractography study of human cortico-pontine projections. *Brain Research, 1307*, 63–71.

Dürr, A., Cossee, M., Agid, Y., Campuzano, V., Mignard, C., Penet, C., … Koenig, M. (1996). Clinical and genetic abnormalities in patients with Friedreich's ataxia. *New England Journal of Medicine, 335*(16), 1169–1175.

Dutka, D. P., Donnelly, J. E., Nihoyannopoulos, P., Oakley, C. M., & Nunez, D. J. (1999). Marked variation in the cardiomyopathy associated with Friedreich's ataxia. *Heart, 81*(2), 141–147.

Egger, K., Clemm von Hohenberg, C., Schocke, M. F., Guttmann, C. R., Wassermann, D., Wigand, M. C., ... Boesch, S. (2014). White matter changes in patients with Friedreich ataxia after treatment with erythropoietin. *Journal of Neuroimaging, 24*(5), 504–508. doi: 10.1111/jon.12050.

Eigentler A., Nauchbauer W., Donnemiller E., Poewe W., Gasser R. W., & Boesch, S. B. (2014). Low bone mineral density in Friedreich ataxia. *Cerebellum, 13*, 549–557.

Evans-Galea, M.V., Carrodus, N., Rowley, S. M., Corben, L. A., Tai, G., Saffery, R., ... Sarsero, J. P. (2012). FXN methylation predicts expression and clinical outcome in Friedreich ataxia. *Annals of Neurology, 71*(4), 487–497. doi: 10.1002/ana.22671.

Evans-Galea, M. V., Lockhart, P. J., Galea, C. A., Hannan, A. J., & Delatycki, M. B. (2014). Beyond loss of frataxin: The complex molecular pathology of Friedreich ataxia. *Discovery Medicine, 17*(91), 25–35.

Fahey, M. C., Cremer, P. D., Swee, T. A., Millist, L., Todd, M. J., White, O. B., ... Delatycki. M.B. (2008). Vestibular, saccadic and fixation abnormalities in genetically confirmed Friedreich ataxia. *Brain, 131*, 1035–1045.

Fielding, J., Corben, L., Cremer, P., Millist, L., White, O., & Delatycki, M. D. (2010). Disruption to higher order processes in Friedreich ataxia. *Neuropsychologia, 48*(1), 235–242.

Folker, J., Murdoch, B., Cahill, L., Delatycki, M., Corben, L., & Vogel, A. (2010). Dysarthria in Friedreich's Ataxia: A perceptual analysis. *Folia Phoniatrica et Logopedica, 62*, 97–103.

Franca, M. C., Jr., D'Abreu, A., Yasuda, C. L., Bonadia, L. C., Santos da Silva, M., Nucci, A., ... Cendes, F. (2009). A combined voxel-based morphometry and 1H-MRS study in patients with Friedreich's ataxia. *Journal of Neurology, 256*(7), 1114–1120. doi: 10.1007/s00415-009-5079-5.

Friedreich, N. (1863). Uber degenerative atrophie der spinalen hinterstrange. *Virchow's Archiv fur Pathologische Anatomie, 27*, 1–26.

Friedreich, N. (1876). Uber ataxie mit besonderer berucksichtigung der herditaren formen. *Virchow's Archiv fur Pathologische Anatomie, 68*, 145–245.

Friedreich, N. (1877). Uber ataxie mit besonderer berucksichtigung der hereditaren formen. *Virchow's Archiv fur Pathologische Anatomie, 70*, 140–152.

Georgiou-Karistianis, N., Akhlaghi, H., Corben, L. A., Delatycki, M. B., Storey, E., Bradshaw, J. L., & Egan, G. F. (2012). Decreased functional brain activation in Friedreich ataxia using the Simon effect task. *Brain Cognition, 79*(3), 200–208. doi: 10.1016/j.bandc.2012.02.011.

Gibilisco, P., & Vogel, A. P. (2013). Friedreich ataxia. *BMJ, 347*, f7062. doi: 10.1136/bmj.f7062.

Ginestroni, A., Diciotti, S., Cecchi, P., Pesaresi, I., Tessa, C., Giannelli, M., ... Mascalchi, M. (2012). Neurodegeneration in Friedreich's ataxia is associated with a mixed activation pattern of the brain. A fMRI study. *Human Brain Mapping, 33*(8), 1780–1791. doi: 10.1002/hbm.21319.

Harding, A. E. (1981). Friedreich's ataxia: A clinical and genetic study of 90 families with an analysis of early diagnostic criteria and intrafamilial clustering of clinical features. *Brain, 104*(3), 589–620.

Hart, R. P., Henry, G. K., Kwentus, J. A., & Leshner, R. T. (1986). Information processing speed of children with Friedreich's ataxia. *Developmental Medicine & Child Neurology, 28*(3), 310–313.

Hart, R. P., Kwentus, J. A., Leshner, R. T., & Frazier, R. (1985). Information processing speed in Friedreich's ataxia. *Annals of Neurology, 17*(6), 612–614.

Hocking, D. R., Corben, L. A., Fielding, J., Cremer, P. D., Millist, L., White, O. B., & Delatycki, M. B. (2014). Saccade reprogramming in Friedreich ataxia reveals impairments in the cognitive control of saccadic eye movement. *Brain Cognition, 87*, 161–167. doi: 10.1016/j.bandc.2014.03.018.

Kelly, M., Bagnall, R. D., Peverill, R. E., Donelan, L., Corben, L., Delatycki, M. B., & Semsarian, C. (2011). A polymorphic miR-155 binding site in AGTR1 is associated with cardiac hypertrophy in Friedreich ataxia. *Journal of Molecular and Cellular Cardiology, 51*(5), 848–854.

Klopper, F., Delatycki, M.B., Corben, L. A., Bradshaw, J. L., Rance, G., & Georgiou-Karistianis, N. (2011). The test of everyday attention reveals significant sustained volitional attention and working memory deficits in Friedreich ataxia. *Journal of International Neuropsychology Society, 17*(1), 196–200. doi: 10.1017/S1355617710001347.

Koeppen, A. H. (2011). Friedreich's ataxia: Pathology, pathogenesis, and molecular genetics. *Journal of Neurological Sciences, 303*(1–2), 1–12. doi: 10.1016/j.jns.2011.01.010.

Koeppen, A. H., & Mazurkiewicz, J. E. (2013). Friedreich ataxia: Neuropathology revised. *Journal of Neuropathology & Experimental Neurology, 72*(2), 78–90. doi: 10.1097/NEN.0b013e31827e5762.

Koeppen, A. H., Davis, A. N., & Morral, J. A. (2011). The cerebellar component of Friedreich's ataxia. *Acta Neuropathologica, 122*(3), 323–330.

Koeppen, A. H., Kuntzsch, E. C., Bjork, S. T., Ramirez, R. L., Mazurkiewicz, J. E., & Feustel, P. J. (2013). Friedreich ataxia: Metal dysmetabolism in dorsal root ganglia. *Acta Neuropathol Commun, 1*, 26. doi: 10.1186/2051-5960-1-26.

Koeppen, A. H., Morral, J. A., Davis, A. N., Qian, J., Petrocine, S. V., Knutson, M. D., … Danhong, L. (2009). The dorsal root ganglion in Friedreich's ataxia. *Acta Neuropathologica, 118*(6), 763–776.

Koeppen, A. H., Morral, J. A., McComb, R. D., & Feustel, P. J. (2011). The neuropathology of late-onset Friedreichs' ataxia. *Cerebellum, 10*(1), 96–103. doi: DOI 10.1007/s12311-010-0235-0.

Koeppen, A. H., Ramirez, R. L., Becker, A. B., Feustel, P. J., & Mazurkiewicz, J. E. (2015). Friedreich ataxia: Failure of GABA-ergic and glycinergic synaptic transmission in the dentate nucleus. *Journal of Neuropathology & Experimental Neurology, 74*(2), 166–176. doi: 10.1097/NEN.0000000000000160.

Labelle, H., Tohme, S., Duhaime, M., & Allard, P. (1986). Natural history of scoliosis in Friedreich's ataxia. *Journal of Bone & Joint Surgery—American Volume, 68*(4), 564–572.

Loose, R., Kaufmann, C., Tucha, O., Auer, D. P., & Lange, K. W. (2006). Neural networks of response shifting: Influence of task speed and stimulus material. *Brain Research, 1090*(1), 146–155.

Lowe, G. C., Corben, L. A., Duncan, R. E., Yoon, G., & Delatycki, M. B. (2015). "Both sides of the wheelchair": The views of individuals with, and parents of individuals with Friedreich ataxia regarding pre-symptomatic testing of minors. *Journal of Genetic Counseling, 24*(5), 732–743. doi: 10.1007/s10897-014-9801-9.

Manto, M., & Lorivel, T. (2011). Cognitive repercussions of hereditary cerebellar disorders. *Cortex, 47*(1), 81–100.

Mantovan, M. C., Martinuzzi, A., Squarzanti, F., Bolla, A., Silvestri, I., Liessi, G., … Angelini, C. (2006). Exploring mental status in Friedreich's ataxia: A combined neuropsychological, behavioural and neuroimaging study. *European Journal of Neurology, 13*, 827–835.

Mascalchi, M. (2013). The cerebellum looks normal in Friedreich ataxia. *AJNR American Journal of Neuroradiology, 34*(2), E22. doi: 10.3174/ajnr.A3480.

Mateo, I., Llorca, J., Volpini, V., Corral, J., Berciano, J., & Combarros, O. (2004). Expanded GAA repeats and clinical variation in Friedreich's ataxia. *Acta Neurologica Scandinavica, 109*(1), 75–78.

Metz, G., Coppard, N., Cooper, J. M., Delatycki, M. B., Durr, A., Di Prospero, N. A., … Meier, T. (2013). Rating disease progression of Friedreich's ataxia by the International Cooperative Ataxia Rating Scale: Analysis of a 603-patient database. *Brain, 136*(pt 1), 259–268. doi: 10.1093/brain/aws309.

Milbrandt, T. A., Kunes, J. R., & Karol, L. A. (2008). Friedreich ataxia and scoliosis. The experience of two institutions. *Journal of Pediatric Orthopaedics, 28*(2), 234–238.

Milne, S. C., Campagna, E. J., Corben, L. A., Delatycki, M. B., Teo, K., Churchyard, A. J., & Haines, T. P. (2012). Retrospective study of the effects of inpatient rehabilitation on improving and maintaining functional independence in people with Friedreich ataxia. *Archives of Physical Medicine & Rehabilitation, 93*(10), 1860–1863.

Milne, S., Campagna, E., Delatycki, M. B., & Corben, L. A. (2013). Rehabilitation for individuals with Friedreich ataxia: A model of comprehensive care. In M. Morris and R. Iansek (Eds.), *Rehabilitation in Movement Disorders*. (pp 185–202). New York: Cambridge University Press.

Montermini, L., Andermann, E., Labuda, M., Richter, A., Pandolfo, M., Cavalcanti, F., … Cocozza, S. (1997). The Friedreich ataxia GAA triplet repeat: Premutation and normal alleles. *Human Molecular Genetics, 6*(8), 1261–1266.

Montermini, L., Richter, A., Morgan, K., Justice, C. M., Julien, D., Castellotti, B., … Pandolfo, M. (1997). Phenotypic variability in Friedreich ataxia: Role of the associated GAA triplet repeat expansion. *Annals of Neurology, 41*(5), 675–682.

Morral, J. A., Davis, A. N., Qian, J., Gelman, B. B., & Koeppen, A. H. (2010). Pathology and pathogenesis of sensory neuropathy in Friedreich's ataxia. *Acta Neuropathologica, 120*(1), 97–108. doi: 10.1007/s00401-010-0675-0.

Mottram, P. M., Delatycki, M. B., Donelan, L., Gelman, J. S., Corben, L. A., & Peverill, R. E. (2011). Early changes in left ventricular long axis function in Friedreich ataxia – Relation with the FXN gene mutation and cardiac structural change. *Journal of the American Society of Echocardiography, 24*(7), 782–789.

Nachbauer, W., Bodner, T., Boesch, S., Karner, E., Eigentler, A., Neier, L., … Delazer, M. (2014). Friedreich ataxia: Executive control is related to disease onset and GAA repeat length. *Cerebellum, 13*(1), 9–16. doi: 10.1007/s12311-013-0513-8.

Nieto, A., Correia, R., de Nobrega, E., Monton, F., & Barroso, J. (2013). Cognition in late-onset Friedreich ataxia. *Cerebellum, 12*(4), 504–512. doi: 10.1007/s12311-013-0457-z.

Nieto, A., Correia, R., de Nóbrega, E., Montón, F., Hess, S., & Barroso, J. (2012). Cognition in Friedreich ataxia. *Cerebellum, 11*(4), 834–844.

Noval, S., Contreras, I., Sanz-Gallego, I., Manrique, R. K., & Arpa, J. (2012). Ophthalmic features of Friedreich ataxia. *Eye (Lond), 26*(2), 315–320. doi: 10.1038/eye.2011.291.

Pagani, E., Ginestroni, A., Della Nave, R., Agosta, F., Salvi, F., De Michele, G., … Mascalchi, M. (2010). Assessment of brain white matter fiber bundle atrophy in patients with Friedreich ataxia. *Radiology, 255*(3), 882–889. doi: 10.1148/radiol.10091742.

Pandolfo, M. (2009). Friedreich Ataxia: The clinical picture. *Journal of Neurology, 256*, 3–8.

Pandolfo, M., & Pastore, A. (2009). The pathogenesis of Friedreich ataxia and the structure and function of frataxin. *Journal of Neurology, 256*(Suppl 1), 9–17.

Parkinson, M. H., Boesch, S., Nachbauer, W., Mariotti, C., & Giunti, P. (2013). Clinical features of Friedreich's ataxia: Classical and atypical phenotypes. *Journal of Neurochemistry, 126 Suppl 1*, 103–117. doi: 10.1111/jnc.12317.

Pastore, A., & Puccio, H. (2013). Frataxin: A protein in search for a function. *Journal of Neurochemistry, 126 Suppl 1*, 43–52. doi: 10.1111/jnc.12220.

Quercia, N., Somers, G. R., Halliday, W., Kantor, P. F., Banwell, B., & Yoon, G. (2010). Friedreich ataxia presenting as sudden cardiac death in childhood: Clinical, genetic and pathological correlation, with implications for genetic testing and counselling. *Neuromuscular Disorders, 20*, 340–342.

Rance, G., Corben, L. A., & Delatycki, M. B. (2012). Auditory pathway changes mirror overall disease progress in individuals with Friedreich ataxia. *Journal of Neurology, 259*(12), 2746–2748. doi: 10.1007/s00415-012-6679-z.

Rance, G., Corben, L., Barker, E., Carew, P., Chisari, D., Rogers, M., … Delatycki, M. (2010). Auditory perception in individuals with Friedreich's ataxia. *Audiology & Neurotology, 15*, 229–240.

Rance, G., Fava, R., Baldock, H., Chong, A., Barker, E., Corben, L., & Delatycki, M. (2008). Speech perception ability in individuals with Friedreich ataxia. *Brain, 131*, 2002–2012.

Reetz, K., Dogan, I., Costa, A. S., Dafotakis, M., Fedosov, K., Giunti, P., … Schulz, J. B. (2015). Biological and clinical characteristics of the European Friedreich's Ataxia Consortium for Translational Studies (EFACTS) cohort: A cross-sectional analysis of baseline data. *Lancet Neurology, 14*(2), 174–182. doi: 10.1016/S1474-4422(14)70321-7.

Regner, S. R., Lagedrost, S. J., Plappert, T., Paulsen, E. K., Friedman, L. S., Snyder, M. L., … Lynch, D. R. (2012). Analysis of echocardiograms in a large heterogeneous cohort of patients with Friedreich ataxia. *The American Journal of Cardiology, 109*(3), 401–405.

Ribaï, P., Pousset, F., Tanguy, M., Rivaud-Pechoux, S., Le Ber, I., Gasparini, F., … Dürr, A. (2007). Neurological, cardiological, and oculomotor progression in 104 patients with Friedreich ataxia during long-term follow-up. *Archives of Neurology, 64*, 558–564.

Salthouse, T. A., & Heddon, T. (2002). Interpreting reaction time measures in between-group comparisons. *Journal of Clinical & Experimental Neuropsychology, 24*(7), 858–872.

Santner, W., Schocke, M., Boesch, S., Nachbauer, W., & Egger, K. (2014). A longitudinal VBM study monitoring treatment with erythropoietin in patients with Friedreich ataxia. *Acta Radiologica Short Reports, 3*(4), 2047981614531573. doi: 10.1177/2047981614531573.

Santos, R., Lefevre, S., Sliwa, S., Seguin, A., Camadro, J., & Lesuisse, E. (2010). Friedreich Ataxia: Molecular mechanisms, redox considerations, and therapeutic opportunities. *Antioxidants & Redox Signaling, 13*(5), 651–690.

Schmahmann, J. D. (2004). Disorders of the cerebellum: ataxia, dysmetria of thought, and the cerebellar cognitive affective syndrome. *Journal of Neuropsychiatry & Clinical Neurosciences, 16*(3), 367–378.

Schmitz-Hübsch, T., du Montcel, S. T., Baliko, L., Berciano, J., Boesch, S., Depondt, C., … Fancellu, R. (2006). Scale for the assessment and rating of ataxia: Development of a new clinical scale. *Neurology, 66*, 1717–1720.

Schulz, J. B., Boesch, S., Bürk, K., Dürr, A., Giunti, P., Mariotti, C., … Pandolfo, M. (2009). Diagnosis and treatment of Friedreich ataxia: A European perspective. *Nature Review Neurology, 5*(4), 222–234.

Seyer, L. A., Galetta, K., Wilson, J., Sakai, R., Perlman, S., Mathews, K., … Lynch, D. R. (2013). Analysis of the visual system in Friedreich ataxia. *Journal of Neurology*. doi: DOI 10.1007/s00415-013-6978-z.

Shapiro, F., & Specht, L. (1993). The diagnosis and orthopaedic treatment of childhood spinal muscular atrophy, peripheral neuropathy, Friedreich ataxia, and arthrogryposis. *Journal of Bone & Joint Surgery—American Volume, 75*(11), 1699–1714.

Silva, C. B., Yasuda, C. L., D'Abreu, A., Cendes, F., Lopes-Cendes, I., & Franca, M. C., Jr. (2013). Neuroanatomical correlates of depression in Friedreich's ataxia: A voxel-based morphometry study. *Cerebellum, 12*(3), 429–436. doi: 10.1007/s12311-012-0424-0.

Stefanescu, M. R., Dohnalek, M., Maderwald, S., Thurling, M., Minnerop, M., Beck, A., … Timmann, D. (2015). Structural and functional MRI abnormalities of cerebellar cortex and nuclei in SCA3, SCA6 and Friedreich's ataxia. *Brain, 138*(Pt 5), 1182–1197. doi: 10.1093/brain/awv064.

Subramony, S. H., May, W., Lynch, D., Gomez, C., Fischbeck, K., Hallett, M., … Ashizawa, T. (2005). Measuring Friedreich ataxia: Interrater reliability of a neurologic rating scale. *Neurology, 64*(7), 1261–1262.

Synofzik, M., Godau, J., Lindig, T., Schols, L., & Berg, D. (2011). Transcranial sonography reveals cerebellar, nigral, and forebrain abnormalities in Friedreich's ataxia. *Neurodegenerative Diseases, 8*(6), 470–475. doi: 10.1159/000327751.

Timmann, D., Drepper, J., Frings, M., Maschke, M., Richter, S., Gerwig, M., & Kolb, F. P. (2010). The human cerebellum contributes to motor, emotional and cognitive associative learning. A review. *Cortex, 46*(7), 845–857.

Trouillas, P., Takayanagi, T., Hallett, M., Currier, R. D., Subramony, S. H., Wessel, K., … Manyam, B. (1997). International Cooperative Ataxia Rating Scale for pharmacological assessment of the cerebellar syndrome. The Ataxia Neuropharmacology Committee of the World Federation of Neurology. *Journal of Neurological Sciences, 145*(2), 205–211.

Tsou, A. Y., Paulsen, E. K., Lagedrost, S. J., Perlman, S. L., Mathews, K. D., Wilmot, G. R., … Lynch, D. R. (2011). Mortality in Friedreich ataxia. *Journal of Neurological Sciences, 307*, 46–49.

Vieira Karuta, S. C., Raskin, S., de Carvalho Neto, A., Gasparetto, E. L., Doring, T., & Teive, H. A. (2015). Diffusion tensor imaging and tract-based spatial statistics analysis in Friedreich's ataxia patients. *Parkinsonism & Related Disorders, 21*(5), 504–508. doi: 10.1016/j.parkreldis.2015.02.021.

Vogel, A. P., Brown, S. E., Folker, J. E., Corben, L. A., & Delatycki, M. B. (2014). Dysphagia and swallowing-related quality of life in Friedreich ataxia. *Journal of Neurology, 261*(2), 392–399. doi: 10.1007/s00415-013-7208-4.

Weidemann, F., Stork, S., Liu, D., Hu, K., Herrmann, S., Ertl, G., & Niemann, M. (2013). Cardiomyopathy of Friedreich ataxia. *Journal of Neurochemistry, 126* (Suppl 1), 88–93. doi: 10.1111/jnc.12217.

White, M., Lalonde, R., & Botez-Marquard, T. (2000). Neuropsychologic and neuropsychiatric characteristics of patients with Friedreich's ataxia. *Acta Neurologica Scandinavica, 102*(4), 222–226.

White, O. B., & Fielding, J. (2012). Cognition and eye movements: Assessment of cerebral dysfunction. *Journal of Neuro-ophthalmology, 32*(3), 266–273. doi: 10.1097/WNO.0b013e3182688230.

Wollmann, T., Barroso, J., Monton, F., & Nieto, A. (2002). Neuropsychological test performance of patients with Friedreich's ataxia. *Journal of Clinical & Experimental Neuropsychology, 24*(5), 677–686.

Zalesky, A., Akhlaghi, H., Corben, L. A., Bradshaw, J. L., Delatycki, M. B., Storey, E., … Egan, G. F. (2014). Cerebello-cerebral connectivity deficits in Friedreich ataxia. *Brain Structure & Function, 219*(3), 969–981. doi: 10.1007/s00429-013-0547-1.

18

FRAGILE X SYNDROME AND OTHER *FMR1*-RELATED CONDITIONS

Esther S. Ginsberg and David J. Amor

Introduction

Fragile X Syndrome (FXS), the most common cause of inherited intellectual disability, is a genetic developmental disorder, normally transmitted matrilineally and characterised by particular physical features, autistic behaviours, attention problems, hyperactivity, social anxiety and distinctive neurocognitive deficits. The condition, also known as Martin-Bell syndrome, is caused by alterations in the *Fragile X Mental Retardation 1* gene (*FMR1*) located on the long arm of the X chromosome (Xq27.3), which disrupt the synthesis of a functional Fragile X Mental Retardation Protein (FMRP), the product of the affected gene. The most frequent alteration is an increase in the number of consecutive cytosine-guanine-guanine (CGG) repeats in a repetitive DNA sequence in the section coding for the mRNA 5' untranslated region (5'UTR). When such tandem repeats exceed approximately 200 units (*full mutation*), epigenetic modifications (cytosine methylation at CpG sites) occur on the expansion mutation and on the gene's promoter, which typically lead to gene silencing and absence of FMRP (Oberle, 1991; Sutcliffe et al., 1992; Verkerk et al., 1991). Some i ndividuals may have "repeat-length mosaicism" (e.g. full mutation plus premutation) or "methylation mosaicism" (methylated full mutation plus unmethylated full mutation), and individuals in either category may have a less severe phenotype and exhibit variable FMRP levels. FMRP, an mRNA-binding protein involved in translational repression, is expressed in several organs, particularly gonads and the nervous system, where it is required for normal neuronal development, synaptic pruning and plasticity. These neuronal processes, altered in FXS, are thought to underlie the neurocognitive phenotype. Males tend to be more severely affected than females, who normally carry an intact copy of *FMR1* in their second X chromosome. However, in females one X chromosome in every cell is largely inactivated epigenetically. Although inactivation is usually random, skewing in favour of either the maternal or paternal chromosome may be present, leading to a proportion of active X chromosomes with a normal *FMR1* gene that diverges from 50 percent. As a consequence of mosaicism and heterogeneity in X-chromosome inactivation ratios, levels of FMRP may differ widely among individuals, leading to the vastly variable expressivity of the phenotype. Higher FMRP levels are associated with a lower impairment of IQ, cognitive and motor abilities and language development (Kau, Reider, Payne, Meyer, & Freund, 2000; Loesch, Huggins, & Hagerman, 2004). Penetrance for the full mutation is reduced for females and virtually complete for males (Monaghan, Lyon, & Spector, 2013), although mosaic males may have normal intelligence and only very subtle phenotypic features. The condition is usually associated with a normal lifespan.

FXS is one of several disorders related to *FMR1* CGG tandem repeat expansions (see Table 18.1). Alleles with repeat numbers in the ranges of 55–200 (*premutation*) and 44–55 ("*grey zone*") have been linked to Fragile X-associated tremor/ataxia syndrome (FXTAS), a progressive neurodegenerative disease, to Fragile X-associated primary ovarian insufficiency (FXPOI), presenting as early menopause, and to a host of psychiatric, behavioural and cognitive complaints (Loesch, Churchyard, Brotchie, Marot, & Tassone, 2005; Loesch et al., 2011). The molecular pathogenesis of premutation phenotypes is distinct from that of full mutations: premutations are associated with *increased* transcription of FMR1, with elevated levels of CGG repeat-containing FMR1 RNA postulated to cause RNA-mediated cell toxicity (Galloway & Nelson, 2009).

TABLE 18.1 Disorders related to *FMR1* tandem repeat expansions

Mutation type	*Number of CGG repeats*	*Methylation status of* FMR1	*Clinical status*	
			Male	*Female*
Grey Zone	45–54	Unmethylated	At low risk of FXTAS	
Premutation	~55–200	Unmethylated	At risk for FXTAS [1]	At risk for POI and FXTAS [1]
Full mutation	>200	Methylated	100% with intellectual disability	Variable: ~half intellectual disability, half normal intellect
Repeat size mosaicism	<200 and >200 in different cell lines	Partial: mixture of methylated and unmethylated cells	Intellectual disability, usually higher functioning than males with full mutation. At risk of FXTAS.	Variable: normal intellect to mild intellectual disability
Methylation mosaicism	>200	Partial: mixture of methylated and unmethylated cells		
Unmethylated full mutation	>200	Unmethylated	Variable: normal intellect to mild intellectual disability. At risk of FXTAS.	

Preliminary considerations

The relationship between the X chromosome and the intellectual disability phenotype was initially identified cytogenetically in the karyotypes of a proband and related family members obtained by culturing leukocytes under specific conditions (Lubs, 1969). A secondary constriction, the "fragile" site (labelled *Fragile X-Chromosome Site A*, FRAXA) was observed in a fraction of the X chromosomes.

Segregation analyses of this X chromosome in multiple pedigrees showed that penetrance of intellectual impairment depended on the position of individuals within the pedigree: normal transmitting males could pass the allele to their daughters who were also non-penetrant for FXS, but their grandsons showed a much higher risk of being affected (Sherman, Morton, Jacobs, & Turner, 1984). This finding, known as the *Sherman paradox* (genetic anticipation), is explained by the instability of the expansion mutation. Premutation alleles are meiotically and mitotically unstable, tending to increase or decrease in size. The risk of meiotic expansion during oogenesis rises with CGG number, while mitotic instability leads to repeat-length mosaicism (Fu et al., 1991; Oberle, 1991). Selection against the full mutation may occur in the male germ line, which accounts for the mainly matrilineal transmission of FXS (Ashley-Koch et al., 1998).

Onset and prevalence

The onset of FXS is related to CGG repeat number in the expanded tract. Individuals positioned at a certain distance from the ancestral carrier in the family pedigree have a higher probability of carrying the full mutation and expressing FXS in childhood. By contrast, *FMR1*-related disorders linked to premutations are of adult onset.

FXS affects all human subpopulations. Clinical prevalence is estimated at 1:4000 males and 1:8000 females (Turner, Webb, Wake, & Robinson, 1996). On the basis of molecular screening of the general population, the full mutation is thought to be carried by 1 in 2500–5000 individuals (Coffee et al., 2009; Fernandez-Carvajal et al., 2009).

Clinical presentation

Physical phenotype

The physical features of FXS are most apparent in postpubertal males and are frequently absent in females and prepubertal males. Importantly, the absence of physical features cannot be used to exclude the diagnosis of FXS and genetic testing for FXS is recommended in all individuals with cognitive impairment.

Newborns and infants have an increased chance of suffering from congenital hip dislocation, club foot, cleft lip and palate, chronic otitis media, inguinal hernia, gastroesophagical reflux, feeding problems, strabismus, nystagmus, hypotonia and seizures (Hersh, Saul, & Genetics, 2011).

FXS has a characteristic facies: long narrow face, prominent forehead and jaw, elongated everted ears, epicanthic folds, prognathism and relative macrocephaly. Ophthalmological problems such as strabismus, hyperopia, astigmatism, high myopia, cataracts, palpebral ptosis, and adult-onset glaucoma are common (Storm, PeBenito, & Ferretti, 1987). Other frequent features, such as hyperextensible finger joints, mitral valve prolapse, aortic dilation, pectus excavatum, scoliosis, high-arched palate, flat feet and soft skin may be related to a dysplasia of the connective tissue (Lachiewicz, Dawson, & Spiridigliozzi, 2000). Macroorchidism, occasionally found in childhood (Lachiewicz & Dawson, 1994), becomes common after puberty. Males with a full mutation can be fertile (Willems et al., 1992), but fertility is reduced due to impaired spermatogenesis and testicular histological anomalies (Johannisson, Rehde, Wendt, & Schwinger, 1987).

Physiological phenotype

Endocrine abnormalities suggestive of alterations in the function of the hypothalamic-pituitary-adrenal (HPA) axis have been reported (Reiss & Dant, 2003). Macroorchidism and precocious puberty in females may be a manifestation of this dysfunction (Moore, Chudley, & Winter, 1990).

An atypical growth-in-stature pattern has been observed in longitudinal data on body height. Relative to the healthy population, children with FXS, particularly males, experience an accelerated growth throughout the preadolescent period followed by a reduced growth rate during adolescence (Loesch, Huggins, & Hoang, 1995).

Sleep and circadian rhythm are compromised, with greater variability in total sleep time and maintenance. Disrupted sleep architecture has been observed in children, who tend to spend less time in bed and experience a lower proportion of REM sleep (Miano et al., 2008). Melatonin levels are, paradoxically, elevated (Gould et al., 2000), possibly in compensation. Mice missing FMRP have normal cell activity in the supra-chiasmatic nucleus (the circadian centre) but altered cyclical abundance patterns of various clock-component mRNAs (Zhang et al., 2008), which points to a possible role of FMRP in daily cycle regulation.

A generally hyper-excitable nervous system, which underlies hyper-arousal, epilepsy, anxiety, hyperactivity and increased sensory sensitivity, is a feature of FXS. Hyper-arousal, assessed by salivary cortisol, is higher in affected children, particularly males. Increased levels of this hormone, secreted in response to stress, have been detected in boys on typical as well as socially challenging days (Hessl et al., 2002). Boys also showed prominent features of social anxiety (gaze aversion, signs of discomfort and avoidance during social interaction with an unfamiliar adult) when socially challenged (Hessl, Glaser, Dyer-Friedman, & Reiss, 2006). Cortisol levels were lower when eye contact was averted, which suggests an association between gaze avoidance and reaction to stress mediated by the limbic-HPA.

Epilepsy affects around 20 percent of FXS patients. Seizures may start and resolve in childhood, implicate the temporal and frontal lobes and respond well to medication (Musumeci, 1999). EEG patterns and seizures are frequently similar to those of benign focal epilepsy of childhood; individuals who are seizure-free may show epileptiform abnormalities in the EEG (Berry-Kravis, 2002).

Anxiety, hyperactivity, hyperarousal and aggression, the latter frequent in males, may be behavioural responses triggered by heightened sensory sensitivity in FXS (Hagerman & Cronister, 1996). Enhanced sensitivity to stimuli of different sensory modalities in FXS has indeed been reported. Miller et al. (1999) measured electrodermal responses, determined by the sympathetic system, to stimuli of different modalities in healthy and affected individuals. Responses were higher in the FXS group, for all sensory modalities, and correlated inversely with FMRP levels.

Neuropsychological phenotype

Full scale intelligence is usually impaired in FXS, more severely in males. Around 15% of affected males have an intelligent quotient (IQ) above 70 (Hagerman, 2006), but only 60% of females carrying a full mutation show mild to moderate mental impairment and 40% have normal intellectual capacity (Willemsen et al., 2003) or even above-average intelligence. Even when IQ is normal, FXS may be linked to specific learning difficulties. Thus, impaired mathematical and visuo-spatial skills have been reported in females (Murphy & Mazzocco, 2008).

Persons with FXS have poor cognitive control, with deficits in inhibition (capacity to limit or suppress responses or processes) and cognitive flexibility (ability to change cognitive sets according to contextual demands). These deficits, suggestive of fronto-striatal compromise, may underlie impulsivity, attention problems, and cognitive and verbal perseveration in FXS.

Similarly, some attention modalities are compromised in FXS. Sustained attention, the ability to remain on task for a relatively long period of time, seems to be intact (Munir, Cornish, & Wilding, 2000b; Sullivan et al., 2007), but selective and divided attention (respectively the capacity to orient to some stimuli and disregard others and the skill to focus on several stimuli at once), may show deficits (Munir et al., 2000b).

Working memory, the temporary storage and manipulation of information needed for complex cognitive activities, was observed to be impaired in boys with FXS, particularly for the recall of non-meaningful information (Hooper et al., 2008; Munir, Cornish, & Wilding, 2000a). Verbal and visuospatial working memory deficits were also detected, more pronounced for tasks demanding higher cognitive control (Lanfranchi, Cornoldi, Drigo, & Vianello, 2009).

Persons with FXS have difficulties in social interaction and communication that stem from language weaknesses, avoidance of eye contact and deficits in theory of mind. Thus, the speech of boys with FXS engaged in dyadic face-to-face conversation features repetitions (phonemes, words or phrases) and tangential language (utterances whose content is not related to the current topic of conversation). These dysfluencies could be attributable to an awareness of social obligations and a desire to communicate, both hindered by anxiety and arousal, a situation that may also accelerate speech and enhance the effects of inhibitory deficits (Sudhalter & Belser, 2001).

Face-to-face conversation usually implies eye contact, which individuals with FXS try to avoid. Functional magnetic resonance imaging studies show atypical patterns of brain activation during exposure to direct gaze (e.g. Watson, Hoeft, Garrett, Hall, & Reiss, 2008). During successive exposure to direct gaze, affected boys exhibit higher activation in the frontal cortex, lower activation in the left insula, and enhanced sensitisation in the left amygdala (Watson et al., 2008). Increased amygdala and insula activation has been observed in anxiety-prone individuals during emotion processing (Stein, Simmons, Feinstein, & Paulus, 2007), which suggests a relation between gaze processing and elevated anxiety in FXS.

Theory of mind (TOM), the ability to attribute mental states to oneself and to others, is affected in FXS. Cornish et al. (2005) detected a specific signature characterised by an inability to dissociate appearance from reality, the latter prevailing in participants' judgments. Grant, Apperly, and Oliver (2007) observed deficits in boys with few and many autistic features, but attributed these deficits to a more basic difficulty with working memory. Losh, Martin, Klusek, Hogan-Brown, and Sideris (2012) identified similar TOM shortfalls in boys with autism and with comorbid FXS/autism, but not with non-comorbid FXS. This suggests that a single network may underlie TOM deficits in both idiopathic and FXS-associated autism.

Comorbidities

FXS is frequently comorbid with Autism Spectrum Disorder (ASD) and Attention Deficit Hyperactivity Disorder (ADHD), both of which are developmental conditions of diverse etiology, diagnosed behaviourally, involving a complex set of dysfunctions.

ASD involves a number of disabilities, such as poor social communication/interaction and restricted/repetitive behaviours. While persons with FXS usually exhibit some autistic traits, such as gaze avoidance or impaired social interaction, only 35% meet the criteria for ASD diagnosis. Conversely, 2.5% – 6% of individuals with a primary diagnosis of ASD may actually have FXS (Hagerman, R. & Hagerman, P., 2002). The comorbid sub-phenotype has more severe cognitive, adaptive and receptive/expressive language deficits than the single conditions. Interestingly, FMRP levels are not associated with autistic traits. This suggests that additional genetic factors may underlie the comorbidity (Hagerman & Harris,

2008). Nevertheless, *FMR1*-associated autism may not be identical to non-syndromic ASD. A comparison of autistic traits in FXS and ASD boys matched for IQ showed that comorbid FXS/ASD occurs with lower impairments in some social, non-verbal and repetitive behaviours, but more manic-hyperactive and general-anxiety behaviours than non-syndromic ASD (Thurman, McDuffie, Hagerman, & Abbeduto, 2014). This discordance is further supported by the observation of different brain anomalies in toddlers affected by each condition (Hazlett et al., 2009).

ADHD, which involves problems with attentional control and/or hyperactivity/impulsivity, affects 36%–93% of patients with FXS (in Sullivan et al., 2007). Impaired inhibition, prominent in FXS, has been postulated as an enabler of hyperactive forms of ADHD through its effect on executive functions (Barkley, 1997). Consequently, this shared inhibition deficit could underlie FXS-ADHD comorbidity. Comorbid ADHD, more frequent in males, follows a lifespan course: hyperactivity increases during childhood and declines with growth, although inattention may persist in adulthood (Tranfaglia, 2011).

Diagnosis

FXS is confirmed by the presence of an epigenetically silenced full-mutation allele in peripheral blood lymphoblasts or lymphocytes through specific polymerase chain reaction protocols and methylation-sensitive Southern blot. For unusual phenotypes, FMRP levels may be determined. In the absence of a full mutation, total or partial gene deletions may be detected by chromosome microarray, and DNA sequencing is performed to identify other *FMR1* anomalies (point-mutations). High-throughput quantitative methylation analysis of the FMR1 gene shows considerable promise for the diagnosis of FXS, including the detection of individuals with methylation mosaicism and repeat-length mosaicism, with methylation levels predictive of FMRP levels and degree of cognitive impairment (Godler et al., 2012; Inaba et al., 2014).

There are no specific clinical rating scales for FXS. The severity of the condition is associated with the extent of gene silencing. Since FMRP levels correlate with intellectual impairment, IQ scores are indicative. Measures of adaptive behaviour, such as the Vineland Adaptive Behaviour Scales (Sparrow, Balla, & Cicchetti, 1984) are associated with FMRP and autistic behaviour in childhood (Hatton et al., 2003).

Clinical vignette

A 4 year old boy was referred to his paediatrician for assessment of developmental delay.

His parents reported that he had walked at age 18 months and started speaking single words from age 3 years. He was observed to be hyperactive and exhibited poor eye contact, temper tantrums and occasional hand flapping. Physical examination was normal, although a relatively large head was noted. Family history revealed that his maternal grandfather had been diagnosed with worsening tremor and a maternal aunt had experienced menopause at age 32 years. Fragile X PCR testing did not detect a normal sized CGG repeat allele, and Southern blot testing showed a methylated full mutation allele of approximately 400 CGG repeats. A Fragile X premutation of approximately 90 repeats was detected in the boy's mother and maternal grandfather.

Further genetics

The FMR1 gene

FMR1 contains 17 *exons* (protein-coding sectors) that are alternatively selected and joined together during mRNA maturation. This combinatorial process, *alternative splicing*, can potentially render 20 different mRNAs, each coding for an FMRP *isoform*, a structurally related but biochemically dissimilar protein (Ashley et al., 1993; Verkerk et al., 1993). Some isoforms show dissimilar mRNA-binding affinities in in-vitro assays (Evans, Blice-Baum, & Mihailescu, 2012) which indicates that modulation of alternative splicing may determine FMRP activity levels in different cells and tissues. Isoform levels may also vary with developmental stage, as evidenced from animal studies (Brackett et al., 2013).

Complexity of the locus

Four genes have been found sharing the *FMR1* locus: *Antisense FMR1* (*ASFMR1*), *FMR4*, *FMR5* and *FMR6*. *ASFMR1*, located in the non-coding strand relative to *FMR1* and overlapping with its CGG repeat region, codes for a polyproline peptide, is upregulated in *FMR1* "grey zone" and premutation alleles and silenced in full mutations (Ladd et al., 2007). Its overexpression has been linked to parkinsonism (Loesch et al., 2011). The other genes are transcribed into long non-coding RNAs (lncRNAs). Relative to *FMR1*, *FMR4* and *FMR6* are antisense, while *FMR5* is sense-oriented (Khalil, Faghihi, Modarresi, Brothers, & Wahlestedt, 2008; Pastori et al., 2014). The biological functions of these lncRNAs are currently unknown. Given the regulatory functions of antisense lncRNAs (Pelechano & Steinmetz, 2013), these non-translatable transcripts could be implicated in self-regulatory circuits that allow *FMR1* to modulate its own transcription, alternative splicing and/or translation.

Unusual cases

A normal phenotype associated with full mutations, surprisingly unmethylated, has been identified in four males without intellectual impairment (e.g. Tabolacci et al.,

2008). Analyses of cell lines established from three of these individuals show unmethylated DNA expansion tracts and promoters, normal transcription of mRNA but reduced translation of FMRP, and histone epigenetic patterns with some marks respectively similar to those in normal and FXS cells. These findings, consistent among the cell lines, point to a common genetic mechanism underlying this epigenetic phenotype, with possible implications for therapies aiming at restoring methylated full mutations to the unmethylated state (Pietrobono et al., 2005; Tabolacci et al., 2008).

Conversely, an FXS-like clinical phenotype has been observed in individuals carrying normal *FMR1* alleles, standard-size mRNA and FMRP levels in lymphocytes (Chiurazzi et al., 1994; Clarke, Mowat, Kooy, Reyniers, & Willemsen, 2004). These FXS phenocopies could emerge from similar alterations caused by different factors in the same genomic and/or proteomic networks. Alternatively, another *FMR1*-related gene may be contributing to the phenotype.

Neuropathology

Development

FXS brains follow an irregular developmental trajectory. In male infants, some regions (caudate nucleus, thalamus, fusiform gyrus and cerebellar vermis) show atypical grey matter volumes while others (orbital gyri, basal forebrain and thalamus) show standard grey matter volumes which increase over time. Likewise, initially large white matter volumes in the striatal prefrontal regions undergo further growth. Early grey matter alterations are postulated to the stem from a genetic effect on developmental stages before birth or soon thereafter, late grey matter anomalies may be the result of defective synaptic pruning, while white matter changes may be due to axonal pathology associated with low FMRP levels (Hoeft et al., 2010).

Fronto-striatal circuitry

Research in clinical and healthy individuals has implicated regions of the frontal lobe and/or the striatum, especially the caudate nucleus, in perseverative behaviours and cognitive flexibility (e.g. Caplan et al., 1990; Monchi, Petrides, Petre, Worsley, & Dagher, 2001). Consistent with this observation, the caudate nucleus, particularly the head, has been found to be enlarged in FXS (e.g. Eliez, Blasey, Freund, Hastie, & Reiss, 2001; Gothelf et al., 2008; Hollander et al., 2005; Laing, Partington, Robinson, & Turner, 1991). Poor performance in tasks demanding inhibition and cognitive flexibility was seen in animal models for FXS with altered synaptic function in the prefrontal cortex (Krueger, Osterweil, Chen, Tye, & Bear, 2011). These findings further support the view that fronto-striatal dysfunction underpins poor response inhibition and cognitive flexibility in FXS.

The striatum has several connecting loops with the cerebral cortex (Seger, 2009). Fronto-striatal connections include those involved in shifting of attention, motor planning and executive functions, all of which are usually impaired in FXS (in Hessl, Rivera, & Reiss, 2004). Since caudate nucleus size normally correlates with IQ, the enlargement in FXS may be indicative of aberrant neuronal organisation (Reiss, Abrams, Greenlaw, Freund, & Denckla, 1995)

Cerebellum

The cerebellar vermis is reduced in FXS, particularly the posterior lobules VI and VII (Mostofsky et al., 1998; Reiss, Aylward, Freund, Joshi, & Bryan, 1991; Reiss, Freund, Tseng, & Joshi, 1991). This anomaly has been related to deficits in visuo-spatial skills, stereotypic behaviours and lower IQ (Gothelf et al., 2008; Hoeft et al., 2008). This link between vermal volumes and visuo-spatial abilities is supported by the observation of a similar association in typically-developed children after radiation treatment on the vermal area (Horská et al., 2010). Given the role of the cerebellar vermis in the execution and regulation of motor behaviour, visual saccades, auditory processing and certain aspects of language, some anomalies in FXS (hyperactivity, repetitive movements, attention deficits, tactile defensiveness, language dysfunction) may be linked to the hypoplasia of this structure (Hessl et al., 2004).

Other anomalies

Reductions have been observed in the volumes of the superior temporal gyrus, which processes complex auditory stimulus including speech, and the amygdala, implicated in emotion processing (Gothelf et al., 2008) and in white matter connectivity in the fronto-striatal pathways and sensory motor tracts (Barnea-Goraly et al., 2003). An enlargement of the thalamus, which relays information to and from the cortex, has been observed in females (Eliez et al., 2001; Gothelf et al., 2008).

Neurochemistry

FMRP at the synapse

The brain tissue of individuals affected by FXS features neurons with an increased number of abnormally long, thin and immature dendritic spines (Irwin, 2001), also observed in *Fmr1*-knockout mice, a consequence of decreased synaptic pruning (Comery et al., 1997). These observations suggest that neuronal dysgenesis and altered synapses underlie the neuropsychological phenotype of FXS.

FMRP controls cytoskeleton structure and function via suppression of the synthesis of Microtubule-Associated Protein 1B (MAP1B). In the absence of FMRP, excess MAP1B enhances microtubule stability, which affects synaptic plasticity (Lu et al., 2004).

Two types of synaptic plasticity depend on protein synthesis: long term potentiation (LTP) and long term depression (LTD). LTP, the increase in synaptic strength resulting from high-frequency stimulation, is important for maintaining emerging synapses, while LTD, the decrease in synaptic strength due to low-frequency stimulation, underlies activity-guided synapse elimination. LTD is triggered by the activation of postsynaptic ionotropic NMDA receptors or metabotropic glutamate receptors of group 1, including mGluR1 and mGluR5.

The observations that mGluR-dependent LTD (but not NMDA-dependent LTD) is enhanced in the hippocampus of *Fmr1* knockout mice, and that the activation of Group1 mGluRs stimulates the synthesis of FMRP in synaptoneurosomes (Huber, Gallagher, Warren, & Bear, 2002; Weiler et al., 1997) are at the basis of the mGluR theory of Fragile X intellectual impairment.

According to this theory, the activation of Group1 mGluRs stimulates the synthesis of proteins that stabilise LTD and of FMRP, which in turn acts as a suppressor of protein synthesis. The fine balance between protein synthesis stimulation and suppression modulates LTD. In the absence of FMRP the balance is tilted toward increased protein synthesis, leading to an exaggerated LTD.

Manifestations of neuronal hyper-excitability, on the other hand, may be associated with deficits in gamma aminobutyric acid (GABA) pathways. GABA is the main neurotransmitter involved in inhibitory postsynaptic potentials (Watanabe, Maemura, Kanbara, Tamayama, & Hayasaki, 2002). Animal models of FXS show low expression of units of the $GABA_A$ ionotropic postsynaptic receptor and of a number of proteins implicated in the GABA pathway (D'Hulst et al., 2009; Gantois et al., 2006). Thus, low FMRP levels may result in diminished GABAergic inhibition leading to increased neuronal excitability.

Treatment

There is no single treatment for FXS. Symptomatic interventions are implemented according to the age and needs of each patient. Feeding difficulties, otitis media, strabismus, mitral valve prolapse and seizures must be monitored in childhood. School-aged children should attend special educational programs to enhance language, social and cognitive skills. Severe anxiety and social phobia are treated with selective serotonin reuptake inhibitors. Psychotic symptoms leading to aggression may respond to antipsychotic medication (Hersh et al., 2011).

Under investigation are therapies that target the molecular imbalances resulting from *FMR1* inactivation. The use of mGluR selective antagonists to counteract excessive LTD has been suggested as a therapeutic tool for FXS (Bear, 2005) and tried in a mouse model with substantial phenotype rectification (Michalon et al., 2012). Preliminary clinical trials in humans assessing the use of fenobam, a selective negative modulator of mGluR5, showed that the medication is well tolerated and can reduce a startle response (Berry-Kravis et al., 2009). Recent developments, however, show that these modulators may be ineffective in older adults (Mullard, 2015).

Another treatment approach is the administration of GABAergic agonists to strengthen the inhibition of GABA-mediated synapses in order to lower neuronal excitability in FXS. Open-label studies on this type of medication are currently under way (Lozano, Hare, & Hagerman, 2014).

Future developments may see drugs targeting specific proteins within the FMRP interactome that become pathogenic when overexpressed in the absence of FMRP (Darnell & Klann, 2013) particular metabolites with altered levels in FXS (Davidovic et al., 2011), or molecules associated with epigenetic gene silencing.

Summary

Fragile X Syndrome is an X-linked inherited disorder associated with intellectual disability, autistic features, behavioural and social challenges and particular physical characteristics. The disorder, transmitted mainly matrilineally, is due to mutations in the *FMR1* gene, the most frequent being the expansion in the number of consecutive CGG repeats in the 5'UTR.

The full mutation (>200 repeats) usually triggers epigenetic changes that suppress gene expression, resulting in absence of *FMRP*, a protein involved in translational repression and neuronal synaptic maturation. Subsequent dysregulation of the FMRP interactome leads to synaptic dysgenesis and exaggerated long-term synaptic depression, thought to underlie the neuropsychological phenotype of FXS. Shorter CGG expansions have been associated with other adult-onset conditions.

While current treatments for FXS are symptomatic, future therapies may target molecular species involved in synapses, the FMRP protein network, the metabolome or epigenetic gene silencing. Under investigation are antagonists of mGluR5 and agonists of GABA receptors, respectively implicated in the exaggerated long-term synaptic depression and in the neuronal hyper-excitability characteristic of FXS.

Abbreviations

5'UTR: 5'untranslated region
ADHD: Attention Deficit Hyperactivity Disorder
ASD: autism spectrum disorder
ASFMR1: anti-sense fragile mental retardation 1, a human gene
C: cytosine
CpG: C phosphate G, a cytosine and guanine separated by one phosphate
EEG: electro-encephalogram

Fmr1: Fragile X mental retardation 1, a mouse gene
FMR1: Fragile X Mental Retardation 1, the human gene involved in Fragile X Syndrome
FMR4: fragile mental retardation 4, a human gene
FMR5: fragile mental retardation 5, a human gene
FMR6: fragile mental retardation 6, a human gene
FMRP: Fragile X Mental Retardation Protein, product of the *FMR1* gene
FRAXA: Fragile X-chromosome site A
FXPOI: Fragile X-associated primary ovarian insufficiency
FXS: Fragile X Syndrome
FXTAS: Fragile X-associated tremor/ataxia syndrome
G: guanine
GABA: gamma aminobutyric acid
HPA: hypothalamic-pituitary-adrenal
IQ: intelligence quotient
LTD: long-term depression
LTP: long-term potentiation
MAP1B: microtubule-associated protein 1B
mGluR: metabotropic glutamate receptor
NMDA receptor: N-methyl-D-aspartate receptor
PCR: polymerase chain reaction
POI: primary ovarian insufficiency
REM sleep: rapid eye movement sleep
TOM: Theory of Mind
Xq: long arm of the X chromosome

Glossary

Allele: Gene variant with a certain minimum frequency in the population.
Alternative splicing: Process that results in a single gene coding for several proteins.
Antisense: Having a sequence of nucleotides which can bind to the coding (sense) sequence.
Cognitive flexibility: Ability to change cognitive sets according to contextual demands.
Dendritic spine: Small membranous process of a dendrite that receives input from a single axon synapse.
Divided attention: Skill to focus on several stimuli at once.
Epigenetic modification: Chemical changes that modify both DNA (without changing the nucleotide sequence) and histone proteins. Common epigenetic modifications are addition of CH_3- (methyl group) to the A and G of DNA, and post-translational addition of methyl, acetyl, phosphates, ubiquitin and other chemical species to histones.
Exon: Nucleotide sequence of a gene that remains present in the mature RNA.
Expressivity: Variability in the phenotype among individuals carrying a particular genotype.
Facies: Distinctive facial features associated with a particular medical condition.

Fenobam: Non-benzodiazepine anxiolytic.
GABA: Gamma amino butyric acid. Neurotransmitter involved in inhibitory action.
Genetic anticipation: Process by which symptoms and signs of a genetic disorder become evident at an earlier age in successive generations.
Glutamate: Neurotransmitter involved in excitatory action.
HPA axis: Hypothalamic – Pituitary – Adrenal axis. Functional set of feedback interactions between these three glands.
Inhibition: Capacity to limit or suppress responses or processes.
Interactome: Entire set of molecular interactions in a cell.
Ionotropic: Receptor made up by an ion-channel pore in the cell membrane.
Isoform: Applied to proteins, any of the different forms of the same protein.
Karyotype: Number of chromosomes and their appearance. This information can be organised to render a clear profile of a person's chromosomes.
Long term depression: Weakening synapses determined by recent patterns of activity which persist over time.
Long term potentiation: Strengthening of synapses determined by recent patterns of activity which persist over time.
Melatonin: Hormone involved in the entrainment of the circadian rhythm of many physiological functions.
Metabolome: Complete set of metabolites in a biological unit.
Metabotropic: Receptor indirectly linked to membrane through signal transduction mechanism (often involving G proteins).
Mosaicism: Presence of two or more populations of cells within an individual with a different DNA or epigenetic genotype.
Non-coding RNA: Functional RNA molecule which is not translated into a protein.
Open-label study: A type of clinical trial where both researchers and participants know what treatments are being administered.
Penetrance: Proportion of individuals carrying a particular gene allele who also express the allele in the phenotype.
Peptide: Chains of amino acids linked by amide bonds.
Phenocopy: Variation in a phenotype caused by environmental conditions that matches a phenotype determined by genetic factors.
Poliproline: Chain of proline (an amino acid) units.
Polymerase chain reaction: Technology used to increase the number of copies of a piece of DNA.
Proband: First affected family member who seeks medical attention.
Promoter: Region of DNA that initiates transcription of a given gene.
Selective attention: Capacity to orient to some stimuli and disregard others.
Selective serotonin reuptake inhibitors: Compounds used as antidepressants.
Southern blot: Method used for the detection of a specific DNA sequence in DNA samples.
Startle response: Alarm response to a sudden stimulus, usually associated with negative affect.
Sustained attention: Ability to remain on task for a relatively long period of time.
Synaptic plasticity: Ability of synapses to strengthen or weaken over time in response to increases or decreases in their activity.
Synaptic pruning: Process of synaptic elimination.

Synaptoneurosome: Composite structure developed as a preparation enriched in synaptosomes (resealed pre-synaptic structures) with attached neurosomes (sealed postsynaptic structures).

Theory of Mind: The ability to attribute mental states to oneself and to others.

Working memory: Temporary storage and manipulation of information needed for complex cognitive activities.

X-chromosome inactivation: Process by which a great part of one of the two X chromosomes in females is transcriptionally silenced.

Further readings

Denman, R. B. (2012). *Modeling Fragile X Syndrome* (First ed.). Dordrecht, Heidelberg, London and New York: Springer.

Fernandez-Carvajal, I., & Aldrige, D. (2011). *Understanding Fragile X Syndrome—A Guide for Families and Professionals*. London and Philadelphia: Jessica Kingsley Publishers.

Hagerman, R. J. & Hagerman, P. (Eds) (2002). *Fragile X Syndrome: Diagnosis, Treatment, and Research*. (Third ed.). USA: John Hopkins University Press.

Iredale, R. (2011). *Growing Up with Fragile X Syndrome: The Road to Marty Campbell*. Fremantle, Australia: Fontaine Press.

Saunders, S. (2002). *Fragile X Syndrome: A Guide for Teachers* (Second ed.). London: David Fulton.

References

Ashley-Koch, A. E., Robinson, H., Glicksman, A. E., Nolin, S. L., Schwartz, C. E., Brown, W. T., ... Sherman, S. L. (1998). Examination of factors associated with instability of the FMR1 CGG repeat. *American Journal of Human Genetics, 63*(3), 776–785.

Ashley, C. T., Sutcliffe, J. S., Kunst, C. B., Leiner, H. A., Eichler, E. E., Nelson, D. L., & Warren, S. T. (1993). Human and murine FMR-1: Alternative splicing and translational initiation downstream of the CGG-repeat. *Nature Genetics, 4*(3), 244–251.

Barkley, R. A. (1997). Behavioral inhibition, sustained attention, and executive functions: Constructing a unifying theory of ADHD. *Psychological Bulletin, 121*(1), 65–94. doi: 10.1037/0033-2909.121.1.65.

Barnea-Goraly, N., Eliez, S., Hedeus, M., Menon, V., White, C. D., Moseley, M., & Reiss, A. L. (2003). White matter tract alterations in fragile X syndrome: Preliminary evidence from diffusion tensor imaging. *American Journal of Medical Genetics. Part B, Neuropsychiatric genetics, 118B*(1), 81–88.

Bear, M. F. (2005). Therapeutic implications of the mGluR theory of fragile X mental retardation. *Genes Brain & Behavior, 4*(6), 393–398. doi: 10.1111/j.1601-183X.2005.00135.x.

Berry-Kravis, E. (2002). Epilepsy in fragile X syndrome. *Developmental Medicine & Child Neurology, 44*(11), 724–728. doi: 10.1111/j.1469-8749.2002.tb00277.x.

Berry-Kravis, E., Hessl, D., Coffey, S., Hervey, C., Schneider, A., Yuhas, J., ... Hagerman, R. (2009). A pilot open label, single dose trial of fenobam in adults with fragile X syndrome. *Journal of Medical Genetics, 46*(4), 266–271. doi: 10.1136/jmg.2008.063701.

Brackett, D. M., Qing, F., Amieux, P. S., Sellers, D. L., Horner, P. J., & Morris, D. R. (2013). *FMR1* transcript isoforms: Association with polyribosomes; regional and developmental expression in mouse brain. *Plos One, 8*(3), e58296. doi: 10.1371/journal.pone.0058296.

Caplan, L. R., Schmahmann, J. D., Kase, C. S, Feldmann, E., Baquis, G., Greenberg, J., … Hier, D. (1990). Caudate infarcts. *Archives of Neurology, 47*(2), 133–143. doi: 10.1001/archneur.1990.00530020029011.

Chiurazzi, P., DeGraaff, E., Ng, J., Verkerk, A. J. M. H., Wolfson, S., Fisch, G. S., …. Oostra, B. A. (1994). No apparent involvement of the FMR1 gene in five patients with phenotypic manifestations of the fragile X syndrome. *American Journal of Medical Genetics, 51*(4), 309–314.

Clarke, N. F., Mowat, D., Kooy, R. F., Reyniers, E., & Willemsen, R. (2004). Fragile X syndrome phenotype with normal FMR1 gene studies. *American Journal of Medical Genetics Part 129A*(3), 326–328. doi: 10.1002/ajmg.a.30194.

Coffee, B., Keith, K., Albizua, I., Malone, T., Mowrey, J., Sherman, S. L., & Warren, S. T. (2009). Incidence of fragile X syndrome by newborn screening for methylated FMR1 DNA. *American Journal of Human Genetics, 85*(4), 503–514. doi: 10.1016/j.ajhg.2009.09.007.

Comery, T. A., Harris, J. B., Willems, P. J., Oostra, B. A., Irwin, S. A., Weiler, I. J., & Greenough, W. T. (1997). Abnormal dendritic spines in fragile X knockout mice: Maturation and pruning deficits. *Proceedings of the National Academy of Sciences of the United States of America, 94*(10), 5401–5404.

Cornish, K., Burack, J. A., Rahman, A., Munir, F., Russo, N., & Grant, C. (2005). Theory of mind deficits in children with fragile X syndrome. *Journal of Intellectual Disability Research, 49*(pt 5), 372–378.

D'Hulst, C., Heulens, I., Brouwer, J., Willemsen, R., De Geest, N., Reeve, S., … Kooy, R. (2009). Expression of the GABAergic system in animal models for fragile X syndrome and fragile X associated tremor/ataxia syndrome (FXTAS). *Brain Research, 1253*, 176–183.

Darnell, J. C., & Klann, E. (2013). The translation of translational control by FMRP: Therapeutic targets for FXS. *Nature Neuroscience, 16*(11), 1530–1536. doi: 10.1038/nn.3379.

Davidovic, L., Navratil, V., Bonaccorso, C. M., Catania, M. V., Bardoni, B., & Dumas, M. E. (2011). A metabolomic and systems biology perspective on the brain of the fragile X syndrome mouse model. *Genome Research, 21*(12), 2190–2202. doi: 10.1101/gr.116764.110.

Eliez, S., Blasey, C. M., Freund, L. S., Hastie, T., & Reiss, A. L. (2001). Brain anatomy, gender and IQ in children and adolescents with fragile X syndrome. *Brain, 124*(pt 8), 1610–1618.

Evans, T. L., Blice-Baum, A. C., & Mihailescu, M. R. (2012). Analysis of the fragile X mental retardation protein isoforms 1, 2 and 3 interactions with the G-quadruplex forming semaphorin 3F mRNA. *Molecular Biosystems, 8*(2), 642–649. doi: 10.1039/c1mb05322a.

Fernandez-Carvajal, I., Walichiewicz, P., Xiaosen, X., Pan, R., Hagerman, P. J., & Tassone, F. (2009). Screening for expanded alleles of the FMR1 gene in blood spots from newborn males in a Spanish population. *The Journal of Molecular Diagnostics, 11*(4), 324–329. doi: http://dx.doi.org/10.2353/jmoldx.2009.080173.

Fu, Y., Kuhl, D., Pizzuti, A., Pieretti, M., Sutcliffe, J., & Richards, S. (1991). Variation of the CGG repeat at the fragile X site results in genetic instability—Resolution of the Sherman paradox. *Cell, 67*(6), 1047–1058.

Galloway, J. N., & Nelson, D. L. (2009). Evidence for RNA-mediated toxicity in the fragile X-associated tremor/ataxia syndrome. *Future Neurology, 4*(6), 785–785. doi: 10.2217/fnl.09.44.

Gantois, I., Vandesompele, J., Speleman, F., Reyniers, E., D'Hooge, R., Severijnen, L. A., … Kooy, R. F. (2006). Expression profiling suggests underexpression of the $GABA_A$ receptor subunit δ in the fragile X knockout mouse model. *Neurobiology of Disease, 21*(2), 346–357. doi: http://dx.doi.org/10.1016/j.nbd.2005.07.017.

Godler, D. E., Slater, H. R., Bui, Q. M., Storey, E., Ono, M.Y., Gehling, F., … Loesch, D. Z. (2012). Fragile X Mental Retardation 1 (FMR1) intron 1 methylation in blood predicts verbal cognitive impairment in female carriers of expanded FMR1 alleles: Evidence from a pilot study. *Clinical Chemistry, 58*(3), 590–598. doi: 10.1373/clinchem.2011.177626.

Gothelf, D., Furfaro, J. A., Hoeft, F., Eckert, M. A., Hall, S. S., O'Hara, R., … Reiss, A. L. (2008). Neuroanatomy of fragile X syndrome is associated with aberrant behavior and the fragile X mental retardation protein (FMRP). *Annals of Neurology, 63*(1), 40–51. doi: 10.1002/ana.21243.

Gould, E. L., Loesch, D. Z., Martin, M. J., Hagerman, R. J., Armstrong, S. M., & Huggins, R. M. (2000). Melatonin profiles and sleep characteristics in boys with fragile X syndrome: A preliminary study. *American Journal of Medical Genetics, 95*(4), 307–315.

Grant, C. M., Apperly, I., & Oliver, C. (2007). Is theory of mind understanding impaired in males with fragile X syndrome? *Journal of Abnormal Child Psychology, 35*(1), 17–28. doi: 10.1007/s10802-006-9077-0.

Hagerman, R. (2006). Lessons from fragile X regarding neurobiology, autism, and neurodegeneration. *Journal of Developmental and Behavioral Pediatrics, 27*(1), 63–74.

Hagerman, R., & Cronister, A. (1996). *Fragile X Syndrome: Diagnosis, Treatment, and Research* (Second ed.). The Johns Hopkins University Press.

Hagerman, R., & Hagerman, P. (2002). The physical and behavioural phenotype. In *Fragile X Syndrome: Diagnosis, Treatment and Research* (Third. ed., pp. 3–109). Baltimore: John Hopkins.

Hagerman, R., & Harris, S. W. (2008). Autism profiles of males with fragile X syndrome. *American Journal of Mental Retardation, 113*(6), 427–438.

Hatton, D. D., Wheeler, A. C., Skinner, M. L., Bailey, D. B., Sullivan, K. M., Roberts, J. E., … Clark, R. D. (2003). Adaptive behavior in children with fragile X syndrome. *American Journal of Mental Retardation, 108*(6), 373–390. doi: doi:10.1352/0895-8017(2003)108<373:ABICWF>2.0.CO;2.

Hazlett, H., Poe, M., Lightbody, A., Gerig, G., MacFall, J., Ross, A., … Piven, J. (2009). Teasing apart the heterogeneity of autism: Same behavior, different brains in toddlers with fragile X syndrome and autism. *Journal of Neurodevelopmental Disorders, 1*(1), 81–90. doi: 10.1007/s11689-009-9009-8.

Hersh, J. H., Saul, R. A., & Genetics., C. O. (2011). Health supervision for children with fragile X syndrome. *Pediatrics, 127*(5), 994–1006. doi: 10.1542/peds.2010-3500.

Hessl, D., Glaser, B., Dyer-Friedman, J., Blasey, C., Hastie, T., Gunnar, M., & Reiss, A. L. (2002). Cortisol and behavior in fragile X syndrome. *Psychoneuroendocrinology, 27*(7), 855–872.

Hessl, D., Glaser, B., Dyer-Friedman, J., & Reiss, A. L. (2006). Social behavior and cortisol reactivity in children with fragile X syndrome. *Journal of Child Psychology & Psychiatry, 47*(6), 602–610. doi: 10.1111/j.1469-7610.2005.01556.x.

Hessl, D., Rivera, S. M., & Reiss, A. L. (2004). The neuroanatomy and neuroendocrinology of fragile X syndrome. *Mental Retardation & Developmental Disabilities Research Reviews, 10*(1), 17–24.

Hoeft, F., Lightbody, A. A., Hazlett, H. C., Patnaik, S., Piven, J., & Reiss, A. L. (2008). Morphometric spatial patterns differentiating boys with fragile X syndrome, typically developing boys, and developmentally delayed boys aged 1 to 3 years. *Archives of General Psychiatry, 65*(9), 1087–1097.

Hoeft, F., Carter, J. C., Lightbody, A. A., Cody Hazlett, H., Piven, J., & Reiss, A. L. (2010). Region-specific alterations in brain development in one- to three-year-old boys with fragile X syndrome. *Proceedings of the National Academy of Sciences, 107*(20), 9335–9339. doi: 10.1073/pnas.1002762107.

Hollander, E., Anagnostou, E., Chaplin, W., Esposito, K., Haznedar, M. M., Licalzi, E., ... Buchsbaum, M. (2005). Striatal volume on magnetic resonance imaging and repetitive behaviors in autism. *Biological Psychiatry, 58*(3), 226–232. doi: 10.1016/j.biopsych.2005.03.040.

Hooper, S. R., Hatton, D., Sideris, J., Sullivan, K., Hammer, J., Schaaf, J., ... Bailey, D. P. (2008). Executive functions in young males with fragile X syndrome in comparison to mental age-matched controls: Baseline findings from a longitudinal study. *Neuropsychology, 22*(1), 36–47.

Horská, A., LaClair, A., Mohamed, M., Wells, C. T., McNutt, T., Cohen, K. J., ... Kates, W. (2010). Low cerebellar vermis volumes and impaired neuropsychologic performance in children treated for brain tumors and leukemia. *American Journal of Neuroradiology, 31*(8), 1430–1437. doi: 10.3174/ajnr.A2114.

Huber, K. M., Gallagher, S. M., Warren, S. T., & Bear, M. F. (2002). Altered synaptic plasticity in a mouse model of fragile X mental retardation. *Proceedings of the National Academy of Sciences, 99*(11), 7746–7750. doi: 10.1073/pnas.122205699.

Inaba, Y., Schwartz, C. E., Bui, Q. M., Li, X., Skinner, C., Field, M., ... Godler, D. E. (2014). Early detection of fragile X syndrome: Applications of a novel approach for improved quantitative methylation analysis in venous blood and newborn blood spots. *Clinical Chemistry, 60*(7), 963–973. doi: 10.1373/clinchem.2013.217331.

Irwin, S. (2001). Abnormal dendritic spine characteristics in the temporal and visual cortices of patients with fragile-X syndrome: A quantitative examination. *American Journal of Medical Genetics, 98*(2), 161–167.

Johannisson, R., Rehde, R. H., Wendt, V., & Schwinger, E. (1987). Spermatogenesis in two patients with the fragile X syndrome. I. Histology: Light and electron microscopy. *Human Genetics, 76*(2), 141–147.

Kau, A. S. M., Reider, E. E., Payne, L., Meyer, W. A., & Freund, L. (2000). Early behavior signs of psychiatric phenotypes in fragile X syndrome. *American Journal on Mental Retardation, 105*(4), 286–299.

Khalil, A. M., Faghihi, M. A., Modarresi, F., Brothers, S. P., & Wahlestedt, C. (2008). A novel RNA transcript with antiapoptotic function is silenced in fragile X syndrome. *Plos One, 3*(1), e1486.doi:101371/journal.pone.0001486.

Krueger, D. D., Osterweil, E. K., Chen, S. P., Tye, L. D., & Bear, M. F. (2011). Cognitive dysfunction and prefrontal synaptic abnormalities in a mouse model of fragile X syndrome. *Proceedings of the National Academy of Sciences of the United States of America, 108*(6), 2587–2592. doi: 10.1073/pnas.1013855108.

Lachiewicz, A., & Dawson, D.V. (1994). Do young boys with fragile-X-syndrome have macroorchidism. *Pediatrics, 93*(6), 992–995.

Lachiewicz, A., Dawson, D. V., & Spiridigliozzi, G. A. (2000). Physical characteristics of young boys with fragile X syndrome: Reasons for difficulties in making a diagnosis in young males. *American Journal of Medical Genetics, 92*(4), 229–236. doi: 10.1002/(sici)1096-8628(20000605)92:4<229::aid-ajmg1>3.0.co;2-k.

Ladd, P. D., Smith, L. E., Rabaia, N. A., Moore, J. M., Georges, S. A., Hansen, R. S., … Filippova, G. N. (2007). An antisense transcript spanning the CGG repeat region of FMR1 is upregulated in premutation carriers but silenced in full mutation individuals. *Human Molecular Genetics, 16*(24), 3174–3187.

Laing, S., Partington, M., Robinson, H., & Turner, G. (1991). Clinical screening score for the fragile X (Martin-Bell) syndrome. *American Journal of Medical Genetics, 38*(2–3), 256–259.

Lanfranchi, S., Cornoldi, C., Drigo, S., & Vianello, R. (2009). Working memory in individuals with fragile X syndrome. *Child Neuropsychology, 15*(2), 105–119. doi: 10.1080/09297040802112564.

Loesch, D., Churchyard, A., Brotchie, P., Marot, M., & Tassone, F. (2005). Evidence for, and a spectrum of, neurological involvement in carriers of the fragile X pre-mutation: FXTAS and beyond. *Clinical Genetics, 67*(5), 412–417. doi: 10.1111/j.1399-0004.2005.00425.x.

Loesch, D., Godler, D. E., Evans, A., Bui, Q. M., Gehling, F., Kotschet, K. E., … Horne, M. (2011). Evidence for the toxicity of bidirectional transcripts and mitochondrial dysfunction in blood associated with small CGG expansions in the FMR1 gene in patients with parkinsonism. *Genetics in Medicine, 13*(5), 392–399.

Loesch, D., Huggins, R., & Hoang, N. (1995). Growth in stature in fragile-X families—A mixed longitudinal-study. *American Journal of Medical Genetics, 58*(3), 249–256.

Loesch, D. Z., Huggins, R. M., & Hagerman, R. J. (2004). Phenotypic variation and FMRP levels in fragile X. *Mental Retardation & Developmental Disabilities Research Reviews, 10*(1), 31–41.

Losh, M., Martin, G. E., Klusek, J., Hogan-Brown, A. L., & Sideris, J. (2012). Social communication and theory of mind in boys with autism and fragile X syndrome. *Frontiers in Psychology, 3*. doi: 10.3389/fpsyg.2012.00266.

Lozano, R., Hare, E. B., & Hagerman, R. J. (2014). Modulation of the GABAergic pathway for the treatment of fragile X syndrome. *Neuropsychiatric Disease & Treatment, 10*, 1769–1779. doi: 10.2147/NDT.S42919.

Lu, R., Wang, H. P., Liang, Z., Ku, L., O'Donnell, W. T., Li, W., … Feng, Y. (2004). The fragile X protein controls microtubule-associated protein 1B translation and microtubule stability in brain neuron development. *Proceedings of the National Academy of Sciences of the United States of America, 101*(42), 15201–15206. doi: 10.1073/pnas.0404995101.

Lubs, H. (1969). A marker X-chromosome. *American Journal of Human Genetics, 21*(3), 231.

Miano, S., Bruni, O., Elia, M., Scifo, L., Smerieri, A., Trovato, A., … Ferri, R. (2008). Sleep phenotypes of intellectual disability: A polysomnographic evaluation in subjects with Down syndrome and Fragile-X syndrome. *Clinical Neurophysiology, 119*(6), 1242–1247. doi: http://dx.doi.org/10.1016/j.clinph.2008.03.004.

Michalon, A., Sidorov, M., Ballard, T. M., Ozmen, L., Spooren, W., … Lindemann, L. (2012). Chronic pharmacological mglu5 inhibition corrects fragile X in adult mice. *Neuron, 74*(1), 49–56. doi: http://dx.doi.org/10.1016/j.neuron.2012.03.009.

Miller, L. J., McIntosh, D. N., McGrath, J., Shyu, V., Lampe, M., Taylor, A. K., … Hagerman, R. J. (1999). Electrodermal responses to sensory stimuli in individuals with fragile X syndrome: A preliminary report. *American Journal of Medical Genetics, 83*(4), 268–279. doi: 10.1002/(sici)1096-8628(19990402)83:4<268::aid-ajmg7>3.0.co;2-k.

Monaghan, K., Lyon, E., & Spector, E. (2013). ACMG Standards and Guidelines for fragile X testing: A revision to the disease-specific supplements to the Standards and Guidelines for Clinical Genetics Laboratories of the American College of Medical Genetics and Genomics. *Genetics in Medicine, 15*(7), 575–586.

Monchi, O., Petrides, M., Petre, V., Worsley, K., & Dagher, A. (2001). Wisconsin card sorting revisited: Distinct neural circuits participating in different stages of the task identified by event-related functional magnetic resonance imaging. *Journal of Neuroscience, 21*(19), 7733–7741.

Moore, P. S. J., Chudley, A. E., & Winter, J. S. D. (1990). True precocious puberty in a girl with the fragile X-syndrome. *American Journal of Medical Genetics, 37*(2), 265–267.

Mostofsky, S. H., Mazzocco, M. M. M., Aakalu, G., Warsofsky, I. S., Denckla, M. B., & Reiss, A. L. (1998). Decreased cerebellar posterior vermis size in fragile X syndrome—Correlation with neurocognitive performance. *Neurology, 50*(1), 121–130.

Mullard, A. (2015). Fragile X disappointments upset autism ambitions. *Nature Reviews Drug Discovery, 14*(3), 151–153. doi: 10.1038/nrd4555.

Munir, F., Cornish, K., & Wilding, J. (2000a). Nature of the working memory deficit in Fragile-X syndrome. *Brain & Cognition, 44*(3), 387–401. doi: 10.1006/brcg.1999.1200.

Munir, F., Cornish, K., & Wilding, J. (2000b). A neuropsychological profile of attention deficits in young males with fragile X syndrome. *Neuropsychologia, 38*(9), 1261–1270.

Murphy, M. M., & Mazzocco, M. M. M. (2008). Mathematics learning disabilities in girls with fragile X or Turner Syndrome during late elementary school. *Journal of Learning Disabilities, 41*(1), 29–46. doi: 10.1177/0022219407311038.

Musumeci, S. (1999). Epilepsy and EEG findings in males with fragile X syndrome. *Epilepsia, 40*(8), 1092–1099.

Oberle, I. (1991). Instability of a 550 base pair DNA segment and abnormal methylation in fragile X-syndrome. *Science, 252*(5009), 1097–1102.

Pastori, C., Peschansky, V. J., Barbouth, D., Mehta, A., Silva, J. P., & Wahlestedt, C. (2014). Comprehensive analysis of the transcriptional landscape of the human FMR1 gene reveals two new long noncoding RNAs differentially expressed in fragile X syndrome and fragile X-associated tremor/ataxia syndrome. *Human Genetics, 133*(1), 59–67. doi: 10.1007/s00439-013-1356-6.

Pelechano, V., & Steinmetz, L. M. (2013). Gene regulation by antisense transcription. *National Reviews Genetics, 14*(12), 880–893. doi: 10.1038/nrg3594.

Pietrobono, R., Tabolacci, E., Zalfa, F., Zito, I., Terracciano, A., Moscato, U., … Neri, G. (2005). Molecular dissection of the events leading to inactivation of the FMR1 gene. *Human Molecular Genetics, 14*(2), 267–277. doi: 10.1093/hmg/ddi024.

Reiss, A., Abrams, M. T., Greenlaw, R., Freund, L., & Denckla, M. B. (1995). Neurodevelopmental effects of the fmr-1 full mutation in humans. *Nature Medicine, 1*(2), 159–167. doi: 10.1038/nm0295-159.

Reiss, A., Aylward, E., Freund, L. S., Joshi, P. K., & Bryan, R. N. (1991). Neuroanatomy of fragile-X-syndrome: The posterior-fossa. *Annals of Neurology, 29*(1), 26–32.

Reiss, A., & Dant, C. C. (2003). The behavioral neurogenetics of fragile X syndrome: Analyzing gene-brain-behavior relationships in child developmental psychopathologies. *Development & Psychopathology, 15*(4), 927–968. doi: 10.1017/s0954579403000464.

Reiss, A. L., Freund, L., Tseng, J. E., & Joshi, P. K. (1991). Neuroanatomy in fragile-x females: The posterior-fossa. *American Journal of Human Genetics, 49*(2), 279–288.

Seger, C. A. (2009). The involvement of corticostriatal loops in learning across tasks, species, and methodologies. In H. J. Groenewegen, P. Voorn, H. W. Berendse, A. B. Mulder & A. R. Cools (Eds.), *The Basal Ganglia IX* (Vol. 58, pp. 25–39). New York: Springer.

Sherman, S. L., Morton, N. E., Jacobs, P. A., & Turner, G. (1984). The marker (X) syndrome: A cytogenetic and genetic-analysis. *Annals of Human Genetics, 48*(JAN), 21–37.

Sparrow, S., Balla, D., & Cicchetti, D. (1984). Vineland Adaptive Behaviour Scales. Circle Pines. MN: American Guidance Service.

Stein, M. B., Simmons, A. N., Feinstein, J. S., & Paulus, M. P. (2007). Increased amygdala and insula activation during emotion processing in anxiety-prone subjects. *American Journal of Psychiatry, 164*(2), 318–327.

Storm, R. L., PeBenito, R., & Ferretti, C. (1987). Ophthalmologic findings in the fragile X syndrome. *Archives of Ophthalmology, 105*(8), 1099–1102. doi: 10.1001/archopht.1987.01060080101036.

Sudhalter, V., & Belser, R. C. (2001). Conversational characteristics of children with fragile X syndrome: Tangential language. *American Journal on Mental Retardation, 106*(5), 389–400.

Sullivan, K., Hatton, D. D., Hammer, J., Sideris, J., Hooper, S., Ornstein, P. A., & Bailey, D. B. (2007). Sustained attention and response inhibition in boys with fragile X syndrome: Measures of continuous performance. *American Journal of Medical Genetics Part B-Neuropsychiatric Genetics, 144B*(4), 517–532. doi: 10.1002/ajmg.b.30504.

Sutcliffe, J. S., Nelson, D. L., Zhang, F. P., Pieretti, M., Caskey, C. T., D., S., & Warren, S. T. (1992). DNA methylation represses *FMR-1* transcription in fragile X syndrome. *Human Molecular Genetics, 1*(6), 397- 400.

Tabolacci, E., Moscato, U., Zalfa, F., Bagni, C., Chiurazzi, P., & Neri, G. (2008). Epigenetic analysis reveals a euchromatic configuration in the FMR1 unmethylated full mutations. *European Journal of Human Genetics, 16*(12), 1487–1498. doi: 10.1038/ejhg.2008.130.

Thurman, A. J., McDuffie, A., Hagerman, R., & Abbeduto, L. (2014). Psychiatric symptoms in boys with fragile X syndrome: A comparison with nonsyndromic autism spectrum disorder. *Research in Developmental Disabilities, 35*(5), 1072–1086. doi: 10.1016/j.ridd.2014.01.032.

Tranfaglia, M. R. (2011). The psychiatric presentation of fragile X: Evolution of the diagnosis and treatment of the psychiatric comorbidities of fragile X syndrome. *Developmental Neuroscience, 33*(5), 337–348.

Turner, G., Webb, T., Wake, S., & Robinson, H. (1996). Prevalence of fragile X syndrome. *American Journal of Medical Genetics, 64*(1), 196–197. doi: 10.1002/(sici)1096-8628(19960712)64:1<196::aid-ajmg35>3.0.co;2-g.

Verkerk, A., Degraaff, E., Deboulle, K., Eichler, E. E., Konecki, D. S., Reyniers, E., … Oostra, B. A. (1993). Alternative splicing in the fragile X-gene FMR1. *Human Molecular Genetics, 2*(4), 399–404.

Verkerk, A., Pieretti, M., Sutcliffe, J. S., Fu, Y. H., Kuhl, D. P. A., Pizzuti, A., … Warren, S. T. (1991). Identification of a gene (FMR-1) containing a CGG repeat coincident with a breakpoint cluster region exhibiting length variation in fragile-X syndrome. *Cell, 65*(5), 905–914.

Watanabe, M., Maemura, K., Kanbara, K., Tamayama, T., & Hayasaki, H. (2002). GABA and GABA receptors in the central nervous system and other organs. *International Review of Cytology, Volume 213*, 1–47. doi: http://dx.doi.org/10.1016/S0074-7696(02)13011-7.

Watson, C., Hoeft, F., Garrett, A. S., Hall, S. S., & Reiss, A. L. (2008). Aberrant brain activation during gaze processing in boys with fragile X syndrome. *Archives of General Psychiatry, 65*(11), 1315–1323.

Weiler, I. J., Irwin, S. A., Klintsova, A. Y., Spencer, C. M., Brazelton, A. D., Miyashiro, K., … Greenough, W. T. (1997). Fragile X mental retardation protein is translated near synapses in response to neurotransmitter activation. *Proceedings of the National Academy of Sciences of the United States of America, 94*(10), 5395–5400.

Willems, P. J., Roy, B.V., De Boulle, K., Vits, L., Reyniers, E., Beck, O., … Oostra, B. (1992). Segregation of the fragile X mutation from an affected male to his normal daughter. *Human Molecular Genetics, 1*(7), 511–515. doi: 10.1093/hmg/1.7.511.

Willemsen, R., Smits, A., Severijnen, L. A., Jansen, M., Jacobs, A., De Bruyn, E., & Oostra, B. (2003). Predictive testing for cognitive functioning in female carriers of the fragile X syndrome using hair root analysis. *Journal of Medical Genetics, 40*(5), 377–379. doi: 10.1136/jmg.40.5.377.

Zhang, J., Fang, Z., Jud, C., Vansteensel, M. J., Kaasik, K., Lee, C. C., … Nelson, D. L. (2008). Fragile X-related proteins regulate mammalian circadian behavioral rhythms. *American Journal of Human Genetics, 83*(1), 43–52. doi: 10.1016/j.ajhg.2008.06.003.

19

CEREBELLAR-FRONTAL-PARIETAL AXIS IN DEVELOPMENTAL DISORDERS

Darren R. Hocking

Introduction and preliminary considerations

The human capacity to maintain task-related goals, selectively attend to relevant stimuli and avoid distraction is unrivaled, and these cognitive processes depend on distinct frontoparietal networks that subserve adaptive control in response to changing task demands. Although the vast majority of studies in developmental disorders have previously focused on the striatum and its functional interaction with dorsolateral prefrontal cortex, it is argued here that the protracted developmental time course of the frontoparietal and cerebellar networks leave these regions particularly vulnerable during atypical development. The frontoparietal attention regions are broadly separated into two distinct networks that either deploy attention that is driven by environmental stimuli (i.e. behaviourally-relevant, salient stimuli), or by the observers' expectations based on goal-directed, top-down selection of stimuli and responses. This network also flexibly interacts with other regions important for the many and varied functions of cognitive or executive control, which are especially relevant in novel, non-practiced situations.

We shall see in this chapter that the process of development is a critical period of rapid skill acquisition, and delay or disruption to specific regions of the cerebellum and its projections to critical cortical regions may be relevant to development of attention and executive control functions that are subject to disruption in developmental disorders. The relatively uniform cytoarchitecture of the cerebellum supports a uniform computational role in forming internal models that enable such cognitive processes to be optimised by modulating activity in the closed-loop circuits connecting the cerebellum with cortical regions. Early damage to *specific* cerebro-cerebellar circuits in children is commonly associated with poorer outcomes and features that share common overlap with Autism Spectrum Disorder (ASD) and

Cerebellar Cognitive Affective Syndrome (Tavano et al., 2007b; Tavano & Borgatti, 2010; Wang, Kloth & Badura, 2014).

Here, we review the evidence that both frontoparietal and cerebellar dysfunction play a critical role in a range of developmental disorders, and discuss the potential contribution of delayed maturation of long-range cerebellar connectivity with cortical regions contributing to disruption among these cognitive functions. We first discuss the uniform neuroanatomical architecture of the cerebellum, and then outline how the timing and functional topography of cerebellar damage/dysfunction may have major impacts on circuits supporting attention, executive functions and affective regulation. We next review the frontoparietal attention network and discuss how differential rates of maturation within attentional networks, as well as other capacity-limited cognitive processes such as spatial working memory, impact upon typical and atypical development. In the following sections, we discuss the importance of mapping intrinsic functional connectivity between frontoparietal regions and other major networks involved in modulation of attention and the maintenance of the physiological baseline of the brain. Given the complex nature and heterogeneity of many developmental disorders, we argue that examination of abnormalities in these large-scale regions at the network level hold the greatest deal of promise in understanding the pathophysiological mechanisms underlying developmental disorders of control.

The cerebellum in developmental disorders of the brain

The cerebellum ("little brain"), classically defined by its role in sensory-motor function, is located at the anterior end of the hindbrain, and is one of the most architecturally elaborate regions in the central nervous system (CNS). Despite the relatively small size of this structure, it contains over half of the neurons in the adult human brain. However, this complex morphology belies its relatively simple cyto-architecture; the cerebellar cortex is uniformly structured into three layers and consists of five major cell types: the inhibitory stellate and basket cells, Golgi and Purkinje neurons and the excitatory granule cells. The three layers comprise an outermost molecular layer of granule cell axons and Purkinje cell dendritic trees, a monolayer of inhibitory Purkinje cells and a layer of excitatory granule cells. The granular layer receives excitatory input from outside the cerebellum, and projects through the Purkinje cell layer, with the majority of Purkinje cells then projecting to neurons in the cerebellar nuclei, which then project to other white matter regions of the brain. The deep cerebellar nuclei (DCN) receive inhibitory inputs from the Purkinje cells and excitatory inputs from mossy fibres coming from pre-cerebellar nuclei, and climbing fibres originating from the inferior olive (Swanson & Contractor, 2004). Thus, the Purkinje cells serve as the sole output of the cerebellar cortex.

At the morphological level, the cerebellum is divided into a series of folds known as lobules, with each primary lobule further divided into sub-lobules. Cerebellar connectivity with the cerebral cortex and the spinal cord serve to broadly define different cerebellar functional areas including anterior (I-V), central (VIa-VII), posterior (VIII-IX) and nodular (X). The anterior lobe (lobules I-V) and lobule VIII encode predominantly sensorimotor information, while lobules VI and VII (including Crus I, Crus II and lobule VIIb) contribute to higher order processes via reciprocal connections with prefrontal and parietal cortices. The posterior vermal lobule VII is involved in affective regulation via cerebellar-limbic circuitry. Thus, the functional topography of the cerebellum is in general agreement with dissociations between anterior sensorimotor and posterior cognitive/emotional processing in the cerebellum (see Stoodley & Schmahmann, 2009; Stoodley, 2012).

The 'classic' symptoms resulting from cerebellar damage involve the control of movement including dysmetria (e.g. hypermetric or hypometric saccades), movement difficulties associated with posture and balance, gait ataxia, speech dysarthria, hypotonia, impaired swallowing (dysphagia), difficulty with alternating movements (dysdiadochokinesis) and intention tremor. It has been shown that there is a functional topography of motor function within the cerebellum that reflects the different demands on sensory inputs (see Manni & Petrosini, 2004, for a review). Moreover, in children following cerebellar damage, the right cerebellar hemisphere is associated with poorer linguistic outcomes, whereas damage to the left cerebellar hemisphere is mainly associated with poorer visuospatial functions; reflecting contralateral connections between the cerebellum and cerebral cortex (Riva & Giorgi, 2000; Scott et al., 2001). Despite the established role of the cerebellum in motor function (see Manto et al., 2012, for a review), the wealth of current evidence suggests that cerebro-cerebellar connections (cortico-ponto-cerebellar and cerebello-thalamo-cortical loops) constitute a prerequisite for the neuroanatomical basis for a role of the cerebellum in non-motor functions. The concept of Cerebellar Cognitive Affective Syndrome (CCAS) has been introduced to describe a constellation of symptoms arising from such lesions of the posterior cognitive and limbic regions, and disruptions to reciprocal cerebellar connections with cerebral association areas and paralimbic cortices (Schmahmann & Sherman, 1998; Stoodley & Schmahmann, 2009). CCAS is characterised by impairments in language, executive function, visuospatial processing, as well as affective dysregulation—notably these symptoms are most relevant to a range of developmental disorders with which this book is concerned.

The developmental course of the cerebellum, which is typically not mature well into the postnatal years, leaves this structure particularly vulnerable during early development with implications for a broad spectrum of developmental disorders. Yet, the cerebellum also reaches maturation during a sensitive period of genetic and environmental vulnerability, with the potential to shape later developing cortical structures. See Becker and Stoodley (2013) and Wang et al. (2014) for excellent reviews of the role of sensitive periods and the cerebellum in ASD. Children with congenital cerebellar malformations present with a clinical profile that shares some overlap with the CCAS seen in adults with subtle yet notable differences, as well as increased ASD-like behavioural features, and in some cases, diagnoses of ASD (Tavano & Borgatti, 2010; Tavano, Fabbro & Borgatti, 2007a; Tavano et al., 2007b):

A. There is a subgroup of children with cerebellar vermal agenesis and diffuse cerebellar hypoplasia who show profound intellectual disability (ID) (with mostly preserved motor skills), severe verbal/non-verbal communication deficits and behavioural features of social withdrawal alongside a restricted pattern of activities and interests, within the diagnostic limits of ASD.
B. A distinct subgroup of children with diffuse cerebellar hypoplasia who show varying degrees of ID (from profound to moderate-to-severe) with extremely rigid and repetitive behaviour. It is not entirely clear why this is true for only a subset of patients, while others display a clinical profile more consistent with the adult CCAS.
C. Children with lesions confined to the cerebellar hemispheres generally show a normal to borderline intellectual profile alongside lower visuomotor and executive skills. The socio-affective and relational skills are relatively preserved, however, with no evidence of specific developmental delay.
D. Joubert syndrome (JS), an autosomal recessive developmental disorder associated with hypoplasia of the cerebellar vermis, is characterised by generally preserved affective regulation and relational functioning, an opposing pattern to that seen in children with cerebellar malformations (CM). A profile of relative strengths in executive and emotional skills alongside relative weaknesses in verbal memory and expressive language skills appears to differentiate the JS from the CM children (Tavano & Borgatti, 2010).

In sum, the impact of congenital cerebellar lesions on developmental delay is most severe when the phylogenetically most ancient cerebellar vermis is affected. In cases of lesions confined to cerebellar hemispheres (with relative preservation of cerebellar vermis), there appears to be a much more favourable outcome in the development of higher-order cognitive abilities, even at an advanced age (Tavano et al., 2007b). This contrasts with the view that the earlier the cerebellar insult, the greater the severity of impairment (see Steinlin, 2007), but rather is indicative of functional compensatory mechanisms that contribute to the considerable variability in cognitive and affective development in children with CM. Finally, damage to the posterior vermis has been shown to contribute to cerebellar mutism involving significant regression of language (Riva and Georgi, 2000); although a detailed discussion of the role of the cerebellum in language is beyond the scope of this review (see Chapter 6, and Mariën et al., 2014, for an excellent review).

Models of the cerebellum in motor and non-motor functions

The existing experimental and clinical observations have provided evidence for a range of different theoretical stances regarding the role of the cerebellum in motor and non-motor functions. Firstly, a prominent theory is that the cerebellum supports information processing by making predictions on the basis of an "internal model" of sensory events (Wolpert, Miall & Kawato, 1998; Ito, 2005). According to this theory, the cerebellum generates predictions of the sensory requirements of anticipated movement, which in turn are fed forward via projections to frontal and temporo-parietal cortices, and then compared against actual sensorimotor input. Thus the "comparator" role of the cerebellum is such that discrepancies between the predicted and actual movement are detected via visual and proprioceptive feedback. There is general consensus that the cerebellum utilises a "forward model", in conjunction with the parietal cortex, to provide prediction of the expected sensory consequences of an action (Blakemore & Sirigu, 2003; Desmurgot & Grafton, 2000).

Second, an alternative theory has been put forward by Ito (2008) who proposed that cerebellar-dependent forward models can be defined by temporal constraints—that is, where predictions require some form of precise temporal representation. Interestingly, children with ADHD show consistent deficits in timing functions (Rubia, Halari, Christakou & Taylor, 2009), which have also been linked to cerebellar connectivity with frontoparietal regions (Hart, Radua, Mataix-Cols & Rubia, 2012) (see frontoparietal circuitry section below).

Third, an alternative hypothesis is that the cerebellum monitors and coordinates the acquisition of sensory information from multiple inputs, such that cerebellar activity should increase with task difficulty (i.e. when better control of sensory input is required) (Bower, 1997a, 1997b). Based on this conceptualisation, the cerebellum itself does not implement motor or timing functions, but rather the cerebellum facilitates the computational efficiency of the temporal coding of sensory information on which these functions depend upon. This perspective is especially relevant for developmental disorders with cerebellar involvement such as ASD, which can be viewed as a behavioural response to a general and overwhelming lack of control over incoming sensory input (Fatemi, 2013).

Fourth, the "sequence detection model" was proposed to describe the role of the cerebellum in detecting change in sequential order information from incoming sensory information (Leggio, Chiricozzi, Clausi, Tedesco & Molinari, 2011; Molinari et al., 1997). There is compelling evidence from various sources to support a cerebellar role in detecting violations in the sequence order of not only somatosensory events (Restuccia, Della Marca, Valeriani, Leggio & Molinari, 2007), but also in visuospatial (Molinari et al., 1997), and cognitive functions (Leggio et al., 2011). Thus, it is proposed that the cerebellum is involved in the detection of the absence/disappearance of an expected/unexpected stimulus, with activity of the cerebellum increasing if a discrepancy-error signal is detected. Intriguingly, the cerebellar role in cognition has been implicated as a pathogenic mechanism in schizophrenia (Andreasen & Pierson,

2008), ASD (Fatemi et al., 2012) and Friedreich ataxia (see Chapter 17), where cerebellar-like sequence detection deficits have been reported (Gidley Larson & Motofsky, 2008; Hocking et al., 2014; Remillard, 2014).

Finally, the cerebellum has been proposed to act as a homeostatic supervisor of ongoing performance in both sensorimotor and higher-order information processing (Schmahmann, 1996). The corollary of this notion of a "Universal Cerebellar Transform" is that damage to the cerebellum is predicted to result in a similar pattern of impairment across all domains in which maintenance of behaviour requires such homeostatic regulation (Schmahmann, 2004). Thus, the "dysmetria of thought" hypothesis provides a unifying conceptual framework in which hypermetric/hypometric features of the motor system can be extended to the non-motor domain. Again, this has considerable relevance for a range of developmental disorders; for example, the illogical thoughts, cognitive dysmetria, lack of empathy/muted emotional responses seen in schizophrenia, and the self-stimulatory, stereotypical/repetitive behaviours, and sensory overload seen in ASD may have a common origin linked to the homeostatic functions of the cerebellum.

To date, there is no unequivocal support for any one of these models of cerebellar function in developmental disorders, and indeed, the precise role of the cerebellum in perceptual, executive, affective, visuospatial and language functions remains controversial and poorly understood. It has been suggested that the formation of internal models within the cerebellum supports implicit/procedural learning via error-driven refinement of closed-loop cerebro-cerebellar circuits involved in a range of cognitive, motor and affective functions (Stoodley, 2016). Alternatively, the role of the cerebellum may be to provide temporally-accurate predictions of future events across motor and non-motor functions (see Courchesne & Allen, 1997). The complex cerebro-cerebellar system of segregated connections between the cerebellum and various brain regions involved in cognition and emotion suggest that the broad range of cerebellar functions may relate to specific connectivity of cerebellar modules, rather than any specific properties of the cerebellar microcircuitry per se. It has been suggested that disruption of the cerebellum acts early in development to shape the structure and function of connecting cortical regions (e.g. frontoparietal circuits) to which it projects (Wang et al., 2014). In the next section, more recent progress in our understanding of the functioning of frontoparietal circuitry will be discussed to provide a conceptual framework for understanding integrated brain regions underlying attention and goal-directed executive processes that provide flexibility to configure information processing in response to changing task demands.

Frontoparietal circuitry in developmental disorders

A network of frontal and parietal brain regions comprising the presumed human homologue of the frontal eye fields (FEF) and the intraparietal sulcus (IPs) extending into the superior parietal lobe (SPL) represent the frontoparietal regions, which are affected in several developmental disorders which are the focus of this book. Functional neuroimaging has provided a powerful tool for many of the cognitive tasks that require frontoparietal activity to be analysed in terms of brain areas they activate, and studies of attention, more specifically top-down attentional orienting or attentional control, have been some of the most extensively examined (Corbetta & Shulman, 2002; Driver, Eimer & Macaluso, 2004; Posner & Fan, 2007). The most influential model has conceptualised attention as comprising three functionally independent attentional networks, which are responsible for a distinct set of cognitive processes, the alerting, orienting and executive control networks (Posner & Petersen, 1990; Petersen & Posner, 2012). It should be noted that these attention networks heavily overlap and interact with the dorsal visual stream, which has been suggested to be more vulnerable during development, which led to the proposal of a "dorsal stream vulnerability hypothesis" across a range of acquired and developmental disorders (Braddick, Atkinson & Wattam-Bell, 2003; Grinter, Mayberry & Badcock, 2010). The dorsal stream performs computations for transforming spatial relationships ('vision for action') and for controlling visually-guided actions, whereas the ventral visual stream performs computations for 'vision for perception' and is involved in recognition of objects and faces (Milner & Goodale, 1995).

These three attention networks have been shown to have some degree of independence based on behavioural, neurophysiological and neuroanatomical studies (see Raz & Buhle, 2006, for a review). We shall see, however, that these neural networks show an interesting developmental time course across childhood, with an increasing independence between the orienting and executive control networks, with significant implications for understanding atypical development of attentional networks (Posner, Rothbart, Sheese & Voelker, 2012; Reuda et al., 2004). Next, we will briefly review the frontoparietal attention network using a framework of functionally independent attentional networks (Posner & Petersen, 1990; Petersen & Posner, 2012), and extend this to an overarching developmental mechanism that implicates frontoparietal regions in typical and atypical cognitive processes reliant on limited-capacity attention networks.

Alerting network

The alerting network is involved in maintaining and adjusting alertness, referred to as sustained attention or vigilance (i.e. maintaining attention on task over time). The neuroanatomy of alerting includes the nuclei of the reticular formation of the brain stem, specifically the locus coeruleus (LC)-norepinephrene system, which projects to the thalamic nuclei and connects with the right frontal and parietal areas, as well as the brain stem. The brain's norepinephrine system is important in inhibiting spontaneous neural activity, and maintaining appropriate levels of alertness in response to sensory input. The anterior cingulate cortex (ACC) and right dorsolateral prefrontal cortex (DLPFC) are involved in voluntary maintenance of alertness by regulating activity in LC via the thalamus. Finally, the right ventral frontoparietal network functions to maintain vigilance and appropriate levels of alertness.

Within a developmental framework, the tonic (i.e. state of general wakefulness) and endogenous phasic (i.e. endogenously controlled level of alertness) components of alertness continue to develop between the ages of 4 and 7 years (Mezzacappa, 2004), although the efficiency and speed of phasic alertness shows a much more protracted developmental course not reaching adult-like performance until age 10 years (Rueda et al., 2004). Finally, in children aged 8 to 12 years, the frontoparietal network, in particular the right hemisphere, fails to activate to the same extent as in adults, suggestive of a developmentally immature top-down modulation process (Konrad et al., 2005). Interestingly, the poorer sustained attention of children with ADHD has been linked to tasks that engage right frontoparietal activity, and has been associated with the dopamine D4 receptor (DRD4) gene and dopamine transporter genotype (DAT1) variants (Bellgrove, Hawi, Kirley, Gill & Robertson, 2005a, Bellgrove et al., 2005b).

Orienting network

The orienting network can be defined as disengaging, shifting and reengaging attention (Posner, Walker, Friedrich & Rafal, 1984). This is important for *selective attention* (i.e. selecting certain types of task-relevant stimuli and ignoring others). Visuospatial orienting can be exogenous, as when eye/head movements accompany shifts in attention, or endogenous, without corresponding eye/head movements. Orienting visual attention may also be based on reflexive (automatic) or voluntary shifts of spatial attention to a localised area. The neural networks responsible for directing spatial attention include posterior brain areas such as SPL, IPs, temporoparietal junction (TPJ), FEF, thalamus and superior colliculus (Corbetta & Shulman, 2002; Mesuam, 1990; Posner & Petersen, 1990). Acetylcholine is the neuromodulator involved in the orienting network, which has been proposed to facilitate the attentional spotlight to ensure rapid attention reorienting (Thiel, Zilles & Fink, 2005). The activation of FEF and IPs has been implicated in the dorsal attention network (DAN), which is involved in goal-directed (top-down) selection for stimuli and responses (Corbetta, Patel & Shulman, 2008; Power et al., 2011). This contrasts with the neural network for stimulus-driven detection of behaviourally relevant stimuli, the ventral attention network (VAN), which involves a right lateralised system comprising the temporoparietal cortex and inferior frontal cortex (IFC) (Corbetta & Shulman, 2002).

The development of overt orienting to exogenous cues is not fully developed in the first two months of infancy; however, newborns by 4 months of age develop an inhibitory pathway, which is responsible for facilitating and suppressing visuospatial orienting, with the ability to disengage visual attention increasing rapidly (Johnson,

1990). Voluntary shifts in visual attention and accuracy of their termination, as well as attention disengagement, continues to increase with age, with orienting efficiency increasing between the ages of 4 and 7 years (Mezzacappa, 2004). When compared to adults, children aged 8 to 12 years show reduced activation of TPJ, an area involved in identifying salient or unexpected stimuli, and recruit additional brain areas (superior frontal gyrus and insula) during performance on orienting tasks, perhaps reflective of immature neural responses and compensatory pathways (Konrad et al., 2005).

Executive control network

The executive control network involves a multidimensional set of functions associated with a range of higher-order cognitive processes including cognitive flexibility; task initiation and response inhibition; planning and organisation; working memory and regulation of emotion and behaviour. Recent studies suggest executive control is not a unitary function but can be broadly fractionated into three separable yet not completed independent components—the ability to shift between mental sets or tasks ('shifting'); selectively attending to stimuli and inhibiting prepotent responses ('inhibition'); and updating and monitoring in working memory ('updating') (Miyake et al., 2000). The neural networks responsible for executive control comprise regions within the prefrontal cortex—orbitofrontal, ventromedial and DLPC—as well as ACC and subcortical regions, including the basal ganglia and cerebellum (Heyder, Suchan & Daum, 2004).

Moreover, neuroimaging studies provide evidence to support the multidimensional nature of executive control; for example, shifting between tasks has been shown to recruit the bilateral medial prefrontal cortex (Crone, Wendelken, Donohu & Bunge, 2005; Rushworth, Walton, Kennerley & Bannerman, 2004); the ability to inhibit responses is thought to rely on right IFC (Aron, Robbins & Poldrack, 2004); and maintaining information in working memory may be mediated largely by the lateral prefrontal cortex (Smith & Jonides, 1999). Dopamine is the central neuromodulator associated with executive control and functioning of the prefrontal cortex. Indeed, children with ADHD who show dopaminergic genetic variation (DAT1) display increased activation of parietal and prefrontal regions during response inhibition tasks (Braet et al., 2011), suggestive of greater effort and recruitment of these regions.

The executive control network undergoes the most protracted course of development relative to the other attention networks (see Diamond, 2002, for a review); however, each of the components of executive control develop at different rates. For example, the ability to shift between tasks does not reach young adult-like performance until early adolescence, whereas some aspects of inhibitory control (e.g. performance on the Stroop task) do not reach maturity until after the age of 15 (Huzianga, Dolan & van der Molen, 2006). When compared to young adults, children aged 8–12 years show less activation of the right inferior frontal gyrus and the left superior parietal cortex during a flanker (conflict) task (Konrad et al., 2005), suggestive of persistent immaturity within frontoparietal networks in children. There is also general support for the multidimensional nature of the executive control network in developmental disorders. For example, core deficits in behavioural flexibility or shifting are accompanied by greater engagement of frontal regions (dorsal cingulate cortex/superior frontal gyrus, left middle frontal, right inferior frontal gyri) in children with ASD (Yerys et al., 2015).

Cross-functional role of frontoparietal regions in cognition

There is increasing evidence in support of the hypothesis that this network of frontal and parietal regions is the most likely candidate for an attention-based mechanism that supports other cognitive functions such as visuospatial working memory (Klingberg, 2006; Nobre et al., 2004). In spite of the support for this attention-based conceptualisation, this view has been challenged by proponents of more traditional models which postulate process-specific modules and domain-specific temporary storage systems in working memory (Baddeley, 2007; Baddeley & Hitch, 1974; Jonides et al., 2008), which can be linked to specific circumscribed brain regions. However, there is increasing evidence to support activation of the DAN (FEF and IPs/SPL) during performance on a range of short-term memory/working memory tasks (see Lückmann, Jacobs & Sack, 2014, for a review), supporting the view that working memory and spatial attention share common neural processes. This is consistent with studies showing impaired spatial working memory performance as the attentional load on visual search increases (Silk, Bellgrove, Wrafter, Mattingley & Cunnington, 2010; Vandenberghe, Molenberghs & Gillebert, 2012), and evidence of increased activity of the IPs during performance on spatial working memory and concurrent visual search tasks (Silk et al., 2010).

This raises an important question: what is the source of this limited-capacity process that is a common feature of both spatial working memory and visual search performance? The IPs play a crucial role in representing a spatial map where the coordinates of spatial locations are integrated to control shifts in spatial attention, and is important for a range of visually-guided actions including directing eye movements, reaching, pointing, grasping and object manipulation (Corbetta & Shulman, 2002). It is therefore conceivable that a shared feature of the maintenance of working memory and top-down attentional control is the function of a saliency map supported by the IPs (Gillebert et al., 2013; Silk et al., 2010). This is analogous to the role of the DAN in directing activity of brain regions based on a saliency map during attentional orienting, which can be extended to working memory. See Astle and Scerif (2011) for an excellent review of individual differences in the interaction between attentional control and visual working memory in typically developing children.

In summary, there is increasing evidence to support overlapping neural processes involved in top-down control of attention and working memory in the adult literature.

What remains unclear, however, is whether or not developmental changes in attentional control drive white matter maturation in frontal and parietal regions associated with developmental improvements in working memory capacity (see Klingberg, 2006). Indeed, this right lateralised frontoparietal network shows a rather protracted course of development into early adulthood (Klingberg, Forssberg & Westerberg, 2002; Kwon, Reiss & Menon, 2002). With the advent of connectivity and large-scale brain network studies, the target for future studies should not simply be investigation of individual nodes in this network, but rather how they operate in ensemble, and perhaps most importantly how this large-scale network changes over developmental time, and across a range of developmental disorders, to which we now turn to in the next section.

Cerebellar frontoparietal connectivity in developmental disorders

Functional and resting-state connectivity studies

New advances in high-field functional neuroimaging techniques have provided a wealth of evidence suggesting that developmental disorders do not solely arise from deficits in specific regions in isolation; rather, it is more likely the product of anomalous connectivity throughout interconnected neural systems. Functional connectivity refers to the temporal correlation between spatially remote neurophysiological signals, as indexed by statistical dependence across these signals in distributed neural networks. It has been suggested that increasing frontoparietal connectivity with age, and maturation of white matter structure, underlies the development of attentional and visuospatial working memory capacity (Edin, Macoveanu, Olesen, Tegnér & Klingberg, 2007; Klingberg et al., 2002; Mabbott, Noseworthy, Bouffet, Laughlin & Rockel, 2006; Scherf, Sweeney & Luna, 2006). Indeed, developmental shifts in frontoparietal connectivity are assumed to relate to changes in specific regions recruited during visuospatial working memory tasks—that is, children recruit limited activation in DLPFC and parietal regions and rely more on ventromedial regions (caudate nucleus, anterior insula) (see also Crone, Wendelken, Donohue & Bunge, 2006), whereas by adolescence activation includes a more diffuse network including DLPFC, ACC, posterior parietal cortex (PPC), anterior insula and even more specialised networks emerging by adulthood (Scherf et al., 2006). These results suggest that, perhaps via synaptic pruning and myelination, refinement of both localised and distal connections may support maturation of frontoparietal connectivity necessary for adult-level cognitive control. This is consistent with increased frontoparietal synaptic connectivity emerging as the strongest predictor of developmental increases in working memory during childhood (Edin et al., 2007). Furthermore, there is evidence of changes in functional connectivity within the DAN with age, specifically reduced anterior IPs connectivity with prefrontal and sensorimotor regions across late childhood and adolescence (Vinette & Bray, 2015). Further disruption or delay in these developmental processes may play an important role in developmental disorders of attention and control, where aberrant functional connectivity of the IPs has been reported, including ASD (Nielsen et al., 2013), ADHD (Tomasi & Volkow, 2012), and Williams syndrome (Meyer-Lindenberg et al., 2004).

Recent emphasis has also been placed on the resting state functional MRI which detects spontaneous fluctuations of the blood oxygen level-dependent (BOLD) signal during a period of task-free resting state. This approach has revealed the presence of large-scale intrinsic connectivity networks (ICNs), each subserving specific cognitive functions; the frontoparietal (central executive) network, default mode network (DMN) and cinguloopercular (salience) network (Dosenbach et al., 2007; Fox et al., 2005; Power et al., 2011). In resting-state connectivity studies, there is a general pattern of increasing *integration* of long-range connectivity with age alongside *segregation* (reduced connectivity with age) with other ICNs (Fair et al., 2007). Importantly, the interregional connectivity of attention networks is incomplete and fragmented in young children (5 to 8 years old) suggestive of less developmental functional connectivity (de Bie et al., 2012). Within this developmental framework of interrelationships between ICNs, a recent hypothesis (Castellanos & Proal, 2012; Sonugal-Barke & Castellanos, 2007) proposes that fluctuations in sustained attention and associated attentional lapses during task performance in ADHD involve (*i*) the default-mode network, an ICN that involves very low frequency coherence within a specific brain network during internal task non-specific cognition during rest, which can persist or intrude into; (*ii*) a range of task-specific ICNs including the DAN, VAN and frontoparietal networks (see Sripada, Kessler & Angstadt, 2014; Tomasi & Volkow, 2012).

Consistent with the importance of dynamic interrelationships between neural regions during resting-state, there is recent evidence in children and adolescents with ASD to indicate increased sensorimotor intrinsic functional connectivity, in the context of reduced cerebellar connectivity with circuits supporting higher order processes (prefrontal and posterior parietal cortices) (Khan et al., 2015). Together these findings lend support to the view that the function of frontoparietal and cerebellar networks is not fully delineated by the activity of its individual components, but is also the outcome of dynamic interrelationships among interconnected neural systems, where parallels are beginning to emerge across a range of neurological and developmental disorders (see Menon, 2011, for a review).

Large-scale brain network studies

More recently developed whole-brain connectomic methods support the view that the brain is functionally organised into large-scale networks, and connectivity within and between these networks change across developmental time (Di Martino et al., 2014). Of the stable ICNs described above, the frontoparietal (central executive) network structure of children (aged 7–9 years) demonstrates continued strengthening of connections with age, which is closely connected to regions within the cinguloopercular (salience) network, but with many adult connections still missing (Fair et al., 2007). With age, there is a strong tendency toward an increase in long-range functional connections and a concomitant reduction in short-range connections within these control networks—that is, segregation and functional integration of information processing streams (Fair et al., 2007).

In line with the importance of connectomic methods for studying large-scale brain networks, there is recent evidence of maturational lag in connections within DMN and its interconnections with the VAN and frontoparietal networks in a large sample of children, adolescents and young adults with ADHD (Sripada et al., 2014, see also Shaw et al., 2007, for diffuse maturation delay in DMN cortical thickness in ADHD). The emergence of the cerebellum as a structure involved in these brain-wide networks (see also Luna et al., 2001) suggests that long-range functional connections between the cerebellum and control networks (fronto-striato-parietal regions) may contribute to the pathophysiology of ADHD (Hong et al., 2014). It is therefore possible that widespread alterations in frontoparietal and cerebellar regions during development of control networks may play a critical role in a range of developmental disorders of control.

Summary

The human capacity for attentional control necessary for adaptive responses to changing task demands is unrivaled, and we have seen in this chapter that these processes depend on distinct frontoparietal and cerebellar networks. The developmental trajectory varies across the three attentional networks (alerting, orienting, executive control) such that developmentally immature top-down modulation (within the DAN network) persists into early adolescence. Yet, the executive control network, which guides adaptive control by integrating external information with internal representations, undergoes the most protracted developmental course, with differing rates of maturation for each individual component of executive control. In developmental disorders, delay or persistent immaturity within these frontoparietal networks may contribute to specific deficits in selective attention, sustained attention and/or attentional control, as well as common processes contributing to spatial attention and visuospatial working memory functions.

Insights emerging from recent advances from the perspective of systems neuroscience have prompted a re-examination of dynamic interrelationships within and among large-scale neural networks. Mapping of intrinsic functional connectivity has revealed distinct frontoparietal (top-down control), default mode and cingulo-opercular (salience) networks, although developmental changes in long-range functional connectivity (segregation) and decreased short-range connections (integration) appear to contribute to mature attention and cognitive control networks. Delay or disruption in connections between ICNs, especially between the frontoparietal, DMN and salience networks may well contribute to attentional lapses, which are a consistent feature of ADHD, and many other developmental disorders associated with attention deficits. The relatively late involvement of the cerebellum into these large-scale brain networks highlight the prolonged maturational changes important for integration of distinct brain regions supporting attention and cognitive control. The inclusion of cerebellar regions in this larger network may be important both to top-down regulation by the prefrontal cortex to other cortical and subcortical circuits, as well as convergence of multimodal sensory information mediated by cerebellar connections to parietal cortex. It is likely that future studies targeting aberrant connectivity within and between widespread, yet anatomically connected, cerebellar-fronto-parietal circuits, will be an important conceptual advance in our understanding of a range of developmental disorders of control.

Abbreviations

ACC: Anterior cingulate cortex
ADHD: Attention Deficit Hyperactivity Disorder
ASD: Autism Spectrum Disorder
BOLD: blood-oxygen level dependent
CCAS: Cerebellar Cognitive Affective Syndrome
CM: Cerebellum malformation
DAN: Dorsal attention network
DAT1: dopamine transporter 1
DLPFC: Dorsolateral prefrontal cortex
DMN: Default-mode network
DRD4: dopamine D4 receptor
FEF: Frontal eye fields
ICN: intrinsic connectivity networks
ID: Intellectual disability
IFC: Inferior frontal cortex
IPs: Intraparietal sulcus
JS: Jobert syndrome
LC: Locus coeruleus
PPC: Posterior parietal cortex
SPL: Superior parietal lobe
TPJ: Temporoparietal junction
VAN: Ventral attention network
WS: Williams syndrome

Further readings

Arnsten, A. M. T., & Rubia, K. (2012). Neurobiological circuits regulating attention, cognitive control, motivation, and emotion: Disruptions in neurodevelopmental psychiatric disorders. *Journal of the American Academy of Child & Adolescent Psychiatry, 51*(4), 356–367.

Becker, E. B., & Stoodley, C. J. (2013). Autism spectrum disorder and the cerebellum. *International Review of Neurobiology, 113*, 1–34.
Castellanos, F. X., & Proal, E. (2012). Large-scale brain systems in ADHD: Beyond the prefrontal-striatal model. *Trends in Cognitive Sciences, 16*(1), 17–26.
Manto, M., Bower, J. M., Conforto, A. B., Delgado-García, J. M., da Guarda, S. N., Gerwig, M., … Timmann, D. (2012). Consensus paper: Roles of the cerebellum in motor control-the diversity of ideas on cerebellar involvement in movement. *Cerebellum, 11*(2), 457–87.
Mariën, P., Ackermann, H., Adamaszek, M., Barwood, C. H., Beaton, A., Desmond, J., … Ziegler, W. (2014). Consensus paper: Language and the cerebellum: An ongoing enigma. *Cerebellum, 13*(3), 386–410.
Wang, S. S., Kloth, A. D., & Badura, A. (2014). The cerebellum, sensitive periods, and autism. *Neuron, 83*(3), 518–532.

References

Andreasen, N. C., & Pierson, R. (2008). The role of the cerebellum in schizophrenia. *Biological Psychiatry, 64*(2), 81–8.
Aron, A. R., Robbins, T. W., & Poldrack, R. A. (2004). Inhibition and the right inferior frontal cortex. *Trends in Cognitive Sciences, 8*(4), 170–7.
Astle, D. E., & Scerif, G. (2011). Interactions between attention and visual short-term memory (VSTM): What can be learnt from individual and developmental differences? *Neuropsychologia, 49*(6), 1435–45.
Baddeley, A. D. (2007). *Working Memory, Thought, and Action*. New York: Oxford University Press.
Baddeley, A. D., & Hitch, G. (1974). Working memory. In G. H. Bower, (ed.), *The Psychology of Learning and Motivation: Advances in Research and Theory*. (pp. 47–89). New York: Academic Press.
Becker, E. B., & Stoodley, C. J. (2013). Autism spectrum disorder and the cerebellum. *International Review of Neurobiology, 113*, 1–34.
Bellgrove, M. A., Hawi, Z., Kirley, A., Gill, M., & Robertson, I.H. (2005a). Dissecting the attention deficit hyperactivity disorder (ADHD) phenotype: Sustained attention, response variability and spatial attentional asymmetries in relation to dopamine transporter (DAT1) genotype. *Neuropsychologia, 43*(13), 1847–57.
Bellgrove, M. A., Hawi, Z., Lowe, N., Kirley, A., Robertson, I. H., & Gill, M. (2005b). DRD4 gene variants and sustained attention in attention deficit hyperactivity disorder (ADHD): Effects of associated alleles at the VNTR and -521 SNP. *American Journal of Medical Genetics. Part B, Neuropsychiatric Genetics, 136B*(1), 81–6.
Blakemore, S. J., & Sirigu, A. (2003). Action prediction in the cerebellum and in the parietal lobe. *Experimental Brain Research, 153*(2), 239–45.
Bower, J. M. (1997a). Control of sensory data acquisition. *International Review of Neurobiology, 41*, 489–513.
Bower, J. M. (1997b). Is the cerebellum sensory for motor's sake, or motor for sensory's sake: The view from the whiskers of a rat? *Progress in Brain Research, 114*, 463–96.
Braddick, O., Atkinson, J., & Wattam-Bell, J. (2003). Normal and anomalous development of visual motion processing: Motion coherence and 'dorsal-stream vulnerability'. *Neuropsychologia, 41*(13), 1769–84.
Braet, W., Johnson, K. A., Tobin, C. T., Acheson, R., McDonnell, C., Hawi, Z., … Garavan, H. (2011). fMRI activation during response inhibition and error processing: The role of

the DAT1 gene in typically developing adolescents and those diagnosed with ADHD. *Neuropsychologia, 49*(7), 1641–50.

Castellanos, F. X., & Proal, E. (2012). Large-scale brain systems in ADHD: Beyond the prefrontal-striatal model. *Trends in Cognitive Sciences, 16*(1), 17–26.

Corbetta, M., & Shulman, G. L. (2002). Control of goal-directed and stimulus-driven attention in the brain. *Nature Reviews Neuroscience, 3*(3), 201–15.

Corbetta, M., Patel, G., & Shulman, G. L. (2008). The reorienting system of the human brain: From environment to theory of mind. *Neuron, 58*(3), 306–24. doi: 10.1016/j.neuron.2008.04.017.

Courchesne, E., & Allen, G. (1997). Prediction and preparation, fundamental functions of the cerebellum. *Learning & Memory, 4*(1), 1–35.

Crone, E. A., Wendelken, C., Donohue, S. E., & Bunge, S. A. (2005). Neural evidence for dissociable components of task-switching. *Cerebral Cortex, 16*(4), 475–86.

Crone, E. A., Wendelken, C., Donohue, S., van Leijenhorst, L., & Bunge, S. A. (2006). Neurocognitive development of the ability to manipulate information in working memory. *Proceedings of the National Academy of Sciences of the United States of America, 103*(24), 9315–20.

de Bie, H. M., Boersma, M., Adriaanse, S., Veltman, D.J., Wink, A.M., Roosendaal, S.D., … Sanz-Arigita, E. J. (2012). Resting-state networks in awake five- to eight-year old children. *Human Brain Mapping, 33*(5), 1189–201.

Desmurget, M., & Grafton, S. (2000). Forward modeling allows feedback control for fast reaching movements. *Trends Cognitive Sciences, 4*(11), 423–431.

Di Martino, A., Fair, D. A., Kelly, C., Satterthwaite, T. D., Castellanos, F. X., Thomason, M.E., … Milham, M. P. (2014). Unraveling the miswired connectome: A developmental perspective. *Neuron, 83*(6), 1335–53.

Diamond, A. (2002). Normal development of prefrontal cortex from birth to young adulthood: Cognitive functions, anatomy and biochemistry. In D.T. Struss, R.T. Knight (Eds.), *Principles of Frontal Lobe Function*. Oxford: Oxford University Press.

Dosenbach, N. U., Fair, D. A., Miezin, F. M., Cohen, A. L., Wenger, K. K., Dosenbach, R. A., … Petersen, S. E. (2007). Distinct brain networks for adaptive and stable task control in humans. *Proceedings of the National Academy of Sciences of the United States of America, 104*(26), 11073–8.

Driver, J., Eimer, M., & Macaluso, E. (2004). Neurobiology of human spatial attention: Modulation, generation, and integration, In N. Kanwisher, & J. Duncan (Eds.), *Attention and Performance XX: Functional BrainImaging of Visual Cognition*. London: Oxford University Press.

Edin, F., Macoveanu, J., Olesen, P., Tegnér, J., & Klingberg, T. (2007). Stronger synaptic connectivity as a mechanism behind development of working memory-related brain activity during childhood. *Journal of Cognitive Neuroscience, 19*(5), 750–60.

Fair, D. A., Dosenbach, N. U., Church, J. A., Cohen, A. L., Brahmbhatt, S., Miezin, F.M., … Schlaggar, B. L. (2007). Development of distinct control networks through segregation and integration. *Proceedings of the National Academy of Sciences of the United States of America, 104*(33), 13507–12.

Fatemi, S. H. (2013). Cerebellum and autism. *Cerebellum, 12*(5), 778–9.

Fatemi, S. H., Aldinger, K. A., Ashwood, P., Bauman, M. L., Blaha, C. D., Blatt, G. J., … Welsh, J.P. (2012). Consensus paper: Pathological role of the cerebellum in autism. *Cerebellum, 11*(3), 777–807.

Fox, M. D., Snyder, A. Z., Vincent, J. L., Corbetta, M., Van Essen, D. C., & Raichle, M.E. (2005). The human brain is intrinsically organized into dynamic, anticorrelated functional networks. *Proceedings of the National Academy of Sciences of the United States of America, 102*(27), 9673–8.

Gidley Larson, J. C., & Mostofsky, S. H. (2008). Evidence that the pattern of visuomotor sequence learning is altered in children with autism. *Autism Research, 1*(6), 341–53.

Gillebert, C. R., Caspari, N., Wagemans, J., Peeters, R., Dupont, P., & Vandenberghe, R. (2013). Spatial stimulus configuration and attentional selection: Extrastriate and superior parietal interactions. *Cerebral Cortex, 23*(12), 2840–54.

Grinter, E. J., Maybery, M. T., & Badcock, D. R. (2010). Vision in developmental disorders: Is there a dorsal stream deficit? *Brain Research Bulletin, 82*(3–4), 147–60.

Hart, H., Radua, J., Mataix-Cols, D., & Rubia, K. (2012). Meta-analysis of fMRI studies of timing in attention-deficit hyperactivity disorder (ADHD). *Neuroscience & Biobehavioral Reviews, 36*(10), 2248–56.

Hétu, S., Grégoire, M., Saimpont, A., Coll, M. P., Eugène, F., Michon, P. E., & Jackson, P.L. (2013). The neural network of motor imagery: An ALE meta-analysis. *Neuroscience & Biobehavioral Reviews, 37*(5), 930–49.

Heyder, K., Suchan, B., & Daum, I. (2004). Cortico-subcortical contributions to executive control. *Acta Psychologica, 115*(2–3), 271–89.

Hocking, D. R., Corben, L. A., Fielding, J., Cremer, P. D., Millist, L., White, O. B., & Delatycki, M. B. (2014). Saccade reprogramming in Friedreich ataxia reveals impairments in the cognitive control of saccadic eye movement. *Brain & Cognition, 87*, 161–167.

Hong, S. B., Zalesky, A., Fornito, A., Park, S., Yang, Y. H., Park, M. H., … Kim, J. W. (2014). Connectomic disturbances in attention-deficit/hyperactivity disorder: A whole-brain tractography analysis. *Biological Psychiatry, 76*(8), 656–63.

Huizinga, M., Dolan, C.V., & van der Molen, M.W. (2006). Age-related change in executive function: Developmental trends and a latent variable analysis. *Neuropsychologia, 44*(11), 2017–36.

Ito, M. (2005). Bases and implications of learning in the cerebellum—Adaptive control and internal model mechanism. *Progress in Brain Research, 148*, 95–109.

Ito, M. (2008). Control of mental activities by internal models in the cerebellum. *Nature Reviews Neuroscience, 9*(4), 304–13.

Johnson, M. H. (1990). Cortical maturation and the development of visual attention in early infancy. *Journal of Cognitive Neuroscience, 2*(2), 81–95.

Jonides, J., Lewis, R. L., Nee, D. E., Lustig, C. A., Berman, M. G., & Moore, K. S. (2008). The mind and brain of short-term memory. *Annual Review of Psychology, 59*, 193–224.

Khan, A. J., Nair, A., Keown, C. L., Datko, M.C., Lincoln, A. J., & Müller, R.A. (2015). Cerebro-cerebellar resting-state functional connectivity in children and adolescents with Autism Spectrum Disorder. *Biological Psychiatry, 78*(9), 625–634. doi: 10.1016/j.biopsych.2015.03.024.

Klingberg, T. (2006). Development of a superior frontal-intraparietal network for visuo-spatial working memory. *Neuropsychologia, 44*(11), 2171–7.

Klingberg, T., Forssberg, H., & Westerberg, H. (2002). Increased brain activity in frontal and parietal cortex underlies the development of visuospatial working memory capacity during childhood. *Journal of Cognitive Neuroscience, 14*(1), 1–10.

Konrad, K., Neufang, S., Thiel, C. M., Specht, K., Hanisch, C., Fan, J., Herpertz-Dahlmann, B., & Fink, G. R. (2005). Development of attentional networks: An fMRI study with children and adults. *Neuroimage, 28*(2), 429–39.

Kwon, H., Reiss, A. L., & Menon, V. (2002). Neural basis of protracted developmental changes in visuo-spatial working memory. *Proceedings of the National Academy of Sciences of the United States of America, 99*(20), 13336–41.

Leggio, M. G., Chiricozzi, F. R., Clausi, S., Tedesco, A. M., & Molinari, M. (2011). The neuropsychological profile of cerebellar damage: The sequencing hypothesis. *Cortex, 47*(1), 137–44.

Lückmann, H. C., Jacobs, H. I., & Sack, A. T. (2014). The cross-functional role of frontoparietal regions in cognition: Internal attention as the overarching mechanism. *Progress in Neurobiology, 116*, 66–86.

Luna, B., Thulborn, K. R., Munoz, D. P., Merriam, E. P., Garver, K. E., Minshew, N. J., … Sweeney, J. A. (2001). Maturation of widely distributed brain function subserves cognitive development. *Neuroimage, 13*(5), 786–93.

Mabbott, D. J., Noseworthy, M., Bouffet, E., Laughlin, S., & Rockel, C. (2006). White matter growth as a mechanism of cognitive development in children. *Neuroimage, 33*(3), 936–46.

Manni, E., & Petrosini, (2004). A century of cerebellar somatotopy: A debated representation. *Nature Reviews Neuroscience, 5*(3), 241–249.

Manto, M., Bower, J. M., Conforto, A. B., Delgado-García, J. M., da Guarda, S. N., Gerwig, M., … Timmann, D. (2012). Consensus paper: Roles of the cerebellum in motor control—The diversity of ideas on cerebellar involvement in movement. *Cerebellum, 11*(2), 457–87.

Mariën, P., Ackermann, H., Adamaszek, M., Barwood, C. H., Beaton, A., Desmond, J., … Xiegler, W. (2014). Consensus paper: Language and the cerebellum: An ongoing enigma. *Cerebellum, 13*(3), 386–410.

Menon, V. (2011). Large-scale brain networks and psychopathology: A unifying triple network model. *Trends in Cognitive Sciences, 15*(10), 483–506.

Mesulam, M. M. (1990). Large-scale neurocognitive networks and distributed processing for attention, language, and memory. *Annals of Neurology, 28*(5), 597–613.

Meyer-Lindenberg, A., Kohn, P., Mervis, C. B., Kippenhan, J. S., Olsen, R. K., Morris, C.A., & Berman, K.F. (2004). Neural basis of genetically determined visuospatial construction deficit in Williams syndrome. *Neuron, 43*, 623–631.

Milner, A. D., & Goodale, M. A. (1995). *The Visual Brain in Action*. New York, Oxford University Press.

Miyake, A., Friedman, N. P., Emerson, M. J., Witzki, A. H., Howerter, A., & Wager, T. D. (2000). The unity and diversity of executive functions and their contributions to complex "Frontal Lobe" tasks: A latent variable analysis. *Cognitive Psychology, 41*(1), 49–100.

Molinari, M., Leggio, M. G., Solida, A., Ciorra, R., Misciagna, S., Silveri, M. C., & Petrosini, L. (1997). Cerebellum and procedural learning: Evidence from focal cerebellar lesions. *Brain, 120* (Pt 10), 1753–62.

Nielsen, J. A., Zielinski, B. A., Fletcher, P. T., Alexander, A. L., Lange, N., Bigler, E. D., … Anderson, J.S. (2013). Multisite functional connectivity MRI classification of autism: ABIDE results. *Frontiers in Human Neuroscience, 7*, 599.

Nobre, A. C., Coull, J. T., Maquet, P., Frith, C. D., Vandenberghe, R., & Mesulam, M. M. (2004). Orienting attention to locations in perceptual versus mental representations. *Journal of Cognitive Neuroscience, 16*(3), 363–73.

Olesen, P. J., Westerberg, H., & Klingberg, T. (2004). Increased prefrontal and parietal activity after training of working memory. *Nature Neuroscience, 7*(1), 75–9.

Petersen, S. E., and Posner, M. I. (2012). The attention system of the human brain: 20 years after. *Annual Review of Neuroscience, 35*, 73–89.

Posner, M. I., & Fan, J. (2007). Attention as an organ system. In J. Pomerantz (Eds), *Neurobiology of Perception and Communication: From Synapse to Society*. Cambridge: De Lange Conference IV. Cambridge University Press.

Posner, M. I., & Petersen, S.E. (1990). The attention system of the human brain. *Annual Review of Neuroscience, 13*, 25–42.

Posner, M. I., Rothbart, M. K., Sheese, B. E., & Voelker, P. (2012). Control networks and neuromodulators of early development. *Developmental Psychology, 48*(3), 827–35.

Posner, M. I., Walker, J. A., Friedrich, F. J., & Rafal, R. D. (1984). Effects of parietal injury on covert orienting of attention. *The Journal of Neuroscience, 4*(7), 1863–74.

Power, J.D., Cohen, A. L., Nelson, S. M., Wig, G. S., Barnes, K. A., Church, J. A., … Petersen, S.E. (2011). Functional network organization of the human brain. *Neuron, 72*(4), 665–78.

Raz, A., & Buhle, J. (2006). Typologies of attentional networks. *Nature Reviews Neuroscience, 7*(5), 367–79.

Remillard, G. (2014). The study of sequence learning in individuals with schizophrenia: A critical review of the literature. *Journal of Neuropsychology, 8*(2), 231–45.

Restuccia, D., Della Marca, G., Valeriani, M., Leggio, M. G., & Molinari, M. (2007). Cerebellar damage impairs detection of somatosensory input changes. A somatosensory mismatch-negativity study. *Brain, 130*(pt 1), 276–87.

Riva, D., & Giorgi, C. (2000). The cerebellum contributes to higher functions during development: Evidence from a series of children surgically treated for posterior fossa tumours. *Brain, 123* (pt 5), 1051–61.

Rubia, K., Halari, R., Christakou A., & Taylor, E. (2009). Impulsiveness as a timing disturbance: Neurocognitive abnormalities in attention-deficit hyperactivity disorder during temporal processes and normalization with methylphenidate. *Philosophical Transactions of the Royal Society of London: Part B, Biological Sciences, 364*(1525), 1919–1931. doi: 10.1098/rstb.2009.0014.

Rueda, M. R., Fan, J., McCandliss, B. D., Halparin, J. D., Gruber, D. B., Lercari, L. P., & Posner, M. I. (2004). Development of attentional networks in childhood. *Neuropsychologia, 42*(8), 1029–40.

Rushworth, M. F., Walton, M. E., Kennerley, S. W., & Bannerman, D. M. (2004). Action sets and decisions in the medial frontal cortex. *Trends in Cognitive Sciences, 8*(9), 410–7.

Sack, A. T. (2009). Parietal cortex and spatial cognition. *Behavioral Brain Research, 202*(2), 153–61.

Sack, A. T., & Schuhmann, T. (2012). Hemispheric differences within the fronto-parietal network dynamics underlying spatial imagery. *Frontiers in Psychology, 28*(3), 214. doi: 10.3389/fpsyg.2012.00214.

Scherf, K. S., Sweeney, J. A., & Luna, B. (2006). Brain basis of developmental change in visuospatial working memory. *Journal of Cognitive Neuroscience, 18*(7), 1045–58.

Schmahmann, J. D. (1996). From movement to thought: Anatomic substrates of the cerebellar contribution to cognitive processing. *Human Brain Mapping, 4*(3), 174–98.

Schmahmann, J. D. (2004). Disorders of the cerebellum: Ataxia, dysmetria of thought, and the cerebellar cognitive affective syndrome. *The Journal of Neuropsychiatry & Clinical Neurosciences, 16*(3), 367–78.

Schmahmann, J. D., & Sherman, J. C. (1998). The cerebellar cognitive affective syndrome. *Brain, 121* (pt 4), 561–79.

Scott, R. B., Stoodley, C. J., Anslow, P., Paul, C., Stein, J. F., Sugden, E. M., & Mitchell, C.D. (2001). Lateralized cognitive deficits in children following cerebellar lesions. *Developmental Medicine & Child Neurology, 43*(10), 685–91.

Shaw, P., Eckstrand, K., Sharp, W., Blumenthal, J., Lerch, J. P., Greenstein, D., … Rapoport, J. L. (2007). Attention-deficit/hyperactivity disorder is characterized by a delay in cortical maturation. *Proceedings of the National Academy of Sciences of the United States of America, 104*(49), 19649–54.

Silk, T. J., Bellgrove, M. A., Wrafter, P., Mattingley, J. B., & Cunnington, R. (2010). Spatial working memory and spatial attention rely on common neural processes in the intraparietal sulcus. *Neuroimage, 53*(2), 718–24.

Smith, E. E., & Jonides, J. (1999). Storage and executive processes in the frontal lobes. *Science, 283*(5408), 1657–61.

Sonuga-Barke, E. J., & Castellanos, F.X. (2007). Spontaneous attentional fluctuations in impaired states and pathological conditions: A neurobiological hypothesis. *Neuroscience and Biobehavioral Reviews, 31*(7), 977–86.

Sripada, C. S., Kessler, D., & Angstadt, M. (2014). Lag in maturation of the brain's intrinsic functional architecture in attention-deficit/hyperactivity disorder. *Proceedings of the National Academy of Sciences of the United States of America, 111*(39), 14259–64.

Steinlin, M. (2007). The cerebellum in cognitive processes: Supporting studies in children. *Cerebellum, 6*(3), 237–41.

Stoodley, C. J. (2012). Cerebellum and cognition: Evidence from functional imaging studies. *Cerebellum, 11*(2), 352–65.

Stoodley, C.J. (2016). The cerebellum and neurodevelopmental disorders. *Cerebellum, 15*(1), 34–37.

Stoodley, C. J., & Schmahmann, J. D. (2009) Functional topography in the human cerebellum: A meta-analysis of neuroimaging studies. *Neuroimage, 44*(2), 489–501.

Swanson, G. T., and Contractor, A. (2004). Recording in the cerebellar slice. *Current Protocols in Neuroscience, Chapter 6*, Unit 6.18, doi: 10.1002/0471142301.ns0618s25.

Tavano, A., & Borgatti, R. (2010). Evidence for a link among cognition, language and emotion in cerebellar malformations. *Cortex, 46*(7), 907–18.

Tavano, A., Fabbro, F., & Borgatti, R. (2007a). Language and social communication in children with cerebellar dysgenesis. *Folia Phoniatrica et Logopaedica, 59*(4), 201–9.

Tavano, A., Grasso, R., Gagliardi, C., Triulzi, F., Bresolin, N., Fabbro, F., & Borgatti, R. (2007b). Disorders of cognitive and affective development in cerebellar malformations. *Brain, 130*(pt 10), 2646–60.

Thiel, C. M., Zilles, K., & Fink, G. R. (2005). Nicotine modulates reorienting of visuospatial attention and neural activity in human parietal cortex. *Neuropsychopharmacology, 30*(4), 810–20.

Tomasi, D., & Volkow, N. D. (2012). Abnormal functional connectivity in children with attention-deficit/hyperactivity disorder. *Biological Psychiatry, 71*(5), 443–50.

Vandenberghe, R., Molenberghs, P., & Gillebert, C. R. (2012). Spatial attention deficits in humans: The critical role of superior compared to inferior parietal lesions. *Neuropsychologia, 50*(6), 1092–103.

Vinette, S. A., & Bray, S. (2015). Variation in functional connectivity along anterior-to-posterior intraparietal sulcus, and relationship with age across late childhood and adolescence. *Developmental Cognitive Neuroscience, 13*, 32–42.

Wang, S. S., Kloth, A. D., & Badura, A. (2014). The cerebellum, sensitive periods, and autism. *Neuron, 83*(3), 518–32.

Wolpert, D. M., Miall, R. C., & Kawato, M. (1998). Internal models in the cerebellum. *Trends in Cognitive Sciences, 2*(9), 338–47.

Yerys, B. E., Antezana, L., Weinblatt, R., Jankowski, K. F., Strang, J., Vaidya, C. J., … Kenworthy, L. (2015). Neural correlates of set-shifting in children with autism. *Autism Research, 8*(4), 386–97.

20
LAST THOUGHTS

John L. Bradshaw, Peter G. Enticott and Nicole J. Rinehart

The late 20th century saw much interest in the basal ganglia and frontostriatal system, while this century may be the turn of the cerebellum, the Last Great Unknown or Terra Incognita. This "little brain" seems to complement the neocortex in both behavioural and evolutionary terms, doing far more than merely coordinating fine movement and balance. It also plays important cognitive roles, again perhaps in terms of coordination and synthesis, pulling together disparate sources of information from various brain regions. Hence the dense and complex interlocking between neocortex and cerebellum. Indeed, while the cerebellum maintains abundant connections with non-motor regions throughout life, it may well also guide the ontogenetic maturation of such circuitry, and during critical developmental periods influence cognitive and socially oriented structures and functions, such as can appear dysfunctional in autism.

Can someone, living in solitary isolation, ever conceivably suffer from a developmental disorder? This thought experiment suggests that unlike other medical or purely neurological syndromes, the nature of societal conventions and expectations, and the interaction of an individual with society, is also crucial. Joan of Arc was a heroine in her time, and likely nowadays would be diagnosed with a psychotic disorder such as schizophrenia. It all depends upon whatever is currently considered desirable, appropriate or acceptable.

Thus, developmental disorders typically lie upon several continua, or spectra, merging with normality at one end of a distribution, and with other developmental disorders at another. Not only may clinicians disagree as to whether an individual's behaviour is or is not pathological, but also, if pathological, as to whether, for example, it lies within the autistic spectrum or that of ADHD. This has led to long-standing disputes as to comorbidity and criteria for diagnosis, a recent example in history being Asperger's disorder that appeared in diagnostic manuals in the 1990s and then was removed in 2013. Such 'movement' of diagnostic labels fuels concern for misdiagnosis, incorrect labelling, stigmatising, and in the case of the removal of Asperger's disorder, under diagnosis of a disorder that has very real and lifelong impacts on the developing individual.

Another consequence can be an apparent increase in prevalence, recently of certain disorders, such as autism and ADHD, an apparent increase stemming in fact from misdiagnosis, an increased awareness or salience, altered criteria, changes in placing cut-offs with normality or with other disorders. This includes such questions as, for example, where the boundary should lie between autism and ADHD, or schizophrenia, or developmental language disorder, or borderline personality disorder or intellectual developmental disorder. Indeed, these syndromes are all behaviourally defined in large part, whatever might be any underlying pathologies; thus, to a large extent diagnosis will always require expert clinical opinion supported by future biomarkers as foreshadowed in this book.

Indeed, diagnostic, prognostic and treatment considerations are not always compatible in defining, describing or managing an apparent dysfunction. The latter may have more than one single cause, genetically, structurally and biochemically, and may therefore manifest as a kind of final common path from various origins. And, conversely, a single genetic, structural or biochemical anomaly may have different clinical manifestations in different individuals. Thus, it is unlikely that a single "magic bullet" will ever treat any one developmental disorder, given the various possible origins and genetic and environmental influences, and the fact that developmental disorders in an individual may evolve and change during life, as society changes and the individual adapts.

Nor is there any gold standard or fixed biomarker for diagnosis, such as the presence of a pathogen. In clinical medicine, the nearest analogue might be hypertension, with its multiple causes and changing criteria for what are acceptable systolic or diastolic pressures. It is ever tempting to appeal to genetics in such contexts. However, it may no longer be appropriate to regard genes just as discrete protein-coding beads on a string, since so much of the genome codes for more than just proteins – and is far from "junk", as once thought – and even where there is protein coding, the elements of DNA can often overlap. Maybe it is no accident that both developmental disorders, and genes themselves, can overlap with fuzzy boundaries. And just as one gene may control several processes, depending upon where and how it is expressed, so too a single disorder may be caused via the interaction of multiple genes.

Despite ever-mounting evidence, from family studies, of the genetic underpinnings of developmental disorders, the probable genetic origins themselves are rarely clear. Apart from certain rare disorders, such as Angelman's syndrome, the above is perhaps particularly true where there are highly variable clinical manifestations or phenotypes, and where they are difficult to distinguish from other, often very similar, disorders.

Judging solely by its presentation, Angelman's syndrome, with its associated ataxia, might qualify for inclusion in this volume as a developmental disorder with cerebellar features. A rare (1 in 20,000) single-gene, autosomal recessive disorder, it is characterised by intellectual disability, developmental delay, speech impairment, seizures, ataxia, frequent inappropriate laughter – all features found in varying combinations in the developmental disorders addressed in this book.

Developmental disorders, unlike Angelman's, are typically a product, as we have seen, of the interaction of genes (themselves no longer seen as completely deterministic) and environment. The latter can alter the behaviour of genes without changing the actual DNA sequences. This phenomenon of epigenetics seems particularly important in the context of developmental disorders. Stress and stressors of various types, and/or their alleviation or absence, may play important mediating roles in which disorder may manifest, and how. However, neither genes nor epigenetics are wholly determinant, even though lifestyle choices, or impacting events, may leave their mark upon the expression of the genes of future generations via methylation, the process that may make a gene less active.

The nature and extent of any genetic contribution, with respect to developmental disorders generally, is becoming clearer with the ability to perform genome-wide associative studies across many thousands of individuals. It is thus possible to identify genetic variation in single nucleotide polymorphisms, and determine the extent of chromosomal variants such as copy-number variations, which can lead to pathological increase or decrease of function. There may be mutations in protein coding, as well as in regulatory processes, themselves possibly subject to environmental influences. However, evidence to date suggests that developmental disorders tend to manifest as an apparent consequence of commonly-occurring variants at a large number of loci, even though any single variant may only have a small effect upon an overall polygenic disease risk.

Such considerations emphasise the fruitlessness of debates, such as the relative importance of mind versus body, nature versus nurture, brain versus behaviour. All interact, with different levels of reductionist explanation and interpretation. For diagnosis and management, measures should be made at all such levels and for all such entities with the recognition, also, that circuits and networks within the brain are no less important than the functioning of specific nodes, centres or regions. And that the brain is itself plastic, continually adapting and changing its circuitry and connections throughout life, in response to events, pressures, trauma and expectations.

An observation, common to a number of chapters in this book, is that comorbidities often largely define the clinical picture of a given disorder, and are often similar across disorders. Thus, ADHD and autism may be one of the most frequent of possible comorbidities, and left untreated, may typically be what most deleteriously affects behaviour. We do not know why ADHD is so often comorbid with autism. Is it because both involve closely adjacent dysfunctions within the frontostriatal system? Or does ADHD moderate an excessively narrow attentional focus in autism, maybe adaptively in a Darwinian sense?

The twin and related questions of comorbidities, and where to place a borderline between any two related disorders, can be usefully addressed via the recent emphasis upon identifying endophenotypes. Thus the latter, occupying a place more proximal to possibly mediating genes than the actual disorders themselves, are well placed both to suggest possible aetiologies, and to taxonomically segregate those developmental disorders.

However, it would still seem that these disorders might stem from particular malfunctions in different regions within the frontostriatal-cerebellar circuitries. Vulnerable individuals may inherit a tendency to a general instability within these networks, with different family members thereby subject to an increased risk for and incidence of any one or more of these disorders, rather than inheriting a particular one.

There remains the question as to why all these disorders, with such strong genetic links, and usually so disadvantageous, persist in the genome rather than being selected out. Maybe in "low doses," or when manifesting particularly in close relatives, they are associated with certain adaptive advantages. Thus, in some ways ADHD may benefit the explorer or soldier who has to maintain hair-trigger awareness and responses, or in modern times we might think of the great entrepreneurs who have documented a history of childhood ADHD. Similarly, the focused obsessionality in autism or Asperger's may advantage the scientist or forensic expert, and a degree of paranoia may be useful to spies, intelligence agents or diplomats. And it is surely no accident that creativity in the arts seems to associate with depression or bipolar disorder. Or is it simply the case that in a system as genetically and structurally complex as the human brain, there are certain weak regions, "fracture zones," where recurrent failures may be expected?

In an affected individual, a function may appear deficient, but in fact may only be developmentally delayed, and poor performance on testing may only be of clinical significance if not accompanied by other more widespread levels of deficit. Indeed, age of first clinical manifestation of a disorder may turn out to be more significant than age at actual testing. Conversely, while there may appear to be preservation of a function, fMRI may often indicate compensatory recruitment of areas other than those normally operating in typically developing children.

One is left with the feeling that often there may be a common biological thread running through many of these disorders, given how they tend to merge and blend with each other. If so, might it be the cause, or the result, of the syndrome's occurrence? Might impairments at different levels of executive function be such a key? Answers, and treatment, might come from new advances in functional imaging and transcranial electrical and magnetic stimulation, likely of an ambulatory nature, such that individuals may be studied, and treated, in far more naturalistic and "ecologically valid" contexts.

We must seek to integrate individual studies of behaviours, disorders, brain anatomy and function into a better and more inclusive, holistic even, understanding of the brain's operation. Each neurone probably participates in many different functions at different times, and each function is likely performed by an orchestra of many neurones, whose members or population may also shift over time.

We conclude by reflecting that with recent major advances in genetics, and foreshadowing of the possibility in the near future of personalized medicine, tailoring intervention and treatments to the individual's possibly quite idiosyncratic personal characteristics, needs and problems, particularly but not exclusively with respect to phenotype, it has become increasingly important to identify likely relevant biomarkers of possible disease subtypes. Such advances in genotypic/phenotypic correlations have coincided with a growing realization, especially in biological psychiatry, that many disorders are far from homogeneous, but may be both conceptually, and usefully, further fractionated along quite a number of dimensions.

A POSTSCRIPT

John L. Bradshaw

A 3-dimensional sculpture can be realised via two fundamentally opposing stratagems or approaches. We can construct the end product by the incremental addition of new elements or components, each of which can themselves be similarly put together; alternatively, like a Michelangelo, we can commence with a uniform, unformed block of marble or metal, and successively subtract unwanted material, until the final, intended end product slowly emerges or is revealed, as if always present, if hidden, within the initial unformed block.

The brain develops along both of these lines. New neurones, connection and circuits are added, typically during early *in utero* phases. Subsequently, maybe during the first few months or years of a baby's existence outside of its mother, inappropriate, unwanted or no longer necessary neurones or connections may be discarded, lost, by a process of developmental or programmed apoptosis or culling. This permits the fine-tuning of an end product – except, of course, that in a much reduced form, unwanted circuits may be silenced by epigenetic processes or lost, or new ones similarly formed or added throughout life, maybe at an ever reducing rate, as a consequence of experiences or environmental demands. Thus, nature may initially control the gross development of the general architecture, and environment may continuously modify the "end" product, in entirely idiosyncratic fashion, different in and peculiar to each individual, throughout his or her life history.

It cannot be contested that the very general architecture of the human brain is largely similar for every individual, with particular neurones, circuits, networks and areas largely responsible for certain brain functions, such as, perhaps, sensory and perceptual processes, cognitive aspects, drives and emotions, motor mechanisms, and in our own highly social species, maybe also social and group behaviour. However, epigenetic amplification or suppression of function can modify the number of processing elements (neurones and connections) and size of regionally specialised areas, as a function of environmental experiences and pressures. For example, originally specialised visual areas can assume auditory or tactual responsibilities in the event of the later occurrence of blindness or deafferentation; brain plasticity as a concept is currently *a la mode*. Apparently specialized regions can increase or decrease in area or volume consequent upon life's experiences.

The nature of human consciousness is currently a "hot topic" of discussion and research. The editors of this book have long been of the view that a necessary, if not sufficient, feature of consciousness is one of modelling. Our *perception* of a current reality, our generation of appropriate *motor* responses, our *cognitive apprehension* of potential strategies, our *emotional* investment in certain general situations, our approach to our understanding of our *social* context or milieu, all involve predictive modelling of possible consequences.

There is a nested hierarchy within the brain of regional specialization, contributing circuits, and neurones and synapses. In such a reductionist context, the individual may also in part be subordinate or subjugated to his or her society, which like a flock of birds or a shoal of fishes, may show new emergent group behaviour, with partial synchronisation of each individual member's behaviour.

Psychiatric pathology can therefore stem from maldevelopment of structure or function, and also from changing societal expectations or norms. Homosexuality is no longer a crime or even an aberration, merely just one thread in the rich fabric of society. This book addresses some of the mechanisms whereby "normal" behaviour may be realised, thwarted, never attained or subsequently lost. It should not be seen as judgemental or prescriptive, or providing a basis, canon or recipe for change to some phantasmagoric or protean ideal.

SUBJECT INDEX

3p21 chromosomal region 120
5-HT1B 122
5-hydroxytryptophan 125
7q11.23 chromosomal region 274
10q24 chromosomal region 120
22q11 deletion syndrome 256

abstract processing 104
Academy of Cognitive Therapy 167
acamprosate 220
acetylcholine 3, 23, 340
Achenbach's Child Behaviour checklist 39
action cortex 21
action potential 49
acute coronary syndrome and depression 161
addiction 208–21; brain stimulation studies 216–19; clinical symptoms 209–10; clinical vignette 211–12; definition 208; genetics and epigenetics 212–14; intrinsic and extrinsic factors 212; neurobiology 214; neuroimaging studies 216, 218–19; neuropsychological studies 216, 217, 218; pharmacological treatment 220–1; prevalence 210; psychiatric comorbidity 210–11; psychological treatment 220; treatment 220–1
Addiction Severity Index (ASI) 210
ADHD. *See* attention deficit hyperactivity disorder (ADHD)
Adolescent and Adults Coordination Questionnaire (AAC-Q) 67
adolescent onset subtype of conduct disorder 141
adoption studies 163; and attention deficit hyperactivity disorder (ADHD) 121
Adult Dyspraxia and Developmental Coordination Disorder Questionnaire (ADC) 67
adynamia 33
affect, definition 157
affective cortico-basal ganglia-thalamo-cortical pathway 179
affective network 17
aggression 139, 141
agrammatism 35
Alcoholics Anonymous (AA) 212
alcohol-induced depressive disorder 212
alcohol use: and attention deficit hyperactivity disorder (ADHD) 123–4; brain stimulation studies 219; dependence 210; and frontal cortex 218–19; and gambling disorder (GD) 233–4; neuroimaging 218–19; neuropsychological studies 218; pharmacotherapies 220–1; prefrontal cortex 218
Alcohol Use Disorders Identification Test (AUDIT) 210
alerting network 23, 339–40
alien-limb syndrome 20
alogia 252
alternative splicing 318
Alzheimer's disease 17
amgydala 164, 280
amphetamines 258

amygdala 6, 320
Angelman's syndrome 51, 354–5
Anger Control Training (ACT) 145
anhedonia 160, 252
anodal stimulation 49, 50
anomia 35
anterior cingulate 5, 71, 164, 199, 215, 216
anterior cingulate cortex (ACC) 126, 180, 182, 219, 339, 343
anterior insula 343
anterior putamen 6
anticholinergic agents 301
anti-convulsant drugs 39
antidepressants 240, 301
antiglutamatergics 182
antihistaminergics 200
antipsychotics 181, 182, 200, 240, 260
antisaccade 297
antisense *FMR1* 318
antisocial personality disorder (ASPD) 213
anxiety: and autism spectrum disorder (ASD) 103; and Williams syndrome (WS) 273
anxiety disorders 177; and depression 162; and gambling disorder (GD) 233–4
anxiolytics 182
anxious distress and depression 157, 160
apathy 20
Apgar scale 39
aphasia 20, 252
Applied Behavioural Analysis (ABA) 282
arcuate premotor area 5
aripiprazole 200, 261
Aristotle 157
arousal network 22–23
arrhythmias in Friedreich ataxia (FRDA) 293
asenapine 260
Asperger's disorder 99, 354, 356
association loop with basal ganglia and brain 5, 6
associative information 1, 3
astrocytoma 30
ataxia 31, 291
atomoxetine 125, 200
ATP2C2 gene 86
attachment disorder 106
attention 339–41; and autism spectrum disorder (ASD) 104; and Fragile X Syndrome (FXS) 315; and Friedreich ataxia (FRDA) 298, 300; and schizophrenia 259–60; and Williams syndrome (WS) 277
attentional bias 236
attention control 22–23
attention deficit hyperactivity disorder (ADHD) 19, 39, 46, 47, 48, 51, 52, 53, 101, 119–30, 340, 345, 354, 355–6; aetiology of 120–1; and autism spectrum disorder (ASD) 102; biomarkers of 126; candidate genes in 121–2; and cerebellum 337; comorbidity 119, 120; comorbidity with conduct disorder and oppositional defiant disorder 143, 146–8; comorbidity with developmental coordination disorder 65–66, 68, 73; comorbidity with language disorder (LD) 84; and drug exposure during pregnancy 124; endophenotypes and 128–30; environmental risk factors 122–5; and exposure to prenatal alcohol 123–4; and exposure to toxins 124–5; and Fragile X Syndrome (FXS) 317; genetic architecture of 121; genetic factors 120–1; and low weight birth 123; and maternal smoking 124; neurochemistry 125; neuroimaging 126–8; and Tourette syndrome 192, 193, 196, 200–1; and Williams syndrome (WS) 273, 279–80
attention difficulties 20
attention networks 22–23
Attention Problems (APs) scale 125
attention process training 39
auditory hallucinations 252
auditory integration therapy 110
auditory processing: and Friedreich ataxia (FRDA) 292–3; and language disorder (LD) 87
Australia 161
Autism Diagnostic Observation Schedule (ADOS) 274
autism spectrum disorder (ASD) 20, 36, 46, 47, 48, 51, 99–110, 333, 336, 344, 354, 355, 356; and attention deficit hyperactivity disorder (ADHD) 102, 120; and cerebellum 337–8; clinical characteristics 100; clinical vignette 101; comorbidity 101–4; comorbidity with language disorder (LD) 84, 85; and conduct disorder and oppositional defiant disorder 147; depression in 104; and developmental coordination disorder 66; diagnostic instruments and clinical rating scales 100–1; and epilepsy 102; and Fragile X Syndrome (FXS) 316–17; genetics and epigenetics 108–9; interventions 109–10; and mental health problems 103–4; and mood disorders 104; neuromotor

profile 107; neuropathology 105–7; neuropsychology 104–5; prevalence 100; and psychosis 104; sleeping and eating problems 102–3; stereotypical movements in 103; and Tourette syndrome 192, 193, 196; and Williams syndrome (WS) 273–4, 276, 282
Autistic Disorder 99
avolition 252

Backward Digit Span Task 87
basal ganglia 1–10, 16, 17, 89, 180, 214, 353; anatomy of 2–9; connecting with the brain 4–6; connections within 3–4; direct pathway connections 3, 7; dopamine functioning within 4; hyperdirect pathway connections 4, 8; indirect pathway connections 4, 7; inputs into 2; and language disorder (LD) 85, 88; modes of function 6–9; outputs from 2–3; proposed roles of 9–10; and schizophrenia 257, 258
basal ganglia-thalamo-cortical loops with basal ganglia and brain 5
basket cells 334
Bayley Scales of Infant Development 39
Beck Depression Inventory (BDI) 163
behavioural parent-management training 145
Benton Facial Recognition Test 276
Benton Line Orientation Test 35
benzodiazepines 182
bereavement and depression 157
"Beyondblue" initiative 161
biomarkers 45–46, 354; for attention deficit hyperactivity disorder (ADHD) 126
bipolar disorder 50, 51
bitemporal standard pulse ECT 168
bizarre delusions 252
black bile 157
blood flow reduced in cerebellar cognitive affective syndrome (CCAS) 32
blood oxygen level-dependent (BOLD) 344
Body Dysmorphic Disorder (BDD) 177
Boston Naming Test 39
botulinum toxin 201
boys. *See* males
brain. *See also* specific parts of the brain: abnormalities and attention deficit hyperactivity disorder (ADHD) 126–8; and addiction 214–15; atypical growth and autism spectrum disorder (ASD) 105; connecting with the basal ganglia 4–6; and depression 164–5; development and circuitry 359–60; inputs from the basal ganglia 2–3; and language disorder (LD) 89–90; neural networks 17–18; stimulation and addiction 216–17; stimulation for depression 167–8; and Tourette syndrome 198–9; volume changes in schizophrenia 257–8
brainstem 3, 7, 18
Brief Psychotic Disorder 251
Bruininks-Oseretsky Test of Motor Proficiency (BOT-2) 66–67

CACNA1C 120
CACNB 120
Cadherin13 gene 122
callous and unemotional traits 141, 142–3
Cambridge Automated Neuropsychological Test Battery (CANTAB) 179
Canadian Problem Gambling Index 234
Cancer Australia 161
candidate gene association studies 52
cannabis 210
cardiac dysfunction in Friedreich ataxia (FRDA) 293
cardiac events and depression 161, 162
catatonia 160, 252
catecholamines 121–2, 165
catechol-O-methyl-transferase (COMT) 213, 255
cathodal stimulation 49, 50
caudal medial dorsal premotor cortex 16
caudate nucleus 1, 2, 5, 6, 89, 319–20
central nervous system (CNS) 45
cerebellar cognitive affective syndrome (CCAS) 29–41, 281, 334, 335, 336; clinical features 34–36; clinical rating scales 39; diagnostic instruments 39; future directions 40; laterality 37; neurophysiology 30, 32; neuropsychiatric symptoms 36–37; neuroscientific explanations of 37–39; onset and prevalence 29–30, 31; and posterior fossa syndrome 33–34; treatment 39–40
cerebellar cortex 334–6
cerebellar-frontal-parietal axis 333–46
cerebellar lateralization 37
cerebellar malformations 333–46
cerebellar mutism 33
cerebellar tumour 30
cerebellar vermis 336
cerebello-thalamo-cortical circuitry 296, 297, 298, 299–300, 335

cerebellum 198, 333, 353; abnormalities and autism spectrum disorder (ASD) 106; affective zone 30; cognitive zone 30; connectivity with cortical regions 334–46; in developmental brain disorders 334–6; and Fragile X Syndrome (FXS) 320; and Friedreich ataxia (FRDA) 292, 297, 298–300; injury to 29–41; internal model functions of 38–39; involvement in developmental coordination disorder 71; lobules of 334–5; models in motor and non-motor functions 337–8; motor zone 30; and schizophrenia 257–8; and Williams syndrome (WS) 280–1
cerebral blood flow 217
cerebral cortex 1, 19
cerebro-cerebellar connections 335
chasing losses 233
checking compulsions 175
chelation therapy 110
Chiari 1 Malformations 30, 32
childhood onset subtype of conduct disorder 141
chlorpromazine 260
cholinesterase inhibitors 109
CHRNA5Asn398Asp 214
chromosome 7, 86
chronic smokers 217–18
cinguloopercular network 23, 344, 345
circadian rhythm and Fragile X Syndrome (FXS) 314
cleaning compulsions 175
clinical neuroscience technologies 45–53; computational modelling 53; genetics 50–51; neuroimaging 46–47; non-invasive brain stimulation 47; repetitive transcranial magnetic stimulation (rTMS) 48; transcranial electrical stimulation (TES) 49–50; transcranial magnetic stimulation (TMS) 47–48
clomipramine 180
clonidine 196, 200, 201
clozapine 261
clumsiness 292
Clumsy Child Syndrome 64
CMIP gene 86
CNTNAP2 gene 86
cocaine: brain stimulation studies 216–17; neuroimaging studies 216; neuropsychological studies 216; prenatal exposure 124; treatment for 221; use and prefrontal cortex 215–17
cognition 9; and behavioural treatment for developmental coordination disorder 72–73; and the cerebellum 337; changes after cerebellar injury 33–34; control in addiction 214–15; control in Tourette syndrome 199–200; deficits in language disorder (LD) 87; dysfunction and depression 164; flexibility 237; and Fragile X Syndrome (FXS) 315; impairments in schizophrenia 259–60; training 262; zone of the cerebellum 30
cognitive behavioural therapy (CBT) 167, 180, 182, 220, 239, 261–2
community level factors in conduct disorder and oppositional defiant disorder 144
comparator role of the cerebellum 337
Competing Language Processing Task 87
Complex Developmental Trauma 256
Comprehensive Behavioural Intervention for Tics (CBIT) 200
compulsions 173–4, 175
compulsive drug-seeking 214–15
computational modelling 53
computed tomography 39
conditioned responses 10
conduct disorder (CD) 139–49, 201, 213; aetiology 144; and attention deficit hyperactivity disorder (ADHD) 120; clinical vignette 139–40; comorbidity 143; description, etiology and epidemiology 140–4; developmental neurobiology 148–9; developmental progression and outcomes 141–2; evidence-based treatment 144–6; neuropsychology 146–9; prevalence 143; treatment 145–6
congenital malformations causing cerebellar cognitive affective syndrome (CCAS) 30, 31
connectivity, functional and structural in Williams syndrome (WS) 281–2
connectome 17, 18, 19
continuous performance test (CPT) 179
contralateral prefrontal cortex 35
control, need for 176
Coping Power 145
coprolalia 191, 193
copropraxia 193
copy number variants (CNVs) 51, 108, 256; and attention deficit hyperactivity disorder (ADHD) 121

corpus callosum 280
cortical inhibition 166
cortical thickness 71
cortico-cortical connections 19
cortico-ponto-cerebellar loops 335
corticostriatal neurons 4
cortico-striatal-thalamic regions 280
cortico-striatal-thalamo-cerebellar circuits 271
cortico-striatal-thalamo-cortical circuits (CSTC) 181–2, 198, 200
cortisol 314
craving 219; and addiction 218
cue-exposure 218
cue reactivity 237–8
CYLN2 275
cytosine-guanine-guanine (CGG) repeats 311–12

D1 receptors 4, 7, 8, 200
D2 dopamine receptor gene 123
D2 receptors 4, 7, 8, 258, 260–1
D3 receptors 7
D4 dopamine receptor gene 122, 124
D4 receptors 7, 126, 340
D5 dopamine receptor gene 122
D5 receptors 7
daily living activities interference 67
DBH 214
decision-making 20, 21, 236–7
declarative memory 88–89
deep brain stimulation (DBS) 168, 199, 201
deep cerebellar nuclei (DCN) 334
deep repetitive transcranial magnetic stimulation (rTMS) 48
default mode network (DMN) 17, 128, 344, 345
delayed sensory feedback 38
Delusional Disorder 251
delusions 252
dementia and depression 161, 164
dentate nucleus (DN) 298, 299
dependence. *See* addiction
deplorization 48, 49
depression 20, 49, 50, 156–68; atypical features 160; and autism spectrum disorder (ASD) 104; brain stimulation 167–8; and catatonia 160; clinical symptomatology 159–61; clinical vignette 163; cognitive correlates of 164; comorbidity 161–2; genetic inheritability 158; genetics and epigenetics 163–4; glutamatergic theory of 165; melancholic features 160; monoamine hypothesis of 165; neurochemistry 165–6; neuropathology 164–5; and obsessive compulsive disorder (OCD) 177; onset and prevalence 157–9; peripartum onset 160; pharmacotherapy 166–7; physical comorbidities 161; psychiatric comorbidities 162; psychotherapy 167; psychotic features 160; rating scales 163; risk factors 158–9; and schizophrenia 254; seasonal pattern of 161; treatment 166–8
de Ruiter, M. B. 237
developmental apraxia 64
developmental clumsiness 64
developmental coordination disorder (DCD) 63–74; clinical symptoms 65; clinical vignette 67–68; comorbidity 65–66, 68; comorbidity with language disorder (LD) 84; diagnostic instruments and clinical rating scales 66–67; genetics and epigenetics 68–69; neuropathology/neurochemistry 70–72; neuropsychology 69–70; onset and prevalence 64–65; treatment 72–73
developmental dyspraxia 64
Development Coordination Disorder Questionnaire (DCDQ-2007) 67
development language disorder 81
diabetes mellitus 293
diachesis 32
diagnosis, mis- or under-, 354
Diagnostic and Statistical Manual (DSM) for Mental Disorders 234
Diagnostic and Statistical Manual of Mental Disorders 4th edition (DSM-IV) 39
Diagnostic Confidence Index (DCI) 195
Diagnostic Interview for Gambling Severity (DIGS) 234
Diagnostic Interview Schedule 234
diets, exclusion 110
diffusion tensor imaging (DTI) 126, 127, 148, 218, 281, 299
Dimensional Obsessive Compulsive Scale (DOCS) 176
direct gaze 316
direct pathway connections in basal ganglia 3, 7
DISC1 255
disinhibited giggling 33
disorganized thinking 252
dizygotic twins. *See* twin studies
DNA methylation 295

dopamine 4, 10, 18, 23, 165, 166, 198, 218, 341; and addiction 214; and attention deficit hyperactivity disorder (ADHD) 121–2, 125; and cocaine use 215–16; and gambling disorder (GD) 235, 239; loss of 8–9; and obsessive compulsive disorder (OCD) 181; release of 7; and schizophrenia 258
dopamine agonists 39, 181, 200
dopamine antagonists 165, 181, 198
dopamine D1 receptor. *See* D1 receptors
dopamine D2 receptor. *See* D2 receptors
dopamine D4 receptor. *See* D4 receptors
dopamine hypothesis of schizophrenia 258
dopamine neurotransmission 217
dopamine receptors 4, 7, 255. *See also* specific subtypes
dopaminergic genes 123
dopaminergic neurons 4
dopaminergic neurotransmission 125, 214, 221
dopaminergic projections 2, 3
dopaminergic system 201
dopamine transporter gene (DAT1) 52, 122, 126, 128, 340, 341
dorsal anterior cingulate cortex 279
dorsal attention network (DAN) 340, 342, 343
dorsal attention system 23
dorsal basal ganglia 1
dorsal root ganglion (DRG) 298–9
dorsal stream vulnerability hypothesis 339
dorsal striatum 2, 3, 4
dorsal visual stream 339
dorsolateral prefrontal cortex (DLPFC) 5, 16, 70, 126, 258, 279, 339–41, 343; cortex circuitry 215, 216–19
dorsolateral prefrontal cortex (DPFC) 181–2
dorsolateral striatum 8, 10
dorsomedial striatum 8, 10
doubt 173–4
Down syndrome 273
DRD1–4, 255
drug dependence. *See also* addiction: definition 208
drug exposure during pregnancy: and attention deficit hyperactivity disorder (ADHD) 124
drug receptors 213
Drug Use Disorders Identification Test (DUDIT) 210
DSM-1 191
DSM-5 64, 67, 82, 99, 140, 141, 157, 159, 191, 210, 231, 251, 252, 253
DSM-IV 64, 231
DSM-IV-TR 99
DTNBP1 255
dual-task costs 279
dysarthria 292
dysbindin 255
dysdiadochokinesis 335
dyslexia comorbidity with language disorder (LD) 84, 85
dysmetria 40, 335
dysmetria of thought hypothesis 338
dysphagia 292, 335
dysplasia 31
dysprosody 35
Dysthymia 157

Early Symptomatic Syndromes Eliciting Neurodevelopmental Clinical Examinations 102
eating disorders: and autism spectrum disorder (ASD) 102–3; and depression 162
echoing speech 252
echolalia 193
echopraxia 193
elastin (ELN) gene 273, 274
electroconvulsive therapy (ECT) 49, 167–8
electroencephalography (EEG) 45, 47, 148, 199, 238, 277
electronic gaming machines 232, 234–5
emotions: regulation 146–7; regulation by cognition 36; and reward centres 164
empathy 147; lack of 142, 143
encephalin 7
endocrine conditions and depression 162
endogenous attention 23
endophenotypes and attention deficit hyperactivity disorder (ADHD) 128–30
entorhinal cortex 5
environment: and polygenic neurodevelopmental disorders 51; and schizophrenia 256; and Tourette syndrome 197
Environmental Stress Hypothesis (ESH) 66
epilepsy 315; and autism spectrum disorder (ASD) 102
ESSENCE 102
ethanol 218
event-related potentials (ERPs) 277
excitatory granule cells 334
excitatory responses 18
exclusion diets 110

executive attention 21
executive control network 22, 23, 341–2
executive dysfunction 34–35, 86, 164
Executive Dysfunction (EF) theory 104, 105
executive functioning 69–70, 146–7, 179, 181, 198, 259; and Friedreich ataxia (FRDA) 295; and Williams syndrome (WS) 277
executive network 23
exogenous attention 23
expressing and grasping complexity 35
expressive language disorder 82
external globus pallidus (GPe) 2, 3, 4, 5, 7, 8, 9
eye movements in Friedreich ataxia (FRDA) 297–8

face processing and Williams syndrome (WS) 276–7
face-to-face conversation 316
facial emotion recognition 147, 149
familial aggregation studies 51–52; and attention deficit hyperactivity disorder (ADHD) 121; and language disorder (LD) 85
family therapy 145
feelings, definition 157
females. *See also* gender differences: and depression 158; and gambling disorder (GD) 232; and obsessive compulsive disorder (OCD) 174; and schizophrenia 254
fenobam 321
fibromyalgia 50
FKBP6 275
fluorescent in-situ hybridization (FISH) 273
fluoxetine 125
fluphenazine 260
FMR1 alleles 319
FMR1 CGG tandem repeat expansions 311–12
FMR1 gene 311–12, 317–19
FMR1 related disorders 311–22
FMR4 318
FMR5 318
FMR6 318
focal electrically administered seizure therapy (FEAST) 168
foetal alcohol syndrome (FAS) 123–4
forbidden thoughts 175
formal thought disorder 252
forward model of the cerebellum 337
FOXP2 gene 86, 89
fractional anisotropy (FA) 72, 127, 148, 281
Fragile X-associated primary ovarian insufficiency (FXPOI) 312
Fragile-X-associated tremor/ataxia syndrome (FXTAS) 312
Fragile X-Chromosome Site A (FRAXA) 313
Fragile X Mental Retardation 1 gene *(FMR1). See FMR1* gene
Fragile X Mental Retardation Protein (FMRP) 311–12, 317, 320–1
Fragile X Syndrome (FXS) 51, 311–22; clinical presentation 313–16; clinical vignette 317–18; comorbidities 316–17; diagnosis 317; genetics 318–19; neurochemistry 320–1; neuropathology 319–20; neuropsychological phenotype 315–16; onset and prevalence 313; physical phenotype 313–14; physiological phenotype 314–15; treatment 321–2
frataxin 294, 297, 298
Friedreich ataxia (FRDA) 291–302, 338; clinical symptoms 292–3; clinical vignette 293–4; cognitive and behavioural implications of 295–6; diagnostic instruments and clinical rating scales 300; genetics 294–5; neuroimaging 299–300; neuropathology 298–9; prevalence, onset, and progression 291–2; treatment 300–1
Friedreich Ataxia Rating Scale (FARS) 298, 300
Friedreich, Nicholaus 291
Frontal Behavioural Inventory 39
frontal cortex 3, 6, 9, 15–24, 177, 198, 280, 319; and addiction 219–20; anatomical connections 16–17; anatomical description 16; attention control 22–23; biochemistry 18; connectivity 17–18; damage to 20–21; development 18–20; and language disorder (LD) 88; roles 21–22
frontal eye fields (FEF) 5, 181, 338, 340
frontal lobes 181; and atypical connectivity 105–6
fronto-cellular brain network 17
fronto-parietal brain network 17
frontoparietal circuitry 23, 106, 277, 333, 338–9, 343–5; in Williams syndrome (WS) 279–80
fronto-parietal disorder 81
fronto-striatal brain network 17
frontostriatal-cerebellar circuitry 356

frontostriatal circuitry 106, 126, 127, 353; and Fragile X Syndrome (FXS) 319–20; and gambling disorder (GD) 237–9; and Williams syndrome (WS) 279–80
frontostriatal cortex 271; and conduct disorder and oppositional defiant disorder 144, 145; impairment 139, 148–9
fronto-striatal-thalamic network 279; and depression 164
fronto-striato-parietal dysfunction 279
fronto-temporal frontal cortex 19
Functional Difficulties Questionnaire (FDQ) 67
functional magnetic resonance imaging (*f*MRI) 46, 47, 126, 127, 180, 198, 219, 237, 279, 299, 300, 316, 344
functional neuroimaging 46, 148–9
fusiform face area (FFA) 280
FXN gene 291, 294

GAA1 allele 294–5
GABA 3, 4, 7, 18, 48, 106, 165–6, 214, 216, 217, 218, 221, 259; and Fragile X Syndrome (FXS) 321
GABAergic agonists 322
GABAergic inhibitory stellate interneurons 16
GABAergic neurons 182
GABAergic processes 48
GABAergic projections 2, 7
Gage, Phineas 139
gait: abnormalities in Williams syndrome (WS) 278–9; instability in Friedreich ataxia (FRDA) 292
gambling disorder (GD) 231–41; clinical symptoms 233; clinical vignette 234–5; comorbidity 233–4; diagnostic instruments and clinical rating scales 234; genetics and molecular genetics 235; neurochemistry 239; neuropathology 237–9; neuropsychology 236–7; onset and prevalence 232; treatment 239–40
γ-aminobutyric acid. *See* GABA
gamma aminobutyric acid. *See* GABA
gender differences. *See also* females; males: and depression 158; and Fragile X Syndrome (FXS) 311; and gambling disorder (GD) 232; and obsessive compulsive disorder (OCD) 174; and schizophrenia 254; and Tourette syndrome 194
gene-environment interactions 123
gene mutations and autism spectrum disorder (ASD) 108–9
generalized anxiety disorder (GAD) 201
general transcription factor II-I genes 274–5
genes 51–52; and additive disorders 213; deletion in Williams syndrome (WS) 274; and language disorder (LD) 86; and schizophrenia 255–6; and Tourette syndrome 197
genetic anticipation 313
genetics 50–53, 354–5; and attention deficit hyperactivity disorder (ADHD) 120–1; and conduct disorder and oppositional defiant disorder 144; and depression 158; and schizophrenia 255–6
genome wide association studies (GWAS) 52, 86, 197; and attention deficit hyperactivity disorder (ADHD) 121, 122; and depression 163–4
Genome-wide Complex Trait Analysis (GCTA) 194
genotype 51
genotype-phenotype in Williams syndrome (WS) 274
Georgiou-Karistianis, N. 300
Gilles de la Tourette, Georges Albert Edouard Brutus 191
Gilles de la Tourette syndrome. *See* Tourette syndrome
Gilles de la Tourette Syndrome-Quality of Life Scale (GTS-QoL) 195
globus pallidus 1, 2
glucose-fructose oxidoreductase domain 1 gene 122
glutamate 18, 48, 165, 214, 216, 217, 218, 221; in schizophrenia 258
glutamate hypothesis of schizophrenia 259
glutamatergic agents 240
glutamatergic pathways in schizophrenia 258–9
glutamatergic STR neurons 182
glutamatergic theory of depression 165
glutamatergic topographic projections into the basal ganglia 2
glutaminergic excitatory pyramidal neurons 16
goal-directed learning 8–10
Golgi neurons 334
GPi/SNr output complex 7
G protein-coupled receptor kinase interacting protein ArfGAP1 (GIT1) 122
grammar difficulties 83

grey matter 19, 148; in addiction 216; in Fragile X Syndrome (FXS) 319; in language disorder (LD) 89; in schizophrenia 257; in Williams syndrome (WS) 279–80
Griffiths Mental Developmental Scales 39
grossly disorganized or abnormal motor behaviour 252
gross motor ability 65
GTF2IRD1 274–5
GTF2IRD2 275
GTF21 274–5
guanfacine 200
guanine-adenine-adenine (GAA) trinucleotide repeats 294–5
guilt, lack of 142, 143

Habit Reversal Therapy (HRT) 200
habitual behaviours 8–10
hair-pulling disorder 177
hallucinations 252
haloperidol 200, 260
Hamilton Rating Scale for Depression (HRSD) 163
Heart Foundation (Australia) 161
Helping the Non-Compliant Child (HNC) 145
high definition transcranial current stimulation (HD-tDCS) 50
hippocampal cortex 5
hippocampus 6, 164–5
Hippocrates 157
hoarding 175, 177
HPA axis 158
Huntington's disease 7, 255, 257
hyperactivity. *See* attention deficit hyperactivity disorder (ADHD)
hyperactivity-impulsivity 119
hyper-arousal in Fragile X Syndrome (FXS) 314
hyperbaric oxygen 109
hyperdirect pathway connections in basal ganglia 4, 8
hyper-reactivity 20
hypersociability 271
hypometabolism 32
hypoperfusion 32, 37
hypothalamus-pituitary-adrenal (HPA) axis 314

idea generation 237
impaired set-shifting 35
impulsivity 125, 213, 215
inactivity and developmental coordination disorder 65
inarticulate sounds 193
inattention 35, 119
incoherent thinking 252
inconsolable crying 33
Incredible Years (IY) 145
indirect pathway connections in basal ganglia 4, 7
inferior frontal cortex (IFC) 340
inferior frontal gyrus (IFG) 22, 71, 89
inferior parietal cortex (IPC) 71, 128
inferior parietal lobule 22
inferior prefrontal cortex 15
inferior temporal gyri 5
inheritability 158; of addiction 213; of depression 163; of gambling disorder (GD) 235; of obsessive compulsive disorder (OCD) 178; of schizophrenia 255–6; of Tourette syndrome 194
inhibitory control 236
inhibitory interference control 21
inhibitory stellate 334
inter-family transmission of obsessive compulsive disorder (OCD) 178
intermediate phenotypes 213
internal globus pallidus (GPi) 2, 3, 4, 5, 7, 8
internal model functions of the cerebellum 38–39
internal modeling of actions 69
International Classification of Diseases 82
International Classification of Diseases (ICD-10) 64, 67, 99, 191, 234
International Classification of Diseases and Health Problems 210
International Cooperative Rating Scale (ICARS) 300
International Society for Interpersonal Psychotherapy 167
interpersonal psychotherapy (IPT) 167
intraprietal sulcus (IPs) 280, 338, 340, 342, 343
intrinsic connectivity networks (ICNs) 344
Iowa Gambling Task (IGT) 236, 238
IQ: and Fragile X Syndrome (FXS) 315, 317; and Williams syndrome (WS) 275–6
iron metabolism in Friedreich ataxia (FRDA) 294
isoform 318

Joan of Arc 353
Joubert syndrome (JS) 336

KE family 86
ketamine 168

language. *See also* verbal ability: comprehension 104; dysfunction 335, 336; and Fragile X Syndrome (FXS) 315–16; impairment 81; and schizophrenia 260; and Williams syndrome (WS) 277
language disorder (LD) 81–91; clinical vignette 83; comorbidity 84–85; diagnostic considerations 82–83; genetics 85–86; neuropathology 89–90; neuropsychology 86–89; prevalence and onset 83–84; therapy 90; treatment 90
Late Onset Friedreich Ataxia (LOFA) 291
late preterm infants 123
lateral dorsal premotor cortex (PMd) 16
lateral habenula 3
lateral orbitofrontal cortex 5, 182
lateral orbitofrontal loop with basal ganglia and brain 5
lateral parietal cortex 128
lateral prefrontal cortex 15, 16, 17, 21
lateral premotor frontal cortex 16
latrophilin 3 (LPHN3) 122
lead and attention deficit hyperactivity disorder (ADHD) 124
Learning Disorder 201
left hemisphere dominant features 37
left superior frontal gyrus (SFG) 71
left ventricle dysfunction in Friedreich ataxia (FRDA) 293
life stressors and depression 158
limbic-frontal network 164
limbic information 1, 3
limbic loop with basal ganglia and brain 5, 6
limbic-prefrontal circuits 148
limited prosocial emotions 143
LIMK1 274, 275
linguistic deficits 35
linkage studies 52; and depression 163
lobules of cerebellum 334–5
long non-coding RNAs (IncRNAs) 318
long-term depression (LTD) 49, 321
long-term potentiation (LTP) 49, 321
low functioning autism 100
low weight birth and attention deficit hyperactivity disorder (ADHD) 123

macroorchidism 314
magnetic resonance imaging (MRI) 39, 45, 148
magnetic seizure therapy (MST) 168
magnetic stimulation 47–48
magnetoencephalography (MEG) 47, 199, 277
Major Depressive Disorder (MDD) 156, 177
Major Depressive Episode (MDE) 159
males. *See also* gender differences: and attention deficit hyperactivity disorder (ADHD) 119; and autism spectrum disorder (ASD) 100; and conduct disorder and oppositional defiant disorder 143; and developmental coordination disorder 65; and Fragile X Syndrome (FXS) 311; and gambling disorder (GD) 232; and obsessive compulsive disorder (OCD) 174, 194; and schizophrenia 254
Martin-Bell syndrome 311
maternal smoking and attention deficit hyperactivity disorder (ADHD) 124
maternal stress and autism spectrum disorder (ASD) 109
McCarron Assessment of Neuromuscular Development (MAND) 66
medial dorsal premotor cortex 16
medial dorsal thalamus 5, 16
medial prefrontal cortex 15, 16, 128
medical conditions and schizophrenia 255
medications for autism spectrum disorder (ASD) 108–9
medulloblastoma 30, 33
melancholia 157, 160. *See also* depression
melatonin 102–3
memory: and language disorder (LD) 87–89; and schizophrenia 259–60; and Williams syndrome (WS) 277–8
memory-guided saccade 297
mental health: and autism spectrum disorder (ASD) 101–4; and developmental coordination disorder 65; and gambling disorder (GD) 233; illness and addiction 211
mentalising 105
mesocorticolimbic circuitry 18, 214, 216, 218
mesolimbic/mesocortical tract 165
mesolimbic reward circuitry 238, 239
metabolic conditions and depression 162
metabotropic glutamate receptor (GRM3) 255
methylation mosaicism 311, 312
methylphenidate 73, 122, 125, 128, 282
mGluR1 321

mGluR5 321
mGluR selective antagonists 321
MHC 255
microstructural abnormality in autism spectrum disorder (ASD) 106
Microtubule-Associated Protein 1B (MAP1B) 320
midbrain dopaminergic neurons 4
midbrain tegmentum 2
middle-frontal cortex 71
mindfulness-based relapse prevention therapy 220
minicolumnar pathology in autism spectrum disorder (ASD) 106
mirror neuron system (MNS) 21–22, 71
modafinil 221
Monetary Incentive Delay Task 238
monoamine hypothesis of depression 165
monoamine oxidase A (MAOA) 213, 215
monoamine oxidase (MAO) inhibitors 167
monoamines 125
monogenic neurodevelopmental disorders 51
monozygotic twins. *See* twin studies
Montgomery-Ashberg Depression Rating Scale (MADRS) 163
Mood Assessment Scale 163
mood congruent psychosis 160
mood, definition 157
mood disorders 50, 301; and autism spectrum disorder (ASD) 103; and gambling disorder (GD) 233–4
mood incongruent psychosis 160
mood stabilizers 182, 240
morphine 182
mortality and attention deficit hyperactivity disorder (ADHD) 119
motivated self-initiated purposeful activities 252
motivational enhancement therapy 239
motivational interviewing (MI) 220, 239
motor behaviour, grossly disorganized or abnormal 252
motor control 9, 37–38
motor cortex 38
motor development and autism spectrum disorder (ASD) 107
motor functioning 335; and language disorder (LD) 85; and models of the cerebellum 337–8; problems 64
motor loop with basal ganglia and brain 5, 6
motor planning 278; internal modeling of 69
Motor tic, obsessions and compulsions, vocal tic evaluation survey (MOVES) 195
motor tics 48, 191, 192, 195. *See also* tics
motor zone of the cerebellum 30
Movement Assessment Battery for Children-2 (MABC) 66–67
movement control 9
movement disorders 7
movement disturbance in autism spectrum disorder (ASD) 107
multiple sclerosis and depression 161
mutism 252
myelination 19

nalmefene 240
naltrexone 213, 220, 240
National Epidemiological Catchment Area (ECA) study 174
National Hospital Interview Schedule (NHIS) 195
National Institute for Health and Clinical Excellence (NICE) 182
National Opinion Research Centre DSM Screen for Gambling Problems (NODS) 234
NCF1 275
need for control 176
negative affectivity 158
negative symptoms of schizophrenia 252
neocortex 18, 353
nervous system hyper-arousal and Fragile X Syndrome (FXS) 314
neural connectivity in autism spectrum disorder (ASD) 106
neurexin 197
Neurexin Transynaptic Connexus 197
neurobiology and conduct disorder and oppositional defiant disorder 148–9
neurodegenerative conditions causing cerebellar cognitive affective syndrome (CCAS) 30, 31
neurodevelopment and obsessive compulsive disorder (OCD) 176–7
neurofeedback 110
neuroimaging 46–47; for addiction 216–19; for attention deficit hyperactivity disorder (ADHD) 126–8; for developmental coordination disorder 70; for Friedreich ataxia (FRDA) 299–300

neurological conditions: and autism spectrum disorder (ASD) 101–2; and depression 162; and Friedreich ataxia (FRDA) 292–3
neuromotor profile in autism spectrum disorder (ASD) 106–7
neuropathology: in autism spectrum disorder (ASD) 106–7; in Fragile X Syndrome (FXS) 319–20; in Friedreich ataxia (FRDA) 298–9; in obsessive compulsive disorder (OCD) 179–80; in Williams syndrome (WS) 279–80
neuropeptides 18
neurophysiology of developmental coordination disorder 69–70
neuropsychiatric symptoms in cerebellar cognitive affective syndrome (CCAS) 36–37
neuropsychology: in autism spectrum disorder (ASD) 104–5; in conduct disorder and oppositional defiant disorder 146–9; in Friedreich ataxia (FRDA) 295–6; in language disorder (LD) 86–89; in obsessive compulsive disorder (OCD) 178–9; in Williams syndrome (WS) 275–6
neuroregulin 1 (NRG1) 255
neuroticism 158
neurotransmitters 18, 23, 198; in attention deficit hyperactivity disorder (ADHD) 121–2, 125; in depression 165; in schizophrenia 258–9
neursocience techniques 45–53
nicotine: brain stimulation studies 218; dependence and gambling disorder (GD) 233; neuroimaging studies 216–17; neuropsychological studies 217; and prefrontal cortex 217
nigrostriatal tract 165
nisoxetine 125
nitric oxide synthase1 (NOS1) 122
NMDAR antagonists 109, 165
NMDA receptors 18, 48, 165, 258–9
N-methyl-D-aspartate receptor. *See* NMDA receptors
noise, sensitivity to 273
non-bizarre delusions 252
non-motor functions and models of the cerebellum 337–8
non-obscene socially inappropriate (NOSI) behaviours 191, 193
nonword repetition 87
noradrenaline 18, 121; and attention deficit hyperactivity disorder (ADHD) 125
noradrenaline transporter 125
noradrenergic activity 165
noradrenergic agents 200
noradrenergic inputs into the basal ganglia 2
norephinephrine 165, 166, 339; and gambling disorder (GD) 235
NRGN 255
nucleus accumbens 2, 5

obsessions 173–4, 175
obsessive-compulsive behaviours (OCB) 194, 196; and Williams syndrome (WS) 273
obsessive compulsive disorder (OCD) 46, 50, 52, 173–83; clinical vignette 177; comorbidity 177–8; frontostriatal circuitry 181–2; genetics 178; neurochemistry 180–1; as neurodevelopmental disorder 176–7; neuropathology 179–80; neuropsychology 178–9; obsessions and compulsions 175; onset and prevalence 174–5; rating scales of severity 175–6; and schizophrenia 255; and Tourette syndrome 193, 194, 196, 200–1; treatment 182–3
Obsessive Compulsive Inventory-Revised (OCI-R) 176
Obsessive Compulsive Personality Disorder (OCPD) 176
obstetic complications and schizophrenia 256
occupational therapy for developmental coordination disorder 72–73
ocular motor control 297–8
oculomotor dysfunction in Friedreich ataxia (FRDA) 292
oculomotor loop with basal ganglia and brain 5, 6
odd gait 107
olanzapine 261
olfactory tubercle 2
omega-3-fatty acids 110
oncology and depression 161, 162
opioid antagonists 240
opioid use 210
oppositional defiant disorder (ODD) 66, 139–49; aetiology 144; and attention deficit hyperactivity disorder (ADHD) 120; clinical vignette 139–40; comorbidity 143; description, etiology and epidemiology 140–4; developmental

neurobiology 148–9; evidence-based treatment 144–6; neuropsychology 146–9; prevalence 143; treatment 144–5
OPRM1 213
optodes 47
optogenetics 52
orbitofrontal cortex (OFC) 16, 149, 180, 181, 198, 238, 280, 341; circuitry 215, 217
orbitomedial frontal cortex 6
orbitomedial prefrontal cortex 18
organophosphate pesticides (OPs) and attention deficit hyperactivity disorder (ADHD) 124
orienting network 22, 23, 340–1
oxytocin 109

Paediatric Autoimmune Neuropsychiatric Disorder Associated with Streptococcus (PANDAS) 180, 197
palilalia 193
palipraxia 193
pallidum 5
panic disorder and schizophrenia 255
parahippocampal place area (PPA) 280
Parent Child Interaction Therapy (PCIT) 144–5
parent-focused interventions for autism spectrum disorder (ASD) 109
parenting and conduct disorder and oppositional defiant disorder 144
Parent Management Training - Oregon (PMTO) 145
Parent Tic Questionnaire (PTQ) 195
parent training 144–5
parietal cortex 17, 22, 23, 35, 198, 271
parkinsonism 318
Parkinson's disease 7, 9, 20–21, 239, 257; and depression 161
paternal age and schizophrenia 256
pedunculopontine tegmental nucleus 3
perfectionism 176
Pergolide 200
peripartum onset of depression 160
perseveration of actions 35
Persistent Depressive Disorders 157
personality change 36
personality disorder 201; and gambling disorder (GD) 234
pharmacological treatments: for developmental coordination disorder 73; for schizophrenia 260–1
pharmacotherapy for depression 161, 166–7
phasic alertness 340
phenotypes 51; intermediate 213
phonic tics 191. *See also* tics
physical aggression 141
physically awkward 64
physical therapy for developmental coordination disorder 72–73
physiological dependence 208–9
pimozide 200
placenta pathology and schizophrenia 256
planning 21, 237; and Williams syndrome (WS) 278
polychlorinated biphenyl (PCBs) and attention deficit hyperactivity disorder (ADHD) 124
polygenic gene model 121
polygenic neurodevelopmental disorders 51
polysubstance use 210
pons 20
positive symptoms for schizophrenia 252
positron emission tomography (PET) 126, 128, 180, 181, 198–9, 216, 218, 219
posterior cerebellum 35
posterior cingulate cortex 128
posterior fossa syndrome 33–34, 39
posterior parietal cortex (PPC) 5, 343
posterior putamen 6
post traumatic stress disorder and schizophrenia 254
postural control 65
precocious puberty 314
prefrontal cortex (PFC) 3, 5, 6, 15, 17, 18, 181, 214–15, 341; and attention deficit hyperactivity disorder (ADHD) 125; and chronic cocaine use 215–16; and chronic nicotine use 217; connections 16; damage to 20; and depression 164–5; regions 148; role of 21
Premenstrual Dysphoric Disorder 157
Premonitory Urge Tics Scale (PUTS) 195
premotor cortex 5, 15, 16, 17; damage to 20–21; roles of 21–22
prenatal exposure: to alcohol and attention deficit hyperactivity disorder (ADHD) 123–4; to infection and schizophrenia 256
preparatory set 21
pre-SMA medial dorsal premotor cortex 16, 22
preterm infants 123
primary motor cortex 3

Probabilistic Response Learning Task 238
Problem Gambling Severity Index (PGSI) 234
Problem Solving Skills training (PSST) 145
Procedural Deficit Hypothesis 88
procedural memory 88, 89
process-oriented treatment for developmental coordination disorder 72
protein-protein interaction network 52
protein synthesis and Fragile X Syndrome (FXS) 321
psuedo-bulbar 36
psychiatric disorders: and attention deficit hyperactivity disorder (ADHD) 120; and depression 162; and substance use disorders 210–11
psychoeducation 200, 262
psychological dependence 208–9
psychological therapy: for obsessive compulsive disorder (OCD) 182–3; for schizophrenia 261–2
psychopharmacology: for autism spectrum disorder (ASD) 109; for depression 164; for Tourette syndrome 200–1; for Williams syndrome (WS) 282
psychosis: and autism spectrum disorder (ASD) 104; and depression 160
psychosocial interventions: for oppositional defiant disorder 144–5; for schizophrenia 261–2
psychosocial stressors and depression 158
psychostimulant drugs 125, 210
psychotherapy for depression 161, 167
psychotic disorder and gambling disorder (GD) 234
pulmonary conditions and depression 162
pure TS 192, 201
Purkinje cells 106, 257, 334
putamen 1, 2, 5, 7

quetiapine 261
Quick Inventory of Depressive Symptomatology (QIDS) 163

raphe nuclei 165
reaction time 296, 297
reading difficulties 85
real orientation therapy 39
reasoning 15
receptive language disorder 82
religiosity and obsessive compulsive disorder (OCD) 174
renal infectious disease and depression 162
reorienting attention 104
repeat-length mosaicism 311, 312
repetitive behaviours 103–4, 252
repetitive Transcranial Magnetic Stimulation (rTMS) 39–40, 46, 48, 168, 216, 219
response inhibition 146–7, 236
response perseveration 147
response selection and Friedreich ataxia (FRDA) 300
reticular activating system 3
Rett syndrome 51
reward and punishment tasks 238
reward circuitry 214
reward processing 9
Rey-Osterreich Complex Figure Test (ROCF) 39, 179
rheumatologic conditions and depression 162
rich-club hubs 17, 18
right hemisphere dominant features 37
risk evaluation 215
risperidone 200, 260, 261
rostral brainstem 165
rostral medial dorsal premotor cortex 16

Scale for Assessment and Rating of Ataxia (SARA) 300
Schizoaffective Disorder 251, 253
schizophrenia 17, 46, 48, 49, 50, 51, 52, 251–63, 337; brain structure in 257–8; clinical symptoms 251–3; clinical vignette 253–4; comorbidity and differential diagnosis 254–5; dopamine hypothesis of 258; environmental factors 256; genetic factors 255–6; glutamate hypothesis of 259; neuropathology 257–60; neuropsychology 259–60; neurotransmitters in 258–9; prevalence and onset 254; treatment 260–2
Schizophrenia Spectrum disorders 251
Schizophreniform Disorder 251
Schizotypal Personality Disorder 251
scoliosis 293
seasonal episodes of depression 161
season of birth and schizophrenia 256
secretin therapy 110
selective attention 340
selective serotonin reuptake inhibitors (SSRIs) 166, 180–1, 182, 201
selfish gene hypothesis 199
sensorimotor cortex 5, 198
sensorimotor information 1, 3, 6
sensory sensitivity in Fragile X Syndrome (FXS) 315

sequence detection model of the cerebellum 337
sequencing impairment 35
serotonergic dysfunction in obsessive compulsive disorder (OCD) 179–81
serotonergic projections into the basal ganglia 2
serotonergic system 164
serotonin 18, 122, 165, 166, 180–1; and gambling disorder (GD) 235; and schizophrenia 258, 259
serotonin 5 HT2a receptor 260
serotoninergic system 201
serotonin/noradrenaline reuptake inhibitors (SNRIs) 166
serotonin reuptake inhibitors (SRIs) 39, 165, 321
serotonin transporter 164, 213
Severity of Dependence Scale 210
Sherman paradox 313
shifting mental tasks 341, 342
Simons Foundation Autism Research Initiative (SFARI) 108
single gene mutations 108
single nucleotide polymorphisms (SNPs) 51, 108, 120, 197
single-photon emission computerized tomography. *See* SPECT
skin-picking disorder 177
SLC6A3 126
SLC6A4 122, 213
sleep: and autism spectrum disorder (ASD) 102–3; and Fragile X Syndrome (FXS) 314
SLI1 gene 86
SLI2 gene 86
SMA medial dorsal premotor cortex 16
smoking cessation 214
smoking expectancy 217–18
smoking, maternal and attention deficit hyperactivity disorder (ADHD) 124
social cognition and conduct disorder and oppositional defiant disorder 147
social skills training 262
society's impact on developmental disorders 353
somatic cell line mutations 108
somatosensory behaviour and basal ganglia 1
South Oaks Gambling Screen (SOGS) 234
spatial attention 340, 342
spatial memory 278
special education problems and Tourette syndrome 192
specific language impairment (SLI) 81, 82
SPECT 32, 39, 128
speech impairment and developmental coordination disorder 66
spinal cord and cerebellum 335
stair and surface stepping 278–9
step descent 278–9
stereotypes and tics in autism spectrum disorder (ASD) 103
sticky fixation 277
stimulus-response habits 10
stress and depression 158
striatal cholinergic interneurons 3
striatum 1, 3, 4, 5, 6, 7, 8, 10, 20, 71, 164, 180, 182, 238, 279, 319–20
stroke: causing cerebellar cognitive affective syndrome (CCAS) 30, 31; and depression 161
Stroop task 39, 179, 198, 236
structural magnetic resonance imaging (sMRI) 126, 216, 217, 218
structural neuroimaging 148
Structured Clinical Interview for DSM-IV (SCID) 39, 210
Structured Clinical Interview for Pathological Gambling 234
STX1A 275
subcortical anomalies and language disorder (LD) 89
subcortical frontal cortex 19
subcortical regions of the brain 23
subcortico-cortico connections 19
substance dependence 209. *See also* addiction; and schizophrenia 254
substance P projections 7
Substance-Related and Addictive Disorders 231
substance specific genes 213
substance use disorders 210; and depression 162
substantia nigra 1
substantia nigra pars compacta (SNc) 2, 3, 4, 7
substantia nigra pars reticulata (SNr) 2, 3, 4, 5, 7, 8
subthalamic nucleus (STN) 1, 2, 4, 7, 8
suicidal ideation 161
suicide and schizophrenia 254
super-conducting detectors and amplifiers (SQUIDS) 47
superior cerebellar peduncles (SCP) 299
superior colliculus 3, 5
superior parietal lobe (SPL) 339
superior temporal gyrus 5, 320

supplementary motor area (SMA) 6, 16, 21, 22, 181
supratentorial regions 32
supravalvular aortic stenosis (SVAS) 274
surgical treatment and cerebellar cognitive affective syndrome (CCAS) 32
sustained attention 339
symmetry obsessions 175
synapses 18, 19; and Fragile X Syndrome (FXS) 320–1
synaptogenesis 18–19
synaptosomal-associated protein 25 (SNA25) 122

task-oriented treatment for developmental coordination disorder 72
TCF4 255
temperamental risk factor for depression 158
temporal cortex 5
temporal gyrus 89
temporal lobe 6
temporal organizing function 21
temporoparietal cortex 340
temporoparietal junction (TPJ) 340, 341
Test of Everyday Attention 298
Test of Visual-Perceptual Skills 39
Tetrabenazine 200
tetrapods and basal ganglia 1
thalamus 5, 7, 9, 16, 17, 180, 182; outputs from 2–3
theory of attention networks 22–23
Theory of Mind (ToM) 104, 147, 315–16
thinking, disorganized or incoherent 252
thioridazine 260
tic disorders 175, 178
tics 191, 192–3, 195, 196. *See also* specific types of tics; and autism spectrum disorder (ASD) 103
Tic Screening Questionnaire 195
Tic Spectrum of Disorders 191
time: passage of 38–39; sense of 21
tobacco 210, 217; exposure and attention deficit hyperactivity disorder (ADHD) 124
tonic alertness 340
topirmamate 200, 221
Tourette syndrome 47, 48, 103, 175, 178, 191–202; clinical symptoms 192–3; clinical vignette 196; comorbidity 193–5; diagnostic instruments and clinical rating scales 195–6; evolutionary/adaptive aspects 199–200; genetic association with attention deficit hyperactivity disorder (ADHD) 194; genetic association with obsessive compulsive disorder (OCD) 194–5; genetics and epigenetics 197–8; neuropathology/neurochemistry 198–9; neuropsychology 198; onset and prevalence 192; treatment 200–1
Tourette Syndrome International Database Consortium 193
Tower of London/Hanoi (TOL/TOH) 179
Tower of London task 237, 278
toxins: and attention deficit hyperactivity disorder (ADHD) 124–5; and depression 162
Trail Making Test 39, 179, 237
transcranial alternating current stimulation (tACS) 50
transcranial direct current stimulation (tDCS) 47, 49–50, 219
transcranial electrical stimulation (TEST) 49–50
transcranial magnetic stimulation (TMS) 47–48, 109, 199, 299
transcranial random noise stimulation (tRNS) 50
traumatic brain injury and depression 161
trichotillomania 177
tricyclic antidepressants (TCAs) 167
Triple P Positive Parenting Program 145
tryptophan hydroxylase (TPH2) 165
TSC1 gene 106
TS-Plus 191, 201
tuberoinfundibular tract 165
tuberous sclerosis 106, 108
twin studies 52, 158, 356; and addiction 212–13; and attention deficit hyperactivity disorder (ADHD) 121; and autism spectrum disorder (ASD) 108; and depression 163; and developmental coordination disorder 68; and language disorder (LD) 86; and obsessive compulsive disorder (OCD) 178; and schizophrenia 255; and Tourette syndrome 197
type A β-haemolytic streptococcal bacteria 180

uncinate fascicle 148
unconditioned responses 10
Universal Cerebellar Transform 338

variable number of tandem repeats (VNTR) 126
variant gene mutations 108

ventral attention network (VAN) 23, 340, 344, 345
ventral attention system 23
ventral basal ganglia 1
ventral frontal cortex 23
ventral pallidum 5
Ventral Pallidum/Substantia Nigra (VP/SN) 182
ventral premotor cortex (PMv) 16, 20–22
ventral stream areas 280
ventral striatum 2, 5, 6, 238
ventral tegmental area (VTA) 2, 3
ventral visual stream 339
ventrolateral prefrontal cortex (VLPFC) 238
ventromedial cortex 341
ventromedial prefrontal cortex (VMPFC) 238, 239
verbal ability 146. *See also* language
verbal fluency 39; deficit 35
verbal memory 278
vermis 30, 320, 336; injury and neuropsychiatric symptoms 36–37
Very Late Onset Friedreich Ataxia (VLOFA) 291
vigilance 339
Vineland Adaptive Behavioral Scale 39, 317
visuomotor integration 278–9
visuospatial dysfunction 35, 335; and Williams syndrome (WS) 274–7
visuospatial orienting 340
vitamin deficiencies and depression 162
vocal tics 191, 192, 195. *See also* tics
voxel-based morphometry (VBM) 279, 281, 299

Weak Central Coherence (WCC) theory 104–5
Wechsler Intelligence Scale for Children (WISC) 146, 179
Wechsler Intelligence Scales for Preschool and Primary School Children 275
Weschler Adult Intelligence Scale-Revised 39
white matter 20, 148; and attention deficit hyperactivity disorder (ADHD) 127; and Fragile X Syndrome (FXS) 319; and Friedreich ataxia (FRDA) 299; and language disorder (LD) 89; and schizophrenia 258
WHO 161
Williams syndrome (WS) 271–83, 344; attention 277; and cerebellum 280–1; clinical vignette 272–3; comorbidity 273; executive functions 277; functional and structural connectivity 281–2; gait features 278–9; genetics 274; memory 277–8; motor planning 278; neuropathology 279–80; neuropsychology 275–6; prevalence 273; treatment 282; visuomotor integration 278; visuospatial, language and face processing 276–7
Williams syndrome (WS) critical region (WSCR) 274
Wisconsin Card Sorting Task 39, 237, 259
working memory 21, 69–70, 87, 88, 341, 342, 343; and Fragile X Syndrome (FXS) 315; and Friedreich ataxia (FRDA) 298; impairment 35
World Health Organization (WHO) 209
World Mental Health Composite International Diagnostic Interview (WMH-CIDI) 210

X chromosomes and Fragile X Syndrome (FXS) 311–13

Yale-Brown Obsessive Compulsive Scale (YBOCS) 175–6
Yale Global Tic Severity Rating Scale (YGTSS) 195
Yale Global Tic Severity Scale 195

ZNF7804A 255
zuclopenthixol 260
Zung Self-rating Depression Scale 163